Antioxidants Handbook

Antioxidants Handbook

Editor: Ned Burnett

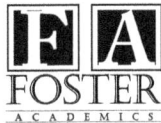

FOSTER
ACADEMICS

www.fosteracademics.com

www.fosteracademics.com

FA
FOSTER
ACADEMICS

Cataloging-in-Publication Data

Antioxidants handbook / edited by Ned Burnett.
        p. cm.
Includes bibliographical references and index.
ISBN 978-1-63242-570-6
1. Antioxidants. 2. Antioxidants--Therapeutic use. 3. Pharmacology.
I. Burnett, Ned.

RM666.A555 A58 2018
615.7--dc23

Foster Academics,
118-35 Queens Blvd., Suite 400,
Forest Hills, NY 11375, USA

ISBN 978-1-63242-570-6 (Hardback)

Contents

Preface

This book has been a concerted effort by a group of academicians, researchers and scientists, who have contributed their research works for the realization of the book. This book has materialized in the wake of emerging advancements and innovations in this field. Therefore, the need of the hour was to compile all the required researches and disseminate the knowledge to a broad spectrum of people comprising of students, researchers and specialists of the field.

Antioxidants are molecules that check the chemical reactions that are caused by free radicals in the human body. They play a significant role in medical science. Antioxidants help in the prevention of cancer by reducing cell damage. They also help to decrease the effects of aging as well as minimize risks of Asperger's syndrome, Alzheimer's disease and Parkinson's disease. This book on antioxidants traces the progress of this field and highlights some of its key concepts and applications. Through this book, the readers would gain knowledge that would broaden their perspective about antioxidants. It will serve as a valuable source of reference for graduate and post graduate students.

At the end of the preface, I would like to thank the authors for their brilliant chapters and the publisher for guiding us all-through the making of the book till its final stage. Also, I would like to thank my family for providing the support and encouragement throughout my academic career and research projects.

Editor

Low Concentration of Quercetin Antagonizes the Cytotoxic Effects of Anti-Neoplastic Drugs in Ovarian Cancer

Na Li[1,9], **Chaoyang Sun**[1,9], **Bo Zhou**[1], **Hui Xing**[2], **Ding Ma**[1], **Gang Chen**[1]*, **Danhui Weng**[1]*

1 Cancer Biology Research Center, Tongji Hospital, Tongji Medical College, Huazhong University of Science and Technology, Wuhan, Hubei, China, **2** Department of Obstetrics and Gynecology, Xiangyang Central Hospital, First Affiliated Hospital of Hubei University of Arts and Science. Xiangyang, Hubei, China

Abstract

Objective: The role of Quercetin in ovarian cancer treatment remains controversial, and the mechanism is unknown. The aim of this study was to investigate the therapeutic effects of Quercetin in combination with Cisplatin and other anti-neoplastic drugs in ovarian cancer cells both *in vitro* and *in vivo*, along with the molecular mechanism of action.

Methods: Quercetin treatment at various concentrations was examined in combination with Cisplatin, taxol, Pirarubicin and 5-Fu in human epithelial ovarian cancer C13* and SKOV3 cells. CCK8 assay and Annexin V assay were for cell viability and apoptosis analysis, immunofluorescence assay, DCFDA staining and realtime PCR were used for reactive oxygen species (ROS)-induced injury detection and endogenous antioxidant enzymes expression. Athymic BALB/c-nu nude mice were injected with C13*cells to obtain a xenograft model for *in vivo* studies. Immunohistochemical analysis was carried out to evaluate the ROS-induced injury and SOD1 activity of xenograft tumors.

Results: Contrary to the pro-apoptotic effect of high concentration (40 µM–100 µM) of Quercetin, low concentrations (5 µM–30 µM) of Quercetin resulted in varying degrees of attenuation of cytotoxicity of Cisplatin treatment when combined with Cisplatin. Similar anti-apoptotic effects were observed when Quercetin was combined with other anti-neoplastic agents: Taxol, Pirarubicin and 5-Fluorouracil (5-Fu). Low concentrations of Quercetin were observed to suppress ROS-induced injury, reduce intracellular ROS level and increase the expression of endogenous antioxidant enzymes, suggesting a ROS-mediated mechanism of attenuating anti-neoplastic drugs. In xenogeneic model, Quercetin led to a substantial reduction of therapeutic efficacy of Cisplatin along with enhancing the endogenous antioxidant enzyme expression and reducing ROS-induced damage in xenograft tumor tissue.

Conclusion: Taken together, these data suggest that Quercetin at low concentrations attenuate the therapeutic effects of Cisplatin and other anti-neoplastic drugs in ovarian cancer cells by reducing ROS damage. Quercetin supplementation during ovarian cancer treatment may detrimentally affect therapeutic response.

Editor: Ruby John Anto, Rajiv Gandhi Centre for Biotechnology, India

Funding: This work was supported by the National Basic Research Program of China (973 Program, 2009CB521808); National Nature and Science Foundation of China (81230038; 81272859; 81025011; 81090414; 81000979; 81101962); Nature and Science Foundation of Hubei Province (2011CBD542); Fundamental Research Funds for the Central Universities (HUST: 2012TS058). The funders had no role in study design, data collection and analysis, decision to publish, or preparation of the manuscript.

Competing Interests: The authors have declared that no competing interests exist.

* Email: gumpc@126.com (GC); weng.dh@gmail.com (DW)

9 These authors contributed equally to this work.

Introduction

Ovarian cancer is the most frequent invasive malignancy of the female genital tract in the United States, with an estimated 22,240 cases diagnosed annually. Approximately 14,030 women die each year from ovarian cancer, representing the most common cause of death among women with gynecological malignancies [1]. Platinum drugs, such as Cisplatin and Carboplatin, are first-line chemotherapeutic agents for the treatment of ovarian cancer. Although most patients display chemosensitivity when beginning therapy, acquired drug resistance has become a major impediment in cancer treatment. The factors that may enhance or suppress the anticancer effect of anti-neoplastic drugs appear to be important in the treatment of ovarian cancer.

Quercetin (3,3′,4′,5,7-pentahydroxyflavone, Quer) belongs to a class of flavonoid compounds, and is in various vegetables, fruits, seeds, nuts, tea, and red wine [2]. It is the major flavonoid in the human diet, with an estimated daily dietary intake of 25 mg in the United States [3]. As a proven antioxidant, Quercetin is recommended to take orally for cancer prevention and health care [4]. In recent years, several studies have noted that Quercetin may act as a potential anticancer drug by enhancing the toxicity of Cisplatin treatment in hepatoma HA22T/VGH and ovarian cancer A2780 cells [5–7]. Nevertheless, there are studies reported that in contrast to high concentrations of the flavonoid decreased cell survival and viability, low concentrations increased total antioxidant capacity of cancer cells and prevent cell death due to cytotoxic drugs such as Cisplatin and 5-Fu in lung cancer A549 and colorectal cancer HCT116 cells [8,9]. The role of Quercetin in ovarian cancer treatment is controversial, and the mechanism of action remains unknown.

Cisplatin and other anti-neoplastic agents lead to increases in intracellular reactive oxygen species (ROS) that may contribute to their therapeutic effect. Antioxidant such as Vitamin C supplements may attenuate the anti-neoplastic activity of drugs that increase ROS [10]. Quercetin is known to reduce intracellular ROS levels in various cell types by promoting the intracellular ROS-scavenging system, which includes modulating detoxifying enzymes, such as superoxide dismutase 1(SOD1) and catalase (CAT). It prompted us to question that whether Quercetin could also negate the cytotoxic effects of anti-neoplastic drugs that increased ROS. The aim of this study was to investigate the effects of Quercetin in combination with Cisplatin and other anti-neoplastic drugs in ovarian cancer cells both *in vitro* and *in vivo*, along with the molecular mechanism of action.

Materials and Methods

Ethics Statement

This study was carried out in strict accordance with the recommendations in the Guide for the Care and Use of Laboratory Animals of the National Institutes of Health. The protocol was approved by the Committee on the Ethics of Animal Experiments of Tongji Medical college, Huazhong University of Science and Technology (Permit Number: S292). All efforts were made to minimize suffering of animals.

Chemicals and reagents

Quercetin (>99% pure), cis-Diammineplatinum(II) dichloride (Cisplatin), Taxol (Paclitaxel) was purchased from Sigma Chemical Co. (St. Louis, MO), dissolved in DMSO, aliquoted, and stored at $-20°C$. Pirarubicin (Zhejiang Hisun Pharmaceutical Co.,Ltd., China) and 5-Fluorouracil (5-Fu) (Shanghai Xudong Haipu Pharmaceutical Co Ltd., China) were dissolved in normal saline.

Cell culture

The human epithelial ovarian cancer cell line C13* [11] is the Cisplatin-resistant clone of ov2008 cell line which was derived from a human ovarian carcinoma. This C13* cell line was a gift from Prof. Rakesh at the Ottawa Regional Cancer Center, Ottawa, Canada [3]. SKOV3 ovarian cancer cell line was obtained from American Type Culture Collection (ATCC). Ovarian cancer cells were cultured in RPMI 1640 medium with 10% fetal bovine serum (FBS) at 37°C with 5% CO_2.

Cell viability

Cell viability was measured with CCK8 assay (cell counting kit-8, Dojindo Molecular Technologies, Tokyo, Japan). Cells were prepared in 96-well cell culture plates at a cellular density of $5×10^3$ cells/well and treated with Quercetin/anti-neoplastic drugs (Cisplatin, taxol, Pirarubicin and 5-Fu) or vehicle (DMSO with the same dilution rate as the drugs) at 37°C for 48 h. The cell monolayer was washed three times with phosphate-buffered saline (PBS) containing 1.2 mM $CaCl_2$ and 0.7 mM $MgCl_2$, then a 1:10 diluted CCK8 solution in RPMI 1640 was added to the cells and incubated for 2 h at 37°C. The results were measured by a microplate reader at 450 nm and expressed as percentages of control values (obtained for cells treated with vehicle).

Annexin V/PI staining

Cells were trypsinized and washed with serum-containing medium. The samples ($5×10^5$ cells) were centrifuged for 5 min at 400×g and the supernatant was discarded. The cells were then stained using an Annexin V-FICT/PI apoptosis kit (keyGEN bioTECH, Nanjing) in accordance with the manufacturer's instructions. The number of apoptotic cells was detected and analyzed using flow cytometry.

Measurement of ROS

ROS was detected using Reactive Oxygen Species Assay Kit (Beyotime, China) according to manufacturer's instructions. After the molecular probe 5-(and-6)-chloromethyl-2′,7′-dichlorodihydrofluorescein diacetate (DCFH-DA) diffuses into cells and is sequestered intracellularly by de-esterification, the subsequent reaction with peroxides generates fluorescent 5-chloromethyl-2′,7′-dichlorofluorescein (DCF). Briefly, following treatment, cells were collected by centrifugation, resuspended in PBS containing 10 μmol/L DCFH-DA, incubated for 20 min at 37°C, washed with PBS to remove excess dye, and then incubated with RPMI medium at 37°C for 10 min, Fluorescence results were obtained using the FL-1 channel of a Becton Dickinson FACSCalibur, and analyzed using CellQuest Software. The percentage of cells displaying increased dye uptake was used to reflect an increase in ROS levels.

Immunofluorescence assay

Briefly, C13* cells were seeded in 24-well cell culture plates containing a sterile glass slide at a cellular density of $2×10^4$ cells/well. After treated with different drugs for 48 h, cells were washed three times with ice-cold PBS, and fixed with 4% paraformaldehyde in PBS for 20 min at room temperature. After blocking with 1% non-fat milk for 2 h, goat anti-8-OHdG and mouse anti-γH2AX antibodies (Millipore) were added to the slides respectively. Following 4 h incubation, the slides were washed 3 times with 0.5% PBS-Tween20 (PBST) and the fluorescein CY3-conjugated secondary mouse anti-goat antibody and FITC-conjugated goat anti-mouse secondary antibody (Sigma-Aldrich) were added at a dilution of 1:100. The cells were incubated for 45 min at 37°C. Finally, the cells were washed as described above and examined with fluorescence microscopy (Olympus, Tokyo, Japan). Five random high power field images were taken of each group, Image J software was used to calculate the numbers of highly positive stained cells.

Real-time Reverse Transcription Polymerase Chain Reaction (RT-PCR)

C13* cells were seeded in 6-well cell culture plates at a density of $5×10^5$ cells/well, and treated with Quercetin and Cisplatin for 48 h. Total RNA was extracted using Trizol (Invitrogen, China). Complementary DNA was synthesized in accordance with the manufacturers protocol (Toyobo, Japan). Real-time PCR amplification was performed on an ABI PRISM 7500 cycler with SYBR reagent (Toyobo, Japan). The thermal cycling conditions were set as given in the instructions included with the cycler, with an annealing temperature of 60°C. Oligonucleotides used for amplification of Superoxide dismutase 1 (SOD1), endonuclease G (ENDOG), cytochrome c (cyto-c), glutathione peroxidase (GPx), catalase (CAT) and uncoupling protein 2 (UCP2) (Table S1) were designed using Primer 5.0 and synthesized by Invitrogen. Quantitative normalization of cDNA was performed using the housekeeping gene glyceraldehyde-3-phosphate dehydrogenase (GAPDH) as an internal control to determine the uniformity of the template RNA for all specimens. For each sample, the expression of the gene of interest was derived from the ratio of their expression to GAPDH expression using the following formula: relative expression $= 2 - (\Delta Ct$ sample $- \Delta Ct$ control), $\Delta Ct = Ct$ gene $- Ct$ GAPDH.

In vivo xenograft studies

The *in vivo* evaluation of Quercetin was carried out using a xenograft model of human C13*cells. Athymic BALB/c-nu nude mice (4–6 weeks old, obtained from Beijing HFK bioscience company, Beijing, China) were housed in a specific pathogen-free room within the animal facilities at the Laboratory Animal Center of University of Tongji Medical College. Animals were allowed to acclimatize to their new environment for one week prior to use. C13* cells (2×10^6) were resuspended in PBS medium with Matrigel basement membrane matrix (BD Biosciences, Bedford, MA) at a 1:1 ratio (total volume 100 μL), then were subcutaneously injected into the flanks of nude mice (day 0). From the 10th day of injection, mice were randomly assigned to 4 treatment groups (n = 8 for each group) and injected intraperitoneally (i.p.) with normal saline (NS), Quercetin (20 mg/kg body weight, daily), Cisplatin (4 mg/kg body weight, every four days), and combined Quercetin and Cisplatin treatment (using the above dosages) for 21 consecutive days. Body weight and tumor mass were measured every 5 days. Tumor volume was determined using a caliper and calculated according to the formula (width$^2 \times$length)/2. Mice were killed by cervical dislocation under anesthesia after three weeks treatment (day 30).

Immunohistochemical analysis

Immunohistochemical studies were performed on the xenograft tumors after they were removed from nude mice. The tumors were fixed in 40 mg/mL paraformaldehyde, paraffin-embedded and cut into 4 μm serial sections. Next, endogenous peroxidases were quenched and the sections were washed carefully with phosphate buffered saline (PBS) three times. The sections were blocked with 2% goat serum and rabbit serum respectively in PBS at 37°C temperature for 45 min, then incubated with mouse anti-SOD1 antibody (1:500 dilution, Abcam) and goat anti-8-OHdG antibody (1:800 dilution, Millipore) overnight at 4°C. Afterwards, the sections were incubated with goat anti- mouse and mouse anti- goat horseradish peroxidase-conjugated secondary antibodies separately and avidin-biotin complex followed by diaminobenzi- dine (Vector ABC, Burlingame, CA, USA). Immersed in 2% ammonia water, haematoxylin was used for counterstaining. Sections were incubated with rabbit and goat IgG serum respectively as negative controls.

Positive 8-OHdG staining was mainly in the nuclei while positive expression of SOD1 was primarily a cytoplasm pattern both in tumor cells rather than in the stromal cells. Because of the intensity of 8-OHdG and SOD1 staining within each section was mostly homogeneous, the immunoreactivity in the samples was semi-quantitatively evaluated using the following criteria: strong positive (scored as 3), strong staining intensity (>90% of cancer cells); moderate positive (scored as 2), moderate staining intensity (>50–89% of positive cells); weak positive (scored as 1), weak staining intensity (>10–49% of positive cells); absent (scored as 0), no staining intensity and no positive or only a few positive cells [12,13]. The staining intensity and proportion of each section stained were calculated using five random high power field images of each group by two independent investigators.

Statistical Analysis

All experiments were performed in triplicate. Data are presented as mean ± standard deviation. Statistical analyses were performed using SPSS19.0. Differences between two groups were compared using the Student's *t* test. The statistical differences between more than two groups were determined by one-way ANOVA analysis followed by post hoc pairwise comparisons. $P < 0.05$ was considered statistically significant.

Results

Quercetin at low concentrations promotes the survival of ovarian cancer C13* cells treated with Cisplatin

Platinum-based chemotherapy is the most important therapy in the treatment of ovarian cancer. To determine the potential role Quercetin may play in Cisplatin resistance in ovarian cancer, C13* cells were exposed to different concentrations of Quercetin, Cisplatin, or a combination of the two. The IC50 of Cisplatin-treated C13* cells was approximately 80 μM (IC50 = 78.8 μM, 95% CI: 72.9– 85.1 μM) (Figure S1A). When C13* cells were treated with 80 μM Cisplatin in combination with increasing doses of Quercetin, we found that the cytotoxicity of Cisplatin was reduced when combining with low concentrations of Quercetin (5 μM to 30 μM), while relative high concentration of Quercetin (100 μM) increased Cisplatin cytotoxicity (Fig. 1A). To determine the antagonistic effect or sensitization of the drugs combination, we calculated the combina- tion index (CI) for the drugs based on Chou and Talalay's theorem [14]. The results showed that low concentrations of Quercetin antagonized the cytotoxic effects of cisplatin in C13* cells, while high concentrations of Quercetin have an additive effect with cisplatin (Table S2). We also carried out combination experiments with a series of different cisplatin concentrations plus fixed concentrations of Quercetin (20 μM), which showed that low concentrations of Quercetin increased C13* cell resistance to cisplatin in varying degrees (Figure S2). Phase-contrast images of C13* cells treated with vehicle control, Cisplatin, or combinations of Quercetin (20 μM, 80 μM) with Cisplatin (80 μM) are shown in Fig. 1B.

To further quantify the apoptotic effects of Quercetin and Cisplatin treatment, C13* cells were stained with Annexin-V FITC and PI, and subsequently analyzed by flow cytometry for cell apoptosis. Obvious decreases in numbers of apoptotic cells were detected for cells treated with Cisplatin and 20 μM Quercetin than with Cisplatin alone (Fig. 1C,1D). Proportions of Annexin V-stained cells were higher in Cisplatin-treated cells than those of cells treated with an additional 20 μM Quercetin.

In order to generalize our conclusions, we carried out CCK8 assays in SKOV3, a commonly used ovarian cancer cell line. The results revealed that low concentrations of Quercetin reduced the cytotoxic effects of Cisplatin in SKOV3 cells (Figure S3).

Quercetin attenuated the therapy effects of different anti-neoplastic drugs in ovarian cancer cells

To examine whether Quercetin attenuate the anti-cancer effects of other anti-neoplastic drugs, we treated C13* cells with three other anti-neoplastic drugs commonly used in ovarian cancer treatment, 5-Fu, Taxol, and Pirarubicin. C13* cells were treated with a series of increasing doses of Quercetin and fixed 5-Fu (5 μM), Taxol (3 μM) and Pirarubicin (3 nM) at approximate concentrations of the IC50 respectively (Figure S1). Similar to the results obtained with Cisplatin, treatment using these drugs in combination with Quercetin resulted in more cell resistance than treatment with anti-neoplastic drugs alone (Fig. 2.) At the concentration of 20 μM, Quercetin showed obvious anti-apoptotic effects against these three drugs. Quercetin showed a low-

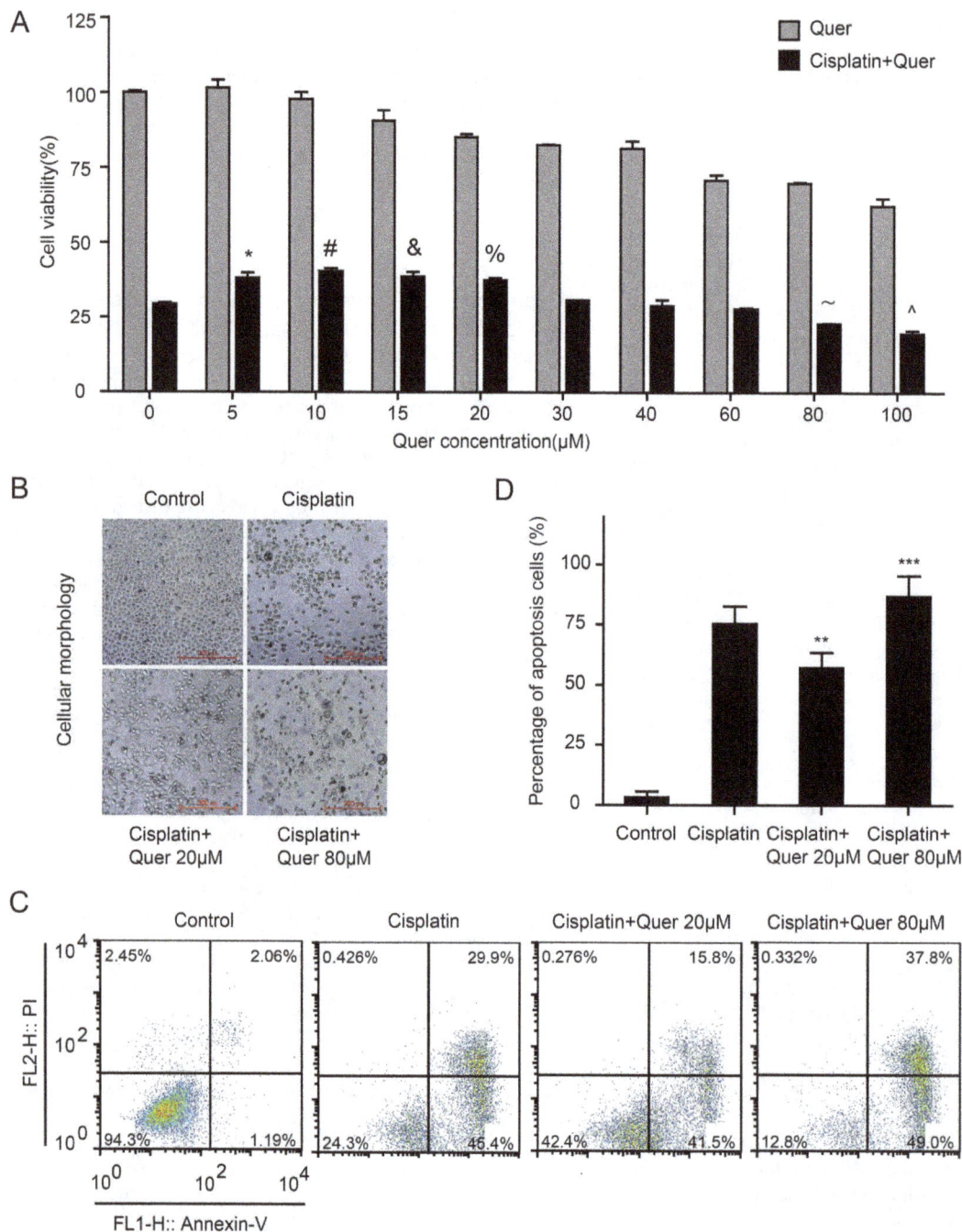

Figure 1. Quercetin in combination with Cisplatin impacts the survival of ovarian cancer C13* cells. (A), Cell viability of groups exposed to different concentrations of Quercetin alone, or combined with 80 μM Cisplatin for 48 hours was measured with CCK8 assay and expressed as percentage of control values. *$P = 0.039$, #$P = 0.009$, &$P = 0.027$, %$P = 0.010$, ANOVA test followed by post hoc pairwise comparisons. (B), Phase-contrast images of C13* cells treated with vehicle control (DMSO with the same dilution rate as the drugs), Cisplatin, or combination of Quercetin(20 μM,80 μM) with Cisplatin (80 μM). (C, D), Cell apoptosis of different treatment groups was detected and analyzed using flow cytometry. Experiments were performed in triplicate (N = 3 per experiment). Group of Cisplatin combined with Quercetin treatment VS. group of Cisplatin treatment, **$P = 0.033$, ***$P = 0.043$, ANOVA test followed by post hoc pairwise comparisons.

concentration-specific protecting effect to ovarian cancer cells treated with 5-Fu (Fig. 2A), similar to the results obtained with Cisplatin. In combination with Taxol or Pirarubicin, however, Quercetin maintained the effect of promoting cells survial against anticancer drugs even at relatively high concentrations (80 μM, 100 μM) (Fig. 2B, 2C).

Quercetin reduced the oxidative injury of ovarian cancer cells caused by Cisplatin

We investigated the mechanism by which Quercetin attenuated the cytotoxic effects of Cisplatin. As previously reported [15], many anti-neoplastic drugs including Cisplatin, lead to increases in intracellular ROS that contribute to their therapeutic effect. We

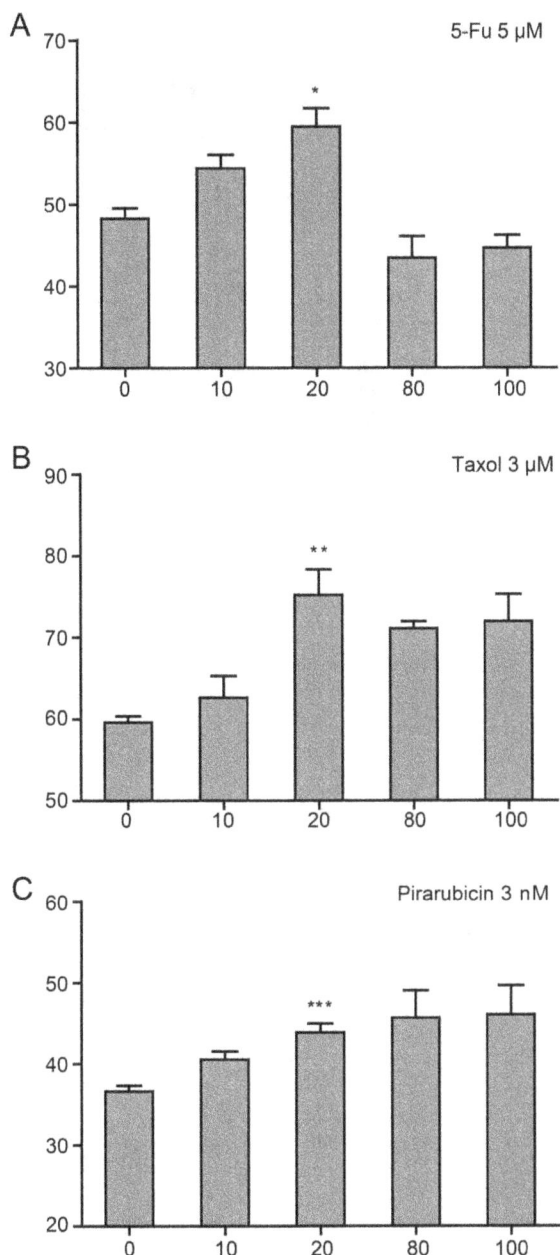

Figure 2. Quercetin in combination with different anti-neoplastic drugs impacts the survival of ovarian cancer C13* cells. (A~C), Cell viability of Quercetin in combination with 5-Fu, Taxol and Pirarubicin was measured with CCK8 assay and expressed as percentage of control values. N = 3 per experiment. Group of Cisplatin combined with Quercetin 20 μM treatment VS. Group of Cisplatin treatment, *P = 0.048, **P = 0.040, ***P = 0.032, Student t-test.

questioned whether Quercetin may alter the ROS-associated injury caused by these drugs. The expression of 8-hydroxydeoxyguanosine (8-OHdG), a marker of oxidative DNA stress and the most frequently detected and studied DNA lesion [16], was estimated by immunofluorescence assay. We also measured the level of total cytotoxic injury by detection of γH2AX, a common marker of DNA damage. The results showed that the fluorescence intensities of both γH2AX and 8-OHdG were much lower in the treatment group of 80 μM Cisplatin combined with low concen-

tration Quercetin (20 μM) than the group of 80 μM Cisplatin alone. Contrary to this, 80 μM Cisplatin with high concentration (60 μM, 100 μM) of Quercetin increased the intensity of fluorescence (Fig. 3A, 3B). Counting of positive cells using Image J software showed that combination treatment with Quercetin (20 μM) had a more obvious decrease of 8-OHdG than that of γH2AX, compared to Cisplatin treatment alone (36.40% and 19.33% respectively) (Fig. 3B). It indicated that low concentrations of Quercetin reduced the oxidative injury of ovarian cancer cells caused by Cisplatin.

Quercetin reduced ROS level of ovarian cancer cells undergoing Cisplatin treatment

To determine whether Quercetin reduced the ROS injury by decreasing intracellular ROS, Reactive Oxygen Species Assay Kit was used to detect intracellular ROS levels of C13* cells in different treatment groups. Compared to cells treated with vehicle control or Cisplatin alone, treatment with an additional 20 μM Quercetin lead to a reduction in intracellular levels of ROS (Fig. 4A, 4C). Quantitative analysis showed that Quercetin (20 μM) treatment gave an obvious reduction in ROS level (mean value 70.4) compared to the control group (mean value 99.05) (P< 0.001) (Fig. 4B, 4D). In agreement with previous results, exposure to Cisplatin caused ovarian cancer C13* cells to accumulate the intracellular ROS, with a mean ROS level of 123.5. In treatment group of Cisplatin combined with Quercetin, this value was reduced to 83.38 (Fig. 4D), even lower than the vehicle control group (99.05) (P<0.001) (Fig. 4B).

Quercetin increased the expression of endogenous antioxidant enzymes in ovarian cancer cells

The results above indicated that Quercetin could reduce intracellular ROS of ovarian cancer cell, so we sought to determine a mechanism of action. The most important antioxidant components of cells against ROS are the endogenous antioxidant enzymes, including Superoxide dismutase 1 (SOD1), endonuclease G (ENDOG), cytochrome c (cyto-c), glutathione peroxidase (GPx), catalase (CAT), and uncoupling protein 2 (UCP2). We measured the expression of endogenous antioxidant enzymes by realtime PCR. Compared to cells treated with vehicle control or Cisplatin alone, treatment combining Cisplatin with 20 μM Quercetin lead to various degrees of increase in the expression of SOD1, ENDOG, cyto-c, GPx, CAT and UCP2 (Fig. 5A~F).

Quercetin promoted ovarian cancer growth with Cisplatin treatment in vivo

We used C13* cells to generate xenograft tumors in athymic nude BALB/c-nu mice to determine whether Quercetin could attenuate the effects of chemotherapy in vivo. As expected, treatment with Cisplatin alone reduced tumor growth compared with vehicle treated mice. Treatment with Quercetin alone slightly suppressed tumor growth compared with normal saline control (tumor volumes of 111.75 mm^3 and 120.51 mm^3 respectively) (P = 0.015). Tumors from mice treated with Cisplatin in combination with Quercetin were approximately 1.8 times larger at day 30 than those treated with Cisplatin alone (P<0.001; Fig. 6A, 6B). Comparing the average weights of tumors removed from mice, we found that tumors treated with combination of Quercetin and Cisplatin (72.53±7.33 mg) were significantly heavier than that treated with Cisplatin alone (41.47±6.72 mg), P<0.001 (Fig. 4D). Further, the combination of Cisplatin and Quercetin treatment

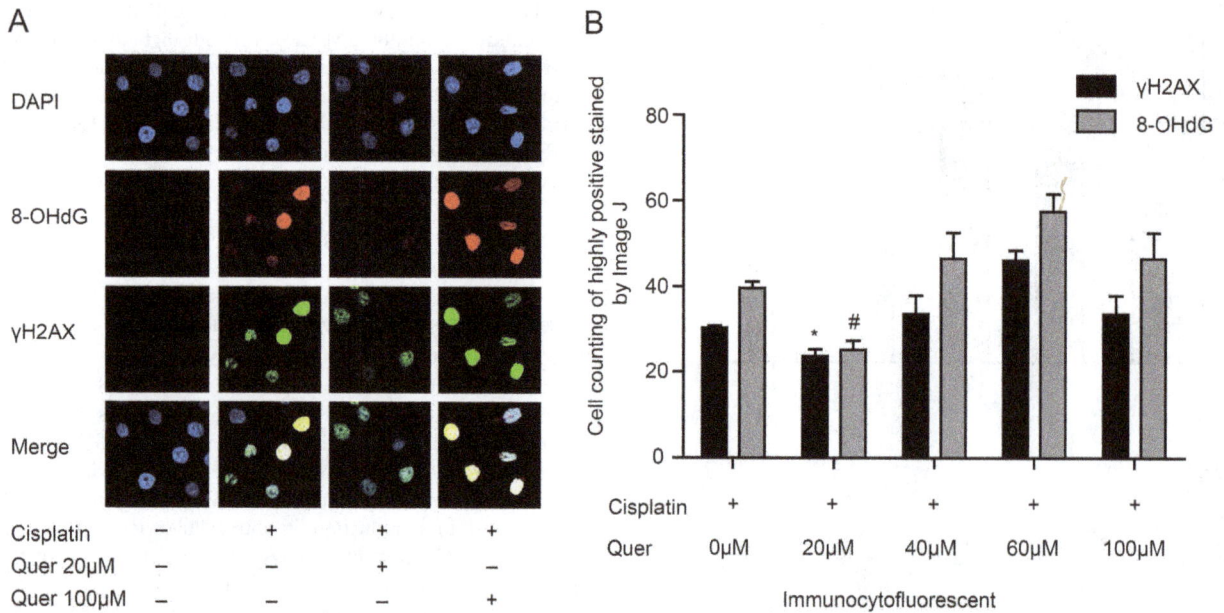

Figure 3. Quercetin reduced oxidative injury of ovarian cancer cells caused by Cisplatin. (A), 8-OHdG and H2AX expression in C13* cells treated with Quercetin in combination with Cisplatin was detected by immunofluorescence assay. (B), Numbers of highly positive stained cells in five random high-power fields were counted by Image J and expressed as percentage of Cisplatin group values. Group of Cisplatin combined with Quercetin 20 μM treatment VS. Group of Cisplatin treatment, N = 3. *P = 0.004, #P = 0.001, Student t-test.

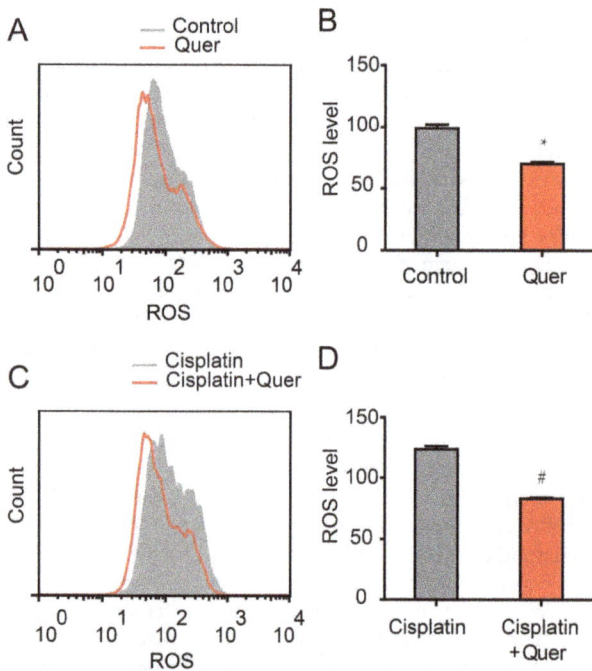

Figure 4. Quercetin reduced ROS level of ovarian cancer cells in combination with Cisplatin treatment. Intracellular ROS levels of C13* cells of different treatment groups were detected by Reactive Oxygen Species Assay using flow cytometry. (A, B) The ROS levels of C13* cells treated by vehicle control or 20 μM Quercetin for 24 hours. (C, D) The ROS levels of C13* cells treated by 80 μM Cisplatin with or without 20 μM Quercetin for 24 hours. N = 3. *P < 0.001, #P < 0.001, Student t-test.

displayed a cancer promoting effect compared to the control group, measured both in tumor size and in tumor weight (Fig. 6C).

Quercetin enhanced the expression of endogenous antioxidant enzyme SOD1 of ovarian cancer cells *in vivo*, and prevented ROS-induced damage

In order to confirm the protective effect against oxidative injury by Quercetin in vivo, immunohistochemical assays were carried out in tumors removed from nude mice xenograft model. 8-OHdG, a marker of oxidative DNA stress, was located mainly in cancer cell nucleus. In tumors treated with vehical or Quercetin alone, 8-OHdG staining showed weak intensity with the scores of 0.4 and 0.6 respectively. In the group treated with Cisplatin alone, almost all cancer cells displayed extremely strong 8-OHdG staining with score 2.8. As expected, mice group treated by Cisplatin in combination with Quercetin had a much lower level of 8-OHdG staining (score 1.6) in tumors than the one treated with Cisplatin alone (Fig. 6D–E).

DNA repair enzymes prevent the accumulation of damaged DNA and antioxidants protect cells against free radicals. We detected SOD1 expression, which is a critical endogenous antioxidant enzyme for tolerating the oxidative stress, to find out if Quercetin affected on the activity of endogenous antioxidant enzyme. Positive expression of SOD1 was primarily a cytoplasm pattern in ovarian cancer cells rather than stromal cells. The antioxidant enzyme SOD1 was highly overexpressed in tumors treated with Quercetin or Cisplatin plus Quercetin (score 2.0 and 2.6 respectively) compared to tumors treated with vehicle or Cisplatin alone (score 1.2 and 0.6 respectively) (Fig. 6D–E). The results indicated that Quercetin enhanced the endogenous antioxidant enzyme SOD1 expression of ovarian cancer cells *in vivo*, and prevented ROS-induced damage.

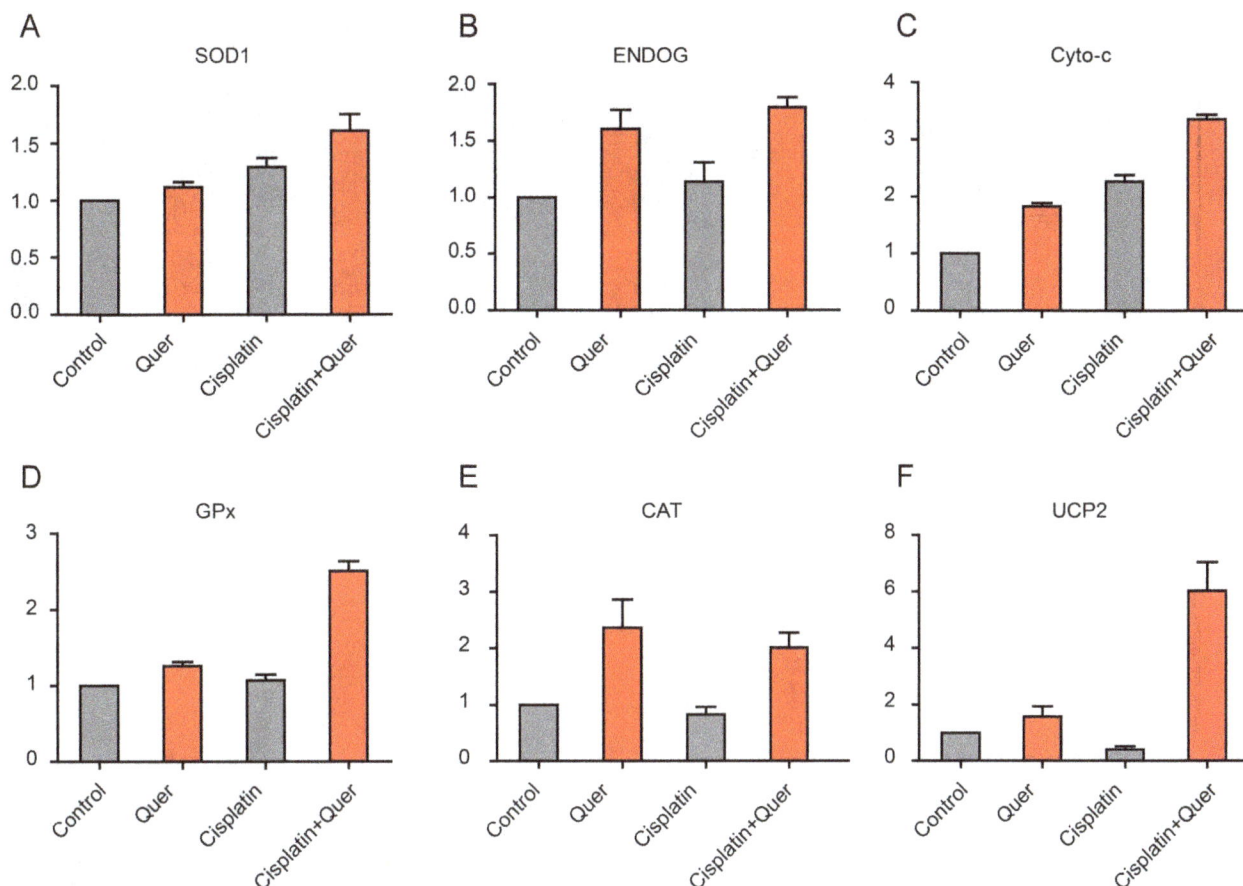

Figure 5. Quercetin increased the expression of endogenous antioxidant enzymes in ovarian cancer cells. (A~F), Expression of antioxidant enzymes of C13* cells was detected by real-time PCR. N = 3.

Discussion

As a classical flavonoid compound, Quercetin is usually recommended to take orally every day for general health care and cancer prevention. Staedler *et al.* found that Quercetin at concentrations of 5 µM and 10 µM could increase the efficacy of 100 µM doxorubicin in breast cancer cells in vitro [17,18], while other researchers came to different conclusions [8,9]. Samuel *et al.* [8] reported that in colorectal and prostate cancer cells, the therapeutic effects of drug in combination with Quercetin were influenced by the effective doses and the p53 status of the cells (the combination of 5-Fu with up to 6 µM Quercetin promoted cologenic survival in p53 null cells while 50 µM Quercetin acted opposite role in p53 wild type cells). In this study, Quercetin at high concentrations, either alone or combined with Cisplatin displayed anti-neoplastic effects in ovarian cancer C13* cells, while low concentration (5 µM–30 µM) of Quercetin appeared to antagonize the cytotoxic effects of anti-neoplastic agents including Cisplatin, 5-Fu, Taxol, and Pirarubicin. We also explored the mechanism of the anti-apoptotic effect of Quercetin when combined with Cisplatin. C13* cells treated with additional 20 µM Quercetin showed a decreased intracellular ROS levels and elevated expression of endogenous antioxidant enzymes including SOD1, ENDOG, cyto-c, GPx, CAT, and UCP2, than cells treated with Cisplatin alone. In a nude mouse xenograft model injected with C13* cells, daily intraperitoneal injection of Quercetin at 40 mg/kg led to a substantial reduction of

therapeutic efficacy of Cisplatin. Tumors in mice treated with Cisplatin in combination with Quercetin displayed enhanced SOD1 expression and decreased 8-OHdG staining than those of mice treated with Cisplatin alone. Overall, our data indicated that administration of Quercetin at low concentrations may antagonize the cytotoxic effects of anti-neoplastic drugs in ovarian cancer cells, and that Quercetin decreased the levels of oxidative injury caused by Cisplatin.

Researchers have not reached a unanimous conclusion about the absorption of Quercetin intake, and taking into account individual differences in absorption and different dosage forms, the plasma concentration after a certain dose of Quercetin taken was not under control. It has been reported that a 100 mg single dose Quercetin taken orally was found to result in a serum concentration of 0.8 mM [19], while aother report showed that a 4 g oral dose of Quercetin led to no measurable Quercetin in either the plasma or urine of healthy volunteers [20]. A recent study showed that, in healthy volunteers supplemented with 50, 100, or 150 mg/day Quercetin orally for 2 weeks, plasma concentrations of Quercetin were 145 nmol/L, 217 nmol/L and 380 nmol/L respectively [21], which were all lower than the low-concentration dosage (20 µM) used for our *in vitro* experiments. It's hard to control the exact plasma concentration of Quercetin for individuals to intake it. As the results of the present study, low concentration of Quercetin may attenuate the therapeutic effects of Cisplatin and some other anti-neoplastic drugs, so Quercetin

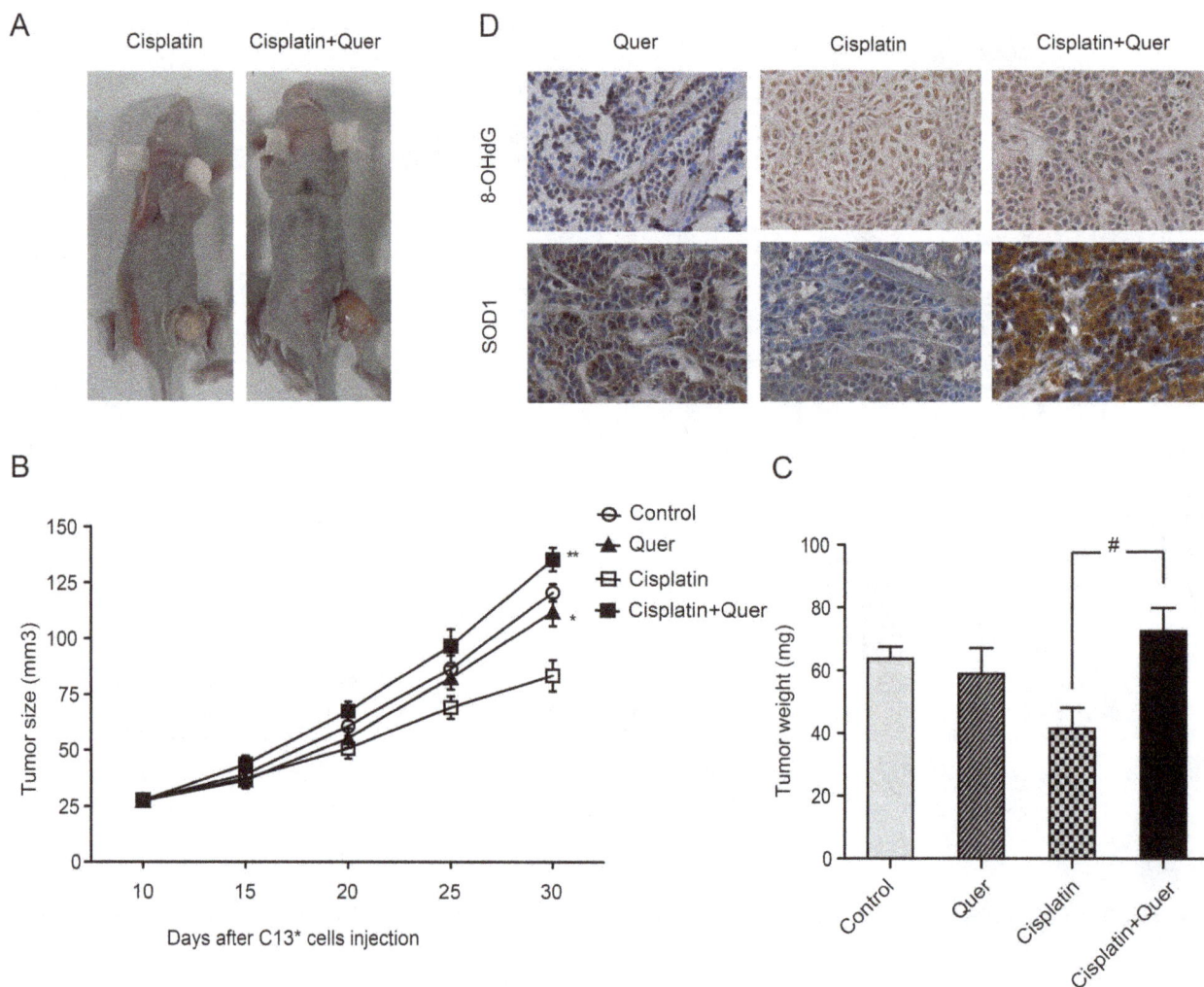

Figure 6. Quercetin in combination with Cisplatin promoted ovarian tumor growth. Mice were injected with NS, 20 mg/kg Quercetin, 4 mg/kg Cisplatin, or Quercetin plus Cisplatin, ip. C13* cell xenografts (2×10^6) were inoculated in the right flank of female athymic nude nu/nu mice. Tumor volumes was determined by a caliper and calculated according to the formula (width2×length)/2. (A), Tumor formation in mice of Cisplatin treatment group and combined with Quercetin group. (B), Average relative tumor growth as analyzed by the increase in tumor volumes for 8 mice per experimental group **Cisplatin plus Quercetin VS. Cisplatin, $P<0.001$; *Quercetin VS. Control, $P=0.015$, ANOVA test followed by post hoc pairwise comparisons; (C), Average tumor weights of each group. #Cisplatin combined with Quercetin VS. Cisplatin, $P<0.001$, ANOVA test followed by post hoc pairwise comparisons; (D), Immunohistochemical analysis of 8-OHdG and SOD1 in xenograft tumors removed from nude mice. (E), The quantification data of the differences in the expression SOD-1 and 8-OHdG, *: $P<0.001$, **:$P<0.001$, ANOVA test followed by post hoc pairwise comparisons.

supplementation in ovarian cancer patients during chemotherapy may be antagonistic to the cytotoxic effects of chemotherapy.

Supporting Information

Figure S1 The IC50 values of C13* cells treated with four anti-neoplastic drugs respectively. Cell viability of C13* cells exposed to a series of concentrations of Cisplatin, 5-Fu, Taxol and Pirarubicin for 48 hours was measured using CCK8 assay and expressed as percentage of control values (A~D).

Figure S2 Quercetin at a low concentration (20 μM) improved C13* cells survival in combination of different concentrations of Cisplatin treatment.

Figure S3 The IC50 value and cell viability of SKOV3 cells exposed to a series of concentrations of Cisplatin for 48 hours was measured using CCK8 assay (A); Cell viability of of SKOV3 cells exposed to different concentrations of Quercetin alone, or combined with 50 μM Cisplatin for 48 hours was measured using CCK8 assay and expressed as percentage of control values (B).

Table S1 Primers used in this study for real-time PCR experiments.

Table S2 The combination indexs of different concentration of Quercetin in combinations with Cisplatin.

Author Contributions

Conceived and designed the experiments: DM GC DW. Performed the experiments: NL CS BZ. Analyzed the data: AL CS HX. Contributed reagents/materials/analysis tools: DM. Wrote the paper: NL GC.

References

1. Siegel R, Naishadham D, Jemal A (2013) Cancer statistics, 2013. CA Cancer J Clin 63: 11–30.
2. Formica JV, Regelson W (1995) Review of the biology of Quercetin and related bioflavonoids. Food Chem Toxicol 33: 1061–1080.
3. Asselin E, Mills GB, Tsang BK (2001) XIAP regulates Akt activity and caspase-3-dependent cleavage during cisplatin-induced apoptosis in human ovarian epithelial cancer cells. Cancer Res 61: 1862–1868.
4. Gates MA, Vitonis AF, Tworoger SS, Rosner B, Titus-Ernstoff L, et al. (2009) Flavonoid intake and ovarian cancer risk in a population-based case-control study. Int J Cancer 124: 1918–1925.
5. Kim JY, Kim EH, Park SS, Lim JH, Kwon TK, et al. (2008) Quercetin sensitizes human hepatoma cells to TRAIL-induced apoptosis via Sp1-mediated DR5 up-regulation and proteasome-mediated c-FLIPS down-regulation. J Cell Biochem 105: 1386–1398.
6. Chang YF, Chi CW, Wang JJ (2006) Reactive oxygen species production is involved in quercetin-induced apoptosis in human hepatoma cells. Nutr Cancer 55: 201–209.
7. Nessa MU, Beale P, Chan C, Yu JQ, Huq F (2011) Synergism from combinations of cisplatin and oxaliplatin with quercetin and thymoquinone in human ovarian tumour models. Anticancer Res 31: 3789–3797.
8. Samuel T, Fadlalla K, Mosley L, Katkoori V, Turner T, et al. (2012) Dual-mode interaction between quercetin and DNA-damaging drugs in cancer cells. Anticancer Res 32: 61–71.
9. Robaszkiewicz A, Balcerczyk A, Bartosz G (2007) Antioxidative and prooxidative effects of quercetin on A549 cells. Cell Biol Int 31: 1245–1250.
10. Heaney ML, Gardner JR, Karasavvas N, Golde DW, Scheinberg DA, et al. (2008) Vitamin C antagonizes the cytotoxic effects of antineoplastic drugs. Cancer Res 68: 8031–8038.
11. Sun C, Li N, Yang Z, Zhou B, He Y, et al. (2013) miR-9 regulation of BRCA1 and ovarian cancer sensitivity to cisplatin and PARP inhibition. J Natl Cancer Inst 105: 1750–1758.
12. Pylvas M, Puistola U, Laatio L, Kauppila S, Karihtala P (2011) Elevated serum 8-OHdG is associated with poor prognosis in epithelial ovarian cancer. Anticancer Res 31: 1411–1415.
13. Lu P, Qiao J, He W, Wang J, Jia Y, et al. (2014) Genome-Wide Gene Expression Profile Analyses Identify CTTN as a Potential Prognostic Marker in Esophageal Cancer. PLoS One 9: e88918.
14. Chou TC (2010) Drug combination studies and their synergy quantification using the Chou-Talalay method. Cancer Res 70: 440–446.
15. Gao S, Chen T, Choi MY, Liang Y, Xue J, et al. (2013) Cyanidin reverses cisplatin-induced apoptosis in HK-2 proximal tubular cells through inhibition of ROS-mediated DNA damage and modulation of the ERK and AKT pathways. Cancer Lett 333: 36–46.
16. Wu LL, Chiou CC, Chang PY, Wu JT (2004) Urinary 8-OHdG: a marker of oxidative stress to DNA and a risk factor for cancer, atherosclerosis and diabetics. Clin Chim Acta 339: 1–9.
17. Staedler D, Idrizi E, Kenzaoui BH, Juillerat-Jeanneret L (2011) Drug combinations with quercetin: doxorubicin plus quercetin in human breast cancer cells. Cancer Chemother Pharmacol 68: 1161–1172.
18. Ramos AM, Aller P (2008) Quercetin decreases intracellular GSH content and potentiates the apoptotic action of the antileukemic drug arsenic trioxide in human leukemia cell lines. Biochem Pharmacol 75: 1912–1923.
19. Hollman PC, van Trijp JM, Mengelers MJ, de Vries JH, Katan MB (1997) Bioavailability of the dietary antioxidant flavonol quercetin in man. Cancer Lett 114: 139–140.
20. Gugler R, Leschik M, Dengler HJ (1975) Disposition of quercetin in man after single oral and intravenous doses. Eur J Clin Pharmacol 9: 229–234.
21. Egert S, Wolffram S, Bosy-Westphal A, Boesch-Saadatmandi C, Wagner AE, et al. (2008) Daily quercetin supplementation dose-dependently increases plasma quercetin concentrations in healthy humans. J Nutr 138: 1615–1621.

2

Induction of Peroxiredoxin 1 by Hypoxia Regulates Heme Oxygenase-1 via NF-κB in Oral Cancer

Min Zhang[1]☉, Min Hou[1]☉, Lihua Ge[1], Congcong Miao[1], Jianfei Zhang[1], Xinying Jing[1], Ni Shi[2], Tong Chen[2]*, Xiaofei Tang[1]*

1 Institute of Dental Research, Beijing Stomatological Hospital and School of Stomatology, Capital Medical University, Beijing, China, 2 Division of Medical Oncology, Department of Internal Medicine, The Arthur G. James Cancer Hospital and Richard J. Solove Research Institute, The Ohio State University, Columbus, Ohio, United States of America

Abstract

Overexpression of peroxiredoxin 1 (Prx1) has been observed in numerous cancers including oral squamous cell carcinoma (OSCC). The precise molecular mechanism of up-regulation of Prx1 in carcinogenesis, however, is still poorly understood. The objective of this study is to investigate the relationship between Prx1 and hypoxia, and potential mechanism(s) of Prx1 in OSCC cell line SCC15 and xenograft model. We treated wild-type and Prx1 knockdown SCC15 cells with transient hypoxia followed by reoxygenation. We detected the condition of hypoxia, production of reactive oxygen species (ROS), and expression and/or activity of Prx1, heme oxygenase 1 (HO-1) and nuclear factor-kappa B (NF-κB). We found that hypoxia induces ROS accumulation, up-regulates Prx1, increases NF-κB translocation and DNA binding activity, and down-regulates HO-1 *in vitro*. In Prx1 knockdown cells, the expression level of HO-1 was increased, while NFκB translocation and DNA binding activity were decreased after hypoxia or hypoxia/reoxygenation treatment. Moreover, we mimicked the dynamic oxygenation tumor microenvironment in xenograft model and assessed the above indices in tumors with the maximal diameter of 2 mm, 5 mm, 10 mm or 15 mm, respectively. Our data showed that tumor hypoxic condition and expression of Prx1 are significantly associated with tumor growth. The expression of HO-1 and NF-κB, and NF-κB DNA binding activity were significantly elevated in 15 mm tumors, and the level of 8-hydroxydeoxyguanosine was increased in 10 mm and 15 mm tumors, compared to those in size of 2 mm. The results from this study provide experimental evidence that overexpression of Prx1 is associated with hypoxia, and Prx1/NF-κB/HO-1 signaling pathway may be involved in oral carcinogenesis.

Editor: Xin-Yuan Guan, The University of Hong Kong, China

Funding: This work was supported by the National Natural Science Foundation (81070836), the Beijing Natural Science Foundation (7102065) and ZYLX201407, Beijing Municipal Administration of Hospital Key Medical Development Project. The funders had no role in study design, data collection and analysis, decision to publish, or preparation of the manuscript.

Competing Interests: The authors have declared that no competing interests exist.

* Email: xftang10@yahoo.com (XFT); tong.chen@osumc.edu (TC)

☉ These authors contributed equally to this work.

Introduction

Oral squamous cell carcinoma (OSCC) is the most common head and neck cancer worldwide. Despite of the advantages of surgery, chemotherapy and radiotherapy, the 5-year survival rate of OSCC has not improved markedly in the past 30 years [1–3]. Metastasis and chemotherapy/radiotherapy resistance are still main concerns in clinical cancer therapy. Hypoxia, a common feature of cancer, promotes tumor cell invasion and metastasis in tumor microenvironment leading to the resistance of tumor cells to chemotherapy and radiotherapy [4,5]. It has been reported that the pathological features including active invasiveness, lymph node metastasis and vascular proliferation are associated with tumor tissue hypoxia in OSCC [6,7]. Exposure to hypobaric hypoxia leads to a significant increase in production of reactive oxygen species (ROS) in animals. The accumulation of ROS induced by hypoxia can result in oxidative stress and tumor progression [8]. The ROS-mediated response can be regulated by antioxidants

and antioxidant enzyme systems, such as superoxide dismutase, catalase and thioredoxin/peroxiredoxin [9].

Peroxiredoxins (Prxs) are a superfamily of multifunctional antioxidant thioredoxin-dependent peroxidases. Peroxiredoxin 1 (Prx1) is a major member in Prxs family and acts as an antioxidant to scavenge ROS in a wide range of organisms. Prx1 is involved in multiple biological conditions/activities including oxidative stress, cell proliferation and cell apoptosis [9]. Prx1 is overexpressed in many malignancies including esophagus, lung, breast and pancreatic cancers. Elevated Prx1 expression is associated with diminished overall survival and poor clinical outcome [10,11]. Overexpression of Prx1 has also been reported in OSCC, but the precise molecular mechanism of Prx1 in oral carcinogenesis remains obscure [12]. The expression of nuclear factor-kappa B (NF-κB) and Heme oxygenase-1 (HO-1) are increased in OSCC [13,14]. Numerous studies showed that NF-κB responses to hypoxia–reoxygenation *in vitro* [15]. NF-κB can be regulated by Prx1, through its initial activation in cytoplasm [16] or by altering the concentration of oxidant leading to the oxidative inactivation of NF-κB [17]. HO-1, a 32-kDa heat shock protein, can catalyze the oxidative degradation of heme to biliverdin, which is subsequently reduced to bilirubin. HO-1 can be induced by hypoxia, heat shock and cytotoxic oxidants [18,19]. HO-1 is one of the targets of NF-κB under stressful conditions [20–23]. Although the mechanism of Prx1 in oxidant stress is not clear, multiple evidences suggest that Prx1 may response to hypoxia and regulate NF-κB pathway cascade. In this study, we investigated the alteration of Prx1 in response to hypoxia and evaluated the potential correlations between Prx1 and NF-κB/HO-1 using oral cancer cell system and xenograft model.

Materials and Methods

Cell culture

Human OSCC cells, SCC15, (ATCC, Manassas, VA) were maintained in DMEM-F12 supplemented with 10% (v/v) fetal bovine serum (FBS) (Gibco, USA) containing 100 units/mL penicillin and 100 µg/mL streptomycin. SCC15 cells were grown at 37°C in an atmosphere of 5% CO_2 and 95% air. To knock down Prx1, SCC15 cells were transfected with Prx1 shRNA Plasmid (Santa Cruza Biotechnology) using Lipofectamine 2000 (Invitrogen, USA) according to the manufacturer's instructions. Control shRNA Plasmid-A (Santa Cruza Biotechnology) was transfected as control. The efficiency of Prx1 shRNA knockdown was determined by qRT-PCR and western blot analyses.

Pimonidazole staining in SCC15 cells

Cells were grown on coverslips for 24 h prior to hypoxia treatment. During hypoxia treatment, cells were put in a hypoxia incubator with gas containing 1% O_2, 5% CO_2 and 94% N_2 at 37°C for different periods of time. 200 µM of pimonidazole was added to the medium and incubated for 30 min. After washed with PBS, cells were fixed with paraformaldehyde (3%) at room temperature for 10 min and subsequently washed again with PBS. After blocked with BSA, coverslips were incubated with hypoxyprobe-1 mouse monoclonal antibody MAB1 (1:100) in the Hypoxyprobe-1 Plus kit (Chemicon Int., Temecula, CA) overnight. A secondary FITC-conjugated anti-mouse antibody was used. Coverslips were mounted and immunostained cells were examined on an Olympus IX71 microscope (Tokyo, Japan).

ROS detection

The production of intracellular ROS in cells was measured with 2′,7′-dichlorodihydrofluorescein diacetate (DCF-DA) using FACS analysis. The SCC15 cells were collected and suspended in 500 µL diluted DCF-DA. The mixture was incubated at 37°C for 20 min and then washed twice with PBS. The samples were analyzed by flow cytometer within 1 h. Data was normalized to the values from controls. The mean DCF fluorescence intensity was measured with excitation at 488 nm and emission at 525 nm. The experiments were performed in triplicate.

Immunofluorescence

Cells grown on coverslips were rinsed with PBS, fixed and permeabilized in acetone at −20°C for 10 min. After incubation with PBS containing 5% BSA for 1 h, monoclonal anti-NF-κB antibody (Cell Signaling Technology, 1:100 in PBS-BSA) was added at 4°C and incubated overnight. Coverslips were washed with PBS, incubated with Alexa Fluor 546 anti-rabbit (Molecular Probes, 1:500) secondary antibody at room temperature for 1 h, and mounted in Dako Cytomation fluorescent mounting medium. Confocal images were collected using a Leica SP2 laser scanning

confocal microscope equipped with UV excitation, an argon laser, a 633/1.32 OIL PH3 CS objective, and a confocal pinhole set at 1 Airy unit. All the confocal images were single optical sections.

Xenograft model

Forty male BALB/c nude mice (Beijing Vital River Laboratories, China) were used to produce tumorigenicity of the SCC15 cells in vivo. The experiment protocol was approved by the local ethical committee for animal use. The SCC15 cells (6×10^6) were suspended in 100 µL of phosphate-buffered saline and were transplanted subcutaneously in the right and left flanks of 4-week old nude mice. The tumor growth was monitored every 3 days after transplantation. The tumors were harvested when the maximal diameter of tumors reached 2 mm, 5 mm, 10 mm or 15 mm, respectively. To label hypoxic cells, the nude mice were injected intraperitoneally with 0.1 mL saline containing pimonidazole hydrochloride (1-[(2-hydroxyl-3-piperidinyl) propyl]-2-nitroimidazole hydrochloride) at a dosage of 60 mg/kg body weight 1 hour before tumor excision. Mice were implemented euthanasia and the tumor specimens were removed and immediately stored in liquid nitrogen for molecular/cellular analysis, or in formalin to make paraffin-embedded tissue blocks. Total 80 tumors were divided into four groups according to the tumor diameter (20 tumors/size).

Pimonidazole staining in tumors

The paraffin-embedded blocks with tumor samples were sectioned for pimonidazole staining. The sections were incubated with primary rabbit anti-pimonidazole antiserum hypoxyprobe-1 MAB1 (dilution: 1:50; Chemicon, USA) at 4°C overnight. To evaluate the condition of hypoxia, five representative light microscopic areas were computed on each section (magnification ×200) and the mean optical density (MOD) was calculated using the Image Pro Plus 7.0 analyzer, MOD = IOD/area.

qRT-PCR analysis

Total RNA was extracted from cultured cells and tumor tissues using TRIzol (Invitrogen Life Technologies, USA) according to the manufacturer's instructions. cDNA was synthesized by reverse transcribing 2 µg RNA with the High-Capacity cDNA Reverse Transcription Kit (Applied Biosystems, USA). One-microliter aliquots of cDNA were used as templates. The FAMTM Dye/MGB probes of Prx1, HO-1 and ß-actin were synthesized by ABI (Assay ID: Prx1, HS0060202; HO-1, HS00015796; human ACTB, 4352935E). For data analysis, the $2^{-\Delta\Delta CT}$ method was used with normalization of data of interested genes to housekeeping gene ß-actin. The experiments were conducted in triplicate.

Western blot analysis

Cells and tumor tissues were lysed in immunoprecipitation assay buffer (50 mM Tris-Cl [pH 7.4], 1% NP40, 150 mM NaCl, 1 mM EDTA, 1 M phenylmethylsulfonyl fluoride, 10 µg each of aprotinin and leupeptin, and 1 mM Na3VO4). After centrifuged at 12,000 g for 30 min, the supernatant was collected and protein concentration was determined using the Lowry method. Equal amounts of protein were separated on 12% SDS-PAGE gels and blotted onto nitrocellulose membranes. The blots were incubated with anti-Prx1 (1:5000, Upstate, USA) and anti-HO-1 (1:2000, Abcam, USA) antibody. Antibody of β-actin (Sigma, St. Louis, MO) was used as a loading control. Immunoreactive bands were detected with horseradish peroxidase-conjugated secondary antibodies and enhanced by chemiluminescence reagents (Amersham

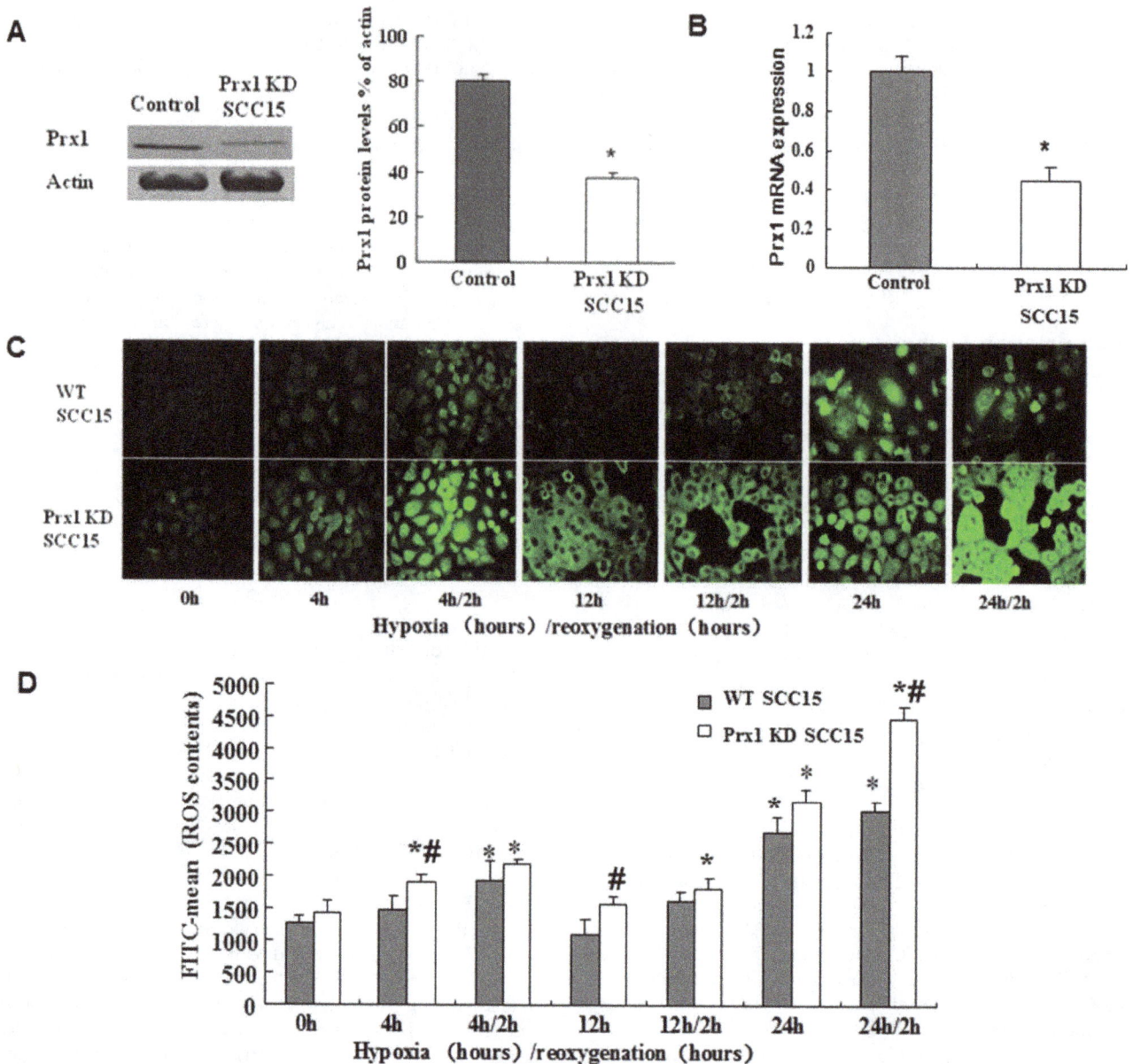

Figure 1. Prx1 knockdown increases hypoxia and intracellular ROS production in SCC15 cells. A, Prx1 protein was significantly decreased by shRNA transfection. B, Prx1 mRNA was significantly reduced by shRNA transfection. C, Pimonidazole staining showed the increased hypoxia status in cells after hypoxia/reoxygenation treatment. D, Intercellular ROS level identified by flow cytometry in cells after hypoxia/reoxygenation treatment. *$P<0.05$ vs. WT SCC15 cells; #$P<0.05$ vs. control hypoxic WT SCC15 cells.

Biosciences, Piscataway, NJ). The experiments were performed in triplicate.

NF-κB DNA binding activity detection

The nuclear protein was extracted from cells and tumor tissues using NE-PER Nuclear and Cytoplasmic Extraction Reagents (Thermo, USA). In brief, cells and tissues were suspended in hypotonic buffer and incubated on ice for 10 min followed by centrifuged at 12,000 g and 4°C for 10 min to precipitate nuclei. After washed in the hypotonic buffer, the nuclei were lysed in a lysis buffer to get the nuclei extracts. NF-κB DNA binding activity was detected using the NF-κB (p65) Transcription Factor Assay Kit (Cayman Chemical Company, USA).

Immunohistochemistry

The paraffin-embedded blocks were sectioned for immunohistochemistry analysis. Sections were treated with 20 mg/L proteinase K (dilution: 1:1000; Sigma-Aldrich, USA) at 37°C for 30 min for antigen retrieval. After blocking the endogenous peroxidase activity with 0.3% hydrogen peroxidase for 15 min, the sections were treated with 8-hydroxydeoxyguanosine (8-OHdG; 1:8000; Abcam, USA) or NF-κB (Cell Signaling Technology, 1:100) primary antibody at 4°C overnight. The slides were incubated in biotinylated secondary IgG antibodies at 37°C for 30 min, and then visualized using DAB for 2–5 min. Mayer's hematoxylin was used to counterstain the sections, which were then dehydrated and mounted. For negative control, PBS was used in place of primary antibodies. The cells with positive staining

A

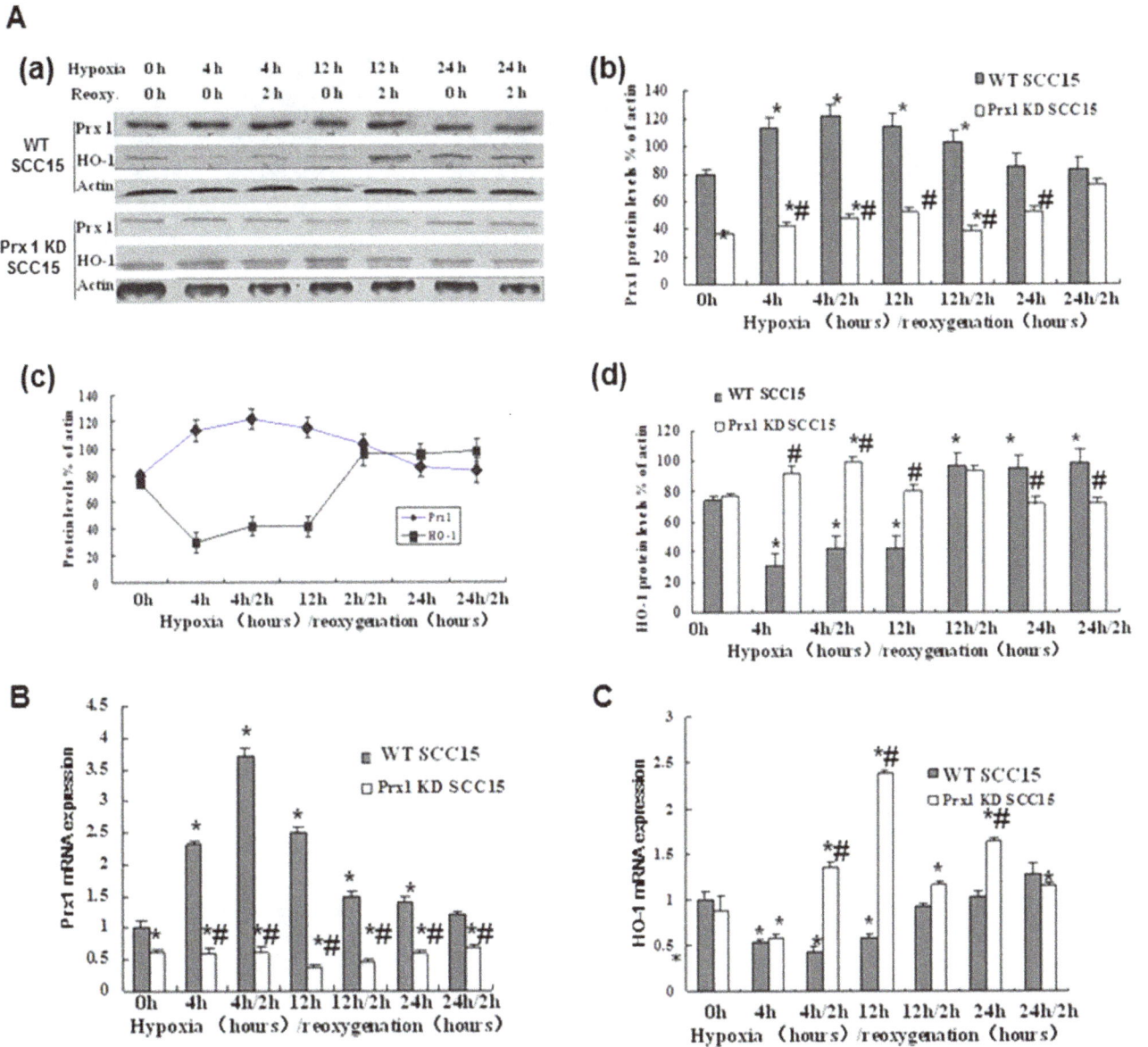

(a) Western blot panels: Hypoxia 0h, 4h, 4h, 12h, 12h, 24h, 24h; Reoxy. 0h, 0h, 2h, 0h, 2h, 0h, 2h. WT SCC15 (Prx1, HO-1, Actin) and Prx1 KD SCC15 (Prx1, HO-1, Actin).

(b) Bar graph — Prx1 protein level % of actin vs Hypoxia (hours)/reoxygenation (hours). ■ WT SCC15, □ Prx1 KD SCC15.

(c) Line graph — Protein level % of actin vs Hypoxia (hours)/reoxygenation (hours). Prx1 and HO-1.

(d) Bar graph — HO-1 protein level % of actin vs Hypoxia (hours)/reoxygenation (hours). ■ WT SCC15, □ Prx1 KD SCC15.

B

Bar graph — Prx1 mRNA expression vs Hypoxia (hours)/reoxygenation (hours). ■ WT SCC15, □ Prx1 KD SCC15.

C

Bar graph — HO-1 mRNA expression vs Hypoxia (hours)/reoxygenation (hours). ■ WT SCC15, □ Prx1 KD SCC15.

Figure 2. Expression of Prx1 and HO-1 in SCC15 cells. A (a), protein expression of Prx-1 and HO-1 detected by Western blot after hypoxia/reoxygenation treatment; A (b and d), Prx1 and HO-1 protein quantitation relative to β-actin; A (c), correlation of Prx-1 and HO-1 after hypoxia/reoxygenation treatment. B and C, mRNA expression of Prx-1 and HO-1 detected by qRT-PCR after hypoxia/reoxygenation treatment. *$P<0.05$ vs. WT SCC15 cells; #$P<0.05$ vs. control hypoxic WT SCC15 cells.

were determined by counting the percentage of stained cells using the Image Pro Plus 7.0 analyzer. A minimum of 1,000 cells were counted for each tumor specimen.

Statistical analysis

The expression levels of Prx1, HO-1, NF-κB and 8-OHdG, and data from ROS production, pimonidazole staining, immunofluorescence and NF-κB DNA binding activity were analyzed and compared using one-way analysis of variance (ANOVA). All statistical analysis was carried out using SPSS Software for Windows 17.0. Differences were considered statistically significant at $P<0.05$. All P values were two-sided.

Results

Prx1 knockdown increases hypoxia and intracellular ROS production

We used shRNA plasmid to knock down Prx1 in SCC15 cells. As shown in Figure 1A and 1B, the levels of Prx1 mRNA and protein expression were reduced to 40–50% by shRNA transfection in SCC15 cells. After Prx1 knockdown, we detected the hypoxic condition in both Prx1 knockdown cells and control cells, which were transfected with empty vector. Our data showed that hypoxic condition was increased by hypoxia or hypoxia/reoxygenation except 12-h hypoxia treatment in control cells (Figure 1C, upper panel). In Prx1 knockdown cells, the hypoxic condition increased more significantly compared to control cells (Figure 1C, lower pannel). The highest hypoxia was observed in

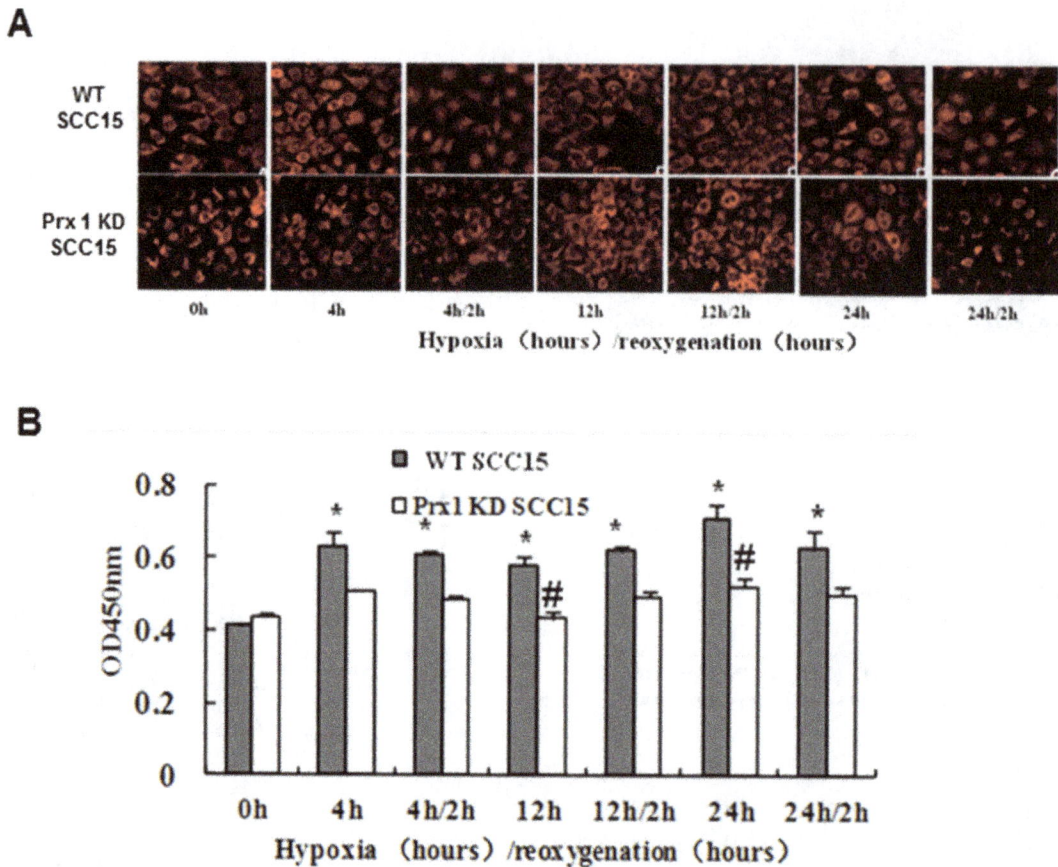

Figure 3. NF-κB DNA binding activity in SCC15 cells. A, Endogenic nuclei expression of NF-κB. B, NF-κB DNA binding activity detected by ELISA. *$P < 0.05$ vs. WT SCC15 cells; #$P < 0.05$ vs. control hypoxic WT SCC15 cells.

Prx1 knockdown cells after 24 h hypoxia/2 h reoxygenation treatment, and 2 h reoxygenation treatment did not decrease the hypoxia level elevated by hypoxia treatment. We also detected the production of intracellular ROS. Similar to hypoxia condition, the production of intracellular ROS was increased by hypoxia treatment except 12 h hypoxia and 12 h hypoxia/2 h reoxygenation treatment (Figure 1D). The accumulation of intracellular ROS is higher in Prx1 knockdown cells compared to it in control cells.

Prx1 negatively regulates HO-1 under hypoxic conditions

In order to determine whether Prx1 was related to HO-1 in SCC15 cells under hypoxic conditions, we assessed the expression levels of Prx1 and HO-1 after hypoxic treatment. As shown in Figure 2A (a, b), the protein expression of Prx1 was increased by hypoxic treatment. However, the protein expression of HO-1 was decreased at initial stages of hypoxia when Prx1 expression was increased, and then increased while Prx1 expression decreased in 12 h hypoxia/2 h reoxygenation, 24 h hypoxia and 24 h hypoxia/2 h reoxygenation, as indicated in Figure 2A (c and d). In 4 h hypoxia/2 h reoxygenation group, the level of Prx1 protein was increased by 50% while HO-1 protein was down-regulated by 30% compared with untreated cells (Figure 2A–b and d). However, in Prx1 knockdown cells, HO-1 was significantly up-regulated after hypoxia or hypoxia/reoxygenantin treatment except for the 24 h group. The protein expression of HO-1 was increased by 30% (Figure 2A–d), and mRNA level was increased by 1.4-fold in Prx1 knockdown SCC15 cells treated with 4 h

hypoxia/2 h reoxygenation compared with untreated cells (Figure 2C). The mRNA expression of Prx1 was increased by 2.7-fold while the expression of HO-1 mRNA was down-regulated by 40% (Figure 2B and 2C).

Prx1 knockdown inhibits NF-κB translocation and DNA binding activity

We detected the endogenic NF-κB expression in cells after hypoxia treatment. We observed an increased nucleus expression of NF-κB in SCC15 cells after treatment, especially in 24 h hypoxia group (Figure 3A, upper panel). Moreover, in Prx1 knockdown cells, NF-κB translocation from cytoplasm to nucleus was decreased compared with control cells (Figure 3A, lower panel). We then detected NF-κB activity in cells after hypoxia treatment. We found that NF-κB p65 DNA binding ability was significantly decreased in Prx1 knockdown cells after hypoxia treatment compared to control cells (Figure 3B).

Hypoxia is associated with tumor growth in xenograft model

To evaluate the change of the hypoxic conditions during the tumor development, we assessed hypoxia in tumors with maximal diameter of 2 mm, 5 mm, 10 mm or 15 mm. As shown in Figure 4A, the small and scattered positive cells were observed in 2 mm tumors. In 5 mm, 10 mm and 15 mm tumors, the hypoxic cells were mainly located at the centers of the cancer nests. The hypoxia in 5 mm, 10 mm and 15 mm tumors was significantly

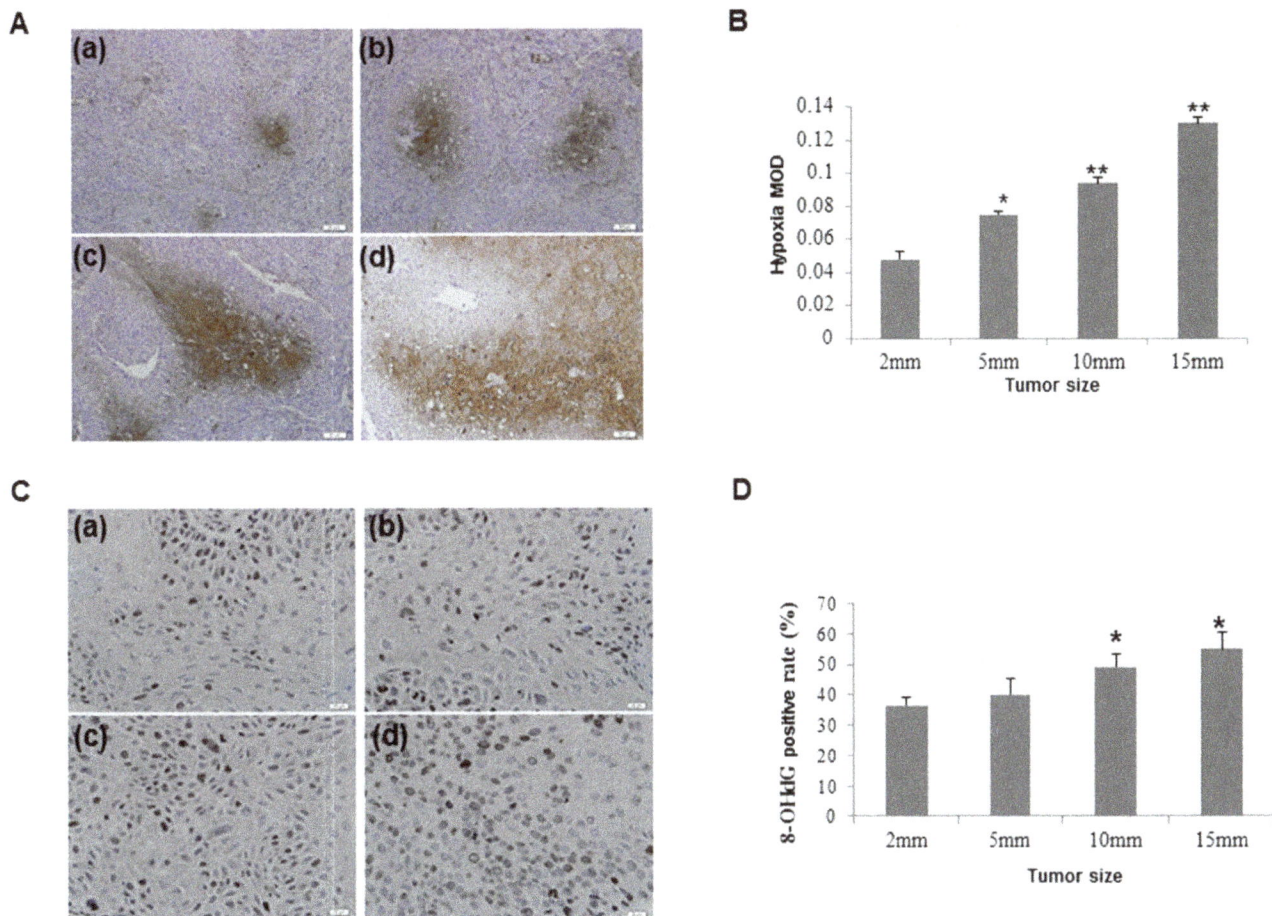

Figure 4. Pimonidazole staining and 8-OHdG expression in xenograft tumors. A, Hypoxia was detected in 2 mm (a), 5 mm (b), 10 mm (c) and 15 mm (d) tumors by pimonidazole staining. B, Hypoxia MOD significantly increases in 5 mm, 10 mm and 15 mm tumors compared to 2 mm tumors. C, 8-OHdG was detected by immunohistochemistry in 2 mm (a), 5 mm (b), 10 mm (c) and 15 mm (d) tumors. D, The level of 8-OHdG was higher in 10 mm and 15 mm tumors compared to 2 mm tumors. $*P<0.05$; $**P<0.01$.

higher than it in 2 mm tumors (Figure 4B). We also detected the level of 8-OHdG to assess the oxidative DNA injury in tumor cells. The expression of 8-OHdG increased from 2 mm to 15 mm tumors (Figure 4C). It was significantly higher in 10 mm and 15 mm tumors compared to 2 mm tumors (Figure 4D).

Overexpression of Prx1 and HO-1 during tumorigenesis in xenograft model

As shown in Figure 5A, the mRNA expression of Prx1 significantly increased in 5 mm, 10 mm and 15 mm tumors compared to 2 mm tumors. The protein expression of Prx1 was also elevated in 10 mm and 15 mm tumors (Figure 5B). Overexpression of HO-1 was observed in 15 mm tumors as indicated in Figure 5C and 5D.

NF-κB translocation and DNA binding activity are increased in xenograft model

NF-κB translocation and DNA binding activity both were elevated when tumor developed. The immunohistochemistry analysis showed that the expression of NF-κB was increased significantly in 15 mm tumors compared to 2 mm tumors (Figure 6A and 6B). Similarly, NF-κB DNA binding activity was significantly elevated in 15 mm tumors than 2 mm tumors (Figure 6C).

Discussion

The overall objective of this study is to explore the role of Prx1 in hypoxia in OSCC. First, we used shRNA to knock down Prx1 in SCC15 cells and then detected Prx1, NF-κB and HO-1 in hypoxia. We also investigated the Prx1 with hypoxia during tumor development in xenograft model. Our data showed that after exposure to hypoxia or hypoxia/reoxygenation, intracellular hypoxia and ROS levels were aggravated. We also found that HO-1 expression was up-regulated in Prx1 knockdown cells, whereas NF-κB translocation and DNA binding activity were decreased. Taken together, these data suggest that the elevated accumulation of ROS induced by hypoxia can up-regulate Prx1, which can activates NF-κB and negatively regulates HO-1 in hypoxia-induced oral cancer cells. Our *in vivo* data showed that overexpression of Prx1 is associated with hypoxia and tumor growth. These results suggest that Prx1/NF-κB/HO-1 signaling pathway may play a key role in carcinogenesis of hypoxia-induced oral cancer.

One of the major functions of Prx1 is thioredoxin-dependent peroxidase activity relying exclusively on the cysteine at the N-terminal region [24]. It scavenges extra ROS as an antioxidant. Hypoxia increases intercellular ROS levels via the mitochondrial electron transport chain. Hypoxia is one of the key factors

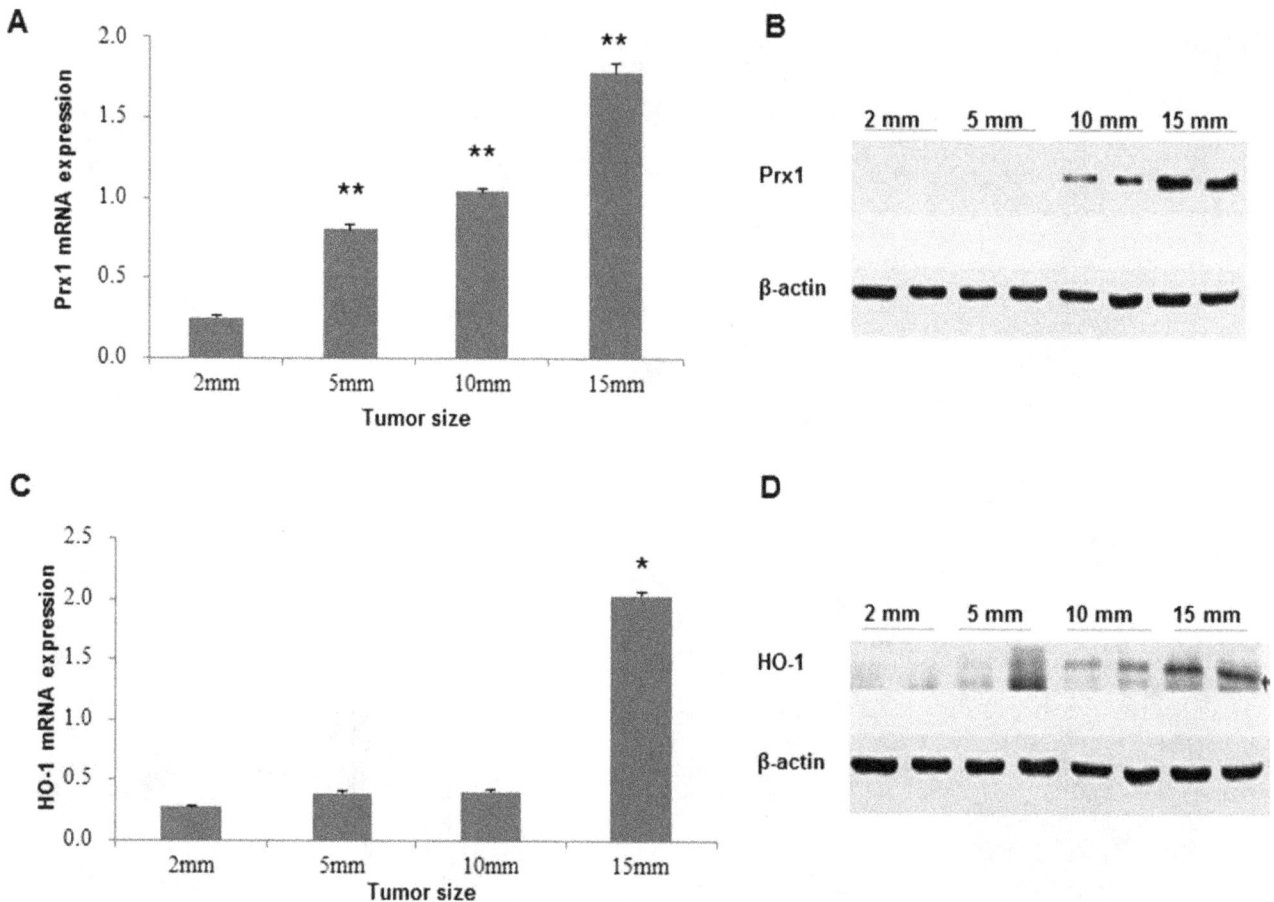

Figure 5. Expression of Prx1 and HO-1 in xenograft tumors. A and C, mRNA expression of Prx1 and HO-1 detected by qRT-PCR. B and D, Protein expression of Prx1 and HO-1 detected by western blot. *$P<0.05$; **$P<0.01$.

influencing tumor initiation and progression through increasing oxidative DNA damage [25]. In recent years, the overexpression of Prx1 was reported to play an important role in many malignancies due to its critical role in pathogenesis of hypoxia. In lung cancer cells, hypoxia/reoxygenation can increase Prx1 expression by activating nuclear factor erythroid 2–related factor 2 (Nrf2), an important transcription factor involved in oxidant stress [26]. The loss of Prx1 expression can enhance the sensitivity to oxidants and therefore, increase ROS production and oxidative DNA damage [27]. In the present study, the mRNA and protein expression of Prx1 was up-regulated in SCC15 cells by either hypoxia (4 h, 12 h) alone or followed by reoxygenation (2 h). In another study reported by Kim et al., Prx1 was only up-regulated by hypoxia/reoxygenation, but not by hypoxia alone [27]. We found that the SCC15 cells are still hypoxic after 2 h reoxygenation treatment, which indicates that Prx1 could still be induced by hypoxia, even after 2 h reoxygenation treatment. Our result suggests that hypoxia is closely related to the overexpression of Prx1 in OSCC. The up-regulation of Prx1 increases the cells' ability to remove extra ROS and protect the tumor cells, which may enhance tumor progression and reduce the efficacies of chemo- and radiotherapies.

A recent study showed that in Hela cells, cytoplasmic Prx1 altered cytoplasmic NF-κB translocation into the nucleus. Nuclear Prx1 regulates NF-κB/DNA binding through elimination of H_2O_2 [23]. Wang et al. reported that Prx1 interacts with NF-κB at the DNA level and presumably modulates its transcriptional activity in breast cancer cells [10]. As a potent antioxidant, HO-1 facilitates tumor progression in a tissue specific manner. Studies have indicated that NF-κB induces expression of HO-1 in tumor tissues [28–31]. Moreover, numerous studies suggested a direct relationship between NF-κB and HO-1, but the function of NF-κB in regulating HO-1 expression in human cells is controversial [32–35]. In this study, our data showed that hypoxia induces Prx1 and NF-κB, and Prx1 regulates HO-1 via activating NF-κB.

Prx1 has been recently identified as an endogenous ligand for toll-like receptor (TLR) ligands [36]. In normoxic conditions, Prx1 can enhance expression of vascular endothelial growth factor (VEGF) via induction of hypoxia-inducible factor 1-alpha promoter activity through Prx1: TLR4 interaction. This process is mediated by NF-κB. NF-κB interacts with the VEGF promoter, however, is not required for Prx1, which suggests that NF-κB can regulate VEGF without Prx1 induction [37]. Prx1 and HO-1 are both characterized as oxidative stress-inducible and heme-related proteins. Prx1 has heme-binding activity. The thiol-specific antioxidant activity of Prx1 can be inhibited by heme. Co-expression or co-induction of Prx1 and HO-1 has been observed in some tissues or cells, indicating that Prx1 and HO-1 proteins may co-localize and interact to exhibit antioxidant activities [15]. Studies have shown that the expression of HO-1 is mainly up-regulated by Nrf2. Nrf2 is also one of the key transcription factors for Prx1 gene expression in hypoxic cancer cells. For the first time, we report that Prx1 and HO-1 could have a negative regulatory relationship in an indirect manner. The precise molecular

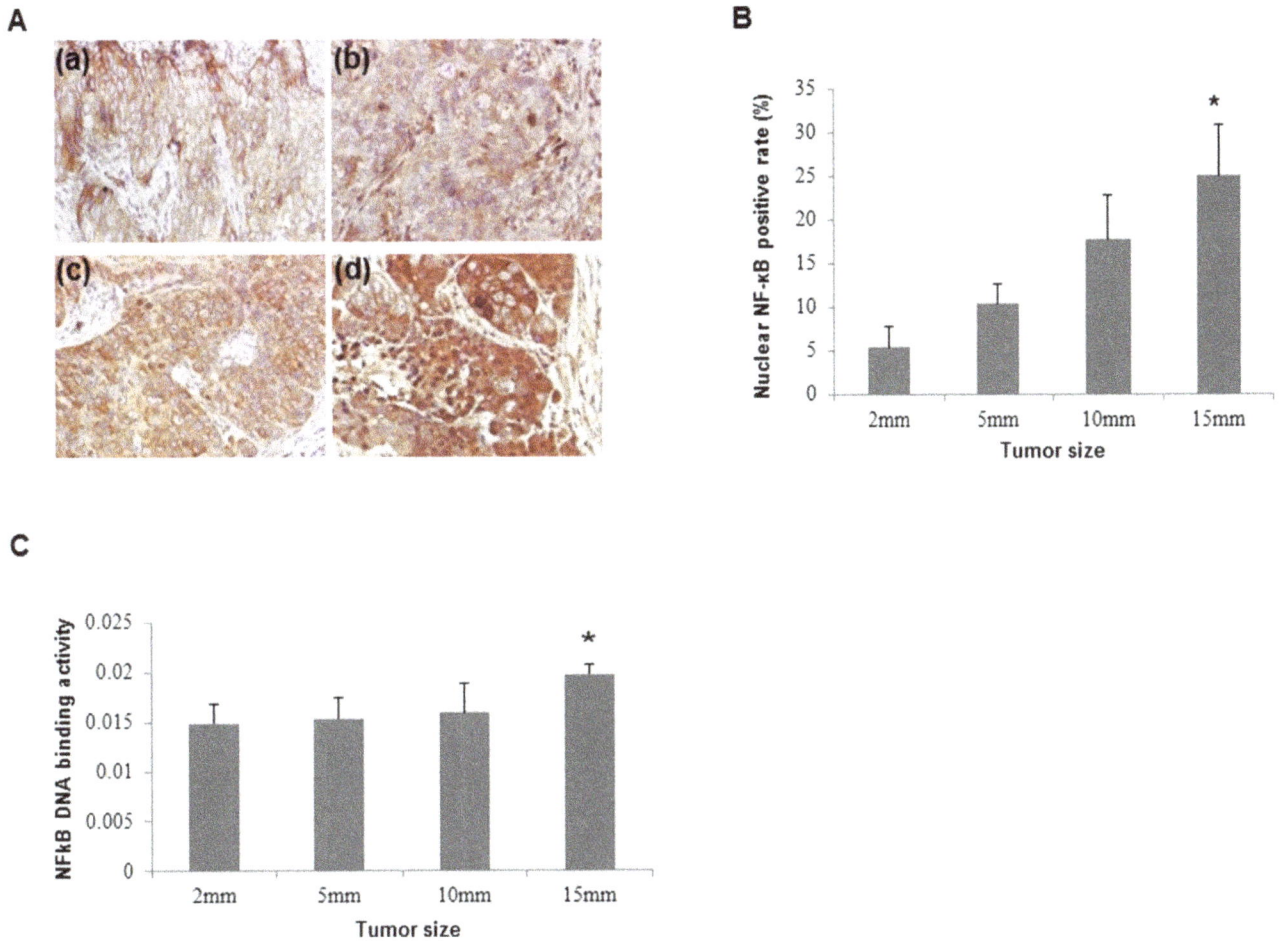

Figure 6. NF-κB expression and DNA binding activity in xenograft tumors. A, NF-κB expression was detected by immunohistochemistry in 2 mm (a), 5 mm (b), 10 mm (c) and 15 mm (d) tumors. B, The percentage of nuclear NF-κB positive cells is significantly increased in 15 mm tumors compared to it in 2 mm tumors. C, NF-κB DNA binding activity was significantly higher in 15 mm tumors compared to 2 mm tumors. *$P<0.05$; **$P<0.01$.

mechanisms, however, needs to be confirmed and investigated in the future study.

In OSCC xenograft model, we found similar results that significant elevation of HO-1 lags behind that of Prx1. Under hypoxic condition and oxidative DNA damage, Prx1 and HO-1 are upregulated and NF-κB DNA binding activity is enhanced. Our data suggests that Prx1 plays antioxidative role by activating NF-κB and regulating HO-1 in hypoxia-related OSCC progression. In conclusion, we found that hypoxia plays an important role in OSCC through regulating Prx1/NF-κB/HO-1 signaling pathway. Our study provides a systemic examination of Prx1 in cell systems and xenograft model of OSCC, each having specific advantages for biomarker research. Further studies on functional role of Prx1 in oral carcinogenesis are warranted. Information from this study may be helpful in developing chemopreventive/therapeutic agents targeting Prx1.

Author Contributions

Conceived and designed the experiments: XFT TC. Performed the experiments: MZ MH. Analyzed the data: XFT TC JFZ NS. Contributed reagents/materials/analysis tools: LHG CCM XYJ. Contributed to the writing of the manuscript: MZ MH XFT TC JFZ NS.

References

1. Warnakulasuriya S (2009) Global epidemiology of oral and oropharyngeal cancer. Oral Oncol 45(4–5): 309–16.
2. Warnakulasuriya S (2009) Causes of oral cancer–an appraisal of controversies. Br Dent J 207: 471–475.
3. Bagan JV, Scully C (2008) Recent advances in Oral Oncology 2007: epidemiology, aetiopathogenesis, diagnosis and prognostication. Oral Oncol 44: 103–108.
4. Miyazaki Y, Hara A, Kato K, Oyama T, Yamada Y, et al. (2008) The effect of hypoxic microenvironment on matrix metalloproteinase expression in xenografts of human oral squamous cell carcinoma. Int J Oncol 32: 145–151.
5. Bussink J, Kaanders JH, van der Kogel AJ (2003) Tumor hypoxia at the microregional level: clinical relevance and predictive value of exogenous and endogenous hypoxic cell markers. Radiother Oncol 67: 3–15.
6. Miyoshi A, Kitajima Y, Ide T, Ohtaka K, Nagasawa H, et al. (2006) Hypoxia accelerates cancer invasion of hepatoma cells by upregulating MMP expression in an HIF-1-alpha-independent manner. Int J Oncol 29: 1533–1539.
7. Munoz-Najar UM, Neurath KM, Vumbaca F, Claffey KP (2006) Hypoxia stimulates breast carcinoma cell invasion through MT1-MMP and MMP-2 activation. Oncogene 25: 2379–2392.
8. Guzy RD, Hoyos B, Robin E, Chen H, Liu L, et al. (2005) Mitochondrial complex III is required for hypoxia-induced ROS production and cellular oxygen sensing. Cell Metab 1: 401–408.

9. Kim YJ, Lee WS, Ip C, Chae HZ, Park EM, et al. (2006) Prx1 suppressed radiation-induced c-Jun NH2 terminal kinase signaling in lung cancer cells through interaction with the glutathione S-transferase Pi/c-Jun NH2-terminal kinase complex. Cancer Res 66: 7136–7142.

10. Neumann CA, Krause DS, Carman CV, Das S, Dubey DP, et al. (2003) Essential role for the peroxiredoxin Prdx1 in erythrocyte antioxidant defence and tumoursuppression. Nature 424: 561–565.

11. Yanagawa T, Omura K, Harada H, Ishii T, Uwayama J, et al. (2005) Peroxiredoxin I expression in tongue squamous cell carcinomas as involved in tumor recurrence. Int J Oral Maxillofac Surg 34: 915–920.

12. Yanagawa T, Iwasa S, Ishii T, Tabuchi K, Yusa H, et al. (2000) Peroxiredoxin1 expression in oral cancer: a potential new tumor marker. Cancer Lett 156: 27–35.

13. Gandini NA, Fermento ME, Salomón DG, Blasco J, Patel V, et al. (2012) Nuclear localization of heme oxygenase-1 is associated with tumor progression of head and neck squamous cell carcinomas. Exp Mol Pathol 93: 237–245.

14. Nakayama H, Ikebe T, Beppu M, Shirasuna K (2001) High expression levels of nuclear factor kappaB, IkappaB kinase alpha and Akt kinase in squamous cell carcinoma of the oral cavity. Cancer 92: 3037–3044.

15. Stanimirovic D, Zhang W, Howlett C, Lemieux P, Smith C (2001) Inflammatory gene transcription in human astrocytes exposed to hypoxia: roles of the nuclear factor-kappaB and autocrine stimulation. J Neuroimmunol 119: 365–376.

16. Jin DY, Chae HZ, Rhee SG, Jeang KT (1997) Regulatory role for a novel human thioredoxin peroxidase in NF-kappaB activation. J Biol Chem 272: 30952–30961.

17. Hansen JM, Moriarty-Craige S, Jones DP (2007) Nuclear and cytoplasmic peroxiredoxin -1 differentially regulate NF-kappaB activities. Free Radic Biol Med 43: 282–288.

18. Bach FH (2005) Heme oxygenase-1: atherapeutic amplification funnel. FASEB J 19: 1216–1219.

19. Otterbein LE, Choi AMK (2000) Heme oxygenase: Colors of defense against cellular stress. Am J Physiol Lung cell Mol Physiol 279: L1029–L1037.

20. Gandini NA, Fermento ME, Salomón DG, Blasco J, Patel V, et al. (2012) Nuclear localization of heme oxygenase-1 is associated with tumor progression of head and neck squamous cell carcinomas. Exp Mol Pathol 93: 237–245.

21. Guo G, Bhat NR (2006) Hypoxia/reoxygenation differentially modulates NF-kappaB activation and iNOS expression in astrocytes and microglia. Antioxid Redox Signal 8: 911–918.

22. Mazza E, Thakkar-Varia S, Tozzi C, Neubauer JA (2001) Expression of hemeoxygenase in the oxygen-sensing regions of the rostral ventrolateral medulla. J Appl Physiol 91: 379–385.

23. Nakaso K, Kitayama M, Mizuta E, Fukuda H, Ishii T, et al. (2000) Co-induction of heme oxygenase-1 and peroxiredoxin I in astrocytes and microglia around hemorrhagic region in the rat brain. Neurosci Lett 293: 49–52.

24. Neumann CA, Fang Q (2007) Are peroxiredoxins tumor suppressors? Curr Opin Pharmacol 7: 375–380.

25. Dos Santos M, Mercante AM, Louro ID, Gonçalves AJ, de Carvalho MB, et al. (2012) HIF1-Alpha Expression Predicts Survival of Patients with Squamous Cell Carcinoma of the Oral Cavity. PLoS One 7: e45228.

26. Kim YJ, Ahn JY, Liang P, Ip C, Zhang Y, et al. (2007) Human Prx1 gene is a target of Nrf2 and is up-regulated by hypoxia/reoxygenation: implication to tumor biology. Cancer Res 67: 546–554.

27. Wang X, He S, Sun JM, Delcuve GP, Davie JR (2010) Selective association of peroxiredoxin 1 with genomic DNA and COX-2 upstream promoterelements in estrogen receptor negative breast cancer cells. Mol Biol Cell 21: 2987–2995.

28. Ruiz-Ramos R, Lopez-Carrillo L, Rios-Perez AD, De Vizcaya-Ruíz A, Cebrian ME (2009) Sodium arsenite induces ROS generation, DNA oxidative damage, HO-1 and c Myc proteins, NF-kappaB activation and cell proliferation in human breast cancer MCF-7 cells. Mutat Res 674: 109–115.

29. Liu PL, Tsai JR, Charles AL, Hwang JJ, Chou SH, et al. (2010) Resveratrol inhibits human lung adenocarcinoma cell metastasis by suppressing heme oxygenase 1-mediated nuclear factor-kappaB pathway and subsequently downregulating expression of matrix metalloproteinases. Mol Nutr Food Res 54 Suppl 2: S196–204.

30. Liu ZM, Chen GG, Ng EK, Leung WK, Sung JJ, et al. (2004) Upregulation of heme oxygenase-1 and p21 confers resistance to apoptosis in human gastric cancer cells. Oncogene 23: 503–513.

31. Rushworth SA, Bowles KM, Raninga P, MacEwan DJ (2010) NF-kappaB-inhibited acute myeloid leukemia cells are rescued from apoptosis by heme oxygenase-1 induction. Cancer Res 70: 2973–2983.

32. Allan ME, Storey KB (2012) Expression of NF-κB and downstream antioxidant genes in skeletal muscle of hibernating ground squirrels, Spermophilus tridecemlineatus. Cell Biochem Funct 30: 166–174.

33. Lee HJ, Lee J, Min SK, Guo HY, Lee SK, et al. (2008) Differential induction of heme oxygenase-1 against nicotine-induced cytotoxicity via the PI3K, MAPK, and NF-kappa B pathways in immortalized and malignant human oral keratinocytes. J Oral Pathol Med 37: 278–286.

34. Lavrovsky Y, Song CS, Chatterjee B, Roy AK (2000) Age-dependent increase of heme oxygenase-1 gene expression in the liver mediated by NF-kappaB. Mech Ageing Dev 114: 49–60.

35. Jeong SI, Choi BM, Jang SI (2010) Sulforaphane suppresses TARC/CCL17 and MDC/CCL22 expression through heme oxygenase-1 and NF-κB in human keratinocytes. Arch Pharm Res 33: 1867–1876.

36. Riddell JR, Bshara W, Moser MT, Spernyak JA, Foster BA, et al. (2011) Peroxiredoxin 1 controls prostate cancer growth through Toll-like receptor 4-dependent regulation of tumor vasculature. Cancer Res 71: 1637–1646.

37. Riddell JR, Maier P, Sass SN, Moser MT, Foster BA, et al. (2012) Peroxiredoxin 1 stimulates endothelial cell expression of VEGF via TLR4 dependent activation of HIF-1α. PLoS One 7: e50394.

3

The Anabolic Androgenic Steroid Nandrolone Decanoate Disrupts Redox Homeostasis in Liver, Heart and Kidney of Male Wistar Rats

Stephan P. Frankenfeld[1], Leonardo P. Oliveira[2], Victor H. Ortenzi[3], Igor C.C. Rego-Monteiro[1], Elen A. Chaves[2], Andrea C. Ferreira[4], Alvaro C. Leitão[1], Denise P. Carvalho[3], Rodrigo S. Fortunato[1]*

1 Laboratório de Radiobiologia Molecular, Instituto de Biofísica Carlos Chagas Filho, Universidade Federal do Rio de Janeiro, Rio de Janeiro, Brazil, **2** Laboratório de Biologia do Exercício, Escola de Educação Física e Desportos, Universidade Federal do Rio de Janeiro, Rio de Janeiro, Brazil, **3** Laboratório de Fisiologia Endócrina Doris Rosenthal, Instituto de Biofísica Carlos Chagas Filho, Universidade Federal do Rio de Janeiro, Rio de Janeiro, Brazil, **4** Polo de Xerém/Laboratório de Fisiologia Endócrina Doris Rosenthal, Instituto de Biofísica Carlos Chagas Filho, Universidade Federal do Rio de Janeiro, Rio de Janeiro, Brazil

Abstract

The abuse of anabolic androgenic steroids (AAS) may cause side effects in several tissues. Oxidative stress is linked to the pathophysiology of most of these alterations, being involved in fibrosis, cellular proliferation, tumorigenesis, amongst others. Thus, the aim of this study was to determine the impact of supraphysiological doses of nandrolone decanoate (DECA) on the redox balance of liver, heart and kidney. Wistar male rats were treated with intramuscular injections of vehicle or DECA (1 mg.100 g^{-1} body weight) once a week for 8 weeks. The activity and mRNA levels of NADPH Oxidase (NOX), and the activity of catalase, glutathione peroxidase (GPx) and total superoxide dismutase (SOD), as well as the reduced thiol and carbonyl residue proteins, were measured in liver, heart and kidney. DECA treatment increased NOX activity in heart and liver, but NOX2 mRNA levels were only increased in heart. Liver catalase and SOD activities were decreased in the DECA-treated group, but only catalase activity was decreased in the kidney. No differences were detected in GPx activity. Thiol residues were decreased in the liver and kidney of treated animals in comparison to the control group, while carbonyl residues were increased in the kidney after the treatment. Taken together, our results show that chronically administered DECA is able to disrupt the cellular redox balance, leading to an oxidative stress state.

Editor: Guillermo López Lluch, Universidad Pablo de Olavide, Centro Andaluz de Biología del Desarrollo-CSIC, Spain

Funding: This work was supported by grants from Fundação Carlos Chagas Filho de Amparo à Pesquisa do Estado do Rio de Janeiro (FAPERJ), Coordenação de Aperfeiçoamento de Pessoal de Nível Superior (CAPES), and Conselho Nacional de Desenvolvimento Científico e Tecnológico (CNPq). The funders had no role in study design, data collection and analysis, decision to publish, or preparation of the manuscript.

* Email: rodrigof@biof.ufrj.br

Introduction

Anabolic-androgenic steroids (AAS) are synthetic molecules similar to the male sex hormone testosterone. The classical therapeutic uses of these substances are the treatment of hypogonadism, bone marrow failure syndromes, bone mineralization and some muscle–wasting disorders [1]. The use of AAS to enhance physical performance or appearance has greatly increased, and individuals usually take doses 10 to 100 fold higher than the therapeutical dose; this abuse can cause many adverse effects [2].

Hepatic structure and function are severely altered by high AAS doses [1–3]. Serum levels of the hepatic enzymes aspartate-aminotransferase, alanine-aminotransferase and lactate-dehydrogenase are increased, and more severe disorders can be induced by high AAS administration, such as peliosis hepatis, hepatocellular hyperplasia and hepatocellular adenoma [1–3]. In the heart, AAS abuse increases the risk of cardiovascular diseases, possibly due to increased total cholesterol and low density protein levels, decreased high density lipoprotein levels, increased blood pressure, thrombosis, myocardial infarction and heart failure [4,5]. The

kidney is also affected: creatinine, blood urine nitrogen and uric acid are increased in AAS-abusers. Moreover, AAS users have a high risk of developing Wilm's tumor, which is otherwise not common in adults [6–8].

Liver, heart and kidney pathophysiology are usually linked to oxidative stress, which is characterized by a disruption of redox signaling and control. Reactive oxygen species (ROS), such as superoxide and hydrogen peroxide (H_2O_2), can be formed by xanthine-oxidase, cytocrome P-450 or mitochondrial electron transport chain, as a by-product, or directly by the NADPH oxidase (NOX) family of enzymes [9]. The NOX family is composed of seven members, NOX1-NOX5 and DUOX1/2, which are differentially expressed among tissues. The physiological roles of NOXs are quite diverse, they act in a wide range of cellular processes, such as cellular proliferation, calcium release and hormonal biosynthesis, but their overexpression is associated with the pathophysiology of various diseases [10]. Intracellular ROS levels are maintained at adequate levels by antioxidant systems that react with these molecules producing less reactive compounds. Catalase and GPx are involved in H_2O_2 detoxification, producing H_2O directly or in a GSH-dependent reaction, while superoxide-dismutase catalyzes the conversion of superoxide to H_2O_2 [11].

As the majority of side effects elicited by AAS have their etiology linked to oxidative stress, the aim of this study was to evaluate the redox balance of AAS target tissues, such as liver, heart and kidney, in rats chronically treated with supraphysiological doses of nandrolone decanoate.

Materials and Methods

Experimental group

Adult male Wistar rats weighing 200–250 g were maintained in an animal room with controlled lighting (12-h light-dark cycle) and temperature (23–24°C). This investigation conforms to the Guide for the Care and Use of Laboratory Animals published by the US National Institutes of Health (NIH Publication No. 85–23, revised 1996) and was approved by the Institutional Committee for Evaluation of Animal Use in Research (Comissão de Ética com o Uso de Animais (CEUA) em Experimentação Científica do Centro de Ciências da Saúde da Universidade Federal do Rio de Janeiro, number: IBCCF 159). The animals were divided into two groups: normal control rats (submitted to vehicle injection; peanut oil with 10% of benzoic alcohol) and rats treated with nandrolone decanoate (Deca Durabolin (50 mg/mL (Organon)) 1 mg.100 g^{-1} b.w. Steroid and vehicle were administered by a single intramuscular injection in the hind limb once a week for 8 wk. We have previously reported that this treatment was effective, decreasing testicular weight and increasing serum testosterone levels in male Wistar rats [12,13]. One week after the last injection, the rats were killed by decapitation, and trunk blood was immediately collected. After collection, the blood was centrifuged (15 min, 3000 g) and serum was collected and stored at −20°C. Liver, kidney and heart were excised, immediately frozen in liquid nitrogen and stored at −80°C. It is important to note that the tissues analyzed here are from the same rats utilized in Frankenfeld et al. (2014) study, in which we shown the effectiveness of the treatment (13).

H_2O_2 generation measurement

H_2O_2 generation was quantified in heart, liver and kidney particulate fractions by the Amplex red/horseradish peroxidase assay (Molecular Probes, Invitrogen), which detects the accumulation of a fluorescent oxidized product. In order to obtain the microsomal fraction, the homogenates from liver, kidney or heart samples were centrifuged at 3000×g for 15 min at 4°C. Then, the supernantant was centrifuged at 100 000×g for 35 min at 4°C and the pellets were resuspended in 0.5 ml 50 mM sodium phosphate buffer, pH 7.2, containing 0.25 M sucrose, 2 mM $MgCl_2$, 5 mg/ml aprotinin and 34,8 mg/ml phenylmethanesulfonyl fluoride (PMSF) and stored at −20°C until H_2O_2 generation measurements, as follows. The microssomal fraction was incubated in 150 mM sodium phosphate buffer (pH 7.4) containing SOD (100 U/ml; Sigma, USA), horseradish peroxidase (0.5 U/ml, Roche, Indianapolis, IN), Amplex red (50 μM; Molecular Probes, Eugene, OR), 1 mM EGTA in the presence or absence of 1 mM NADPH. The fluorescence was immediately measured in a microplate reader (Victor X4; PerkinElmer, Norwalk, CT) at 30°C, using excitation at 530 nm and emission at 595 nm [14]. Specific NADPH Oxidase activity was calculated by the differences between the activities in the presence and absence of NADPH.

The specific enzymatic activity was expressed as nanomoles H_2O_2 per hour per milligram of protein (nmol.h^{-1}.mg^{-1}). Protein concentration was determined by the Bradford assay [15].

Real-time polymerase chain reaction analysis

Total RNA was extracted from the heart using the RNeasy Fibrous Tissue Mini Kit (Qiagen, Valencia, California), and RNeasy Plus Mini Kit (Qiagen, Valencia, California) was used for liver and kidney tissues, following the manufacturer's instructions. After DNAse treatment, reverse transcription was followed by real-time polymerase chain reaction (PCR), as previously described (16). GAPDH was used as an internal control. The specific oligonucleotides listed in Table 1, were purchased from Applied Biosystems (Foster City, California).

Antioxidant enzymes activity

Heart, liver and kidney samples were homogenized in 5 mM Tris-HCl buffer (pH 7.4), containing 0.9% NaCl (w/v) and 1 mM EDTA, followed by centrifugation at 750×g for 10 minutes at 4°C. The supernatant aliquots were stored at −70°C. Catalase activity was assayed following the method of Aebi (1984) and was expressed as units per milligram of protein (U.mg^{-1}) [17]. Glutathione peroxidase (GPx) activity was assayed by following NADPH oxidation at 340 nm in the presence of an excess of glutathione reductase, reduced glutathione and tert-butyl hydroperoxide as substrates [18], and expressed as nmol of oxidized NADPH per milligram of protein (nmol.mg^{-1}). Total superoxide dismutase activity was determined by reduction of cytochrome C at 550 nm [19].

Measurement of total protein reduced thiol and carbonyl residues

The oxidative damage of the studied tissues was determined by the measurement of total protein reduced thiols and carbonyl residues. Total reduced thiols were determined in a spectrophotometer (Hitachi U-3300) using 5,5-dithionitrobenzoic acid (DTNB). Thiol residues react with DTNB, cleaving the disulfide bond to give 2-nitro-5-thiobenzoate (NTB$^-$), which ionizes to the NTB^{2-} di-anion in water at neutral and alkaline pH. The NTB^{2-} was quantified in a spectrophotometer by measuring the absorbance at 412 nm, and was expressed as nmol of reduced DTNB/mg protein [20]. Protein carbonyl residues was evaluated based on a reaction with dinitrophenylhidrazine (DNPH), as previously described by Levine et al. [21], by absorbance at 370 nm, using a molar absorption coefficient of 22,000 $M^{-1}cm^{-1}$, and was expressed as carbonyl derivates (carbonyl nmol/mg protein).

Serum transaminases

Serum transaminases AST/OGT (Aspartate Aminotransferase/ Oxalacetic Glutamic Transaminase) and ALT/TGP (Alanine Aminotransferase/Glutamic Pyruvic Transaminase) were measured by commercially available kits (Laborlab, No. 00300 and No. 00200, respectively).

Statistical analyses

The results are expressed as the mean ± SEM. All data were analyzed by unpaired t test using the Graphpad Prism software (version 5, Graphpad Software, Inc., San Diego, USA). A value of p≤0.05 was considered statistically significant.

Results

NADPH Oxidase activity and mRNA levels

H_2O_2 generation was significantly greater in liver and heart tissues of the treated animals, as shown in figures 1A and 1C,

Table 1. Primers used for the Real-Time Polymerase Chain Reaction Assay.

	Forward	Reverse	Tm (°C)	Gene accession number (Ensembl)	Product size	Position of the primer
NOX1	AACTGGCTGTACTGCTTG	ATTCGTCCATCTCTTGTTCCAG	79.93	NM_053683	198	Forward: 15553–15570 (24383) Reverse: 17230–17251 (24383)
NOX2	CCATTCACACCATTGCACATC	CGAGTCACAGCCACATACAG	79.99	NM_023965	181	Forward: 536–556 (3556) Reverse: 757–776 (3556)
NOX4	TCCATCAAGCCAAGATTCTGAG	GGTTTCCAGTCATCCAGTAGAG	78.33	NM_053524	362	Forward: 165909–165928 (179656) Reverse: 178835–178854 (179656)
DUOX1	GATACCCAAAGCTGTACCTCG	GTCCTTGTCACCCAGATGAAG	81.76	NM_153739	196	Forward: 30616–30626 (34361) Reverse: 32106–32126 (34361)
DUOX2	TGCTCTCAACCCCAAAGT	TCTCAAACCAGTAGCGATCAC	84.35	NM_024141	191	Forward: 5181–5198 (18941) Reverse: 5891–5911 (18941)
GAPDH	TGATTCTACCCACGGCAAGT	AGCATCACCCATTTGATGT	81.30	NM_017008	124	Forward: 2929–2948 (5076) Reverse: 3113–3132 (5076)

A) LIVER

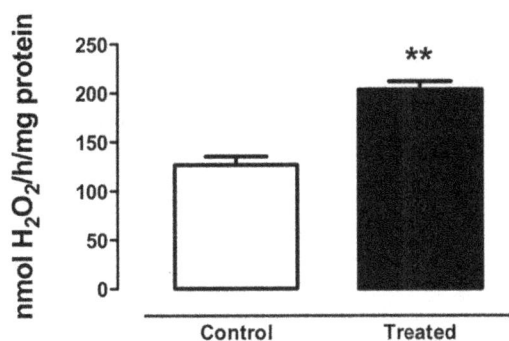

B) KIDNEY

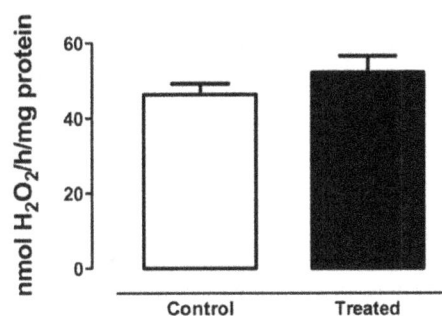

C) HEART

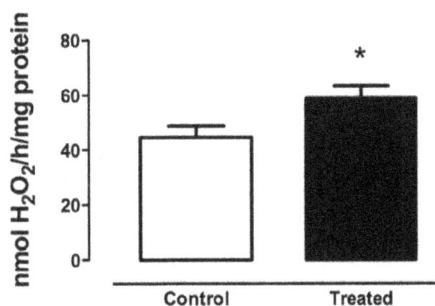

Figure 1. NADPH Oxidase activity in liver (A), kidney (B), and heart (C) of rats treated with Deca Durabolin (50 mg.mL^{-1} Organon, 1 mg/100 g bw, im), once a week, for 8 weeks. H_2O_2 production was determined in the microssomal fraction by the Amplex Red/Horseradish Peroxidase assay. Data were obtained with 10 animals from at least two independent experiments and are shown as mean ± SEM. * $p < 0.05$; ** $p < 0.001$.

A) LIVER

B) HEART

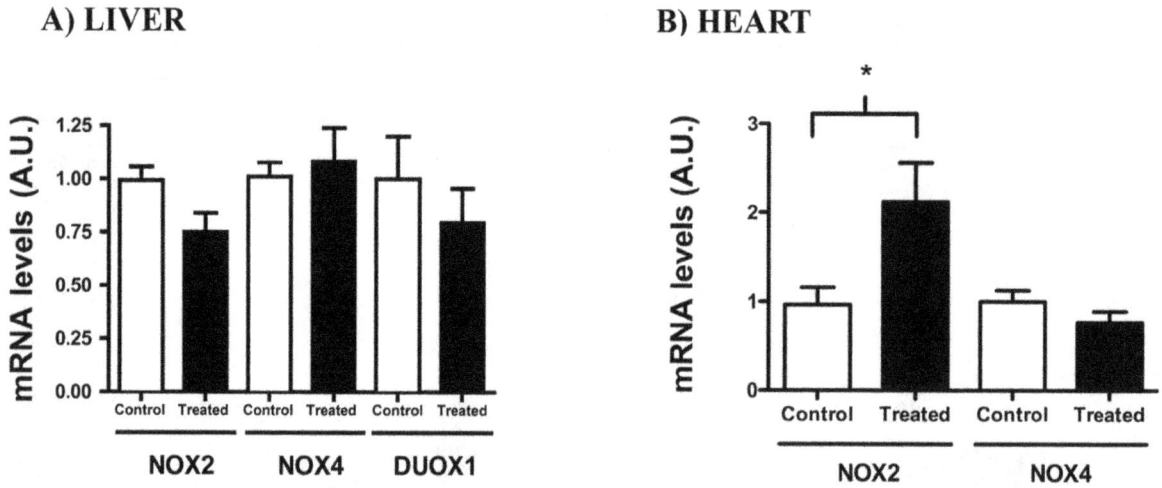

Figure 2. NADPH Oxidases mRNA levels in liver (A) and heart (B) of rats treated with Deca Durabolin (50 mg.mL^{-1} Organon, 1 mg/ 100 g bw, im), once a week, for 8 weeks. mRNA levels were determined by real-time PCR and was expressed relative to the control group. Data were obtained with 10 animals from at least two independent experiments and are shown as mean $\pm$ SEM. * $p < 0.05$.

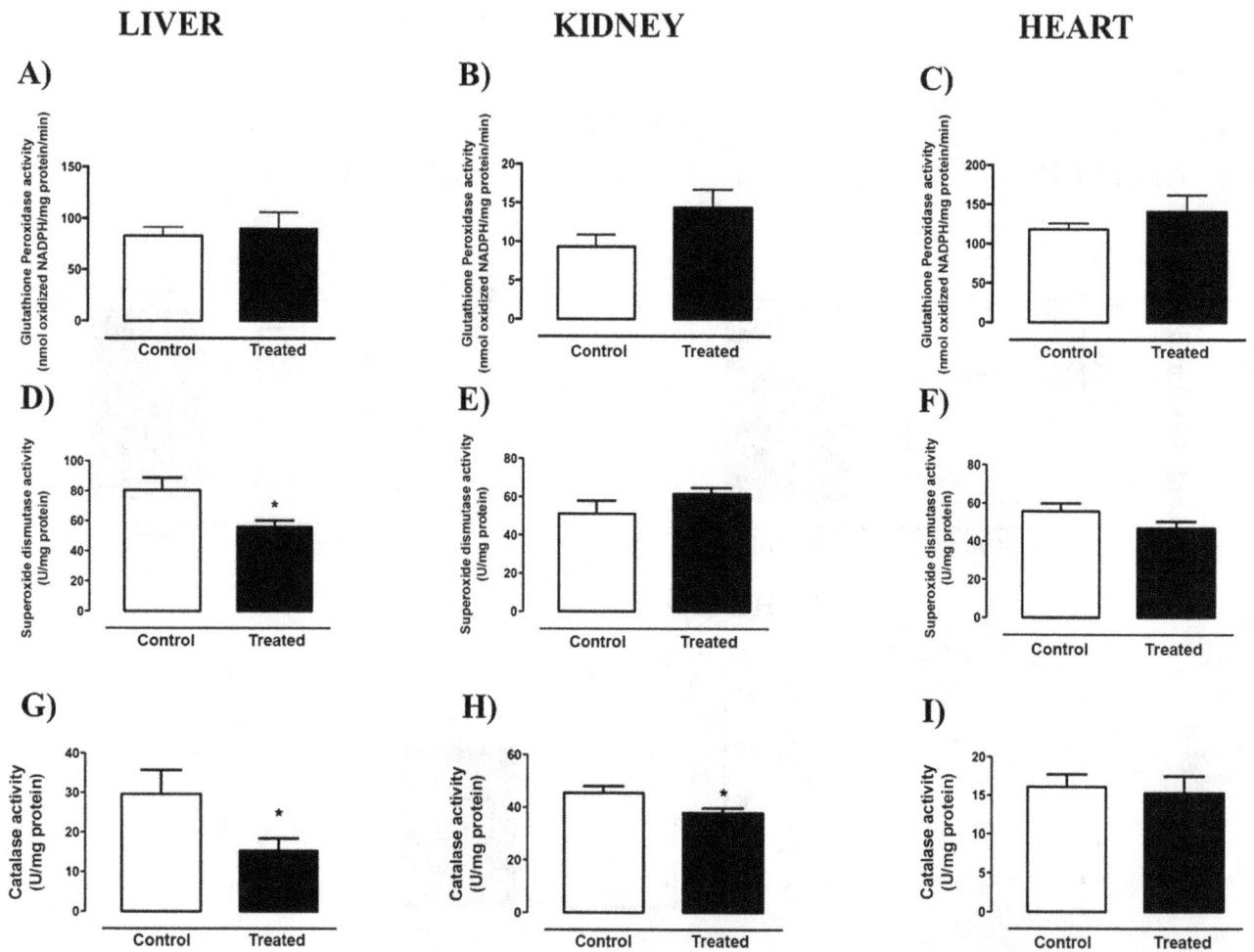

LIVER   KIDNEY   HEART

Figure 3. Antioxidant enzymes activities of rats treated with Deca Durabolin (50 mg.mL^{-1} Organon, 1 mg/100 g bw, im), once a week, for 8 weeks. Glutathione Peroxidase (A,B,C), Superoxide Dismutase (D,E,F) and Catalase (G,H,I) activities were measured in liver, kidney and heart homogenates, respectively, by spectrophotometry. Data were obtained with 6 animals from at least two independent experiments and are shown as mean $\pm$ SEM. * $p < 0.05$.

A) LIVER

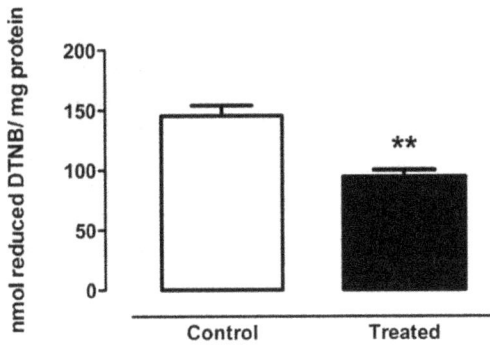

B) KIDNEY

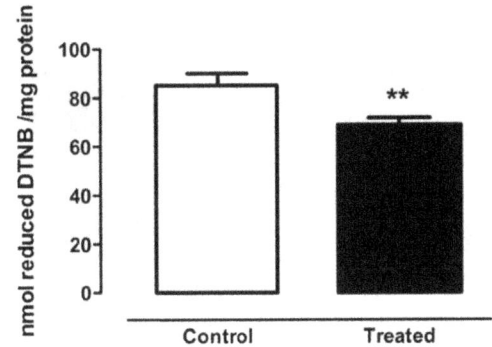

C) HEART

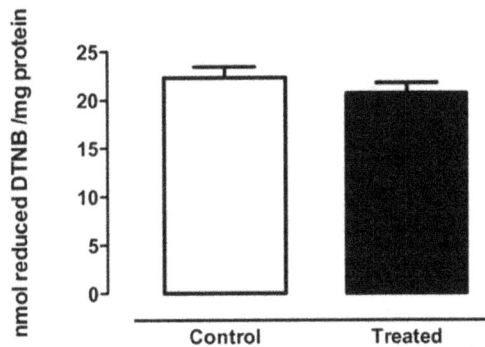

Figure 4. Reduced thiol content of liver (A), kidney (B), and heart (C) of rats treated with Deca Durabolin (50 mg.mL^{-1} Organon, 1 mg/100 g bw, im), once a week, for 8 weeks. Total sulfhydryl groups were measured by the reaction of thiols with DTNB, evaluated in a spectrophotometer at 412 nm. Data were obtained with 6 animals from at least two independent experiments and are shown as mean ± SEM. * $p < 0.05$; **$p < 0.001$.

respectively. No significant differences were found in kidney tissue (Fig. 1B).

In order to evaluate the source of the higher H_2O_2 generation, we evaluated the mRNA expression of the NOX enzymes in the heart and the liver. While NOX 1, 2, 4 and DUOX 1 and 2 are found in the liver, NOX1, NOX2, NOX4 are expressed in the cardiovascular system. NOX2 mRNA levels were higher in the heart of the treated group in comparison to its control, but no differences were found in hepatic NOX2 and DUOX1 mRNA nor in the levels of the NOX4 mRNA in heart and liver (Fig. 2A–B). In our conditions, we could not detect the mRNA of NOX1 and DUOX2 in the liver and NOX1 in the heart.

Antioxidant enzymes activity

Hepatic SOD (Fig. 3D) and Catalase (Fig. 3G) activities of the treated animals were decreased in comparison to the control group, but there was no change in GPx activity (Fig. 3A). In the kidney, the nandrolone treatment only decreased the catalase activity (Fig. 3H), and no differences in the cardiac antioxidant enzymes activities were found.

Biomarkers of oxidative stress

Thiol residues are mainly found in proteins and in low-molecular-mass metabolites such as the highly abundant glutathione (GSH), and can be reversibly oxidized by ROS to nitrosothiols or sulfenic acids, decreasing its cellular levels. On the other hand, carbonyl groups can be formed by the oxidation of proteins by ROS. As shown in figure 3, the protein thiol residues were significantly decreased in liver (Fig. 4A) and kidney (Fig. 4B) of the treated rats, but no changes were found in the heart (Fig. 4C). In the kidney, protein carbonyl content was significantly higher in the treated group as compared to its control (Fig. 5B), but no differences were found in the heart (Fig. 5C) or liver (Fig. 5A).

Serum transaminases profile

No differences were seen between groups on the serum activity of AST/TGO (C = 58.41±3.77 U/L, n = 10; T = 58.93±3.51 U/L, n = 10) and ALT/TGP (C = 12.53±1.03 U/L, n = 10; T = 10.13±0.748 U/L, n = 10).

A) LIVER

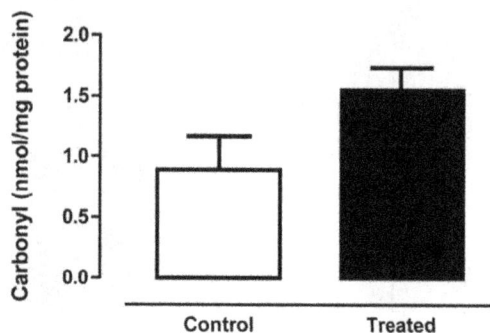

B) KIDNEY

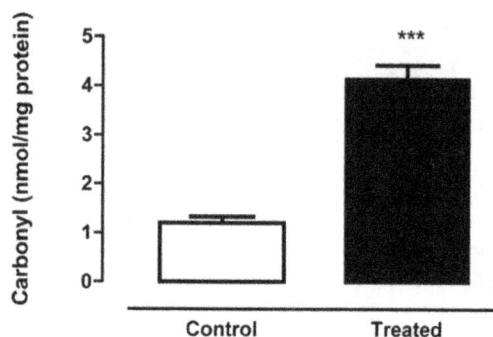

C) HEART

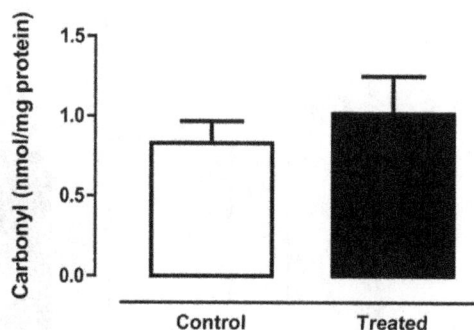

Figure 5. Protein carbonyl content of liver (A), kidney (B), and heart (C) of rats treated with Deca Durabolin (50 mg.mL^{-1} Organon, 1 mg/100 g bw, im), once a week, for 8 weeks. Protein carbonyl content was evaluated based on a reaction with dinitrophenylhidrazine (DNPH), evaluated in a spectrophotometer at 370 nm. Data were obtained with 6 animals from at least two independent experiments and are shown as mean ± SEM. * $p<0.05$; **$p<0.001$.

Discussion

ROS are normally produced by virtually all cells of living organisms, and are able to act in the redox-dependent regulation of different cellular functions, including response to stressors, angiogenesis, cell proliferation and other [22]. In order to maintain intracellular ROS at adequate levels, antioxidant systems react with these molecules producing less reactive compounds. Conceptually, an imbalance between pro-oxidant compounds and antioxidant defenses leads to oxidative stress, but this concept has recently been redefined as the "disruption of redox signaling and control" [11]. ROS molecules can avidly react with cellular constituents. Thus, an increase in its generation or a decrease in its detoxification leads to increased ROS availability that can cause oxidative modifications of DNA, proteins, and lipids. These structural changes in biomolecules can alter cellular function and processes, and play an important role in a range of common diseases and degenerative conditions [11]. As the liver is the major organ involved in the drug metabolization, and the kidneys are responsible for its excretion, these organs are generally affected by high doses of AAS. On the other hand, the effects of AAS on the heart are well documented by us and others [23–25]. As a large body of evidence shows a role of oxidative stress in liver, kidney

and heart dysfunction, we investigated if nandrolone decanoate, the most used AAS by bodybuilders and recreational athletes, could interfere in the redox balance of these tissues.

The most prominent changes caused by nandrolone decanoate treatment were seen in the liver. While NOX activity was increased, the antioxidant enzymes SOD and catalase were decreased after the nandrolone treatment. Moreover, total reduced thiol residues were decreased in nandrolone-treated rat liver. Pey et al. (2003) reported an increase in lipid peroxidation, as well as SOD, GPx and catalase activities in the liver of rats treated with stanozolol (a non-sterified) for 8 weeks, and concluded that in their model the overproduction of ROS exceeded the increase of antioxidant enzymes, leading to lipid peroxidation, but ROS generation was not evaluated [26]. Although the meaning of these results is in the same direction of our findings, there is a discrepancy in antioxidant enzymes activity found in our two studies, which could be due to differences in the AAS and dose utilized. The decreased levels of total hepatic reduced thiol residues in the treated rats suggest an increase in oxidative stress, since excess ROS can react with reduced thiols oxidizing them. Liver NOX2 and NOX4 mRNA levels were unaffected by the treatment, but the activity of these enzymes is not only affected by their mRNA/protein expression, but also by other factors such as protein association and activation by intracellular pathways [10]. So, our hypothesis is that NOX activity is increased, without changes in its expression. The kidney redox balance was also affected by AAS treatment, judging by the increase in protein carbonyl content and decrease of total reduced thiol residues, and diminished catalase activity. No significant changes were observed in the renal NOX activity, but we cannot exclude ROS overproduction by other enzymes, since we measured the activity of NOX enzymes. Cardiac antioxidant enzymes were not affected by treatment, but NOX2 mRNA levels and H_2O_2 production were higher after nandrolone decanoate administration. Utilizing the same treatment protocol, we have reported no differences in rat heart antioxidant enzymes, such as SOD, GPx and catalase, after nandrolone decanoate administration [27]. Interestingly, although we detected increased ROS production in the heart from DECA-treated animals, the reduced thiol residue level and protein carbonyl content were not changed. Thus, we may speculate that there was an increase in antioxidant defense mechanisms, other than modulation of SOD, GPx and/or catalase activities.

Our results clearly show that supraphysiological doses of nandrolone decanoate administered chronically are able to disrupt redox metabolism in the studied tissues, characterizing an oxidative stress state. A link between oxidative stress and DNA damage has been well demonstrated, but the subcellular localization where ROS are generated is crucial in this process [28]. NOX enzymes are transmembrane proteins and can be located at nuclear membrane, near to DNA, increasing the possibility of its damage [10]. Recently, Pozzi et al. (2012) evaluated the DNA damage elicited by nandrolone decanoate in liver, heart, kidney and peripheral blood in rats utilizing a single dose of 5 or 15 mg/Kg b.w. They used the alkaline comet assay, which detects DNA single and double strand breaks and alkali-labile lesions, and found an increased DNA damage in the liver and heart with the lower

and higher dose, but only the higher dose increased DNA damage in the kidney, with values much lower than the other studied tissues [29]. Our results suggest that through the increase in ROS availability, nandrolone decanoate exposure can also lead to DNA damage, but more studies are necessary to elucidate this question. In fact, oxidative stress is implicated not only in carcinogenesis, but also in the pathogenesis of a wide range of diseases that can affect liver, heart, kidney and other tissues. AAS abuse is involved in liver tumor development and inflammation, cardiac autonomic dysfunction and hypertrophy, in addition to mesangial matrix accumulation and increased heat shock proteins in the kidney [23,30,31]. Interestingly, all dysfunctions cited above can be caused by an increase in ROS availability, and NOX enzymes seem to play an important role in those processes. In conclusion, we demonstrated that supraphysiological doses of nandrolone decanoate are able to disrupt redox balance in liver, heart and kidney. Many diseases are linked to oxidative stress, so we believe that this study helps to clarify the physiological changes caused by the abuse of this and related drugs, which increased notably in the past three decades. Besides, our results contribute to elucidate AAS side effects in order to warn AAS abusers about the problems associated with this practice.

Acknowledgments

We are indebted to Dra. Doris Rosenthal for her assistance in English edition and extensive discussion.

Author Contributions

Conceived and designed the experiments: DPC ACL ACF RSF. Performed the experiments: SPF LPO VHO ICCR EAC. Analyzed the data: SPF EAC RSF. Contributed reagents/materials/analysis tools: ACL DPC ACF RSF. Wrote the paper: RSF ACF.

References

1. Shahidi NT (2001) A Review of chemistry, biological action, and clinical applications of anabolic-androgenic steroids. Clinical Therapeutics 23: 1355–1390.
2. Yersalis CE, Bahrke MS (1995) Anabolic-androgenic steroids. Sports Med 19: 326–340.
3. Saborido A, Molano F, Megías A (1993) Effect of training and anabolic-androgenic steroids on drug metabolism in rat liver. Medicine and Science in sports exercise 25: 815–822.
4. Sullivan ML, Martinez CM, Gennis P, Gallagher EJ (1998) The cardiac toxicity of anabolic steroids. Prog Cardiovasc Dis 41:1–15.
5. American Academy of Pediatrics (1997) Committee on Sports Medicine and Fitness. Adolescents and anabolic steroids: a subject review. Pediatrics 99: 904–908.
6. Mochizuki RM, Richter KJ (1998) Cardiomyopathy and cerebrovascular accident associated with anabolic-androgenic steroid use. Phys Sportsmed 16: 109–114.
7. Juhn M (2003) Popular sports supplements and ergogenic aids. Sports Med 33: 921–939.
8. Joyce JA (1991) Anesthesia for athletes using performance-enhancing drugs. AANA J 59:139–144.
9. Aguirre J, Lambeth JD (2010) Nox enzymes from fungus to fly to fish and what they tell us about Nox function in mammals. Free Radic Biol Med 49: 1342–1353. doi: 10.1016/j.freeradbiomed.2010.07.027.
10. Berdad K, Krause KH (2007) The NOX family of ROS-generating NADPH oxidases: physiology and pathophysiology. Physiol Rev 87: 245–313.
11. Jones DP (2008) Radical-free biology of oxidative stress. Am J Physiol Cell Physiol 295: C849–C868. doi: 10.1152/ajpcell.00283.2008.
12. Fortunato RS, Marassi MP, Chaves EA, Nascimento JH, Rosenthal D, et al. (2006) Chronic administration of anabolic androgenic steroid alters murine thyroid function. Med Sci Sports Exerc. 38:256–261.
13. Frankenfeld SP, de Oliveira LP, Ignacio DL, Coelho RG, Mattos MN, et al. (2014) Nandrolone decanoate inhibits gluconeogenesis and decreases fasting glucose in Wistar male rats. J Endocrinol 220:143–153. doi: 10.1530/JOE-13-0259.
14. Fortunato RS, Lima de Souza EC, Ameziane-el Hassani R, Boufraqech M, Weyemi U, et al. (2010) Functional consequences of dual oxidase-thyroperox-idase interaction at the plasma membrane. J Clin Endocrinol Metab 95: 5403–5411. doi: 10.1210/jc.2010-1085.
15. Bradford MM (1976) A rapid and sensitive method for the quantitation of microgram quantities of protein utilizing the principle of protein-dye binding. Anal Biochem 72: 248–254.
16. Schmittgen TD, Livak KJ (2008) Analyzing real-time PCR data by the comparative CT method. Nat Protoc 3: 1101–1108.
17. Aebi H (1984) Catalase in vitro. Methods Enzymol 105:121–126.
18. Flôhé L, Günzler WA (1984) Assays of glutathione peroxidase. Methods Enzymol 105: 114–121.
19. Crapo JD, McCord JM, Fridovich I (1977) Preparation and assay of superoxide dismutases. Methods Enzymol 3: 382–393.
20. Ellman GL (1959) "Tissue sulfhydryl groups". Arch Biochem Biophys 82: 70–77.
21. Levine RL, Garland D, Oliver CN, Amici A, Climent I, et al. (1990) Determination of carbonyl content in oxidatively modified proteins Meth Enzymol 186: 464–478.
22. Giorgio M, Trinei M, Migliaccio E, Pelicci PG (2007) Hydrogen peroxide: a metabolic by-product or a common mediator of ageing signals? Nat Rev Mol Cell Biol 8: 722–728.
23. Do Carmo EC, Fernandes T, Koike D, Da Silva ND Jr, Mattos KC, et al. (2011) Anabolic steroid associated to physical training induces deleterious cardiac effects. Med Sci Sports Exerc 43: 1836–1848. doi: 10.1249/MSS.0b013e318217e8b6.
24. Maior AS, Carvalho AR, Marques-Neto SR, Menezes P, Soares PP, et al. (2012) Cardiac autonomic dysfunction in anabolic steroid users. Scand J Med Sci Sports 23: 548–555. doi: 10.1111/j.1600-0838.2011.01436.x.
25. Marques Neto SR, Silva AD, Santos MC, Ferraz EF, Nascimento JH (2013) The blockade of angiotensin AT (1) and aldosterone receptors protects rats from synthetic androgen-induced cardiac autonomic dysfunction. Acta Physiol (Oxf). 208: 166–171. doi: 10.1111/apha.12056.
26. Pey A, Saborido A, Blázquez I, Delgado J, Megías A (2003) Effects of prolonged stanozolol treatment on antioxidant enzyme activities, oxidative stress markers, and heat shock protein HSP72 levels in rat liver. J Steroid Biochem Mol Biol 87: 269–277.

27. Chaves EA, Pereira-Junior PP, Fortunato RS, Masuda MO, de Carvalho AC, et al. (2006) Nandrolone decanoate impairs exercise-induced cardioprotection: role of antioxidant enzymes. J Steroid Biochem Mol Biol. 99: 223–230.

28. Gorgoulis VG, Vassiliou LV, Karakaidos P, Zacharatos P, Kotsinas A, et al. (2005) Activation of the DNA damage checkpoint and genomic instability in human precancerous lesions. Nature 434: 907–913.

29. Pozzi R, Fernandes KR, Moura CFG, Ferrari RAM, Fernandes KPS, et al. (2013) Nandrolone decanoate induces genetic damage in multiple organs of rats. Arch Environ Contam Toxicol 64: 514–518. doi: 10.1007/s00244-012-9848-2.

30. Neri M, Bello S, Bonsignore A, Cantatore S, Riezzo I, et al. (2011) Anabolic androgenic steroids abuse and liver toxicity. Mini Rev Med Chem 11: 430–437.

31. D'Errico S, Di Battista B, Di Paolo M, Fiore C, Pomara C (2011) Renal heat shock proteins over-expression due to anabolic androgenic steroids abuse. Mini Rev Med Chem 11: 446–450.

4

Neuronal Cellular Responses to Extremely Low Frequency Electromagnetic Field Exposure: Implications Regarding Oxidative Stress and Neurodegeneration

Marcella Reale[1]*, **Mohammad A. Kamal**[2], **Antonia Patruno**[3], **Erica Costantini**[1], **Chiara D'Angelo**[1], **Miko Pesce**[3], **Nigel H. Greig**[4]*

1 Department of Experimental and Clinical Sciences, University "G. d'Annunzio, Chieti, Italy, 2 King Fahd Medical Research Center, King Abdulaziz University, Jeddah, Kingdom of Saudi Arabia, 3 Department of Medicine and Aging Science, University 'G. d'Annunzio' of Chieti-Pescara, Chieti, Italy, 4 Drug Design and Development Section, Translational Gerontology Branch, Intramural Research Program, National Institute on Aging, National Institutes of Health, Baltimore, Maryland, United States of America

Abstract

Neurodegenerative diseases comprise both hereditary and sporadic conditions characterized by an identifying progressive nervous system dysfunction and distinctive neuopathophysiology. The majority are of non-familial etiology and hence environmental factors and lifestyle play key roles in their pathogenesis. The extensive use of and ever increasing worldwide demand for electricity has stimulated societal and scientific interest on the environmental exposure to low frequency electromagnetic fields (EMFs) on human health. Epidemiological studies suggest a positive association between 50/60-Hz power transmission fields and leukemia or lymphoma development. Consequent to the association between EMFs and induction of oxidative stress, concerns relating to development of neurodegenerative diseases, such as Alzheimer disease (AD), have been voiced as the brain consumes the greatest fraction of oxygen and is particularly vulnerable to oxidative stress. Exposure to extremely low frequency (ELF)-EMFs are reported to alter animal behavior and modulate biological variables, including gene expression, regulation of cell survival, promotion of cellular differentiation, and changes in cerebral blood flow in aged AD transgenic mice. Alterations in inflammatory responses have also been reported, but how these actions impact human health remains unknown. We hence evaluated the effects of an electromagnetic wave (magnetic field intensity 1mT; frequency, 50-Hz) on a well-characterized immortalized neuronal cell model, human SH-SY5Y cells. ELF-EMF exposure elevated the expession of NOS and O_2^-, which were countered by compensatory changes in antioxidant catylase (CAT) activity and enzymatic kinetic parameters related to CYP-450 and CAT activity. Actions of ELF-EMFs on cytokine gene expression were additionally evaluated and found rapidly modified. Confronted with co-exposure to H_2O_2-induced oxidative stress, ELF-EMF proved not as well counteracted and resulted in a decline in CAT activity and a rise in O_2^- levels. Together these studies support the further evaluation of ELF-EMF exposure in cellular and in vivo preclinical models to define mechanisms potentially impacted in humans.

Editor: Brandon K Harvey, National Insttitute on Drug Abuse, United States of America

Funding: This work was supported by grants from the Italian MIUR to M. R. and A. P., the King Fahd Medical Research Center, King Abdulaziz University for M. A. K., and the Intramural Research Program, National Institute on Aging, National Institutes of Health for N. H. G. The funders had no role in study design, data collection and analysis, decision to publish, or preparation of the manuscript.

Competing Interests: The authors have declared that no competing interests exist.

* Email: mreale@unich.it (MR); greign@grc.nia.nih.gov (NG)

Introduction

Neurodegenerative diseases are characterized by a slow and progressive loss of neurons within the central nervous system (CNS). They generally occur in later life, are often associated with deficits in brain function (e.g., memory and cognition, or movement – depending on the predominant neuronal population impacted) and are defined as hereditary and sporadic conditions; with the majority of being non-familial [1–3]. There are hundreds of disorders that could be described as neurodegenerative diseases. Many are rare, a few are common and include Alzheimer's disease (AD), Parkinson's disease (PD), amyotrophic lateral sclerosis (ALS), multiple sclerosis, Huntington's disease (HD) and multiple system atrophy (MSA), and these, particularly when combined together, represent one of the most critical health concerns currently impacting developed countries. Neurodegenerative diseases often extend over a decade prior to death, but the actual onset of neurodegeneration may silently precede clinical manifestations by numerous years; for AD by as much as two or three decades [4,5]. Specific environmental factors and lifestyle are considered to play a key role in the pathogenesis of neurodegenerative disorders [6–8]. These can occur during early life and remain quiescent [9,10].

Previous studies have reported that exposure to extremely low-frequency electromagnetic fields (ELF-EMF) can alter animal behavior, cerebral blood flow in aged AD transgenic mice, and modulate gene expression, cell differentiation and survival of neural cell populations [11–13]. An elevated risk of neurodegenerative diseases has been reported in some subjects with occupational exposure to ELF-EMF at magnetic field levels comparable with those present in some residential areas (0.2–5.0 µT). In general, however, epidemiological studies have largely failed to find strong positive associations between neurodegenerative disease occurrence and EMF exposure [14,15]. This could be due to multiple issues that include (i) the wide variability of exposure levels between individuals, (ii) the heterogeneic characteristics and small number of subjects studied, (iii) the intensity and time of EMF exposure, (iv) the target cell phenotype evaluated and, in particular, (v) the selection and appropriateness of endpoints appraised. In light of these considerations, there is strong rationale to evaluate mechanisms via which EMFs may impact neuronal processes to focus epidemiological studies and support the selection of defined future endpoints.

Albeit that human data bears the most direct relevance to human disease, its interpretation is often difficult. Developing and testing hypotheses is generally more easily undertaken in cellular studies. Additionally, their much reduced cost and relative ease of manipulation can allow evaluation of the role of specific environmental factors, either alone or in combination with other agents, on key cellular targets considered central to neurodegenerative disease development. In relation to molecular events potentially impacted by ELF-EMF, live, adult human neurons are not readily available. However, as a valuable alternative, human SH-SY5Y cells express a neuronal phenotype and represent a well characterized immortalized line that, although removed from the *in vivo* system, provide the opportunity to study responses in human rather than rodent neural cells [15].

A large body of evidence supports a direct contribution of inflammation in the development and progression of neurodegeneration [16]. In this regard, a wide range of inflammatory markers, either absent or minimally expressed in the healthly population, have been found present in AD, MS, PD, HD, ALS and MSA [17–22]. Additionally, oxidative stress, marked by lipid peroxidation, nitration, reactive carbonyls, and nucleic acid oxidation, is perhaps the earliest feature of neurodegeneration [23,24] and occurs in vulnerable neurons preceding any defining classical pathology.

Within all aerobic cells, and particularly for highly metabolic neurons, the processes involved in energy production and respiration inevitably generate reactive oxiygen and nitrogen species (ROS and RNS, respectively), which represent a wide range of small signaling molecules with highly reactive unpaired valence electrons. Oxidative stress occurs when ROS/RNS production exceeds the abilities of resident antioxidant defense mechanisms to sequester free radical intermediates, which consequently escape to then damage major macromolecules [23,24]. For example, the presence of the reactive peroxynitrite has been observed in acute and chronic active MS lesions, and nitric oxide metabolites, lipid peroxidation products are reported significantly elevated in the serum of patients with MS [25]. A pronounced increase in NO levels has been described in ALS [26], and oxidative stress is a common downstream mechanism by which nigral dopamine neurons are damaged in PD [27]. ROS is additionally generated by the activation of several inflammatory enzymes, for example the expression of inducible nitric oxide synthase (iNOS) is under the transcriptional control of a variety of inflammatory cytokines, and the expression of proinflammatory mediators appears to be redox sensitive [28,29].

The fine control of inflammatory mediator levels appears to be critical to neuronal homeostasis and health. As an example, a deficiency in neuronal TGF-β signaling promotes neurodegeneration and AD [30], whereas augmented TGF-β can act as an anti-inflammatory cytokine and has potential neuroprotective action in AD and following a CNS insult [31,32]. Interleukin 18 (IL-18)

exerts proinflammatory effects by inducing gene expression and synthesis of cytokines, chemokines and adhesion molecules, whereas its natural inhibitor, IL-18 binding protein (Il-1BP), operates as a key negative feedback mechanism to both balance and limit the impact of inflammation [33]. Likewise, the actions of microglial cells are regulated at a number of stages, such as at the level of their movement by the monocyte chemoattractant protein (CCL2/MCP-1) [34–36].

In the current study, we investigated the impact of an electromagnetic wave (magnetic field intensity, 1mT; frequency, 50 Hz) on SH-SY5Y cell cultures in relation to oxidative stress, with a focus on select mechanisms to balance oxidative damage and inflammation. This well characterized cellular model possesses a number of physiological systems that have parallels to human neurons to provide potential insight into cellular cascades that, by exposure to ELF-EMF, may lead towards neurodegeneration.

Materials And Methods

Cell culture

The neuroblastoma cell line, SH-SY5Y (Sigma-Aldrich, St Louis, MO, USA), was grown in Dulbecco's modified Eagle's medium (DMEM) containing 10% foetal bovine serum and a mixture of streptomycin/penicillin. Cultures were maintained at $37°C$ in a humidified atmosphere of 5% CO_2. On a weekly basis, SH-SY5Y cells were detached and seeded into dishes or multiwell plates and, on reaching 60–70% confluency, cells were continuously exposed to a 50-Hz ELF-EMF at a flux density of 1 mT (r.m.s.) produced by an electromagnetic generator located on a grid to allow air circulation within the central part of its solenoid. Control, non-exposed cell cultures were grown simultaneously. Specifically, cells were placed in a different incubator and cultured under the same conditions and times as ELF-EMF exposed cells. At the end of incubation, both exposed and non-exposed cells were harvested using trypsin-EDTA. Their viability was evaluated by Trypan blue dye exclusion and they were counted in a Burker chamber. In preliminary studies responses to ELF-EMF appeared independent of cell density in challenged cells, and cell density remained similar between challenged and unchallenged cells.

Magnetic field exposure system and exposure conditions of cell cultures

The experimental setup and ELF-EMF exposure system have been previously described [37]. Briefly, an oscillating magnetic field (AC MF) consisted of: (i) a sinusoidal signal 50 Hz waveform generator (Agilent Technologies model 33220A, Santa Clara, CA, USA); (ii) a power amplifier (NAD electronics Ltd., model 216, London, UK); (iii) an oscilloscope (ISO-TECH model ISR658, Vicenza, Italy) dedicated to monitoring output signals from a Gaussmeter (MG-3D, Walker Scientific Inc., Worcester, MA, USA) and the AC MF generator; (iv) a 160 turn solenoid (22 cm length, 6 cm radius, copper wire diameter of 1.25×10^{-5} cm) that generated a horizontal magnetic field. This solenoid was placed inside the exposure incubator. The achieved MF intensity (1 mT (rms)) was continuously monitored using a Hall-effect probe connected to the Gaussmeter. The environmental magnetic noise inside the incubator was related to the geomagnetic field (≈ 40 µT) and to the 50 Hz disturbance associated with the working incubator (≈ 7 µT (rms).

Cell cultures were maintained in a 5% CO_2 atmosphere and at a temperature of $37 \pm 0.3°C$. For ELF-EMF challenge, cells were placed within the central region of the solenoid that was characterized by the greatest field homogeneity (98%) to thereby receive continuous exposure to steady-state 50-Hz ELF-EMF for defined times up to 24 hr; thereafter, cell were immediately harvested for the outcome analyses described below. In addition, a further digital thermometer (HD 2107.2, Delta OHM, Padova, Italy) was placed inside the solenoid directly alongside the cell cultures to record local temperature variations, and the temperature of the cell medium was recorded using a specially designed thermoresistor (HD 9216; Delta OHM, Padova, Italy). No significant temperature changes were observed associated with application of the ELF field ($\Delta T = 0.1°C$). This lack of a thermal effect on cells maintained at $37°C$ is in accord with the known non-thermal nature of ELF interactions with biological molecules [15,37]. Any low-level Joule heating was efficiently dissipated by the incubator's fan mechanism as Dt was $<0.1308°C$ in the medium of exposed cells.

Analyses of NOS activity

At defined times, ELF-EMF exposed and unexposed (control) cells were immediately analysed for NOS activity. This was assayed by measuring the conversion of L-[2,3-^{3}H]arginine to L-[2,3-^{3}H]citrulline in HaCaT cell homogenates. Briefly, 1 µl of radioactive arginine, L-(2,3,4,5)-[^{3}H]Arginine Monohydrochloride 64 Ci/mM, 1 µCi/ µl (Amersham, Arlington Heigths, IL, USA), 5 µl NADPH 10 mM, and 5 µl CaCl$_2$ 6 mM (Calbiochem, San Diego, CA, USA) were added to each sample, which then were incubated for 30 min at room temperature. Thereafter, the reaction was stopped by the addition of 400 µl stop-buffer (50 mM HEPES, pH 5.5, and 5 mM EDTA). Unreacted arginine was removed by the addition of equilibrated cationic exchange resin (Dowex AG50WX-8, Sigma-Aldrich). After centrifugation, the radioactivity, corresponding to L-[^{3}H]-citrulline in the eluate, was measured by liquid scintillation spectrometry and expressed as pmol^{3}H/min/mg.

Determination of O_2^-

Production of O_2^- was determined spectrophotometrically (Hewlett Packard 8452 A, Palo Alto, CA, USA) by monitoring the reduction of ferricytochrome c (Type VI, Sigma-Aldrich) at 550 nm, as described by Pritchard and colleagues [38]. Briefly, ferricytochrome c (50 µmol/L) was added to cuvettes containing cells and PBS (final volume 1 mL), either in the presence or absence of superoxide dismutase (SOD, 350 U/ml) and subsequent changes in absorbance were followed for 10 min. Rates of O_2^- production were calculated on the basis of the molar extinction coefficient of the reduced ferricytochrome c [e = 21000 cm^{-1} (mol/L)$^{-1}$]. Cell counts were used to calculate results as nmol $O_2^-/10^6$ cells/min.

Measurement of catalase (CAT) activity

CAT activity was measured spectrophotometrically as previously described [39]. The decomposition of H_2O_2 was monitored continuously at 240 nm. The assay mixture, in a final volume of 3 ml, contained 10 mM potassium phosphate buffer, 10 mM H_2O_2 and 10 µg of protein enzymatic extract. CAT units were defined as 1 µmole H_2O_2 decomposed/min at $25°C$.

RNA extraction and RT-PCR analysis

Total RNA was extracted from SH-SY5Y cell cultures using TRIzol reagent (Invitrogen, Life Technologies, Paisley, UK) according to the manufacturer's protocol. The RNA concentration was estimated by measuring its absorbance at 260 nm using a Bio-Photometer (Eppendorf, Milano, Italy), and RNA samples were kept frozen at $-80°C$ until use. Purified RNA was electrophoresed on a 1% agarose gel to assess the integrity of the purified RNA.

One µg of RNA was reverse transcribed into cDNA using a Quantitect reverse transcription kit (Qiagen, Milano, Italy), according to the manufacturer's instructions. Polymerase chain reaction (PCR) was performed using the mRNA/cDNA specific cytokine primer pairs (Table 1). All PCR reactions were performed in a PCR-thermocycler (Eppendorf, Milano, Italy). The program utilized for PCR amplification was as follows: an initial period of 5 min at $95°C$, followed by a variable number of cycles of 30 s denaturation at $95°C$, 30 s annealing at $60°C$ and finally 30 s of extention at $72°C$. The programme was terminated with a period of 10 min at $72°C$. To be within the exponential phase of the semi-quantitative PCR reaction, the appropriate number of cycles was newly established for every set of samples. Products were separated by gel electrophoresis on 2% agarose gels and visualized by ethidium bromide staining. All gels were scanned and the percent adjusted volume intensities of all of the RT-PCR products were determined using a Bio-Rad gel documentation system (Bio-Rad, Hercules, CA, USA).). Mean ± SD intensities were calculated for all PCR experiments.

Cell viability

Cell viability was determined by quantitative colorimetric MTT assay (Sigma-Aldrich) using 96-well microplates immediately following ELF-EMF and control (no exposure) challenge. Briefly, 50 ul of the MTT-labeling reagent, at a final concentration of 0.5 mg/ml, was added to each well at the end of the dexamethasone/folic acid period, and the plate was then placed in a humidified incubator ($37°C$, and 5% CO2 and 95% air (v/v)) for an additional 2 hr period. Thereafter, the production of formazan was read at 540 nm λ using a standard 96-well plate reader. The intensity of the color produced was proportional to the number of living SH-SY5Y cells.

Statistical analysis

Band intensities of RT- PCR were quantified by a densitometer and expressed as relative values to the controls. Data are expressed as means ± SD from three or more independent experiments. For statistical analysis, quantitative data were analyzed by Student t test, with appropriate corrections in the case of multiple comparisons. Differences are considered significant at $p < 0.05$.

Results

ELF-EMF does not impact cell morphology and viability

Human SH-SY5Y cultures were subjected to ELF-EMF 50 Hz, 1.0 mT exposure and their cell morphology and proliferation rate were compared to unexposed control cells. Figure 1 illustrates representative images of exposed and control cultures at both 6 and 24 hr. No differences in cell morphology were evident at either time. Additionally, as quantitatively evaluated by MTT assay at 24 hr as well as by image analysis, the cellular proliferation rate was not influenced by the presence of ELF-EMFs; with exposed and unexposed cultures possessing comparable cell numbers.

ELF-EMF elevates NOS activity

NOS activity, determined by measuring the conversion of L-[2,3-^{3}H]arginine to L-[2,3-^{3}H]citrulline, was increased in SH-SY5Y cells exposed to ELF-EMF. As shown in Figure 2, this elevation was significant across all times evaluated (1, 3, 6 and 24 hr), and proved greatest at 1 hr (3.2-fold rise) versus later times (3 hr: 1.9-fold, 6 and 24 hr: 1.7-fold elevation).

Table 1. Sequences of the oligonucleotide primers utilized in the reverse transcriptase polymerase chain reaction.

Gene	Forward Primer Sequence [5'-3']	Reverse Primer Sequence [5'-3']	Primer size
RPS18	CTTTGCCATCACTGCCATTAAG	TCCATCCTTTACATCCTTCTGTC	199 bp
IL18	CAGTCAGCAAGGAATTGTCTC	GAGGAAGCGATCTGGAAGG	139 bp
IL18BP	CAACTGGACACCAGACCTCA	AGCTCAGCGTTCCATTCAGT	235 bp
TGFβ1	AACAATTCCTGGCGATACCTC	GTAGTGAACCCGTTGATGTCC	197 bp
MCP1	AACTGAAGCTCGCACTCTCG	GAGTGAGTGTTCAAGTCTTCGG	327 bp

Effect of ELF-EMF on antioxidant enzyme catalase (CAT) activity

The impact of ELF-EMF-exposure on CAT activity in SH-SY5Y cells was evaluated. As illustrated in Figure 3, under basal conditions CAT activity remained largely unaltered over 1, 3 and 6 hr of incubation, but became elevated by 24 h (2.9-fold vs. 1 hr value). By contrast, the exposure of SH-SY5Y cells to ELF-EMF resulted in significantly heightened CAT activity levels by 6 hr (2.3-fold vs. both the basal level at 6 hr, and the 1 hr level post ELF-EMF exposure).

Table 2 provides key parameters characterizing the kinetics of CAT activity in SH-SY5Y cells exposed and unexposed to ELF-EMF. Exposure induced a modest increase (23%) in total velocity υ of CAT enzyme that was accompanied by a moderate (2.2-fold) rise in the υ_{min} value. The rate of decrease ($\downarrow^{®}$) in the CAT reaction was found to be elevated in the presence of ELF-EMF (3.3-fold), and the time at which maximum activity was recorded (pT) in response to ELF-EMF exposure occurred at 16.5 hr compared to 13.5 hr for controls (Table 2).

Effect of ELF-EMF on cytochrome P450 (CYP-450) activity

Oxidative stress appears to a primary factor contributing to neuronal dysfunction [23,40,52]. As the levels of O_2^- production represents an index of free radical and ROS production, we evaluated the cellular redox state by NADPH oxidase activity using the cytochrome c reduction assay method. Assessment of the effect of ELF-EMF-exposure on CYO 450 activity in SH-SY5Y cells showed that ELF-EMF increased CYP 450 activity and, consequently, O_2^- production at all times studied (Fig. 4), with the greatest increase (62%) occurring after 6 hr of exposure.

A rise (21%) in the total velocity of CYP-450 was measured in response to ELF-EMF exposure, which was accompanied by a significant elevation in the rate of increase ($\uparrow^{®}$) of the enzymatic reaction by 2.4-fold (Table 3). ELF-EMFS exposure did not significantly impact the υ_{min} value. However, the rate of decrease ($\downarrow^{®}$) in CYP-450 enzymatic activity was heightened (5.3-fold) in response to ELF-EMF exposure. The time required for CYP-450 activity to peak was shorter, 15.8 vs. 18.8 hr in ELF-EMF exposed and unexposed cultures, respectively, and this peak activity was elevated from 8.1 to 13.95 (1.7-fold) by exposure (Table 3).

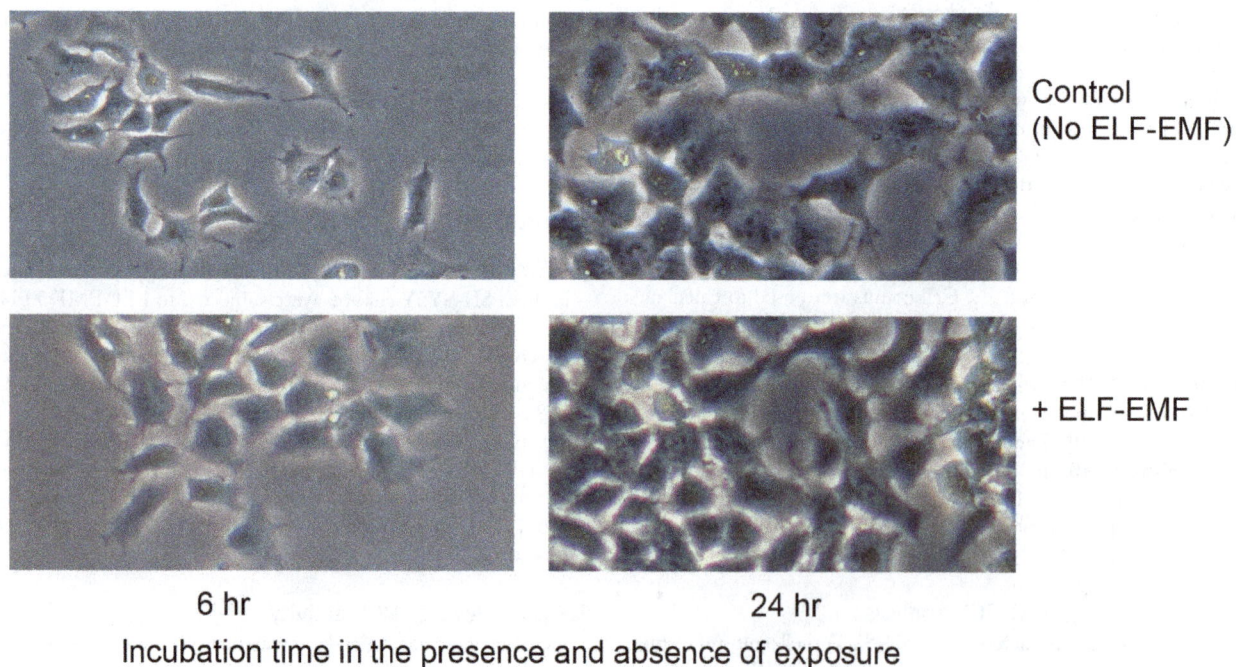

Control (No ELF-EMF)

+ ELF-EMF

6 hr   24 hr

Incubation time in the presence and absence of exposure

Figure 1. ELF-EMF (1 mT (rms), 50 Hz) exposure did not impact phenotypic expression, growth or viability of human SH-SY5Y cells. Representative phase contrast images of proliferative SH-SY5Y cells in culture medium with 10% FBS (400× magnification), grown for 6 and 24 hr the presence and absence of ELF-EMFs. Not shown, cell proliferation was not influenced by the presence of ELF-EMF, as determined by MTT assay at 6 and 24 hr.

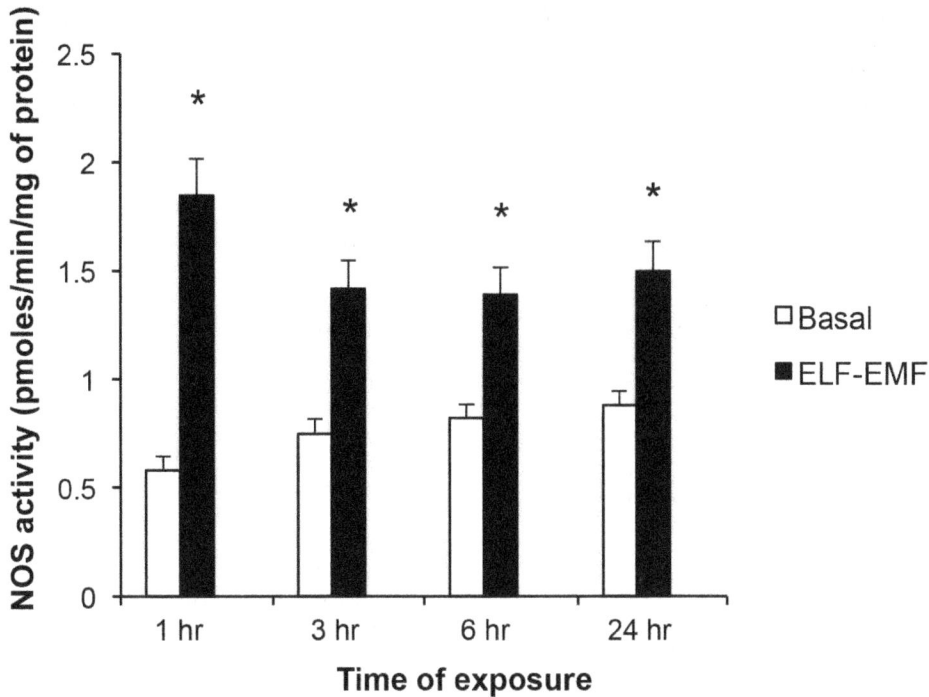

Figure 2. ELF-EMF exposure induced a rapid and sustained elevation in NOS activity. NOS enzymatic activity, determined by measuring the conversion of L-[^{3}H]arginine to L-[^{3}H]citrulline, is expressed in picomoles per minute per milligram of protein. Each value represents the mean $\pm$ s.d. of different experiments performed in triplicate (*p<0.05).

Effect of ELF-EMF exposure on H$_2$O$_2$-treated SH-SY5Y cells line

In light of excessive production of ROS resulting in neuronal damage [23,24], initial blockade of its generation may prove protective for neurons [40]. To explore whether ELF-EMF may impact the homeostatic capability of neural cells, SH-SY5Y cultures were exposed to H$_2$O$_2$ in the presence and absence of ELF-EMF. An initial dose-response evaluation of H$_2$O$_2$ on SH-SY5Y cell viability was performed to identify a subtoxic concentration that would not induce cell death. From this

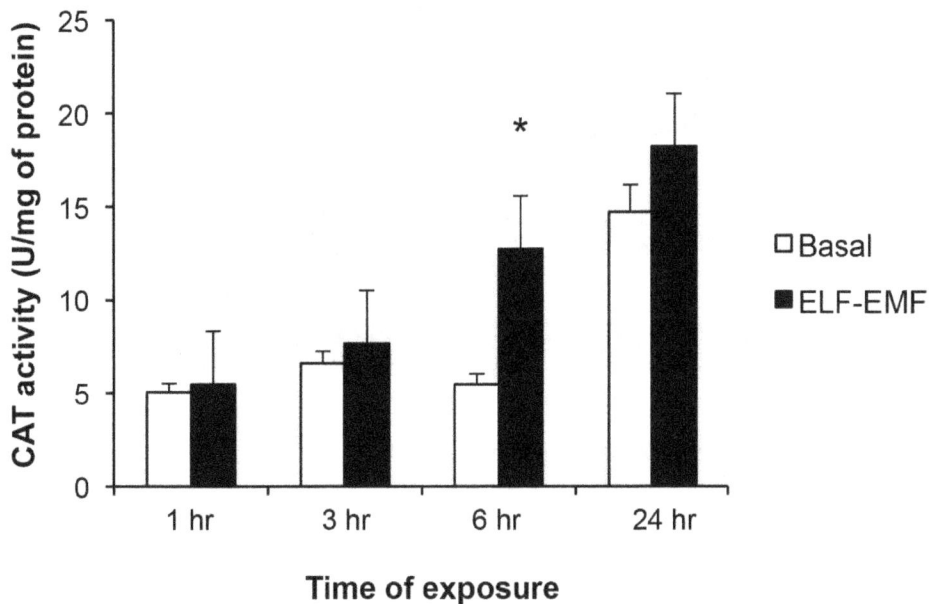

Figure 3. ELF-EMF exposure induced a time-dependent elevation in Catylase (CAT) activity: CAT activity was normalized with respect to the total protein content of cell lysates and expressed as units per mg of protein. Each value was the mean $\pm$ s.d. of three independent experiments performed in triplicate (*p<0.05).

Table 2. Kinetic constants characterizing the impact of ELF-EMF exposure on antioxidant enzyme catalase (CAT) activity in human SH-SY5Y neuronal cultures.

	Total υ	↑ ®	υ$_{min}$	↓ ®	pT (hr)	pυ
Basal	467±6.0	2.0±0.32	1.7±1.3	2.45	13.5	31.2
+ ELF-EMF	575±8.7	1.5±0.12	3.7±0.49	8.0	16.5	26.2

υ = activity; ↑ ® = Upward υ rate; υ$_{min}$ = minimum initial activity; ↓ ® = downward υ rate; pT = peak time; pυ = peak activity.

100 μM H_2O_2 was then used in subsequent experiments. This H_2O_2 challenge induced a significant rise in CAT activity and O_2- production in SH-SY5Y cells over a 24 hr incubation period (p< 0.05 versus control cells not subjected to H_2O_2 (not shown)). As illustrated in Figure 5, co-exposure of cells to ELF-EMF and H_2O_2 induced a decline in CAT activity per unit protein (26% reduction (p<0.05) together with a modest rise in O_2- (9% rise (trend)) with respect to cells treated with H_2O_2 alone (Fig. 5). Hence, ELF-EMF exposure of H_2O_2-treated cells may increase the cell oxidative activity.

Effect of ELF-EMF on expression of cyto/chemokines in SH-SY5Y cells

To characterize the impact of ELF-EMF on early ongoing cellular processes, gene transcription of select cyto/chemokines was evaluated in the presence and absence of ELF-EMF exposure. RT-PCR experiments were performed using specific primers and the density of each band was divided by that of its respective β-actin band for normalization, with the resulting value expressed as a relative intensity (Fig. 6). An increase in the expression of TGFβ (1.5-fold, p<0.05) and IL-18BP (4.2-fold, p<0.05) was observed after 24 hr exposure to ELF-EMF, whereas the expressions of IL-18 and MCP-1 were not statistically significantly affected (Fig. 6).

Discussion

ELF-EMFs are a form of energy, characterized by wavelength or frequency, that are associated with the use of electrical power that generates a magnetic field at a frequency of 50 Hz and a flux density that primarily ranges between 0.2 and 5 mT. The magnetic flux density selected for our study, 1 mT, is 2- and 10-fold the reference levels proposed by the European Community for occupational and general public exposure, respectively. This 1 mT flux density is one of the most studied intensities in medical research focused to elucidate the biological actions of ELF-EMF, consequent to its human translational relevance [41] as during recent years there has been heightened public concern of the impact of ELF-EMFs, associated with both industrial and domesitic use, on human health and welfare. Epidemiological studies have highlighted childhood leukemias, adult primary brain tumors as well as breast cancer, the potential for miscarriage and neurodegenerative disorders [42–44]. In large part, past studies have been fraught by limited exposure assessment and other methodological limitations [43], making ELF-EMF epidemiological data interesting but difficult to interpret and then act upon. Whereas the occurrence of some chronic diseases are relatively uncommon (ALS, HD) and have long latency periods for known risk factors, for others – all be they abundant (AD, PD) - their etiologies remain poorly understood [1,2], which confounds the observation of potential associations, particularly when relying on mortality records [43,44]. Nevertheless, the World Health

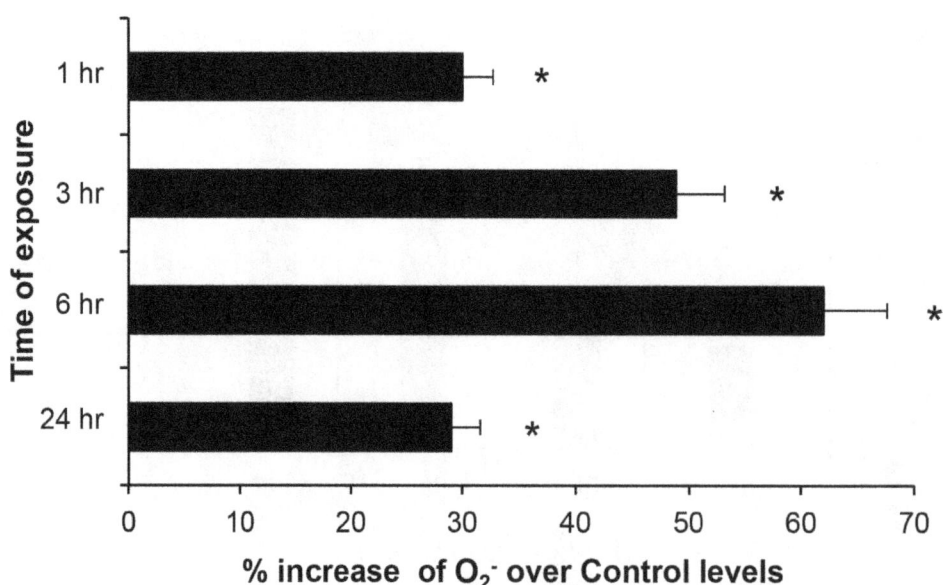

Figure 4. ELF-EMF exposure time-dependently increased O_2^- production: O_2^- production in ELF-EMF exposed SH-SY5Y cells was evaluated by the cytochrome c reduction assay method and expressed as % increase with respect to non exposed SH-SY5Y cells (*p<0.05).

Table 3. Kinetic constants characterizing the impact of ELF-EMF exposure on cytochrome P450 (CYP-450) activity in human SH-SY5Y neuronal cultures.

	Total υ	$\uparrow$ [®]	υ_{min}	$\downarrow$ [®]	pT (hr)	pυ
Basal	287.8±14.2	0.34±0.05	3.3±0.20	0.096	18.8	8.1
+ ELF-EMF	348.8±10	0.80±0.097	3.9±0.38	0.506	15.8	13.95

υ = activity; $\uparrow$ [®] = Upward υ rate; υ_{min} = minimum initial activity; $\downarrow$ [®] = downward υ rate; pT = peak time; pυ = peak activity.

Organization [45,46] and International Programme on Chemical Safety [47] have issued precautions against ELF-EMFs, resulting in exposure level limits being recommended. In parallel with this, there has been increased focus to understand potential mechanisms via which ELF-EMFs may mediate their actions at a cellular level to guide future epidemiological and in vivo research.

The etiology of neurodegenerative diseases is most often multifactorial, and genetic polymorphisms, increasing age as well as environmental cues are primary risk factors [1,2]. Although different neuronal cell populations are affected across diverse neurodegenerative disorders, hallmark protein modification (whether extracellular amyloid plaques and intracellular neurofibrillary tangles as in AD, or α-synuclein as in PD) is a common feature that supports both differential disease diagnosis and provides a mechanistic basis to gauge disease progression [48,49].

It is becoming increasingly clear that, particularly for chronic neurodegenerative disorders occurring late in life, a complex combination of risk factors can initiate disease development and modify proteins with physiological functions into ones with pathological roles via a number of defined mechanisms [50]. A common denominator in the occurrence of diverse pathogenic mechanisms is oxidative stress accompanied by redox dysregulation [51,52,23,40], which have a role in metabolic and mitochondrial dysfunction, excitocity, calcium handling impairment, glial cell dysfunction and neuroinflammation. Each of these can influence one another at multiple different levels, and hence

oxidative stress can both be secondary to them as well as have a primary part in their initiation. Such oxidative stress derives from two primary sources, from chronic ROS creation that is routinely generated from the mitochondrial electron transport chain during normal cellular function [53], and from acute, high levels of ROS generation resulting from nicotinamide adenine dinucleotide phosphate (NADPH) oxidase, particularly associated with the activation of the innate immune system within the CNS [51]. In both circumstances, oxidative stress results when imbalance between ROS production and the clearance of chemically reactive species by endogenous antioxidant enzymes and reducing agents occurs. Environmental factors such as ELF-EMFs, stressors, or disease that augment the former or lower the latter can amplify and drive the process. Thus, in practical terms, oxidative stress is determined by excessive exposure to oxidant molecules when there is insufficient availability of antioxidant mechanisms [23], with the resulting ROS oxidizing vulnerable cellular constituents, including proteins, nucleic acids and lipids, inducing microglial activation, inducing pro-inflammatory and suppressing anti-inflammatory cytokines and related signaling pathways, and ultimately causing both synaptic and neuronal damage and dysfunction. In this regard, the neuronal properties of SH-SY5Y human neuroblastoma cells, together with their pronounced sensitivity to oxidative stress and inflammation, make these cells a valuable model to study a number of neurological pathologies at the molecular, morphological and physiological level.

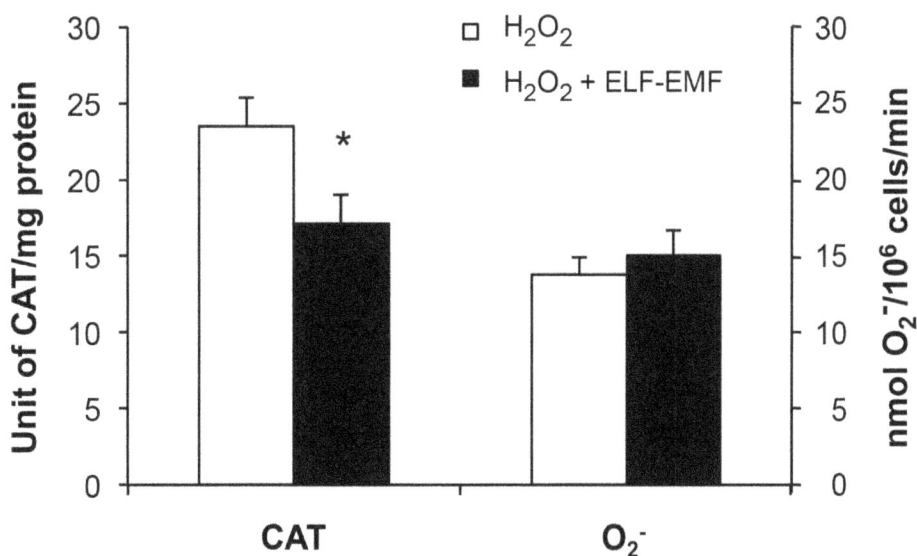

Figure 5. ELF-EMF exposure in the presence of coincident oxidative stress induced a decline in CAT activity. Both CAT activity (normalized to total protein content of cell lysates and expressed as units per mg of protein) and O_2^- production (evaluated by the cytochrome c reduction assay and expressed as nmol $O_2^-/10^6$ cells/min) were quantified in the presence and absence of pre-existing oxidative stress (100 µM H_2O_2) at 24 hr. Each value was the mean ± s.d. of three independent experiments performed in triplicate (*p<0.05).

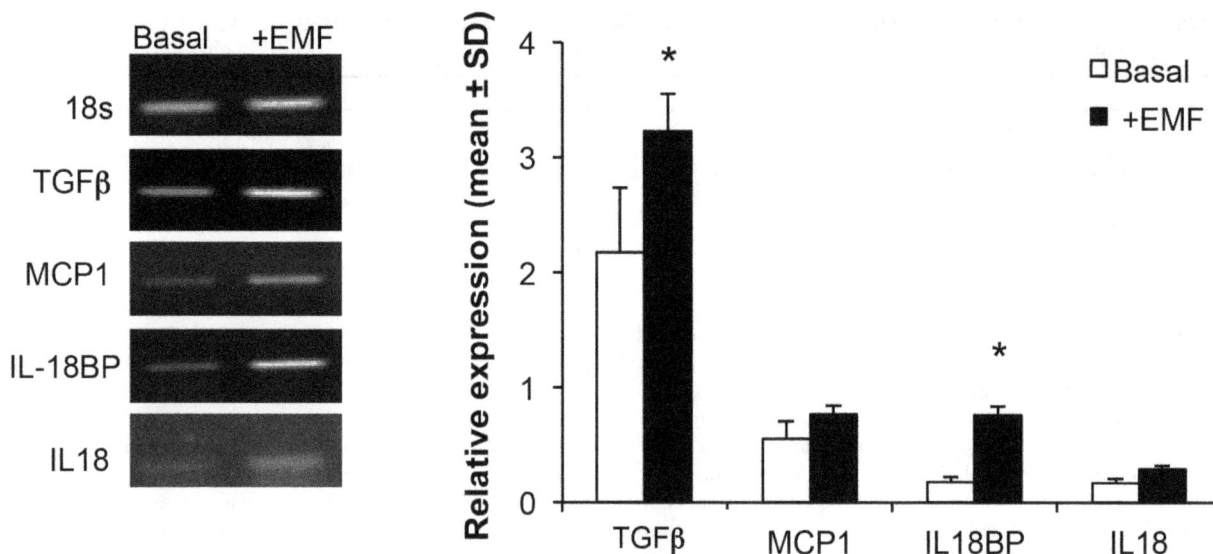

Figure 6. ELF-EMF exposure significantly heightens TGFβ, IL-18 expression. The intensities of bands for TGFβ, IL-18, IL-18BP and MCP-1 are normalized to the GAPDH signals. The expression values are the mean ± S.D. of 2 replicate PCR reactions on RNA isolated from three independent experiments (*p<0.05).

Previous studies have demonstrated that the cellular effects of ELF-EMFs depend, in large part, on their intensity and exposure time, as well as on the phenotype of the cellular target and interactions with intracellular structures [43,54]. In SH-SY5Y cell cultures and a number of other cell types exposed to ELF-EMF, genes involved in the stress response, cell growth and differentiation or protein metabolism have been reported to be generally down-regulated, whereas genes involved in Ca^{2+} metabolism, the PI3-kinase pathway, trascription and it's modulation by splicing are up-regulated [41,54–61]. Such actions are reported to often be accompanied by changes in cell growth and oxidative balance [41,54,61]. In our experimental conditions, timed continuous ELF-EMF (1 mT (rms)), 50 Hz) exposure likewise impacted cellular oxidative status, causing an early rise in NOS activity and O_2^- levels in SH-SY5Y cells. Within a short duration, this was counteracted by a compensatory increase in the antioxidant capacity of CAT to, thereby, provide the potential to more effectively scavenge any prospective ELF-EMF-mediated ROS over-production; thus avoiding oxidative ELF-EMF-induced cellular damage. In this regard, NOS activity peaked following 1 hr of ELF-EMF exposure and, thereafter, its level declined and remained approximately constant (Fig. 2). Accompanying this, a rise in CAT activity was observed after 6 hr of ELF-EMF exposure (Fig. 3) that was associated with enzyme kinetic changes (Table 2). In light of this, ELF-EMF exposure time-dependently elevated the rate of cellular O_2^- production (Fig. 4), which peaked at 6 hr (162% of control values) and, thereafter, declined toward the baseline value. Hence ELF-EMF exposure can be considered to induce an "activated" cellular state, wherein the enhanced generation and the release of free radicals is offset by a compensatory modulation of antioxidant defences, leading to an absence of negative effects on cell growth and viability.

The kinetic evaluation of the catalyzed antioxidant processes proved useful in elucidating the pattern of influence of ELF-EMF exposure. Data presented in the current study indicates that a range of kinetic constants, such as total activity, rate of increase, decrease in enzymatic activities, peak time and specific activity of enzymes are both amenable to rapid change and influenced by

ELF-EMF exposure. Furthermore, key mediators of the inflammatory response, likewise, appear receptive to swift modulation. This is exemplified by an ELF-EMF-induced elevation in the expression of IL-18BP, which provides a signal for terminating the IL-18 mediated inflammatory response, and a rise in TGF-β that can act as an anti-inflammatory cytokine and has shown neuroprotective effects under conditions relevant to AD and following CNS insult [31,32]. In contrast, 24 hr ELF-EMF exposure insignificantly affected the expression of MCP-1, involved in the neuroinflammatory processes associated with diseases characterized by neuronal degeneration [62,63], or of IL-18, likewise, a key player in neuroinflammation and degeneration [64,33,34].

Albeit our results on cytokine expression, despite differences in experimental conditions, are in line with several ELF-EMF exposure studies [44], they are not in accord with ones reporting ELF-EMF promotion of cellular neurodifferentiation, as exemplified by neurite extension and number [65,41]. Although our ELF-EMF exposure condition induced an early rise in NOS and O_2^-, and adaptive cellular changes in CAT activity, it did not exert any cytotoxic or phenotypic changes, as confirmed by the fact that cell morphology and proliferation were unaltered after 6 and 24 hr ELF-EMF (Fig. 1).

In synopsis, we found SH-SY5Y cells useful in the evaluation of neuronal ELF-EMF mediated actions. An ELF-EMF exposure of 1mT proved well tolerated and without relevant action on cellular survival and metabolism, but significantly impacted the balance of oxidative stress and gene transcription of select inflammatory cytokines. This latter result provides impetus to undertake evaluation of a more complete list of genes that are time-dependently up- and down-regulated by ELF-EMF exposure to elucidate its modulatory actions. Our results suggest that adaptive mechanisms can rapidly offset exposure in unchallenged neuronal cultures to maintain homeostasis. However, confronted with existing oxidative stress, as induced by co-exposure to H_2O_2 (Fig. 5), the susceptibility of neuronal cells to free radicals and challenge to maintain homeostasis proved greater. H_2O_2-induced stress in cells co-exposed to continuous ELF-EMF proved to be not well counteracted, resulting in a reduction of CAT activity and a rise in O_2^- levels. Hence, in accord with Falone and colleagues [41], contiuuous ELF-EMF exposure reduced cell tolerance towards simultaneous oxidative challenges, and may aid our understanding of the role of concurrent environmental agent challenges in the development of neurodegenerative diseases.

It is important to note, however, that studies by others [66–68] have demonstrated that ELF-EMF exposure, in the form of transcranial magnetic stimulation (60-Hz, 0.7 mT) applied to rats for 2 hr twice daily, can prove neuroprotective. Administered prior to and after a toxic insult to the brain, for example systemic injection of 3-nitropropionic acid to induce an animal model of HD [69], ELF-EMF can mitigate oxidative damage, elevate neurotrophic protein levels in brain and ameliorate behavioral deficits [66–68], as well as potentially augment neurogenesis [70]. Such studies reiterate that the level and timing of exposure are critical factors impacting outcome measures, and can be potentially scheduled to optimize endogenous compensatory mechanisms following an adverse challenge.

Further studies designed to evaluate the actions of ELF-EMF under multiple conditions, including chronic or sporadic exposure in combination with common stressors pertinent to real life, appear warranted and may both aid our understanding of the true biological impact of ELF-EMF and scientifically anchor proposed exposure limits.

Acknowledgments

The authors dedicate this paper to the memory of their friend and colleague Giovina Vianale.

Author Contributions

Conceived and designed the experiments: MR AP EC CA MP. Performed the experiments: MR AP EC CA MP. Analyzed the data: MR MK EC CA NG. Contributed reagents/materials/analysis tools: AP MP. Contributed to the writing of the manuscript: MR MK NG. Figures: MR NG.

References

1. Bossy-Wetzel E, Schwarzenbacher R, Lipton SA (2004) Molecular pathways to neurodegeneration. Nat Med. 10 Suppl:S2–9.
2. Bertram L, Tanzi RE (2005) The genetic epidemiology of neurodegenerative disease. J Clin Invest. 115(6):1449–57.
3. Moreno-Gonzalez I, Soto C (2012) Natural animal models of neurodegenerative protein misfolding diseases. Curr Pharm Des. 18(8):1148–58.
4. Mullard A (2012) Sting of Alzheimer's failures offset by upcoming prevention trials. Nature Rev. Drug Discov. 11: 657–60.
5. Becker RE, Greig NH, Giacobini E, Schneider LS, Ferrucci L (2014) A new roadmap for drug development for Alzheimer's disease. Nat Rev Drug Discov. 13(2):156.
6. Brown RC, Lockwood AH, Sonawane BR (2005) Neurodegenerative diseases: An overview of environmental risk factors. Environmental Health Perspectives 113: 1250–6.
7. Cannon JR, Greenamyre JT (2011) The Role of environmental exposures in neurodegeneration and neurodegenerative diseases. Toxicological Sciences 124: 225–50.
8. Kraft AD, Harry GJ (2011) Features of microglia and neuroinflammation relevant to environmental exposure and neurotoxicity. Int. J. Environ. Res. Public Health 8: 2980–18.
9. Lahiri DK, Maloney B, Basha MR, Ge YW, Zawia NH (2007) How and when environmental agents and dietary factors affect the course of Alzheimer's disease: the "LEARn" model (latent early-life associated regulation) may explain the triggering of AD. Curr Alzheimer Res. 4(2):219–28.
10. Lahiri DK, Maloney B, Zawia NH (2009) The LEARn model: an epigenetic explanation for idiopathic neurobiological diseases. Mol Psychiatry. 14(11):992–1003
11. Luukkonen J, Liimatainen A, Hoyto A, Juutilainen J, Naarala J (2011) Pre-exposure to 50 Hz magnetic fields modifies menadione-induced genotoxic effects in human SH-SY5Y neuroblastoma cells. PLoS One 6: e18021.
12. Piacentini R, Ripoli C, Mezzogori D, Azzena GB, Grassi C (2008) Extremely low-frequency electromagnetic fields promote in vitro neurogenesis via upregulation of Ca(v)1-channel activity. J Cell Physiol 215: 129–39.
13. Arendash GW, Mori T, Dorsey M, Gonzalez R, Tajiri N, et al. (2012) Electromagnetic treatment to old Alzheimer's mice reverses beta-amyloid deposition, modifies cerebral blood flow, and provides selected cognitive benefit. PLoS One 7: e35751
14. Sonnier H, Kolomytkin O, Marino A (2003) Action potentials from human neuroblastoma cells in magnetic fields. Neuroscience Letters 337: 163–6.
15. Del Vecchio G, Giuliani A, Fernandez M, Mesirca P, Bersani F, et al. (2009) Effect of Radiofrequency Electromagnetic Field Exposure on In Vitro Models of Neurodegenerative Disease. Bioelectromagnetics 30: 564–72.
16. Tweedie D, Sambamurti K, Greig NH (2007) TNF-alpha inhibition as a treatment strategy for neurodegenerative disorders: new drug candidates and targets. Curr Alzheimer Res. 4(4):378–85.
17. Reale M, Iarlori C, Feliciani C, Gambi D (2008) Peripheral chemokine receptors, their ligands, cytokines and Alzheimer's disease. J Alzheimer's Dis. 14 (2): 147–59.
18. Reale M, De Angelis F, Di Nicola M, Capello E, Di Ioia M, et al. (2012) Relation between Pro-inflammatory Cytokines and Acetylcholine Levels in Relapsing-Remitting Multiple Sclerosis Patients. Int J Mol Sci. 13(10):12656–64.
19. Reale M, Iarlori C, Thomas A, Gambi D, Perfetti B, et al. (2009) Peripheral cytokines profile in Parkinson's disease. Brain, Behavior Immunity 23(1):55–63.
20. Reale M, Kamal MA, Velluto L, Gambi D, Di Nicola M, et al. (2012) Relationship between Inflammatory Mediators, Aβ Levels and APOE Genotype in Alzheimer's Disease. Curr Alzheimer Res. 9(4):447–57.
21. Moreau C, Devos D, Brunaud-Danel V, Defebvre L, Perez T, et al. (2005) Elevated IL-6 and TNF-alpha levels in patients with ALS: inflammation or hypoxia? Neurology 65: 1958–60.
22. Poloni M, Facchetti D, Mai R, Micheli A, Agnoletti L, et al. (2000) Circulating levels of tumour necrosis factor-alpha and its soluble receptors are increased in the blood of patients with amyotrophic lateral sclerosis. Neurosci Lett 287: 211–4.
23. Bonda DJ, Wang X, Perry G, Nunomura A, Tabaton M, et al. (2010) Oxidative stress in Alzheimer disease: A possibility for prevention. Neuropharmacology 59: 290–4.
24. Stefani IC, Wright D, Polizzi KM, Kontoravdi C (2012) The role of ER stress-induced apoptosis in neurodegeneration. Curr Alzheimer Res. 9(3):373–87.
25. Ortiz GG, Macias-Islas MA, Pacheco-Moises FP, Cruz-Ramos JA, Sustersik S, et al. (2009) Oxidative stress is increased in serum from Mexican patients with relapsing-remitting multiple sclerosis. Dis. Markers 26: 35–9.
26. Taskiran D, Sagduyu A, Yüceyar N, Kutay FZ, Pögün S (2000) Increased cerebrospinal fluid and serum nitrite and nitrate levels in amyotrophic lateral sclerosis. Int J Neurosci 101: 65–72
27. Blandini F (2013) Neural and immune mechanisms in the pathogenesis of Parkinson's disease. J Neuroimmune Pharmacol. 8(1):189–201.
28. Korhonen R, Lahti A, Kankaanranta H, Moilanen E (2005) Nitric oxide production and signaling in inflammation. Curr. Drug Targets Inflamm. Allergy 4: 471–9.
29. Vaz AR, Silva SL, Barateiro A, Fernandes A, Falcão AS, et al. (2011) Pro-inflammatory cytokines intensify the activation of NO/NOS, JNK1/2 and caspase cascades in immature neurons exposed to elevated levels of unconjugated bilirubin. Exp Neurol. 229(2):381–90.
30. Tesseur I, Zou K, Esposito L, Bard F, Berber E, et al. (2006) Deficiency in neuronal TGF-beta signaling promotes neurodegeneration and Alzheimer's pathology. J Clin Invest. 116: 3060–9.
31. Battista D, Ferrari CC, Gage FH, Pitossi FJ (2006) Neurogenic niche modulation by activated microglia: transforming growth factor beta increases neurogenesis in the adult dentate gyrus. Eur J Neurosci. 23(1): 83–93.
32. Ren RF, Hawver DB, Kim RS, Flanders KC (1997) Transforming growth factor-β protects human hNT cells from degeneration induced by β-amyloid peptide: involvement of the TGF-β type II receptor. Mol Brain Res. 48: 315–22.
33. Dinarello CA, Novick D, Kim S, Kaplanski G (2013) Interleukin-18 and IL-18 Binding Protein. Front Immunol. 4: 289.
34. Sutinen EM, Pirttilä T, Anderson G, Salminen A, Ojala JO (2012) Pro-inflammatory interleukin-18 increases Alzheimer's disease-associated amyloid-β production in human neuron-like cells. J Neuroinflammation. 9: 199.
35. Reale M, Greig NH, Kamal MA (2009) Peripheral chemo-cytokine profiles in Alzheimer's and Parkinson's diseases. Mini Rev Med Chem. 9(10):1229–41.
36. Bose S, Cho J (2013) Role of chemokine CCL2 and its receptor CCR2 in neurodegenerative diseases. Arch Pharm Res. 36(9):1039–50.
37. Vianale G, Reale M, Amerio P, Stefanachi M, Di Luzio S, et al. (2008) Extremely Low Frequency Electromagnetic Field (ELF-EMF) enhances human keratinocyte cell growth and decreases pro-inflammatory chemokines production. Brit J Dermatol 158(6):1189–96.
38. Pritchard KA Jr, Groszek L, Smalley DM, Sessar WC, Wu M, et al. (1995) Native low-density lipoprotein increases endothelial cell nitric oxide synthase generation of superoxide anion. Circ Res 77: 510–518.
39. Aebi HE (1974) Methods of Enzymatic Analysis. In: Bergmayer HU, editor. Chemie. 2nd Edition, Vol. 2. Weinheim: F.R.G. 673–84.
40. Su B, Wang X, Nunomura A, Moreira PI, Lee HG, et al. (2008) Oxidative stress signaling in Alzheimer's disease. Curr Alzheimer Res. 5(6):525–32.

41. Falone S, Grossi MR, Cinque B, D'Angelo B, Tettamanti E, et al. (2007) Fifty hertz extremely low-frequency electromagnetic field causes changes in redox and differentiative status in neuroblastoma cells. Int J Biochem Cell Biol. 39(11):2093–106.

42. Lacy-Hulbert A, Metcalfe JC, Hesketh R (1998) Biological responses to electromagnetic fields. FASEB J 12(6): 395–420.

43. Feychting M, Ahlbom A, Kheifets L (2005) EMF and health. Ann Rev Public Health 26: 165–189.

44. Consales C, Merla C, Marino C, Benassi B (2012) Electromagnetic fields, oxidative stress, and neurodegeneration. Int J Cell Biol. 2012: 683897.

45. WHO (2007) "Electromagnetic fields and public health. Exposure to extremely low frequency fields," Fact Sheet no. 322, WHO, Geneva, Switzerland. < http://www.who.int/peh-emf/publications/facts/fs322/en/> viewed May 16, 2014>

46. WHO (2007) (Environmental Health Criteria 238), Extremely Low Frequency Fields, vol. 35, WHO, Geneva, Switzerland. <http://www.who.int/peh-emf/publications/Complet_DEC_2007.pdf> viewed May 16, 2014.

47. International Programme On Chemical Safety (1984) Environmental Health Criteria 35. Extremely Low Frequency (ELF) Fields <http://www.inchem.org/documents/ehc/ehc/ehc35.htm - PartNumber:9> viewed May 16, 2014.

48. Jack CR Jr, Knopman DS, Jagust WJ, Petersen RC, Weiner MW, et al. (2013) Tracking pathophysiological processes in Alzheimer's disease: an updated hypothetical model of dynamic biomarkers. Lancet Neurol. 12(2):207–16.

49. Saracchi E, Fermi S, Brighina L (2013) Emerging candidate biomarkers for Parkinson's disease: a review. Aging Dis. 5(1):27–34.

50. Moreno-Gonzalez I, Soto C (2011) Misfolded protein aggregates: mechanisms, structures and potential for disease transmission. Semin Cell Dev Biol. 22(5):482–7.

51. von Bernhardi R, Eugenín J (2012) Alzheimer's disease: redox dysregulation as a common denominator for diverse pathogenic mechanisms. Antioxid Redox Signal. 16(9):974–1031.

52. Bonda DJ, Castellani RJ, Zhu X, Nunomura A, Lee HG, et al. (2011) A novel perspective on tau in Alzheimer's disease. Curr Alzheimer Res. 8(6):639–42.

53. Barja G (1998) Mitochondrial free radical production and aging in mammals and birds. Ann N Y Acad Sci 854: 224–238.

54. Eleuteri AM, Amici M, Bonfili L, Cecarini V, Cuccioloni M, et al. (2009) 50 Hz extremely low frequency electromagnetic fields enhance protein carbonyl groups content in cancer cells: effects on proteasomal systems. J Biomed Biotechnol. 2009: 834239.

55. Simkó M, Mattsson MO (2004) Extremely low frequency electromagnetic fields as effectors of cellular responses in vitro: possible immune cell activation. J Cell Biochem. 93(1):83–92.

56. Reale M, De Lutiis MA, Patruno A, Speranza L, Felaco M, et al. (2006) Modulation of MCP-1 and iNOS by 50-Hz sinusoidal electromagnetic field. Nitric Oxide. 15(1):50–7.

57. Patruno A, Amerio P, Pesce M, Vianale G, Di Luzio S (2010) Extremely low frequency electromagnetic field (elf-emf) modulate iNOS, eNOS and Cox-2 expressions in the human keratinocyte cell line hacat: potential therapeutical effects in wound healing. Brit J Dermatol 162: 258–66.

58. Patruno A, Tabrez S, Amerio P, Pesce M, Vianale G, et al. (2011) Kinetic Study on the Effects of Extremely Low Frequency Electromagnetic Field on Catalase, Cytochrome P450, Inducible Nitric Oxide Synthase in Human HaCaT and THP-1 Cell Lines. CNS Neurol Disord Drug Targets. 10(8):936–44.

59. Sunkari VG, Aranovitch B, Portwood N, Nikoshkov A (2011) Effects of a low-intensity electromagnetic field on fibroblast migration and proliferation. Electromagnet Biol Med 30(2): 80–5.

60. Antonini RA, Benfante R, Gotti C, Moretti M, Kuster N, et al. (2006) Extremely low-frequency electromagnetic field (ELF-EMF) does not affect the expression of alpha3, alpha5 and alpha7 nicotinic receptor subunit genes in SH-SY5Y neuroblastoma cell line. Toxicol Lett. 164(3):268–77

61. Martínez-Sámano J, Torres-Durán PV, Juárez-Oropeza MA, Verdugo-Díaz L (2012) Effect of acute extremely low frequency electromagnetic field exposure on the antioxidant status and lipid levels in rat brain. Arch Med Res. 43(3):183–9.

62. Gerard C, Rollins BJ (2001) Chemokines and disease. Nature Immunology 2 (2): 108–115.

63. Azizi G, Khannazer N, Mirshafiey A (2014) The potential role of chemokines in Alzheimer's disease pathogenesis. Am J Alzheimers Dis Other Demen. [Epub ahead of print]

64. Bossù P, Ciaramella A, Salani F, Vanni D, Palladino I, et al. (2010) Interleukin-18, from neuroinflammation to Alzheimer's disease. Curr Pharm Des. 16(38):4213

65. Lisi A, Ledda M, Rosola E, Pozzi D, D'Emilia E, et al. (2006) Extremely low frequency electromagnetic field exposure promotes differentiation of pituitary corticotrope-derived AtT20 D16V cells. Bioelectromagnetics 27: 641–51.

66. Tasset I, Medina FJ, Jimena E, Agüera E, Gascón F, et al. (2010) Neuroprotective effects of extremely low-frequency electromagnetic fields on a Huntington's disease rat model: effects on neurotrophic factors and neuronal density. Neuroscience 209: 54–63.

67. Tasset I, Pérez-Herrera A, Medina FJ, Arias-Carrión O, Drucker-Colín R, et al. (2013) Extremely low-frequency electromagnetic fields activate the antioxidant pathway Nrf2 in a Huntington's disease-like rat model. Brain Stimul. 6: 84–6.

68. Túnez I, Drucker-Colín R, Jimena I, Medina FJ, Muñoz Mdel C, et al. (2006) Transcranial magnetic stimulation attenuates cell loss and oxidative damage in the striatum induced in the 3-nitropropionic model of Huntington's disease. J Neurochem. 97: 619–30.

69. Túnez I, Santamaría A (2009) Model of Huntington's disease induced with 3-nitropropionic acid. Rev Neurol, 48: 430–434.

70. Arias-Carrión O, Verdugo-Díaz L, Feria-Velasco A, Millán-Aldaco D, Gutiérrez AA, et al. (2004) Neurogenesis in the subventricular zone following transcranial magnetic field stimulation and nigrostriatal lesions. J Neurosci Res. 78: 16–28.

5

Oxidative Stress Is Associated with an Increased Antioxidant Defense in Elderly Subjects: A Multilevel Approach

Gemma Flores-Mateo[1,2]*, Roberto Elosua[3,4], Teresa Rodriguez-Blanco[5], Josep Basora-Gallisà[1,2], Mònica Bulló[2,6], Jordi Salas-Salvadó[2,6], Miguel Ángel Martínez-González[7], Ramon Estruch[2,8], Dolores Corella[2,9], Montserrat Fitó[2,10], Miquel Fiol[2,11], Fernando Arós[12], Enrique Gómez-Gracia[13], Isaac Subirana[4,5], José Lapetra[14], Valentina Ruiz-Gutiérrez[2,15], Guillermo T. Sáez[2,16], Maria-Isabel Covas[2,10] for the PREDIMED Study Investigators[¶]

1 Unitat de Suport a la Recerca Tarragona-Reus, Institut Universitari d'Investigació en Atenció Primària Jordi Gol (IDIAP Jordi Gol), Tarragona, Spain, 2 CIBER Fisiopatología Obesidad y Nutrición (CIBEROBN), Madrid, Spain, 3 Epidemiology and Cardiovascular Genetics Research Group, Institut Municipal d'Investigació Mèdica (IMIM), Barcelona, Spain, 4 CIBER de Epidemiología y Salud Pública (CIBERESP), Madrid, Spain, 5 Institut Universitari d'Investigació en Atenció Primària Jordi Gol (IDIAP Jordi Gol), Barcelona, Spain, 6 Human Nutrition Unit, School of Medicine, University Rovira i Virgili, Reus, Spain, 7 Department of Preventive Medicine and Public Health, University of Navarra-Osasunbidea, Servicio Navarro de Salud, Pamplona, Spain, 8 Department of Internal Medicine, Hospital Clinic, Institut dInvestigacions Biomèdiques August Pi Sunyer (IDIBAPS), Barcelona, Spain, 9 Department of Preventive Medicine and Public Health, University of Valencia, Valencia, Spain, 10 Cardiovascular Risk and Nutrition Research Unit, Institut Municipal d'Investigació Mèdica (IMIM), Barcelona, Spain, 11 Institute for Health Sciences Investigation, IdISPa, Palma de Mallorca, Spain, 12 Department of Cardiology, Hospital Txangorritxu, Vitoria, Spain, 13 Department of Epidemiology, School of Medicine of Malaga, Malaga, Spain, 14 Department of Family Medicine, Primary Care Division of Sevilla, San Pablo Health Center, Sevilla, Spain, 15 Instituto de la Grasa, CSIC, Sevilla, Spain, 16 Department of Biochemistry and Molecular Biology, Faculty of Medicine, Service of Clinical Analysis, Doctor Peset University Hospital, University of Valencia, Valencia, Spain

Abstract

Background: Studies of associations between plasma GSH-Px activity and cardiovascular risk factors have been done in humans, and contradictory results have been reported. The aim of our study was to assess the association between the scavenger antioxidant enzyme glutathione peroxidase (GSH-Px) activity in plasma and the presence of novel and classical cardiovascular risk factors in elderly patients.

Methods: We performed a cross-sectional study with baseline data from a subsample of the PREDIMED (PREvención con DIeta MEDiterránea) study in Spain. Participants were 1,060 asymptomatic subjects at high risk for cardiovascular disease (CVD), aged 55 to 80, selected from 8 primary health care centers (PHCCs). We assessed classical CVD risk factors, plasma oxidized low-density lipoproteins (ox-LDL), and glutathione peroxidase (GSH-Px) using multilevel statistical procedures.

Results: Mean GSH-Px value was 612 U/L (SE: 12 U/L), with variation between PHCCs ranging from 549 to 674 U/L (Variance = 1013.5; $P<0.001$). Between-participants variability within a PHCC accounted for 89% of the total variation. Both glucose and oxidized LDL were positively associated with GSH-Px activity after adjustment for possible confounder variables ($P = 0.03$ and $P = 0.01$, respectively).

Conclusion: In a population at high cardiovascular risk, a positive linear association was observed between plasma GSH-Px activity and both glucose and ox-LDL levels. The high GSH-Px activity observed when an oxidative stress situation occurred, such as hyperglycemia and lipid oxidative damage, could be interpreted as a healthy defensive response against oxidative injury in our cardiovascular risk population.

Editor: Luis Eduardo Soares Netto, Instituto de Biociencias - Universidade de São Paulo, Brazil

Funding: This study was funded by the Spanish Ministry of Health (Networks G03/140, RD06/0045 and by the research grants PI040233, PI070240 and Miguel Servet SNS Contract CP06/00100 of the Instituto de Salud Carlos III). The CIBER Fisiopatología de la Obesidad y Nutrition and the CIBER Epidemiología y Salud Pública are initiatives of the Instituto de Salud Carlos III, Madrid, Spain, and the European Union (FEDER). The funders had no role in study design, data collection and analysis, decision to publish, or preparation of the manuscript.

Competing Interests: The authors have declared that no competing interests exist.

* Email: gflores@idiapjgol.org

¶ Membership of the PREDIMED Study Investigators is provided in the Acknowledgments.

Introduction

Coronary heart disease (CHD) is a major cause of morbidity and mortality in the developed world [1]. Atherosclerosis, characterized by the accumulation of cholesterol deposits in large and medium-sized arteries, is the most common pathologic process underlying cardiovascular disease and is often clinically manifested as coronary, cerebrovascular, and/or peripheral arterial disease [2]. An imbalance between antioxidant and oxidant-generating system that leads to oxidative stress has been proposed in the pathogenesis of atherosclerosis [2]. In particular, the oxidation of low density lipoproteins (LDL) by free radicals plays a central role in the formation, progression, and rupture of atherosclerotic plaques [2].

Mammalian cells are, however, protected from free radicals by a wide range of antioxidants such as the scavenger antioxidant enzymes [3]. Glutathione peroxidase is the general name for a family of multiple isozymes that catalyze the reduction of H_2O_2 or organic hydroperoxides to water or the corresponding alcohols using reduced glutathione (GSH) as an electron donor. In mammals, 8 glutathione peroxidases (GPx1–GPx8) have been identified to date, including both selenium-containing GPxs (GPx1–4 and 6) and their non-selenium congeners (GPx5, 7 and 8) [4].

Oxidative stress elicits an induction of antioxidant enzymes, as reported in a recent systematic review [5]. However, most studies were done in animal models; studies that have analyzed this association in humans have reported conflicting results [6–15].

The aim of the present study was to assess the association between the scavenger antioxidant enzyme glutathione peroxidase (GSH-Px) activity in plasma and novel and classical cardiovascular risk factors in elderly individuals at high risk for cardiovascular disease.

Methods

Study design

A cross-sectional study with baseline data from a subsample of the PREDIMED (PREvención con DIeta MEDiterránea) study was performed. The PREDIMED study is a large, parallel-group, multicenter, randomized, controlled, clinical trial aimed at assessing the effects of the traditional Mediterranean diet (TMD) on the primary prevention of cardiovascular disease (www. predimed.es and www.predimed.org). The PREDIMED detailed protocol of the study has been previously published [16].

Subjects

Of the 7,447 participants aged 55 to 80 years from 8 Spanish PHCCs who were randomized to the PREDIMED study groups, 1,069 were randomly selected a posteriori for plasma measurements of glutathione peroxidase-1 activity and included in the present study. Inclusion criteria were the presence of diabetes or at least 3 CHD risk factors: current smoking; hypertension (systolic blood pressure ≥140 mm/Hg, diastolic blood pressure ≥90 mm/Hg, or treatment with antihypertensive drugs); dyslipidemia (high-density lipoprotein [HDL] cholesterol <40 mg/dL for men and <50 mg/dL for women, LDL cholesterol>160 mg/dL, or treatment with cholesterol-lowering drugs); overweight or obesity (body mass index (BMI)>25 kg/m^2), or family history of premature CHD. Exclusion criteria were history of cardiovascular disease, any severe chronic illness, drug or alcohol addiction, history of allergy or intolerance to olive oil or nuts, or low predicted likelihood of changing dietary habits according to the

stages of change model. Individual eligibility was based on a screening visit by the primary care physician.

Baseline assessments

The baseline examination included the administration of 3 types of questionnaire: 1) a validated food frequency questionnaire [17] and an assessment of the degree of adherence to the TMD, assigning a value of 0 or 1 to each of 14 questionnaire items [18], with energy and nutrient intake calculated from Spanish food composition tables [19]; 2) the Minnesota Leisure Time Physical Activity Questionnaire, which has been validated for its use in Spanish men and women [20,21]; and 3) a 47-item general questionnaire assessing life-style, health conditions, smoking habits, sociodemographic variables, history of illness, and medication use. Weight and height were measured with calibrated scales and a wall-mounted stadiometer, respectively. Waist circumference was measured midway between the lowest rib and the iliac crest using an anthropometric tape. Trained personnel measured blood pressure in triplicate with a validated semi-automatic sphygmomanometer (Omron HEM-705CP, The Netherlands) with the patient in a seated position after a 5-minute rest.

Laboratory analysis

Biological samples were obtained after an overnight fast, coded, shipped to central laboratories, and frozen at −80°C until the assay. Plasma glucose and lipid analyses were performed in a PENTRA-400 autoanalyzer (ABX-Horiba Diagnostics, Montpellier, France). Soluble HDL cholesterol was measured by an accelerator selective detergent method (ABX-Horiba Diagnostics, Montpellier, France) and LDL cholesterol was calculated by the Friedewald equation whenever triglycerides were <3.4 mmol/L. Quality control was performed with UNITY External Quality Assessment (BIO-RAD, Hercules, CA, USA). Circulating oxidized LDL (ox-LDL) plasma levels were measured by a commercial enzyme-linked immunoabsorbent assay (Mercodia AB, Uppsala, Sweden). Intra- and inter-assay coefficients of variation were 2.8% and 7.3%, respectively. Plasma GSH-Px activity (GSH-Px; EC 1.11.1.9) was measured by a Paglia and Valentine [22] modification method using cumene hydroperoxide (Ransel RS 505, Randox Laboratories, Crumlin, UK) as a glutathione oxidant. Intra- and inter-run imprecision were 3.6% and 5.43%, respectively.

Statistical analyses

Participants were divided into quintiles of plasma GSH-Px concentration based on the sample distribution. We ensured that the result was not due to multiple comparisons, so we conducted the Holm adjustment [23,24]. This method is just as simple and generally applicable as the Bonferroni method, but much more powerful [25,26].

We applied multilevel statistical procedures [27] to investigate both the association between individual cardiovascular risk factors and GSH-Px and to what extent differences between PHCTs may account for any variation in the outcomes. We modeled individuals (level-1 units) as nested within 8 PHCTs (level-2 units). We modeled the continuous outcome (GSH-Px) using the multilevel linear regression to allow for within-center correlation, applying the Full Maximum likelihood method of estimation. Initially, we examined whether there was a variation between Spanish PHCTs in GSH-Px activity by fitting an unconditional model with no predictors at any level, only the intercept and random errors at the individual and PHCT levels. The second model estimated the effect of individual (level 1) covariates on the outcome and whether these effects varied by PHCT (i.e., we allowed for level-2 random effects). We confirmed the appropriateness of modeling continuous variables as linear (fractional polynomials method).

All statistical tests were 2-sided at the 5% significance level. Analyses were carried out using the HLM for Windows multilevel package, version 10.1, Stata/SE version 9.1 (Stata Corp.).

Research ethics

The study followed the principals contained in the Helsinki Declaration and successive revisions and the standards of good clinical practice. The protocol was approved by the Committee on Clinical Research Ethics (CEIC) of the Institut d'Investigació en Atenció Primària (IDIAP) Jordi Gol, and participants signed an informed consent. Data confidentiality was guaranteed according to the pertinent laws of Spain (Ley Orgánica de Protection de Datos de Carácter Personal, 15/1999, December 1).

Results

Of the 1,060 included participants, 577 (54.4%) were female. The mean age was 66.7 (SD: 8.0) years. GSH-Px activity showed a normal distribution. Plasma glucose and ox-LDL levels increased across GSH-Px quintiles ($P<0.05$). (Table 1).

Table 2 shows the results of both the unconditional and the adjusted model for the association between GSH-Px and cardiovascular risk factors. From the results of the unconditional model, the GSH-Px mean value was 612 U/L (SE: 12 U/L), with a significant variation between PHCCs, ranging from 549 to 674 U/L (Variance = 1013.5; $P<0.001$). The variation in the mean level of GSH-Px was 15 times greater within PHCCs than between PHCCs (Variance = 15266.6; $P<0.001$). Thus, 93.8% of the variability in GSH-Px activity was between participants within centers rather than between PHCCs. The adjusted model (Table 2) showed a reduction in the mean GSH-Px value to 577 U/L (SE: 50 U/L), with a range of variation between PHCCs from 499 to 656 U/L. Results of this model showed that glucose and oxidized LDL were significantly positively associated with GSH-Px activity ($P<0.05$).

Discussion

This study assessed the association between GSH-Px activity and classical and novel cardiovascular risk factors in an elderly population with high cardiovascular risk. We identified a positive association between plasma GSH-Px activity and glucose and ox-LDL levels. The associations were moderately strong and linear,

Table 1. Participant characteristics by quintiles of serum glutathione peroxidase activity (U/L).

	Quintile 1	Quintile 2	Quintile 3	Quintile 4	Quintile 5	P value for trend*
	<507	507567	567–618	618–685	>685	
	(n = 213)	(n = 219)	(n = 212)	(n = 215)	(n = 210)	
Age (years)	67.1±9.2	66.2±8.8	67.5±7.9	66.6±6.7	66.3±7.1	1.000
Sex (female), n (%)	122 (57.1)	116 (52.5)	123 (58.6)	113 (53.3)	107 (50.7)	1.000
Current smokers, n (%)	46 (21.8)	48 (22.4)	46 (22.1)	37 (17.5)	30 (14.5)	1.000
Diabetes, n (%)	94 (44.3)	99 (45.6)	96 (45.7)	112 (52.8)	118 (56.5)	0.076
Hypertension, n (%)	170 (79.7)	177 (81.1)	172 (82.2)	180 (84.8)	160 (76.8)	1.000
Systolic blood pressure (mmHg)	156±61	159±61	153±20	158±54	157±62	1.000
Diastolic blood pressure (mmHg)	88±63	89±63	84±11	89±56	89±64	1.000
Medication use, n (%)						
Antihypertensive agents	153 (73.2)	154 (74.0)	151 (73.7)	156 (75.7)	139 (67.8)	1.000
Lipid-lowering agents	78 (37.3)	96 (46.2)	89 (43.4)	84 (40.8)	95 (46.6)	1.000
Insulin	13 (6.2)	14 (6.8)	7 (3.4)	21 (10.3)	17 (8.3)	1.000
Oral hypoglycemic agents	57 (27.1)	55 (26.4)	55 (26.8)	68 (33.2)	71 (34.6)	0.435
Aspirin or other antiplatelet agents	52 (24.8)	40 (19.1)	43 (20.7)	63 (30.4)	49 (19.8)	1.000
Waist circumference (cm)	107.6±88.8	104.3±62.9	101.6±53.7	97.8±10.3	98.3±11.1	0.468
EEPA leisure time (kcal/day)	224±181	237±195	277±250	273±253	267±240	0.216
Glucose (mg/dL)	117±34	118±35	119±34	125±40	126±39	0.042
Cholesterol (mg/dL)						
Total	203±30	205.8±32.3	209.2±31.2	210.8±35.6	207.5±35.0	0.480
High density lipoprotein (HDL)	50.4±10.5	50.7±10.0	53.2±10.0	52.6±10.7	52.3±10.2	0.288
Low density lipoprotein (LDL)	126±26	128±27	131±26	133±28	130±29	0.216
LDL/HDL cholesterol ratio	2.52±0.62	2.56±0.59	2.51±0.58	2.59±0.61	2.52±0.58	1.000
Triglycerides (mg/dL)	132±63	133±62	124±53	124±55	122±65	0.435
Oxidized LDL (U/L)	70±24	74±26	74±26	76±26	78±27	0.042

Abbreviations: EEPA, daily energy expenditure in leisure-time physical activity. Data are shown as mean ±SD, median (interquartile range), or percentage.
* P value for trend adjusted for multiple testing using Holm correction [24]. One-factor analysis of variance, nonparametric Kruskal Wallis test, and chi-square test were used as appropriate.

Table 2. Fixed and random parameters from a multilevel linear regression model of GSH-Px activity.

	Adjusted Beta coefficient[a]	Standard Error	P value
UNCONDITIONAL MODEL			
Fixed parameters			
Intercept	612	12.43	<0.001
Random parameters[b]	Estimate		P
PHCC-level Variance	1013.51		<0.001
Individual-level Variance	15266.61		
ADJUSTED MODEL			
Fixed parameters			
Intercept	577	50.07	<0.001
Glucose (mg/dl)	0.31	0.13	0.021
Sex (female vs. male)	−9.27	10.34	0.370
Age (years)	−0.53	0.54	0.330
EEPA leisure time (kcal/day)	0.02	0.02	0.251
Smoking (current smoking vs. nonsmoker)	−19.50	11.88	0.101
Insulin (treatment vs. no treatment)	24.66	18.17	0.175
Oral hypoglycemic agents (use vs. no use)	10.36	11.58	0.371
Oxidized LDL (mg/dL)	0.47	0.20	0.017
LDL/HDL cholesterol	2.23	8.23	0.786
Waist circumference (cm)	−0.10	0.08	0.224
Random parameters[b]	Estimate		P
PHCC-level Variance	1600.17		<0.001
Individual-level Variance	14640.03		

Abbreviations: EEPA, daily energy expenditure in leisure-time physical activity. PHCC, primary health care center.
[a]Adjusted β, regression coefficient of the association between each variable in the model and GSH-Px activity, controlling for the other variables in the model.
[b]Random parameters are multilevel measures of outcome variation. PHCC was considered as random.

and persisted after adjustment for age, sex, and other possible confounders.

Although several studies have reported an association between cardiovascular risk factors and GSH-Px, they included small sample sizes and report contradictory results [6–15]. Furthermore, the results shown were either unadjusted [7,8,10–13] or adjusted only by age or sex [6,9,14,15]. Whereas several studies examined the association between GSH-Px activity and diabetes and reported lower serum GSH-Px activity in patients with type 2 diabetes than in non-diabetic participants [6,7,14], other studies found increased GSH-Px activity in diabetic patients, compared to control group [9,15]. Finally, one study found no significant difference in GSH-Px activity between three study groups (diabetic patients with and without hypertension and pre-diabetic patients) [8]. In other results, two of these studies reported a positive relationship between BMI and the antioxidant activity of GSH-Px [9,12], another study found significantly lower erythrocyte GSH-Px activity in obese women compared to normal weight women [10], and one study found no significant differences in GSH-Px activity between patients with essential hypertension and age- and sex-matched healthy controls older than 65 years [13].

The biological oxidative effects of reactive oxygen species (ROS) on lipids, DNA, and proteins are controlled by a wide spectrum of exogenous antioxidant mechanisms, such as vitamins and phenolic compounds in diet, and also by endogenous antioxidants such as the scavenger enzymes, among them GSH-Px [28]. Hyperglycemia is a situation in which ROS are generated [29]. In turn, ROS production induces GSH-Px generation at DNA transcriptional

level [30]. Thus, high GSH-Px activity may result from a preservation of the enzyme by a high antioxidant status (with low generation of ROS) or from increased GSH-Px production stimulated by ROS. Therefore, GSH-Px activity may serve as an indicator of the balance between oxidative status and the bioscavenging of ROS by antioxidants. In the present study we measured the *in vivo* ox-LDL as a marker of oxidative stress in order to examine the relationship between oxidative stress or damage and GSH-Px antioxidant enzyme activity. In our cardiovascular risk population, mean (± standard deviation) ox-LDL values (74±26 U/L) were higher than those obtained in a healthy population (49±22 U/L) using the same method and antibodies as in our study [31]. The positive linear relationship obtained between GSH-Px and both glucose and ox-LDL in our population would be compatible with enhanced production of GSH-Px when oxidative status is increased.

Induction of GSH-Px activity has been proposed as the mechanism by which preconditioning exerts protection in myocardial infarction [30]. In addition, overexpression of intracellular GSH-Px in transgenic animal models has shown to prevent postischemic free radical injury [32]. Cardiovascular risk factors present in our population, such as hypertension, diabetes, hyperlipidemia, and obesity, have been previously linked to oxidative stress and oxidative damage [33,34]. In this population, the fact that a high GSH-Px activity is observed when an oxidative stress situation occurs, such as hyperglycemia and lipid oxidative damage, could be interpreted as a healthy defensive response against the oxidative injury.

In our study, 93.8% of the in the variability GSH-Px activity was due to variability among participants within PHCCs rather than differences between PHCCs. After accounting for individual characteristics, the individual variability was reduced to 90.1%. It can hardly be expected that factors such as presence of genetic variants or selenium levels (a GSH-Px cofactor) influence GSH-Px activity [35]. In selenium-deficient patients, selenium supplementation increases enzymatic antioxidant activity such as GSH-Px and decreases lipid peroxidation [36]. The major sources of selenium are plant foods, meat, and seafood, but the selenium content of foods varies geographically depending on soil and water concentrations and the use of selenium-containing fertilizers [37]. Selenium intake in southern Spain has been reported to be above the Recommended Dietary Allowance (RDA) [38]. However, it is unknown whether selenium intake varies among Spanish populations and whether this could explain part of the variability found within PHCCs in our Spanish population.

The potential of selenoproteins such as selenium-containing GPxs (GPx1–4 and 6) to protect against oxidative stress led to the expectation that selenium would also be protective against type 2 diabetes and other cardiovascular risk factors. However, more recent findings form observational studies and randomized clinical trials have raised concerns that high selenium exposure may lead to type 2 diabetes, insulin resistance, or hyperlipidemia [39]. Additional evidence is needed to provide new insights into the role of selenium and of specific selenoproteins in human biology, especially to clarify the underlying mechanisms linking selenium to chronic disease endpoints. Further epidemiological studies and randomized clinical trials across populations with a different selenium status should be conducted to determine the causal effect of selenoproteins on the development of cardiovascular risk factors and diseases.

This study has strengths and limitations. A strength is its large sample size, geographically widespread within Spain. In addition, the study was carefully conducted using standardized protocols. The multilevel methodological approach allowed us to control for clustering within the PHCCs, thus assessing both the individual independent factors that may influence outcomes and whether there was variability in the plasma GSH-Px activity across PHCCs.

One of the limitations of our study is its cross-sectional design, which can identify associations but not causality. Moreover, cross-sectional studies are notably subject to confounding; for this reason, the analysis was adjusted for possible confounding factors. A large cross-sectional study such as this one contributes to the establishment of new hypotheses for large prospective studies and clinical trials. The relationship between selenoproteins such as GSH-Px and cardiovascular risk factors is undoubtedly complex. Future studies should genotype participants and investigate the potential interactions between genotype, selenium intake or status, and selenoproteins. Besides, they should explore whether other individual factors or contextual features (such as factors linked to

geographical or environmental characteristics of PHCTs) may account for variation in the GSH-Px values.

Our study focused on an elderly population and cannot be extrapolated to a general population. Another potential limitation is that a survival bias could have underestimated the association between GSH-Px activity and cardiovascular risk factors. It is possible that subjects with diabetes, obesity, or hypertension and low GSH-Px activity may have died or developed a cardiovascular disease, and therefore could not be included in our study. Moreover, we could not take into account the duration and control of diabetes in our analyses because these data were not available.

In conclusion, a positive linear association was observed between plasma GSH-Px activity and glucose and ox-LDL levels in an elderly population with high cardiovascular risk. The high GSH-Px activity observed when an oxidative stress situation occurs, such as hyperglycemia and lipid oxidative damage, would be compatible with an increase in antioxidant defenses against oxidative injury in our cardiovascular risk population. Further epidemiological studies and randomized clinical trials are needed to assess the impact of selenoproteins on the development of cardiovascular risk factors and diseases and the cause-effect relationships between hyperglycemia, oxidative status, and GSH-Px in elderly populations at high cardiovascular risk.

Acknowledgments

The authors thank Carlos III Institute PI13/01848 and the participants for their enthusiastic collaboration, the PREDIMED personnel for excellent assistance and the personnel of all affiliated primary care centres.

The PREDIMED Study Investigators are: Hospital Clinic, Institut d'Investigacions Biomèdiques August Pi i Sunyer, Barcelona, Spain: C. Viñas, R. Casas, J.M. Baena, M. Oller, J. Amat, I. Duaso, Y. García, C. Iglesias, and J. Benavent. University of Navarra, Primary Care Division Centres, Pamplona, Spain: A. Sánchez-Tainta, E. Toledo, P. Buil-Cosiales, M. Serrano-Martínez, J. Díez-Espino, A. García-Arellano, I. Zazpe, J. Basterra-Gortari, University Rovira i Virgili, Reus, Spain: R. González, C. Molina, M. Guasch-Ferré, A. Díaz-López, M. Sorli, J. García-Roselló, J. Basora, J. Fernández-Ballart. Institute de Recerca Hospital del Mar, Barcelona, Spain: S. Tello, J. Vila, M. Fitó, H. Schröder, R Flores-Mateo, G. University Hospital of Alava,Vitoria, Spain: F. Aros. del Hierro, J.Algorta. University of Málaga, Málaga, Spain: R. Benítez Pont, M. Bianchi Alba, J.Fernández-Crehuet Navajas, E. Gómez-Gracia. Department of Family Medicine, Primary Care Division of Sevilla, Sevilla, Spain: F.J. García, P. Roman, J.M. Santos, J. Lapetra. University of Las Palmas de Gran Canaria, Las Palmas, Spain: J. Álvarez-Pérez, E. Díez Benítez, I. Bautista Castaño, A. Sánchez-Villegas.

The lead author of The Predimed Study is Ramon Estruch: restruch@clinic.ub.es.

Author Contributions

Conceived and designed the experiments: MAM-G JS-S RE DC MF FA EG-G JL VR-G GTS MIC. Analyzed the data: GFM TR-B IS. Wrote the paper: GFM MFitó RE JBG MB MIC. Approved the final version of the article to be published: All authors.

References

1. Lopez AD, Mathers CD, Ezzati M, Jamison DT, Murray CJ (2006) Global and regional burden of disease and risk factors, 2001: systematic analysis of population health data. Lancet 367: 1747–1757.
2. Stocker R, Keaney JF Jr (2004) Role of oxidative modifications in atherosclerosis. Physiol Rev 84: 1381–1478.
3. Huang H, Mai W, Liu D, Hao Y, Tao J, et al. (2008) The oxidation ratio of LDL: a predictor for coronary artery disease. Dis Markers 24: 341–349.
4. Brigelius-Flohe R, Maiorino M (2013) Glutathione peroxidases. Biochim Biophys Acta 1830: 3289–3303.
5. Karunakaran U, Park KG (2013) A systematic review of oxidative stress and safety of antioxidants in diabetes: focus on islets and their defense. Diabetes Metab J 37: 106–112.
6. Kesavulu MM, Rao BK, Giri R, Vijaya J, Subramanyam G, et al. (2001) Lipid peroxidation and antioxidant enzyme status in Type 2 diabetics with coronary heart disease. Diabetes Res Clin Pract 53: 33–39.
7. Likidlilid A, Patchanans N, Poldee S, Peerapatdit T (2007) Glutathione and glutathione peroxidase in type 1 diabetic patients. J Med Assoc Thai 90: 1759–1767.
8. Bandeira SM, Guedes GS, da Fonseca LJ, Pires AS, Gelain DP, et al. (2012) Characterization of blood oxidative stress in type 2 diabetes mellitus patients: increase in lipid peroxidation and SOD activity. Oxid Med Cell Longev 2012: 819310.
9. Taheri E, Djalali M, Saedisomeolia A, Moghadam AM, Djazayeri A, et al. (2012) The relationship between the activates of antioxidant enzymes in red

blood cells and body mass index in Iranian type 2 diabetes and healthy subjects. J Diabetes Metab Disord 11: 3.

10. Amirkhizi F, Siassi F, Djalali M, Shahraki SH (2014) Impaired enzymatic antioxidant defense in erythrocytes of women with general and abdominal obesity. Obes Res Clin Pract 8: e26–e34.

11. Baez-Duarte BG, Mendoza-Carrera F, Garcia-Zapien A, Flores-Martinez SE, Sanchez-Corona J, et al. (2014) Glutathione Peroxidase 3 Serum Levels and GPX3 Gene Polymorphisms in Subjects with Metabolic Syndrome. Arch Med Res 45:375–382.

12. Ferro FE, de Sousa Lima VB, Soares NR, de Sousa Almondes KG, Pires LV, et al. (2011) Parameters of metabolic syndrome and its relationship with zincemia and activities of superoxide dismutase and glutathione peroxidase in obese women. Biol Trace Elem Res 143: 787–793.

13. Rybka J, Kupczyk D, Kedziora-Kornatowska K, Pawluk H, Czuczejko J, et al. (2011) Age-related changes in an antioxidant defense system in elderly patients with essential hypertension compared with healthy controls. Redox Rep 16: 71–77.

14. Harani H, Otmane A, Makrelouf M, Ouadahi N, Abdi A, et al. (2012) [Preliminary evaluation of the antioxidant trace elements in an Algerian patient with type 2 diabetes: special role of manganese and chromium]. Ann Biol Clin (Paris) 70: 669–677.

15. Likidlilid A, Patchanans N, Peerapatdit T, Sriratanasathavorn C (2010) Lipid peroxidation and antioxidant enzyme activities in erythrocytes of type 2 diabetic patients. J Med Assoc Thai 93: 682–693.

16. Martinez-Gonzalez MA, Corella D, Salas-Salvado J, Ros E, Covas MI, et al. (2012) Cohort profile: design and methods of the PREDIMED study. Int J Epidemiol 41: 377–385.

17. Martin-Moreno JM, Boyle P, Gorgojo L, Maisonneuve P, Fernandez-Rodriguez JC, et al. (1993) Development and validation of a food frequency questionnaire in Spain. Int J Epidemiol 22: 512–519.

18. Schroder H, Fito M, Estruch R, Martinez-Gonzalez MA, Corella D, et al. (2011) A short screener is valid for assessing Mediterranean diet adherence among older Spanish men and women. J Nutr 141: 1140–1145.

19. Mataix J. (2003) Tabla de composición de alimentos [Food composition tables]. Granada: University of Granada.

20. Elosua R, Marrugat J, Molina L, Pons S, Pujol E (1994) Validation of the Minnesota Leisure Time Physical Activity Questionnaire in Spanish men. The MARATHOM Investigators. Am J Epidemiol 139: 1197–1209.

21. Elosua R, Garcia M, Aguilar A, Molina L, Covas MI, et al. (2000) Validation of the Minnesota Leisure Time Physical Activity Questionnaire In Spanish Women. Investigators of the MARATDON Group. Med Sci Sports Exerc 32: 1431–1437.

22. Paglia DE, Valentine WN (1967) Studies on the quantitative and qualitative characterization of erythrocyte glutathione peroxidase. J Lab Clin Med 70: 158–169.

23. Aickin M, Gensler H (1996) Adjusting for multiple testing when reporting research results: the Bonferroni vs Holm methods. Am J Public Health 86: 726–728.

24. Holm S (1979) A simple sequantially rejective multiple test procedure. Scand J Stat 6: 65–70.

25. Levin B (1996) On the Holm, Simes, and Hochberg multiple test procedures. Am J Public Health 86: 628–629.

26. Wright S (1992) Adjusted p-values for simultaneous inference. Biometrics 48: 1005–1013.

27. Goldstein (2003) Multilevel Statistical Models. 3rd edition. London: Arnold.

28. Gutteridge JM (1995) Lipid peroxidation and antioxidants as biomarkers of tissue damage. Clin Chem 41: 1819–1828.

29. Ceriello A, Taboga C, Tonutti L, Quagliaro L, Piconi L, et al. (2002) Evidence for an independent and cumulative effect of postprandial hypertriglyceridemia and hyperglycemia on endothelial dysfunction and oxidative stress generation: effects of short- and long-term simvastatin treatment. Circulation 106: 1211–1218.

30. Zhou X, Zhai X, Ashraf M (1996) Direct evidence that initial oxidative stress triggered by preconditioning contributes to second window of protection by endogenous antioxidant enzyme in myocytes. Circulation 93: 1177–1184.

31. Covas MI, Nyyssonen K, Poulsen HE, Kaikkonen J, Zunft HJ, et al. (2006) The effect of polyphenols in olive oil on heart disease risk factors: a randomized trial. Ann Intern Med 145: 333–341.

32. Mital R, Zhang W, Cai M, Huttinger ZM, Goodman LA, et al. (2011) Antioxidant network expression abrogates oxidative posttranslational modifications in mice. Am J Physiol Heart Circ Physiol 300: H1960–H1970. ajpheart.01285.2010 [pii]. doi:10.1152/ajpheart.01285.2010

33. Guxens M, Fito M, Martinez-Gonzalez MA, Salas-Salvado J, Estruch R, et al. (2009) Hypertensive status and lipoprotein oxidation in an elderly population at high cardiovascular risk. Am J Hypertens 22: 68–73.

34. Weinbrenner T, Cladellas M, Isabel CM, Fito M, Tomas M, et al. (2003) High oxidative stress in patients with stable coronary heart disease. Atherosclerosis 168: 99–106.

35. Jablonska E, Gromadzinska J, Reszka E, Wasowicz W, Sobala W, et al. (2009) Association between GPx1 Pro198Leu polymorphism, GPx1 activity and plasma selenium concentration in humans. Eur J Nutr 48: 383–386.

36. Monget AL, Richard MJ, Cournot MP, Arnaud J, Galan P, et al.(1996) Effect of 6 month supplementation with different combinations of an association of antioxidant nutrients on biochemical parameters and markers of the antioxidant defence system in the elderly. The Geriatrie/Min.Vit.Aox Network. Eur J Clin Nutr 50: 443–449.

37. Shamberger RJ (1980) Selenium in the drinking water and cardiovascular disease. J Environ Pathol Toxicol 4: 305–308.

38. Navarro-Alarcon M, Cabrera-Vique C (2008) Selenium in food and the human body: a review. Sci Total Environ 400: 115–141.

39. Stranges S, Navas-Acien A, Rayman MP, Guallar E (2010) Selenium status and cardiometabolic health: state of the evidence. Nutr Metab Cardiovasc Dis 20: 754–760.

6

Probing the *In Vitro* Cytotoxicity of the Veterinary Drug Oxytetracycline

Zhenxing Chi[1,2]*, Rutao Liu[3], Hong You[1,2], Shanshan Ma[2], Hao Cui[2], Qiang Zhang[2]

1 State Key Laboratory of Urban Water Resource and Environment, Harbin Institute of Technology, Harbin, PR China, **2** School of Marine Science and Technology, Harbin Institute of Technology at Weihai, Weihai, PR China, **3** School of Environmental Science and Engineering, Shandong University, Jinan, PR China

Abstract

The study investigated the effect of oxytetracycline (OTC) on the anti-oxidative defense system, the structure (hemolysis rate and morphology) and function (ATP enzyme activity) of human red blood cells (hRBCs) to investigate the possible toxic mechanism of OTC to hRBCs. The experimental results indicate that OTC can cause a decline in the function of the antioxidant defense system of hRBCs, resulting in oxidative stress. OTC can bring about morphological changes to hRBCs, and further leads to hemolysis, when the concentration of OTC is over 8×10^{-5} M (about 164 µg/ml). At a low OTC concentration, below 4×10^{-5} M (82 µg/ml), OTC can enhance the activity of ATP enzyme of hRBCs, known as hormesis. However, at a high concentration, above 4×10^{-5} M (about 82 µg/ml), the ATP enzymatic activity was inhibited, affecting the function of hRBCs. The estalished mechanism of toxicity of OTC to hRBCs can facilitate a deeper understanding of the toxicity of OTC in vivo.

Editor: Nukhet Aykin-Burns, University of Arkansas for Medical Sciences; College of Pharmacy, United States of America

Funding: State Key Laboratory of Urban Water Resource and Environment, HIT (2013DX09); China Postdoctoral Science Foundation funded project (2013M540297); Natural Scientific Research Innovation Foundation in Harbin Institute of Technology (HIT.NSRIF.2014126); NSFC (21277081); The Cultivation Fund of the Key Scientific and Technical Innovation Project, Ministry of Education of China (708058); Independent innovation program of Jinan (201202083); Independent innovation foundation of Shandong University natural science projects (2012DX002). The funders had no role in study design, data collection and analysis, decision to publish, or preparation of the manuscript.

Competing Interests: The authors have declared that no competing interests exist.

* Email: Zhenxingchi@gmail.com

Introduction

Oxytetracycline (OTC, structure shown in Fig. 1), a type of tetracycline antibiotics with broad-spectrum antibiotic activity [1], [2], is extensively applied for therapeutic purposes in humans as well as an antibiotic and growth promoter in intensive farming systems and aquaculture [3]. Effective therapy should be obtained when plasma OTC concentrations are above 4 µg/ml declared by the National Committee for Clinical Laboratory Standards (NCCLS) to achieve that the target bacteria are not resistant to OTC [4]. At the therapy dose of 20 mg/kg, the maximum serum concentration of OTC can reach 4.10 µg/ml for calves [5]. For different animals, the peak concentration and terminal half-life of OTC in blood can be achieved 4~16 hours and 21~63 hours after administration, respectively [6–10]. OTC concentrations in plasma can be kept at or above 0.5 µg/ml (minimum inhibitory concentration) for approximately 6 days [11].

The bioavailability of OTC is low [3], so the ingested OTC in animal body is metabolized partially and the residual OTC is excreted and released into soils, surface water and groundwater [3], [12]. OTC has been detected at nanogram to low-microgram per liter levels in wastewater effluents and natural waters [13]. OTC can bioaccumulate in various organisms including invertebrates and fish in food chain and enter human bodies by water drinking and food intake such as milk, meat and eggs (at nanogram to microgram per liter levels) [14–16], posing a threat to human health [13]. OTC can also be taken up by blood cells [17]. The Joint FAO/WHO Expert Committee of Food Additives and Contaminants (JECFA), at its 50th Meeting in 1998, established a group acceptable daily intake (ADI) of 0~0.03 mg kg^{-1} body weight for the tetracyclines (oxytetracycline (OTC), tetracycline (TC) and chlortetracycline (CTC)), alone or in combination. The committee also recommended maximum residue limits (MRLs) of 100 µg L^{-1} in milk and muscle of all food-producing species [18], [19].

The toxicity of OTC residues in the environment including animal food, soils, surface and ground water, has attracted widespread attention [1], [2], [20], [21]. OTC can inhibit the antibody levels in fish (dose rate equivalent to 75 mg/kg body weight/day) [22], induces DNA damage in carp kidney cells (exposure dose 250 mg/l) [23], has teratogenic effects on carp embryos (exposure dose 127.5~364.1 mg/l) [24], interacts with cytoplasmic protein synthesis (incubation with 100~500 µg/ml of OTC) [25], and induce blood disorder in Juvenile Nile Tilapia *Oreochromis niloticus* (fish fed with 1.25% OTC and above) [26]. OTC also has effect on the secretion kinetics of the rat exocrine pancreas and can lead to the decrease in trypsin level in male wistar rats (OTC dose 30 mg/kg/d) [27], [28].

Red blood cells (RBCs), also referred to as erythrocytes, are the most abundant cells in the bloodstream [29]. The primary function of RBCs is to transport oxygen from the lungs to various parts of the body [30]. In addition, RBCs are also a key player in getting waste carbon dioxide from the tissues to the lungs of the body where it is expelled [30], and regulate blood pH [31]. However, intake of hazardous substances may result in injury of RBCs, affecting its functions.

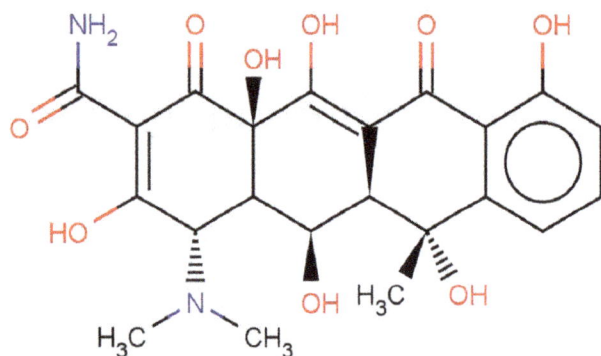

Figure 1. Molecular structure of OTC.

OTC can cause significant reductions in several blood parameters including erythrocyte, hematocrit, and hemoglobin values, for Juvenile Nile Tilapia *Oreochromis niloticus* [26]. However, the effect of OTC on the anti-oxidative defense system of RBCs is still unknown. The changes in the activities of anti-oxidative defense system have been regarded as one of the toxic mechanisms of many hazardous substances. We also have little knowledge about the influence of OTC on the structure and function of RBCs. In this work, we investigated the toxicity indexes of OTC to human red blood cells (hRBCs) including the antioxidant capacity, the hemolysis rate and morphology (structure), and the ATP enzyme activity (function). We consider the work as a worst case scenario in view of the common concentration of OTC residues in the environment. The study is helpful for understanding the effect of OTC on hRBCs during the blood transportation process and its toxicity in vivo.

Materials and Methods

2.1. Reagents and apparatus

EDTA dipotassium salt dihydrate (Tianjin Kermel Chemical Reagent Co., Ltd.) stabilized human blood samples were freshly obtained from Hospital of Shandong University (Jinan).

A stock solution of OTC (1.0×10^{-3} M) was prepared by dissolving 0.0497 g oxytetracycline hydrochloride (Sigma) in 100 ml of saline solution.

2,3-naphthalenedicarboxaldehyde (NDA) was obtained from Nippon Kasei Chemical Co., Ltd. Glutaraldehyde (Tianjin Kermel Chemical Reagent Co., Ltd.) was used as fixative. Isoamyl acetate was obtained from Tianjin Chemagent Research Co., Ltd. PBS buffer (10x, pH 7.4) was purchased from Shanghai Biocolor BioScience & Technology Company. All other reagents were of analytical grade.

All UV-visible absorption spectra and absorption value were measured on a UV-2450 spectrophotometer (SHIMADZU, Kyoto, Japan). Automatic balance centrifuge (LDZ4-2, Jiangsu Jintan Medical Instrument Factory) was used for centrifugation. Vortex mixer (vortex-6) was purchased from Kylin-Bell Lab Instruments Co., Ltd. Digital dry bath incubator (HB-100, Hangzhou Bioer Technology Co., Ltd) was used to control temperature of the samples.

2.2. Ethics statement

The study was approved by the Ethics Committee of Hospital of Shandong University (Jinan). Written informed consent was obtained from all study participants.

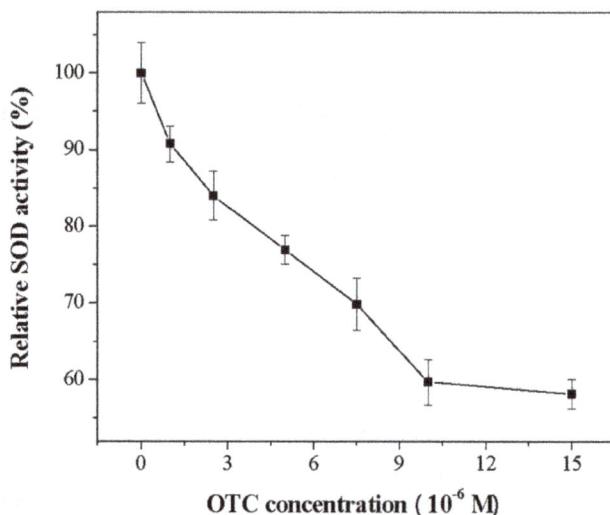

Figure 2. Effect of OTC on SOD activity of hRBCs. Data represent the mean ± SD of three independent experiments.

2.3. Determination of the activities of SOD, CAT and GSH-Px

SOD is a potent protective enzyme that can selectively scavenge $O_2^{\cdot -}$ by catalyzing its dismutation to H_2O_2 and molecular oxygen (O_2) to protect the cells from being injured [32]. CAT catalyzes the degradation of H_2O_2 to H_2O and O_2: $2H_2O_2 \rightarrow 2H_2O + O_2$ [33]. The GSH-Px is an important enzyme extensively existing in vivo, which can specifically catalyze the reduction of H_2O_2 by GSH to protect the integrity of the structure and function of the membrane. With the activities of SOD, CAT and GSH-Px as the indicators, we studied the effect of OTC on the antioxidant defense of hRBCs.

2.3.1. SOD activity determination. Test principle: super-oxide anion radical ($O_2^{\cdot -}$), produced in xanthine and xanthine oxidase reaction systems, can oxidize hydroxylamine to nitrite, which shows violet under the effect of color reagent. The absorbance can be measured with visible or UV-vis spectrophotometer. When the measured sample contains superoxide

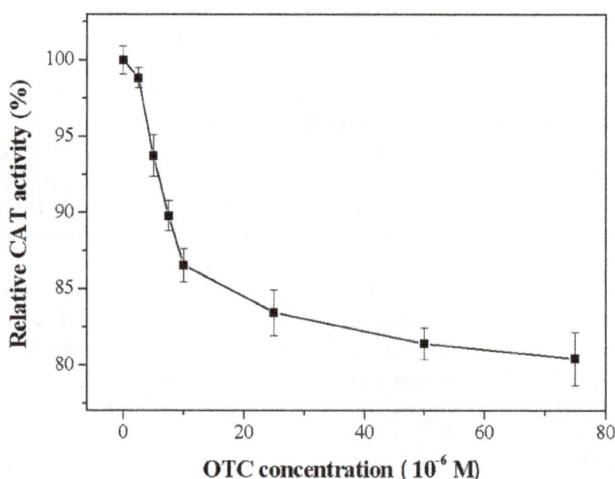

Figure 3. Effect of OTC on CAT activity of hRBCs. Data represent the mean ± SD of three independent experiments.

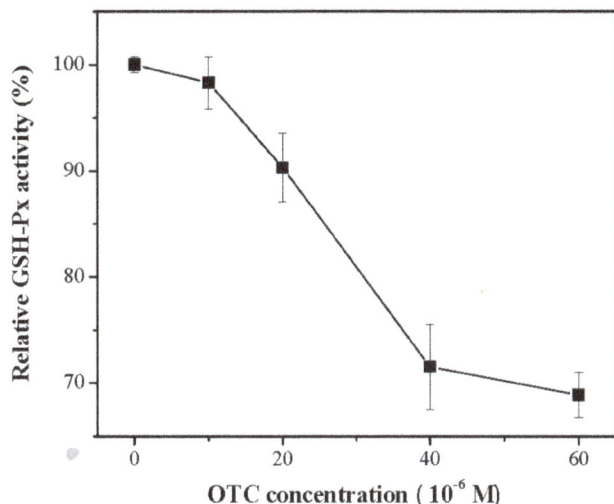

Figure 4. Effect of OTC on GSH-Px activity of hRBCs. Data represent the mean ± SD of three independent experiments.

dismutase (SOD), its specific inhibition of $O_2^{\cdot-}$ can reduce the formation of nitrite, the absorbance value is lower than that of the control with colorimetry. The SOD activity was determined by utilizing the SOD detection kit (Nanjing Jiancheng Bioengineering Institute).

The freshly obtained blood sample (1 ml) was added to 2 ml of PBS, mixed by vortexing, and then the hRBCs were isolated from serum by centrifugation at 2000 rpm for 5 min. After being washed two times with 2 ml of PBS solution, the purified hRBCs were diluted to 2 ml with PBS. 0.2 ml of the diluted cell suspension was added to 0.8 ml OTC solutions of different concentrations and mixed by vortexing, then incubated for 3 hours under gentle shaking. Following incubation, the samples were centrifuged (2000 rpm×5 min), and the supernatant was discarded and the pellet was resuspended in 1 ml PBS. The SOD activity of the sample was measured according to the procedure of the detection kit. The relative SOD activity was calculated using the following formula [34]:

$$\text{Relative SOD activity} = (A_{\text{control}} - A_1)/(A_{\text{control}} - A_0) \times 100\%$$

Where A_{control} is the absorbance of the control tube, A_1 and A_0 are the absorbances of the testing tube of RBCs with and without OTC, respectively.

2.3.2. CAT activity determination. Test principle: the decomposition of hydrogen peroxide (H_2O_2) by catalase (CAT) can be rapidly stopped by ammonium molybdate. The residual H_2O_2 interacts with ammonium molybdate to produce a yellowish complex. The amount formed can be determined at 405 nm to calculate the CAT activity.

The freshly obtained blood sample (1 ml) was washed three times with 2 ml PBS by centrifugation for 5 min at 2000 rpm. The purified hRBCs were diluted to 10 ml with PBS. 0.2 ml of the diluted cell suspension was mixed with 0.8 ml OTC solutions of different concentrations by vortexing, and then incubated for 3 hours under gentle shaking. Following incubation, the samples were centrifuged (2000 rpm×5 min), and the supernatant was discarded and the pellet was resuspended in 0.3 ml ultrapure water to achieve hemolysis. The hemolytic blood was used to measure the CAT activity according to the procedure of the detection kit (Nanjing Jiancheng Bioengineering Institute).

2.3.3. GSH-Px activity determination. Test principle: glutathione peroxidase (GSH-Px) can promote the reaction of H_2O_2 with reduced glutathione (GSH) to produce H_2O and GSSG. The GSH-Px activity can be expressed by the speed of the enzymatic reaction, detected by the consumption of GSH. In the experiment, the GSH-Px activity was determined by utilizing the GSH-Px detection kit (Nanjing Jiancheng Bioengineering Institute) with spectrophotometry method.

The freshly obtained blood sample (1 ml) was washed, diluted, incubated with OTC and centrifuged according to the procedure in Section 2.3.2. The supernatant was discarded and the pellet was resuspended in 1 ml ultrapure water to achieve hemolysis. 0.2 ml of the hemolytic blood was used to measure the GSH-Px activity according to the procedure of the detection kit (Nanjing Jiancheng Bioengineering Institute).

2.4. Determination of GSH

Test principle: GSH is an important nonenzymatic antioxidant. It participates in the maintaining of redox equilibrium which may alleviate cellular oxidative injury. In this work, NDA was used to label the intracellular GSH of hRBCs. Nonfluorescent NDA can readily penetrate the cell membrane, interacting with the nonfluorescent GSH to produce a green fluorescent GSH-NDA derivative [35]. The fluorescence intensity of GSH-NDA derivative was directly proportional to the intracellular content of GSH by fluorescence image analysis. NDA can react concomitantly with the amino and thiol groups of GSH, and no additional nucleophile reagent is required [36]. So the bifunctional reaction is rapid, nonenzymatic, and highly selective [36].

The freshly obtained blood sample (1 ml) was washed, diluted, incubated with OTC and centrifuged according to the procedure

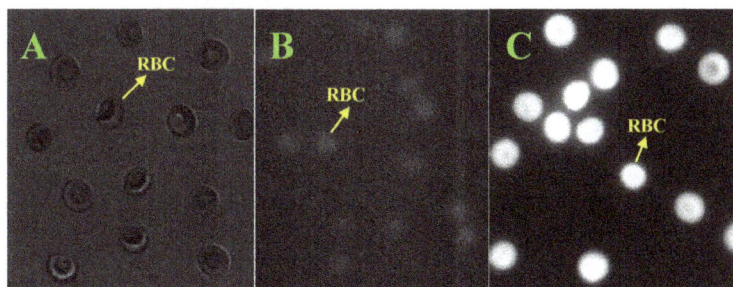

Figure 5. Optical and fluorescence images of hRBCs at 60× magnification (GSH derivatized by NDA). A and B are the hRBCs under bright field and epifluorescence illumination condition, respectively. C is the derived hRBCs under epifluorescence illumination condition.

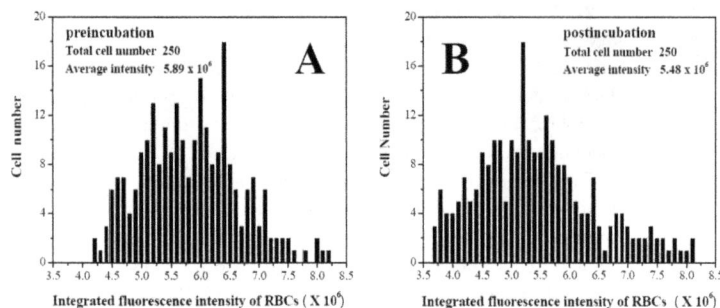

Figure 6. The distribution map of integrated fluorescence intensity (representing glutathione content) of hRBCs. A, hRBCs only; B, hRBCs incubating with 6×10^{-5} mol L^{-1} OTC.

in Section 2.3.2. The supernatant was discarded and the pellet was resuspended in 1 ml PBS. For the determination of GSH, 0.3 ml cell suspension was incubated with 100 µl 0.02 mol/L NDA solution and 0.6 ml PBS for 0.5 hour in the dark at room temperature. 0.05 ml of the suspension was placed on the no-clean cover glass for investigation (24×50 mm, Citotest Labware Manufacturing Co., Ltd).

An inverted microscope (Model IX81, Olympus, Tokyo, Japan) equipped with a 10×objective (PlanApo, Olympus, Tokyo, Japan), a mercury lamp, a mirror unit consisting of 470–490 nm excitation filter (BP470–490), a 505 nm dichromatic mirror (DM 505), a 510–550 nm emission filter (BA510–550) and a 16-bit thermoelectrically cooled EMCCD (Cascade 512B, Tucson, AZ, USA) were used for epifluorescence measurements. The derivatized GSH was excited with a 470–490 nm light ray through the objective. The fluorescence emitted by these molecules was collected by the same objective and the fluorescence images were acquired by the EMCCD. Image acquisition was controlled by the MetaMorph software (Universal Imaging, Downingtown, PA, USA). The micrographs of hRBCs without derivatization were observed by the inverted microscope under bright field and epifluorescence illumination conditions.

2.5. Determination of Malondialdehide (MDA)

Test principle: MDA is the degradation product of lipid peroxidation which can indicate the level of oxidative stress. It can condense with TBA to form a coloured MDA-TBA complex, with the maximum absorption peak at 532 nm that can be measured by visible absorption spectrophotometry.

The freshly obtained blood sample (1 ml) was washed, diluted, incubated with OTC and centrifuged according to the procedure in Section 2.3.1. The supernatant was discarded and the pellet was resuspended in 1 ml ultrapure water to achieve hemolysis. 0.1 ml of the hemolytic blood was used to measure the MDA concentration according to the procedure of the detection kit (Nanjing Jiancheng Bioengineering Institute).

2.6. Hemolysis assay

The freshly obtained blood sample (1 ml) was washed, diluted and mixed with OTC according to the procedure in Section 2.3.2. RBC incubation with ultrapure water and PBS were used as the positive and negative controls, respectively. All the sample tubes were kept in static condition at room temperature for 3 h. Finally, the mixtures were centrifuged at 2000 rpm for 5 min, and 500 µl of supernatant of all samples was diluted with 2.5 ml ultrapure water. The absorbance values of the diluted supernatants (3 ml) at

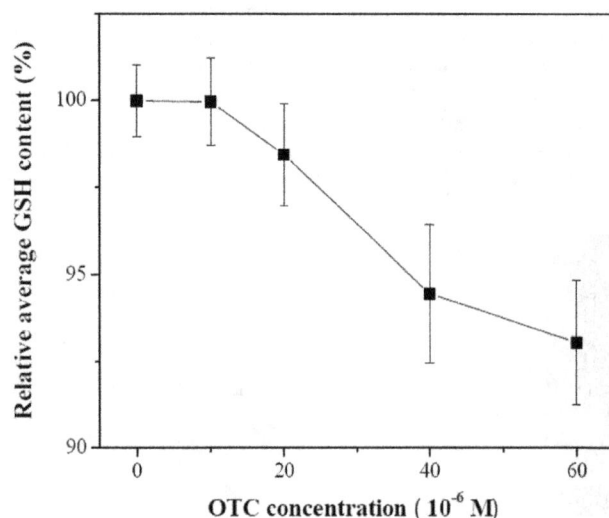

Figure 7. Effect of OTC on GSH content of hRBCs. Data represent the mean ± SD of three independent experiments.

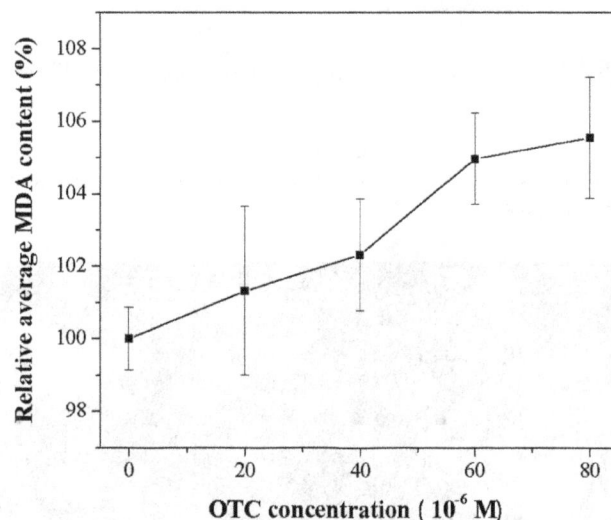

Figure 8. MDA content of hRBCs under different OTC concentrations. Data represent the mean ± SD of three independent experiments.

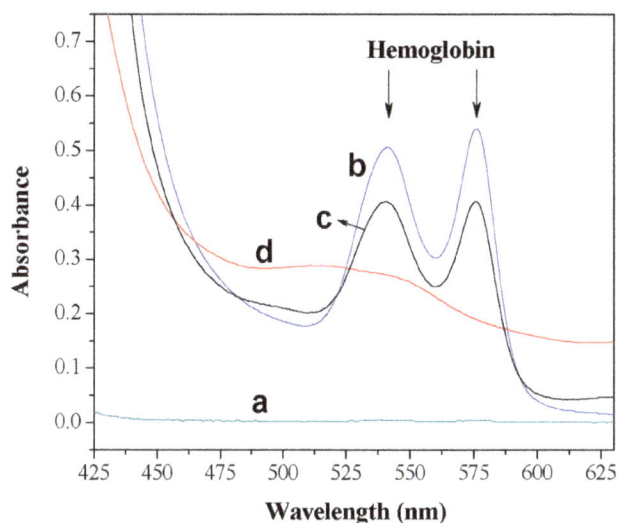

Figure 9. Absorption spectra. (a) supernatant for the hRBCs suspension after centrifugation; (b) hemolysate (incubated with ultrapure water); (c) supernatant for the hRBCs incubated with 1.1×10^{-4} mol/L OTC after centrifugation; (d) hemolysate incubated with 4×10^{-4} mol/L OTC. a, b, c and d have the same number of hRBCs obtained from the same blood sample.

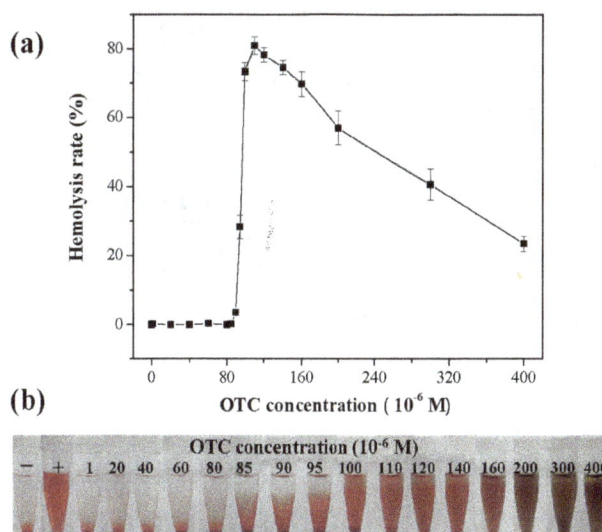

Figure 10. Hemolysis rate (a) and photographs of hemolysis (b) of hRBCs incubated with OTC. (a) hRBCs incubated with OTC at different concentrations ranging from 1 to 4×10^{-4} mol L^{-1} for 3 h. Data represent the mean $\pm$SD from at least three independent experiments. (b) The presence of red hemoglobin in the supernatant indicates damaged hRBCs. D.I. water (+) and PBS (−) are used as positive and negative control, respectively.

540 nm were determined by the UV-2450 spectrophotometer [37]. The hemolysis rate of hRBCs was calculated using the following formula [38]:

$$\text{Hemolysis rate} = (A_{sample} - A_{negative})/(A_{positive} - A_{negative}) \times 100\%$$

Where A_{sample}, $A_{positive}$ and $A_{negative}$ are the absorbances of sample, the positive and negative controls, respectively.

2.7. Scanning electron microscopy (SEM) studies of hRBCs

The freshly obtained blood sample (1 ml) was washed according to the procedure in Section 2.3.1. The purified hRBCs were diluted by 25 times with PBS. 0.2 ml of the diluted cell suspension was incubated with 0.8 ml OTC solutions of different concentrations for 3 hours under gentle shaking. Following incubation, the samples were centrifuged (2000 rpm×5 min) and the supernatant was discarded. Fixation was performed by addition of 2.5% glutaraldehyde and 12 h incubation. The fixed samples were washed with 0.1 M phosphate buffer for more than 3 h. Then, the sample was fixed in osmium tetroxide (1%) for 1~1.5 h and washed in double-distilled water for 2 h. Dehydration was done with increasing concentrations of ethanol (50%, 70%, 80%, 90% and 100%) twice. The ethanol was displaced by isoamyl acetate (100%) for 15 min (twice). Finally, the sample was dried with the conventional critical point drying method, platinum-coated with ion sputtering coater (Eiko, IB-5) and then observed with a scanning electron microscope (Hitachi, S-570) to investigate the effect of OTC on the morphology of hRBCs.

2.8. ATPase activity assay determination

ATPase is an important enzyme existing in the membrane of cells in vivo [39]. It functions in maintaining ionic and osmotic balance inside and outside the cell, maintaining transmembrane electrochemical gradients, and in cellular energy metabolism [39],

[40]. The reduction in ATPase activity can result in the disorder of the functions, which affects the normal function of cells [39], [40]. For example, a rise in internal Na^+, K^+ or Ca^{2+}, Mg^{2+} ions of RBCs can cause changes in cell shape and volume, increase in cellular rigidity and hemolysis. ATPase can cause the decomposition of ATP into ADP and inorganic phosphorus. The activity of ATPase can be determined by measuring the amount of inorganic phosphorus.

The freshly obtained blood sample (1 ml) was washed with PBS, incubated with OTC, and then centrifuged according to the procedure in Section 2.3.1. The supernatant was discarded and the pellet was resuspended in 0.5 ml ultrapure water to achieve hemolysis. 0.2 ml of the hemolytic blood was used to measure the ATPase activity according to the procedure of the detection kit (Nanjing Jiancheng Bioengineering Institute).

2.9. Statistical analysis

Data are from three independent experiments and presented as mean $\pm$ SD in the study of the effect of OTC on the activities of SOD, CAT, GSH-Px and ATPase, content of GSH and MDA, and hemolysis rate of hRBCs.

Results and Discussion

3.1. Effects of OTC on antioxidant capacity of hRBCs

Radicals are present in tissues in vivo as free and bound forms. The bound radical is necessary for normal physiological activity. However, the free radical is highly reactive, easily combining with electrons from tissue macromolecules to achieve more stability through electron pairing. In toxicology, there is interest in free radicals and reactive oxygen species (ROS), which can be produced by the normal metabolism of cells or by the exogenous factors (e.g. smoking, radiation, dust). ROS are free radicals and non-free radical oxygen-containing molecules that have higher chemical reactivity than ground state molecular oxygen [41], including species such as $O_2 \cdot^-$, hydroxyl radicals ($\cdot OH$), nitric

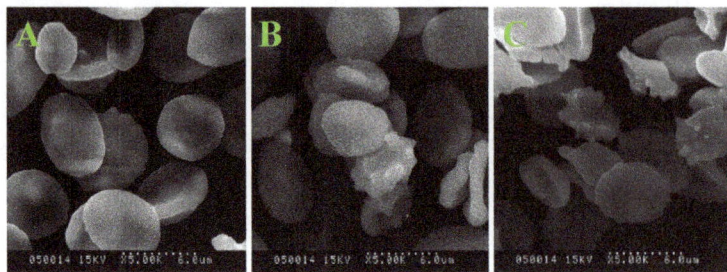

Figure 11. Scanning electron micrographs of hRBCs incubated in PBS containing OTC. The OTC concentration for A, B and C is 0, 1.0×10^{-5} mol L^{-1} and 5.0×10^{-5} mol L^{-1}, respectively.

oxide (NO·), singlet oxygen ($^1O_2$) and H_2O_2 [32]. ROS, within physiological concentrations, play an important role in regulating the body's normal physiological functions such as apoptosis, gene expression and signal transduction [42]. However, when free radicals and antioxidative processes are not balanced, that is, when the production of ROS exceeds the scavenge ability of the body's defense system, or the damaged body's defense system can not function properly, free radicals can produce oxidative stress, inducing the oxidation of biological macromolecules (nucleic acids, proteins, lipids et al), damage to the structure and function of cells, and diseases such as pulmonary fibrosis, epilepsy, hypertension and atherosclerosis [43], [44]. Antioxidants, being mainly natural molecules, can prevent the uncontrolled formation of ROS or inhibit reactions of ROS with biological structures. Enzymes such as SOD, CAT and GSH-Px provide the main antioxidant defense [45]. There must be a balance between the three enzymes to remove ROS from the body properly [46]. As non-enzymatic defense, the role of dietary supplements such as GSH, vitamins (C, E) and carotenoids, is also very important to control oxidative injury [33], [47]. In this section, we studied the effect of OTC on the antioxidant defense of hRBCs including SOD, CAT, GSH-Px and GSH.

In the experiments, SOD activities decreased with increasing OTC concentrations ranging from 0 to 1.5×10^{-5} M and decreases by 41.85% at OTC concentration 1.5×10^{-5} M

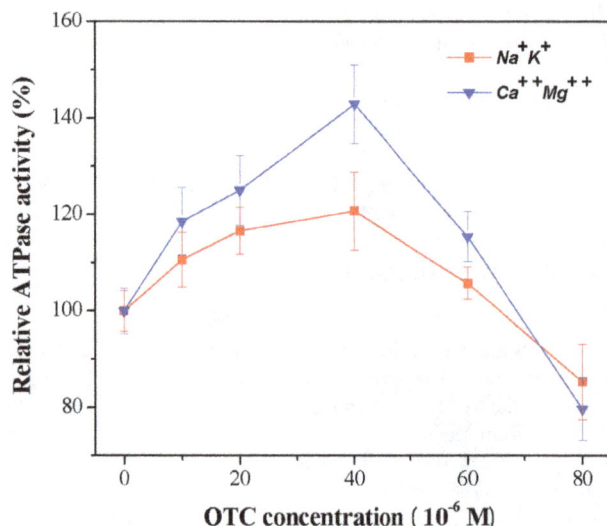

Figure 12. Effect of OTC on ATPase activity of hRBCs. Data represent the mean ± SD of three independent experiments.

(Fig. 2). CAT activity also decreased as OTC concentration increased from 0 to 7.5×10^{-5} M. 19.58% reduction in CAT activity was observed at OTC concentration 7.5×10^{-5} M (Fig. 3). For GSH-Px, the activity also deceased at increasing OTC concentrations (0–6×10^{-5} M) (Fig. 4), and was only 68.89% of the initial concentration when exposed to 6×10^{-5} M OTC.

NDA was used to probe the content of GSH in hRBCs. Fig. 5A shows the hRBCs under bright field. When observed under epifluorescence illumination condition, the cell without derivation with NDA had a very weak fluorescence (Fig. 5B). However, the derived hRBCs exhibited a strong fluorescence (Fig. 5C). The integrated fluorescence intensity of the hRBCs in Fig. 5B is only about 0.6%~0.7% of that of the derived hRBCs in Fig. 5C, so it is negligible. Therefore, the GSH content can be represented by the integrated fluorescence intensity of the derived hRBCs (Fig. 5C). To investigate the influence of OTC on the GSH concentration in hRBCs, 250 hRBCs were selected for every different OTC concentration used. Fig. 6 shows the distribution map of integrated fluorescence intensity. With increasing OTC concentration, the GSH concentration decreased (Fig. 7). At OTC concentration 6×10^{-5} M, GSH content reduced to 93% of the initial concentration (5.48×10^6 compared to 5.89×10^6 average fluorescence intensity).

Exposure of hRBCs to OTC resulted in decreased antioxidant activity of enzymes including SOD, CAT and GSH-Px, and non-enzymatic defenses such as GSH, which all scavenge ROS [32]. So, OTC can reduce antioxidant capacity of hRBCs, which may predispose cells to oxidative injury [48]. To confirm this, we determined the effect of OTC on the concentration of MDA in hRBCs, which is a marker of lipid peroxidation induced by oxidative injury [49], [50]. From Fig. 8, we can seen that MDA content in hRBCs increased with increasing OTC concentrations ranging from 0 to 8×10^{-5} M. 5.5% increment in MDA content was observed at OTC concentration 8×10^{-5} M.

In conclusion, OTC can reduce the antioxidant capacity of hRBCs and induce lipid peroxidation, causing oxidative injury.

3.2. Impact of OTC on the hemolytic activity of hRBCs

In the process of lipid peroxidation in the cell membrane by ROS, membrane fluidity and permeability is altered, affecting cellular structure and function. When RBCs are destroyed, known as hemolysis, contents of the RBCs are released into the bloodstream and can accumulate, causing health problems that can occur suddenly at any time [51], [52], including kidney failure and serious blood clots, which may cause damage to important organs of the body such as the liver, brain, and lung [53]. So, it is very important to investigate the effect of toxic substances on the hemolytic activity of RBCs. The hemolysis caused by toxic substances, which can be expressed as the leakage of hemoglobin, is reflective of membrane damage to the RBCs [38]. After centrifugation, the supernatant from unhemolyzed hRBCs has no absorbance at the range of 425 to 625 nm (Fig. 9). However, the released hemoglobin from damaged hRBCs has two absorption peaks at about 540 nm and 576 nm (Fig. 9). In this research, the absorbance values at 540 nm were used to evaluate the hemolysis rate of hRBCs [37].

To determine if OTC produces hemolysis of hRBCs, hRBCs were exposed to OTC solutions at concentrations ranging from 0 to 4×10^{-4} M for 3 h. The experimental result (Fig. 10a) showed that when the OTC concentration was lower than 8×10^{-5} M, OTC did not induce hemolysis and no hemoglobin was observed in the supernatant, as seen in Fig. 10b, indicating that hRBCs can preserve itself from hemolysis. Hemolysis of hRBCs increased significantly with increasing OTC concentrations starting at a concentration of 8×10^{-5} M, based on the increase in hemoglobin concentrations in the supernatant (Fig. 10b). When the OTC concentration was 1.1×10^{-4} M, hemolysis was 80.99%, however, at higher OTC concentrations (above 1.1×10^{-4} M), hemolysis declined with increasing OTC. The phenomenon was not caused by the oxidation of hemoglobin to methemoglobin, because the absorption peak of methemoglobin at 630–631 nm did not appear in the experimental result. According to our previous study [54], OTC can bind into the central cavity of the hemoglobin molecule. So, we think that OTC interacts with the released hemoglobin, causing the absorbance to decrease. The experimental result that the absorbance of the hemolysate at 540 nm declined after the addition of OTC verified our conclusion.

In conclusion, at lower OTC concentrations ($\leq 8 \times 10^{-5}$ M), hRBCs are protected from membrane hemolysis. OTC has hemolytic activity at a concentration greater than 8×10^{-5} M.

3.3. Effect of OTC on the morphology of hRBCs

Under physiological conditions, the normal hRBCs have a biconcave discoid shape (discocyte) ~8 μm in diameter, consisting of a lipid bilayer membrane filled with aqueous hemoglobin solution [55], [56]. The effect of OTC on hRBC morphology was investigated by SEM. At the concentration of 1.0×10^{-5} M, OTC produced spicule formation on the hRBC membrane (acanthocyte, Fig. 11B) compared with the control hRBCs (Fig. 11A). At a higher concentration of 5.0×10^{-5} M, hRBCs became more deformed, with more cytoplasmic projections (Fig. 11C). The morphological alterations of hRBCs can ultimately lead to the destruction of the cells [57], which explains the observed high hemolytic activity of OTC. According to the bilayer-couple hypothesis [58], shape changes arise from the intercalation of OTC in either the outer or the inner monolayer of the RBC

membrane. The lipid bilayer is the main permeability barrier of membrane, so the structural perturbation induced by OTC will affect its permeability, and thus may affect the function of ion channels, receptors, and enzymes immersed in the membrane lipid [59].

3.4. Influence of OTC on the ATPase activity of hRBCs

ATPase is an important enzyme existing in the membrane of cells in vivo [39]. It functions in maintaining ionic and osmotic balance inside and outside the cell, maintaining transmembrane electrochemical gradients, and in cellular energy metabolism [39], [40].

In this section, we investigated the influence of OTC on the activity of (Na^+, K^+)-ATPase and (Ca^{2+}, Mg^{2+})-ATPase. From Fig. 12, we found that both the activity of (Na^+, K^+)-ATPase and (Ca^{2+}, Mg^{2+})-ATPase increased with increasing OTC concentrations ranging from 0–4×10^{-5} M. At an OTC concentration of 4×10^{-5} M, the activity increased to 120.67% and 142.86% of the initial level for (Na^+, K^+)-ATPase and (Ca^{2+}, Mg^{2+})-ATPase, respectively. However, at higher OTC concentration, the activity decreased. Inhibition rates of 16.67% and 22.25% were observed at the OTC concentration of 4×10^{-5} M for the activity of (Na^+, K^+)-ATPase and (Ca^{2+}, Mg^{2+})-ATPase, respectively.

In summary, At a low concentration of OTC, the ATPase activity increased, known as hormesis. However, at a higher concentration, OTC can inhibit the activity of ATPase, affecting cell function, which verifies the analysis of the experimental results of the antioxidant capacity determination and morphology investigation of hRBCs under different concentrations of OTC (3.1 and 3.3).

Conclusions

The research systemically studied the effect of OTC on the antioxidative defense system, the structure (hemolysis rate and morphology) and function (ATP enzyme activity) of hRBCs. The experimental results indicated that OTC can cause a decline in the function of the antioxidant defense system of hRBCs, enhancing the lipid peroxidation, which further result in the change of morphology and ATP enzyme activity of hRBCs. The established possible toxic mechanism of OTC to hRBCs can facilitate a deeper understanding of the toxicity of OTC in vivo.

Author Contributions

Conceived and designed the experiments: ZC RL. Performed the experiments: ZC. Analyzed the data: ZC SM QZ. Wrote the paper: ZC HY HC.

References

1. Boleas S, Alonso C, Pro J, Fernandez C, Carbonell G, et al. (2005) Toxicity of the antimicrobial oxytetracycline to soil organisms in a multi-species-soil system (MS.3) and influence of manure co-addition. J Hazard Mater 122: 233–241.
2. Ferreira CS, Nunes BA, Henriques-Almeida JM, Guilhermino L (2007) Acute toxicity of oxytetracycline and florfenicol to the microalgae Tetraselmis chuii and to the crustacean Artemia parthenogenetica. Ecotoxicol Environ Saf 67: 452–458.
3. Rigos G, Nengas I, Alexis M, Troisi GM (2004) Potential drug (oxytetracycline and oxolinic acid) pollution from Mediterranean sparid fish farms. Aquat Toxicol 69: 281–288.
4. Doi AM, Stoskopf MK, Lewbart GA (1998) Pharmacokinetics of oxytetracycline in the red pacu (Colossoma brachypomum) following different routes of administration. J Vet Pharmacol Ther 21: 364–368.
5. Brentnall C, Cheng Z, McKellar QA, Lees P (2013) Pharmacokinetic-pharmacodynamic integration and modelling of oxytetracycline administered alone and in combination with carprofen in calves. Res Vet Sci 94: 687–694.
6. Girardi C, Re G, Farca AM, Dacasto M, Ferrero E, et al. (1990) Blood kinetics of sulfamonomethoxine and oxytetracycline following intrauterine spray injection in dairy cows. Pharmacol Res 22: 79–86.

7. Reja A, Moreno L, Serrano JM, Santiago D, Soler F (1996) Concentration-time profiles of oxytetracycline in blood, kidney and liver of tench (Tinca tinca L) after intramuscular administration. Vet Hum Toxicol 38: 344–347.
8. Nouws JF, Vree TB (1983) Effect of injection site on the bioavailability of an oxytetracycline formulation in ruminant calves. Vet Quart 5: 165–170.
9. Uno K (1996) Pharmacokinetic study of oxytetracycline in healthy and vibriosis-infected ayu (Plecoglossus altivelis). Aquaculture 143: 33–42.
10. Roncada P, Ermini L, Schleuning A, Stracciari GL, Strocchia A (2000) Pharmacokinetics and residual behaviour in milk of oxytetracycline in cows following administration of uterine pessaries. J Vet Pharmacol Ther 23: 281–285.
11. Sun Y, Peng Y, Aksornkoae N, Johnson JR, Boring JG, et al. (2002) Controlled release of oxytetracycline in sheep. J Control Release 85: 125–134.
12. Kong WD, Zhu YG, Liang YC, Zhang J, Smith FA, et al. (2007) Uptake of oxytetracycline and its phytotoxicity to alfalfa (Medicago sativa L.). Environ Pollut 147: 187–193.
13. Ye Z, Weinberg HS, Meyer MT (2007) Trace analysis of trimethoprim and sulfonamide, macrolide, quinolone, and tetracycline antibiotics in chlorinated

drinking water using liquid chromatography electrospray tandem mass spectrometry. Anal Chem 79: 1135–1144.

14. Blobel H, Burch CW (1960) Oxytetracycline concentrations in blood serums and milk secretions of cows following intravenous or intramammary treatment. Jour Amer Vet Med Assoc 137: 701–704.

15. Dinsmore RP, Stevens RD, Cattell MB, Salman MD, Sundlof SF (1996) Oxytetracycline residues in milk after intrauterine treatment of cows with retained fetal membranes. J Am Vet Med Assoc 209: 1753–1755.

16. Virolainen N, Pikkemaat M, Elferink J, Karp M (2008) Rapid detection of tetracyclines and their 4-epimer derivatives from poultry meat with bioluminescent biosensor bacteria. J Agric Food Chem 56: 11065–11070.

17. Gabler WL (1991) Fluxes and accumulation of tetracyclines by human blood cells. Res Commun Chem Pathol Pharmacol 72: 39–51.

18. Loke ML, Jespersen S, Vreeken R, Halling-Sorensen B, Tjornelund J (2003) Determination of oxytetracycline and its degradation products by high-performance liquid chromatography-tandem mass spectrometry in manure-containing anaerobic test systems. J Chromatogr B Analyt Technol Biomed Life Sci 783: 11–23.

19. Mamani MCV, Reyes FGR, Rath S (2009) Multiresidue determination of tetracyclines, sulphonamides and chloramphenicol in bovine milk using HPLC-DAD. Food Chem 117: 545–552.

20. Jiao S, Zheng S, Yin D, Wang L, Chen L (2008) Aqueous oxytetracycline degradation and the toxicity change of degradation compounds in photoirradiation process. J Environ Sci (China) 20: 806–813.

21. Li K, Yediler A, Yang M, Schulte-Hostede S, Wong MH (2008) Ozonation of oxytetracycline and toxicological assessment of its oxidation by-products. Chemosphere 72: 473–478.

22. Lunden T, Miettinen S, Lonnstrom LG, Lilius EM, Bylund G (1998) Influence of oxytetracycline and oxolinic acid on the immune response of rainbow trout (Oncorhynchus mykiss). Fish Shellfish Immun 8: 217–230.

23. Qu MM, Sun LW, Chen J, Li YQ, Chen YG, et al. (2004) Toxicological characters of arsanilic acid and oxytetracycline. J Agro-Environ Sci 23: 240–242.

24. Li ZL, Chen HG, Xu Y, Kong ZM (2006) Toxicological effects of three veterinary drugs and feed additives on fish. J Ecol Rural Environ 22: 84–86.

25. De Jonge HR (1973) Toxicity of tetracyclines in rat-small-intestinal epithelium and liver. Biochem Pharmacol 22: 2659–2677.

26. Omoregie E, Oyebanji SM (2002) Oxytetracycline-induced blood disorder in juvenile Nile tilapia Oreochromis niloticus (Trewavas). J World Aquacult Soc 33: 377–382.

27. Hobusch D, Putzke HP (1971) Effect of oxytetracycline (OTC) on the secretion kinetics of the rat exocrine pancreas. Exp Pathol (Jena) 5: 298–307.

28. Lorenzo C, del Olmo Martinez ML, Pastor L, Almaraz A, Belmonte A, et al. (1999) Effects of oxytetracycline on the rat exocrine pancreas. Int J Pancreatol 26: 181–188.

29. Wennmalm A, Benthin G, Petersson AS (1992) Dependence of the metabolism of nitric oxide (NO) in healthy human whole blood on the oxygenation of its red cell haemoglobin. Br J Pharmacol 106: 507–508.

30. D'Alessandro A, Righetti PG, Zolla L (2009) The red blood cell proteome and interactome: an update. J Proteome Res 9: 144–163.

31. Selwyn MJ, Dawson AP, Stockdale M, Gains N (1970) Chloride-hydroxide exchange across mitochondrial, erythrocyte and artificial lipid membranes mediated by trialkyl- and triphenyltin compounds. Eur J Biochem 14: 120–126.

32. Herken H, Uz E, Ozyurt H, Sogut S, Virit O, et al. (2001) Evidence that the activities of erythrocyte free radical scavenging enzymes and the products of lipid peroxidation ape increased in different forms of schizophrenia. Mol Psychiatr 6: 66–73.

33. Mecocci P, Polidori MC, Troiano L, Cherubini A, Cecchetti R, et al. (2000) Plasma antioxidants and longevity: a study on healthy centenarians. Free Radic Biol Med 28: 1243–1248.

34. Xiong J, Hu S, Li J, He S, Feng L (2013) Influence of strong electric field on MDA and SOD of rice under atmosphere pressure. J Phys: Conf Ser 418: 1–7.

35. Gao N, Li L, Shi Z, Zhang X, Jin W (2007) High-throughput determination of glutathione and reactive oxygen species in single cells based on fluorescence images in a microchannel. Electrophoresis 28: 3966–3975.

36. Parmentier C, Wellman M, Nicolas A, Siest G, Leroy P (1999) Simultaneous measurement of reactive oxygen species and reduced glutathione using capillary electrophoresis and laser-induced fluorescence detection in cultured cell lines. Electrophoresis 20: 2938–2944.

37. Shcharbin D, Pedziwiatr E, Blasiak J, Bryszewska M (2010) How to study dendriplexes II: Transfection and cytotoxicity. J Control Release 141: 110–127.

38. Lin YS, Haynes CL (2010) Impacts of Mesoporous Silica Nanoparticle Size, Pore Ordering, and Pore Integrity on Hemolytic Activity. J Am Chem Soc 132: 4834–4842.

39. Cantley LC, Jr., Resh MD, Guidotti G (1978) Vanadate inhibits the red cell (Na+, K+) ATPase from the cytoplasmic side. Nature 272: 552–554.

40. Skou JC, Esmann M (1992) The Na,K-ATPase. J Bioenerg Biomembr 24: 249–261.

41. Ben Othmen L, Mechri A, Fendri C, Bost M, Chazot G, et al. (2008) Altered antioxidant defense system in clinically stable patients with schizophrenia and their unaffected siblings. Prog Neuropsychopharmacol Biol Psychiatry 32: 155–159.

42. Mates JM, Segura JM, Perez-Gomez C, Rosado R, Olalla L, et al. (1999) Antioxidant enzymatic activities in human blood cells after an allergic reaction to pollen or house dust mite. Blood Cells Mol Dis 25: 103–109.

43. Papaharalambus CA, Griendling KK (2007) Basic mechanisms of oxidative stress and reactive oxygen species in cardiovascular injury. Trends Cardiovasc Med 17: 48–54.

44. Wadsworth RM (2008) Oxidative stress and the endothelium. Exp Physiol 93: 155–157.

45. Roversi FM, Galdieri LC, Grego BH, Souza FG, Micheletti C, et al. (2006) Blood oxidative stress markers in Gaucher disease patients. Clin Chim Acta 364: 316–320.

46. Hachul de Campos H, Brandao LC, D'Almeida V, Grego BH, Bittencourt LR, et al. (2006) Sleep disturbances, oxidative stress and cardiovascular risk parameters in postmenopausal women complaining of insomnia. Climacteric 9: 312–319.

47. Gokalp O, Uz E, Cicek E, Yilmaz HR, Ozer MK, et al. (2006) Ameliorating role of caffeic acid phenethyl ester (CAPE) against isoniazid-induced oxidative damage in red blood cells. Mol Cell Biochem 290: 55–59.

48. Aruoma OI (1998) Free radicals, oxidative stress, and antioxidants in human health and disease. J Am Oil Chem Soc 75: 199–212.

49. Das S, Vasisht S, Das SN, Srivastava LM (2000) Correlation between total antioxidant status and lipid peroxidation in hypercholesterolemia. Curr Sci India 78: 486–487.

50. Skaper SD, Fabris M, Ferrari V, Carbonare MD, Leon A (1997) Quercetin protects cutaneous tissue-associated cell types including sensory neurons from oxidative stress induced by glutathione depletion: Cooperative effects of ascorbic acid. Free Radical Bio Med 22: 669–678.

51. Rother RP, Bell L, Hillmen P, Gladwin MT (2005) The clinical sequelae of intravascular hemolysis and extracellular plasma hemoglobin - A novel mechanism of human disease. Jama-J Am Med Assoc 293: 1653–1662.

52. Hill A, Richards SJ, Hillmen P (2007) Recent developments in the understanding and management of paroxysmal nocturnal haemoglobinuria. Brit J Haematol 137: 181–192.

53. Hillmen P, Young NS, Schubert J, Brodsky RA, Socie G, et al. (2006) The complement inhibitor eculizumab in paroxysmal nocturnal hemoglobinuria. New Engl J Med 355: 1233–1243.

54. Chi ZX, Liu RT, Yang BJ, Zhang H (2010) Toxic interaction mechanism between oxytetracycline and bovine hemoglobin. J Hazard Mater 180: 741–747.

55. Manrique-Moreno M, Suwalsky M, Villena F, Garidel P (2010) Effects of the nonsteroidal anti-inflammatory drug naproxen on human erythrocytes and on cell membrane molecular models. Biophys Chem 147: 53–58.

56. Hammer M, Schweitzer D, Michel B, Thamm E, Kolb A (1998) Single scattering by red blood cells. Appl Opt 37: 7410–7418.

57. Zhao Y, Sun X, Zhang G, Trewyn BG, Slowing, II, et al. (2011) Interaction of mesoporous silica nanoparticles with human red blood cell membranes: size and surface effects. ACS Nano 5: 1366–1375.

58. Sheetz MP, Singer SJ (1974) Biological membranes as bilayer couples. A molecular mechanism of drug-erythrocyte interactions. Proc Natl Acad Sci U S A 71: 4457–4461.

59. Suwalsky M, Novoa V, Villena F, Sotomayor CP, Aguilar LF, et al. (2009) Structural effects of Zn(2+) on cell membranes and molecular models. J Inorg Biochem 103: 797–804.

7

Altered Mitochondrial Function and Oxidative Stress in Leukocytes of Anorexia Nervosa Patients

Victor M. Victor[1,2,3]*, Susana Rovira-Llopis[1,2,3], Vanessa Saiz-Alarcon[4], Maria C. Sangüesa[4], Luis Rojo-Bofill[4], Celia Bañuls[1,2,3], Rosa Falcón[1,2,3], Raquel Castelló[1,2,3], Luis Rojo[4,5], Milagros Rocha[1,2,3], Antonio Hernández-Mijares[1,2,3,6]*

1 Foundation for the Promotion of Healthcare and Biomedical Research in the Valencian Community (FISABIO), Valencia, Spain, 2 Service of Endocrinology, University Hospital Doctor Peset, Valencia, Spain, 3 Institute of Health Research INCLIVA, University of Valencia, Valencia, Spain, 4 Psychiatry Service, University Hospital La Fe, Department of Medicine, University of Valencia, Valencia, Spain, 5 Research Group CIBER CB/06/02/0045, CIBER actions, Epidemiology and Public Health, University of Valencia, Valencia, Spain, 6 Department of Medicine, University of Valencia, Valencia, Spain

Abstract

Context: Anorexia nervosa is a common illness among adolescents and is characterised by oxidative stress.

Objective: The effects of anorexia on mitochondrial function and redox state in leukocytes from anorexic subjects were evaluated.

Design and setting: A multi-centre, cross-sectional case-control study was performed.

Patients: Our study population consisted of 20 anorexic patients and 20 age-matched controls, all of which were Caucasian women.

Main outcome measures: Anthropometric and metabolic parameters were evaluated in the study population. To assess whether anorexia nervosa affects mitochondrial function and redox state in leukocytes of anorexic patients, we measured mitochondrial oxygen consumption, membrane potential, reactive oxygen species production, glutathione levels, mitochondrial mass, and complex I and III activity in polymorphonuclear cells.

Results: Mitochondrial function was impaired in the leukocytes of the anorexic patients. This was evident in a decrease in mitochondrial O_2 consumption ($P<0.05$), mitochondrial membrane potential ($P<0.01$) and GSH levels ($P<0.05$), and an increase in ROS production ($P<0.05$) with respect to control subjects. Furthermore, a reduction of mitochondrial mass was detected in leukocytes of the anorexic patients ($P<0.05$), while the activity of mitochondrial complex I ($P<0.001$), but not that of complex III, was found to be inhibited in the same population.

Conclusions: Oxidative stress is produced in the leukocytes of anorexic patients and is closely related to mitochondrial dysfunction. Our results lead us to propose that the oxidative stress that occurs in anorexia takes place at mitochondrial complex I. Future research concerning mitochondrial dysfunction and oxidative stress should aim to determine the physiological mechanism involved in this effect and the physiological impact of anorexia.

Editor: Siyaram Pandey, University of Windsor, Canada

Funding: This study was financed by grants PI12/1984, PI13/1025 and PI13/073 from FIS and co-funded by the European Regional Development Fund of the European Union (FEDER), CIBERehd CB06/04/0071 and PROMETEO 2010/060. V.M.V. and M.R. are recipients of contracts from the Ministry of Health of the Valencian Regional Government and Carlos III Health Institute (CES10/030 and CP10/0360, respectively). S.R. is recipient of a predoctoral fellowship from Carlos III Health Institute (FI11/00637). The funders had no role in study design, data collection and analysis, decision to publish, or preparation of the manuscript.

Competing Interests: The authors have declared that no competing interests exist.

* Email: Victor.Victor@uv.es (VMV); hernandez_antmij@gva.es (AHM)

Introduction

Eating disorders are an increasingly frequent pathology that usually affects young women [1] and whose risk factors are varied and complex [2,3]. Three clinical subtypes of anorexia have been recognised: anorexia nervosa, bulimia nervosa and eating disorders not otherwise classified (EDNOS), which include atypical or incomplete forms of the first two subtypes [4].

Anorexia nervosa (AN), the most severe of the three subtypes, is characterised by a significant and deliberate loss of weight, a distorted perception of one's body and a pathological fear of being fat [4]. It is often a chronic condition, especially in patients that have required hospital treatment [5], and is currently one of the most frequent disorders among adolescents [6]. Mortality is high [7], and associated physical complications are common, particularly those of a cardiovascular nature [8].

Peripheral polymorphonuclear leukocytes (PMN) are inflammatory cells that, once activated, can release molecules that contribute to inflammation, endothelial impairment and oxidative stress. They also generate excessive amounts of ROS, which are harmful to cells, as they can initiate lipid peroxidation and apoptosis [9]. These effects of ROS are neutralised by the complex antioxidant system developed by organisms. In this context, it has been reported that PMN are contributors to the underlying oxidative stress present in inflammatory diseases and related to mitochondrial dysfunction [10–11]. However, their function and redox state in AN patients have not yet been determined.

Mitochondria are an important source of the ROS generated by different complexes, particularly complexes I and III [12–13]. For example, in a study performed using a mouse model of anorexia (anx/anx strain), different symptoms were related with mitochondrial impairment in complex I, including poor feeding, neurodegeneration and muscle weakness [14–15].

The present study highlights an impairment of mitochondrial function in a population of anorexic patients. This impairment was evident in a decrease in mitochondrial O_2 consumption, mitochondrial membrane potential ($\Delta\Psi_m$) and glutathione (GSH) levels, and an increase in ROS production. In addition, we observed a reduction of leukocyte mitochondrial mass and an impairment of mitochondrial complex I activity in this patient population.

Materials and Methods

Study design

The present multi-centre, cross-sectional case-control study was performed exclusively in Caucasian women. First, the patient/volunteer completed a questionnaire about her menstruation, eating habits, self-perception, influence on life of eating behaviour, binges, regulation of body weight and purging behaviour, and medication. Subsequently, anthropometrical measurements and blood pressure were recorded. A fasting blood sample was taken from all subjects.

Subjects

Twenty female AN patients with an age range of 16 to 34 (21.2 ± 5.9) years were recruited at the Eating Disorders Unit of the La Fe University Hospital, Valencia. Patients were diagnosed according to the F 50.0 Anorexia nervosa criteria [307.1] of the Diagnostic and Statistical Manual of Mental Disorders (version DSM IV TR): i.e. BMI <18 Kg/m². The presence of known somatic causes of malnutrition and other diseases that could have had a bearing on a subject's physical condition were ruled out by consulting the patient's medical history.

The control group consisted of twenty healthy women with an age range of 17 to 33 (23.6 ± 2.8) years, and which were pair-matched with the patients according to age. Controls were recruited at the Outpatient's Department of the Endocrinology Service of the Dr. Peset University Hospital in Valencia. Eating disorders, recent alterations in body weight, obesity and other metabolic disturbances that could interfere with the study's objectives were ruled out.

Exclusion criteria were pregnancy or lactation, galactorrhea or any endocrine or systemic disease that could affect reproductive physiology, organic, malignant, haematological, infectious or inflammatory disease, diabetes mellitus, a history of cardiovascular disease and the taking of lipid-lowering or antihypertensive drugs. None of the controls was taking antioxidant supplements at the time. The study was conducted according to the guidelines laid down in the Declaration of Helsinki, and all procedures were approved by the Ethics Committee of the University Hospital Dr Peset. Written informed consent was obtained from all the participants.

A parent or guardian provided written informed consent on behalf of children/minors included in the study.

Body variables and anthropometrical methods

The following anthropometrical parameters were recorded as specified: height was evaluated with a stadiometer with a variation of 0.4 cm; weight was measured using electronic scales with a variation of 0.05 kg and a capacity of up to 220 kg; BMI was evaluated by dividing weight in kilograms by height² (m); blood pressure was evaluated by using a sphygmomanometer. Waist and hip circumferences were also measured.

Laboratory methods

Blood was collected from the antecubital vein at 8–10 a.m, following 12 hours of fasting. Glucose levels were measured using enzymatic techniques and a Dax-72 autoanalyzer (Bayer Diagnostic, Tarrytown, New York, USA). Insulin was measured by an enzymatic luminescence technique. Samples for insulin were processed immediately and frozen until analysis in order to avoid haemolysis. Insulin resistance was calculated according to homeostasis model assessment (HOMA) using baseline glucose and insulin: HOMA = (fasting insulin ($\mu U/ml$) ×fasting glucose (mmol/L)/22.5.

Total cholesterol and triglycerides were measured by means of enzymatic assays, and HDLc concentrations were recorded using a direct method with a Beckman LX-20 autoanalyzer (Beckman Coulter, La Brea, CA, USA). The intraserial variation coefficient was <3.5% for all determinations. LDLc concentration was calculated using the Friedewald method. Non-HDLc concentra-

Table 1. Baseline characteristics and anthropometric data for the women participating in the study.

	Controls (n = 20)	Anorexia nervosa (n = 20)	p-value
Age (years)	23.6±2.8	21.2±5.9	0.210
Weight (kg)	56.8±3.6	40.3±4.1	<0.001
BMI (kg/m²)	20.6±0.6	15.3±0.9	<0.001
Waist circumference (cm)	72.0±4.3	63.4±3.6	<0.001
Systolic blood pressure (mmHg)	107±8	97±9	0.010
Diastolic blood pressure (mmHg)	66±7	65±7	0.833

Comparison between anorexic patients and controls using an unpaired Student's t-test. Data are expressed as mean ± SD. n = 20.

Table 2. Endocrine parameters in anorexia nervosa (AN) patients and healthy control subjects.

	Controls	Anorexia nervosa	p-value
Total cholesterol (mg/dl)	178.6±30.1	192.1±43.3	0.378
LDLc (mg/dl)	105.5±21.5	106.9±37.6	0.910
HDLc (mg/dl)	61.7±10.7	71.2±14.8	0.079
Triglycerides (mg/dl)	56 (46,61.5)	71 (38.5,87.5)	0.368
Apolipoprotein AI (mg/dl)	158.5±25.6	140.1±29.2	0.117
Apolipoprotein B (mg/dl)	74.8±12.8	73.5±26.3	0.884
Glucose (mg/dl)	80.4±8.9	75.0±6.0	0.083
Insulin (μIU/ml)	6.50±1.98	2.54±1.66	<0.001
HOMA-IR	1.29±3.77	0.49±0.39	<0.001

Data are expressed as mean ± SD, except for triglycerides, which are represented as medians and IQ range. Values of serum triglyceride concentrations were normalized using a log transformation. Comparison between anorexic patients and controls using an unpaired Student's t-test. n = 20.

tion was determined based on the difference between total cholesterol and HDLc. Apolipoprotein AI (Apo AI) and B (Apo B) were calculated by immunonephelometry (Dade Behring BNII, Marburg, Germany) with an intra-assay variation coefficient of < 5.5%.

Cells

Human polymorphonuclear leukocytes (PMNs) were obtained from blood samples treated with citrate and incubated with dextran (3%, 45 min). The supernatant was released over Fycoll-Hypaque and centrifuged for 25 min at 250 g. The pellet was resuspended in lysis buffer and centrifuged at room temperature (100 g, 5 min), and was then washed and resuspended in Hank's Balanced Salt Solution (HBSS). PMNs were then counted in a Scepter 2.0 cell counter (Millipore, MA, USA).

Measurement of O_2 consumption, membrane potential ($\Delta\Psi m$) and mitochondrial mass

PMNs were resuspended (5×10^6 cells/mL) in HBSS medium and placed in a gas-tight chamber. A Clark-type O_2 electrode (Rank Brothers, Bottisham, UK) was employed to evaluate mitochondrial O_2 consumption [16]. Sodium cyanide (10^{-3} mol/l), a mitochondrial complex IV inhibitor, was used as a negative control. Measurements were recorded using the Duo.18 data-device (WPI, Stevenage, UK). Rate of O_2 consumption (V_{O2max}) was calculated with the Graph Pad programme. The fluorescent dye tetramethylrhodamine methyl ester (TMRM, 5×10^{-6} mol/L) was used to assess $\Delta\Psi_m$. Mitochondrial mass was measured using the fluorescent dye 10-N-nonyl acridine orange (NAO, 5×10^{-6} mol/L), which binds to cardiolipin independently of $\Delta\Psi_m$ [17]. When evaluated by means of the trypan blue exclusion test and Scepter 2.0 cell counter (Millipore, MA, USA), cell viability was found to be unaltered.

Measurement of ROS production and GSH content

Total ROS production was evaluated by fluorometry using a Synergy Mx plate reader (BioTek Instruments, Winooski, VT) following incubation (30 min) with 5×10^{-6} mol/l of the fluorescent probe 2′,7′-dichlorodihydrofluorescein diacetate (DCFH-DA, 5×10^{-6} mol/L; excitation 485/emission 535 nm), as described elsewhere [16]. GSH content was calculated following incubation (30 min) with the fluorochrome 5-Chloromethylfluorescein Diacetate (CMFDA, 2.5×10^{-6} mol/L; excitation 492/emission 517 nm). In short, cells were seeded on 96-well plates, washed

with phosphate-buffered saline and incubated with CMFDA diluted in phosphate-buffered saline. After 15 min at 37°C, fluorescence intensities were measured. Levels of ROS and intracellular GSH were expressed as arbitrary fluorescence units.

Mitochondrial Respiratory Chain Enzyme Activities

Cell pellets containing approximately 10×10^6 cells were harvested, resuspended in 0.5 ml of Buffer A (20 mM MOPS, 0.25 M sucrose), centrifuged at 5000 g for 3 minutes at 4°C, resuspended in Buffer B (20 mM MOPS, 0.25 M sucrose, 1 mM EDTA), centrifuged at 10000 g for 3 minutes at 4°C and resuspended in 200 μL of 10 mM KH_2PO_4 (pH 7.4). Protein extracts where sonicated for 10 seconds in an Ultrasons cleaner (JP Selecta S.A., Barcelona, Spain). The protein concentration of each sample was determined by the BCA method, as described by the supplier (Pierce, Rockford, IL).

NADH oxidation was evaluated in a cuvette at 340 nm in a dual beam U-2800 spectrophotometer at 30°C. 35 μg of sample were added to 1000 μL of reaction buffer containing 20 mM KH_2PO_4 pH 8, 200 μM NADH, 1 mM NaN_3 and 0.1% BSA. First, a baseline rate was recorded for 2 min. in the absence of the substrate. Ubiquinone was then added to a final concentration of 100 μM and the rate of NADH oxidation was recorded for 3 min. NADH oxidation is produced by mitochondrial Complex I and other cellular NADH dehydrogenases. In order to determine Complex I activity, rotenone, an inhibitor of Complex I, was added to a final concentration of 5 μM and the rate of NADH oxidation was determined for another 3 min. Complex I activity was calculated by subtracting the rotenone-insensitive NADH oxidation rate in its linear phase from the total NADH oxidation rate in its linear phase. Complex III activity was measured by cytochrome C reduction at 550 nm at 30°C. 20 μg of protein were added to 1000 μL of reaction buffer containing 50 mM KH_2PO_4 pH 7.5, 2 mM NaN_3, 0.1%, BSA, 50 μM cytochrome C and 50 μM decylubiquinone, with and without 10 μg/ml antimycin A. Complex III activity was calculated by subtracting the antimycin A-insensitive cytochrome C reduction rate from the total cytochrome C reduction rate in the absence of antimycin A. The activity of the mitochondrial respiratory chain complexes was expressed as nmol min^{-1} mg protein^{-1} and converted to a % of that of controls. Residual activity of the different respiratory chain complexes in the presence of specific inhibitors was always less than 10% that of controls. Human U937 leukocytic cells treated previously with rotenone (10 μM for 12 h) or antimycin A (10 μM

A. Oxygen consumption

B. Membrane potential

C. Mitochondrial mass

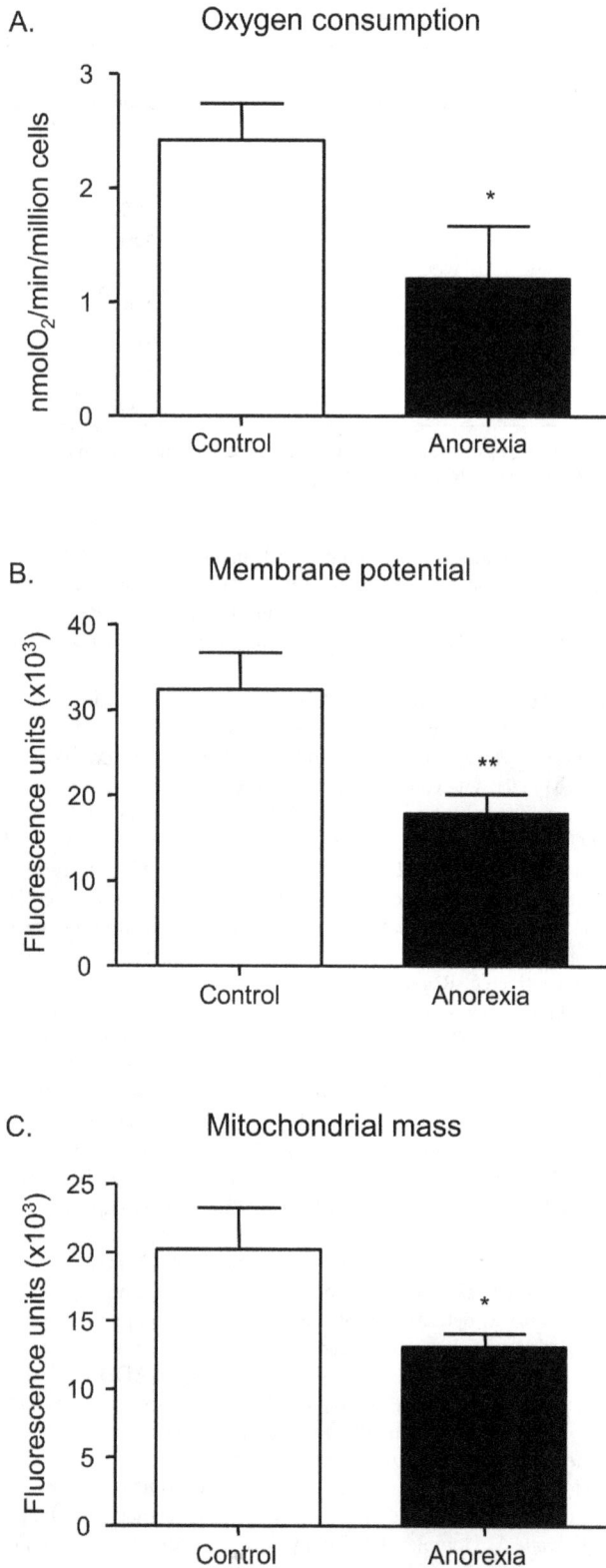

Figure 1. Effect of anorexia on O$_2$ consumption (A) rate, measured as nmol O$_2$/min/million cells, on membrane potential (B), measured by TMRM fluorescence, and on mitochondrial mass (C), measured by NAO fluorescence. n = 20 per group. *P<0.05 and **P<0.01 vs. control.

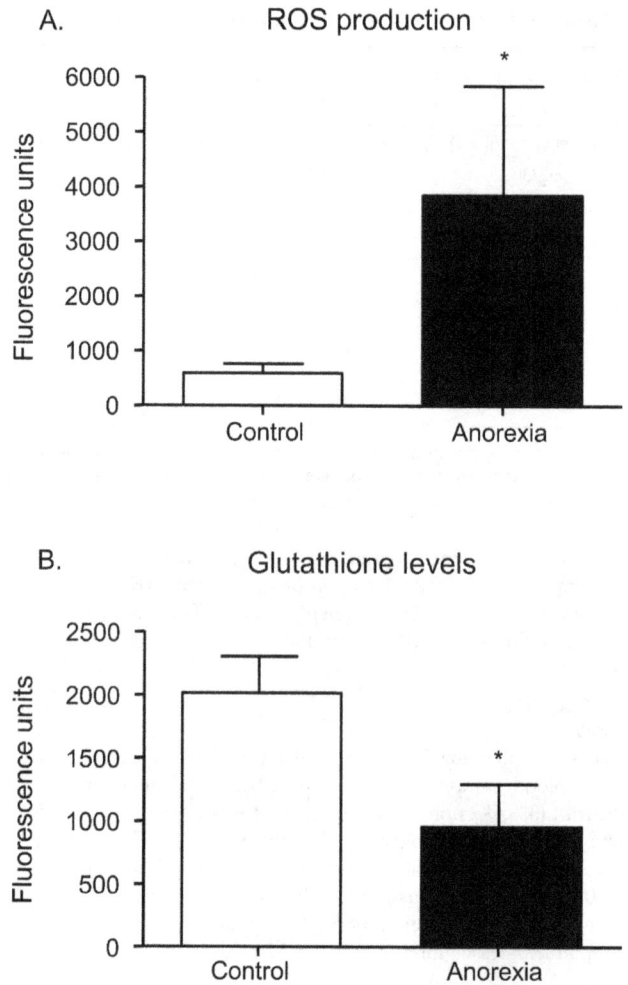

A. ROS production

B. Glutathione levels

Figure 2. Effect of anorexia on ROS production (A), measured by DCFH fluorescence, and on GSH content (B), measured by CMFDA fluorescence. n = 20 per group. *P<0.05 vs. controls.

for 2 h) were used as controls for complex I and complex III inhibition, respectively.

Drugs and solutions

Sodium cyanide, trypan blue, MOPS, BSA, Coenzyme Q1, rotenone, sodium azide (NaN$_3$), cytochrome C, antimycin A, decylubiquinone and HBSS were purchased from Sigma-Aldrich (Sigma Chem. Co., St. Louis, MO, USA). NADH was purchased from Roche Applied Science (Mannheim, Germany). Dextran was provided by Fluka (St. Louis, MO, USA). DCFH-DA was provided by Calbiochem (San Diego, CA, USA). PBS, TMRM, CMFDA and NAO were supplied by Invitrogen (Eugene, OR, USA). Ficoll-Paque TM Plus was purchased from GE Healthcare (Little Chalfont, Buckinghamshire, UK).

Statistical analyses

Statistical analysis was performed with SPSS 17.0 software (SPSS Statistics Inc., Chicago, IL, USA). Continuous variables were expressed as mean and standard deviation (SD) or as median or 25th and 75th percentiles for parametric and non-parametric data, respectively. Patient and control data were compared using a Student's t test for parametric independent samples or a Mann-Whitney U-test for non-parametric samples. Pearson's correlation

A.   Complex I activity

B.   Complex III activity

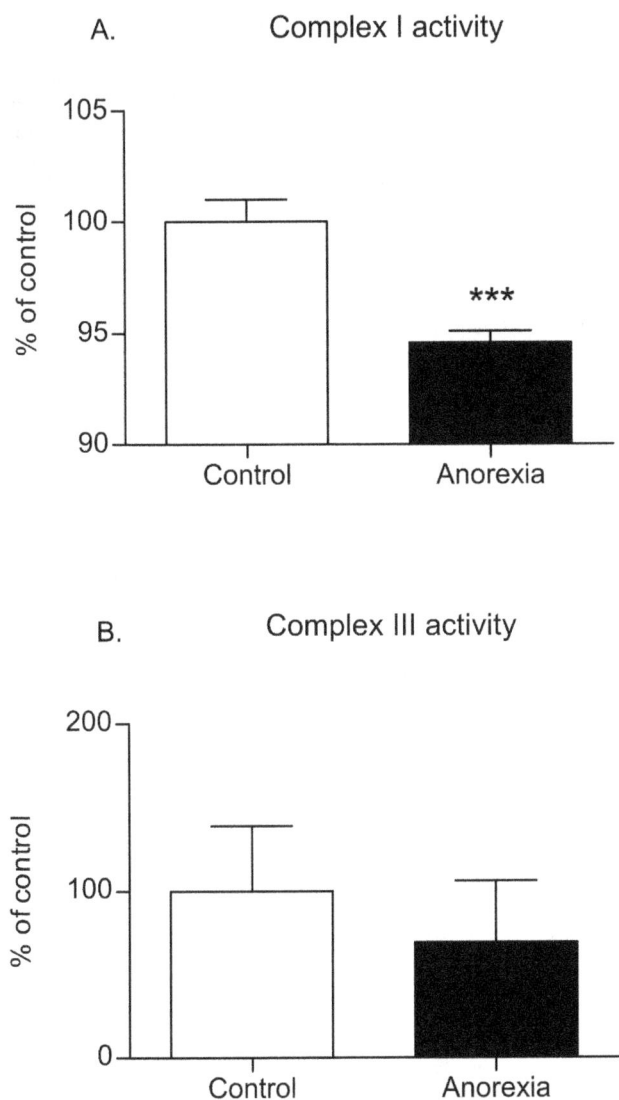

Figure 3. Effect of anorexia on mitochondrial complex I activity (A), measured as the NADH oxidation rate at 340 nm, and on complex III activity (B), measured as the cytochrome C reduction rate at 550 nm. Specific inhibitors for complexes I and III, rotenone and antimycin A, respectively, were employed to ensure the specificity of the assay. n = 8 per group. ***P<0.001 *vs.* control.

or Spearman's correlation coefficients was employed to measure the strength of the association between two variables for parametric and non-parametric data, respectively. All the tests used a confidence interval of 95% and differences were considered significant when P<0.05.

Results

Anthropometric, metabolic and clinical characteristics

The anthropometric characteristics of control subjects and anorexic patients can be seen in Table 1, which shows lower (P<0.001) weight, BMI and waist circumference among the latter. Systolic blood pressure was also lower (P<0.05) in anorexic patients.

Endocrine parameters in anorexic patients and their respective controls are shown in Table 2. Decreases in insulin levels (P<

0.001) and HOMA-IR (P<0.001) were observed in the anorexic group. When assessing potential correlations between BMI and lipid parameters in the anorexic women, it was found that BMI and weight were not associated with any of the parameters analysed (CT, LDLc, HDLc and triglycerides). In contrast, BMI correlated with total cholesterol (r = −0.295; p = 0.027) and HDLc (r = −0.323, p = 0.015) when the whole population was considered (controls and patients).

Mitochondrial O_2 consumption, $\Delta\Psi m$ and mitochondrial mass

A Clark electrode with an O_2-tight chamber was used to evaluate the rate of mitochondrial O_2 consumption in PMNs from the blood of both anorexic patients and controls. O_2 consumption proved to be mitochondrial, since the presence of sodium cyanide inhibited O_2 consumption (95–99%; not shown). The rate of O_2 consumption was lower in anorexic patients than in controls (Fig. 1A, P<0.05). Both TMRM (P<0.01) and NAO (P<0.05) fluorescence were diminished in anorexic patients (P<0.05), the former indicating a reduction in $\Delta\psi_m$ (Fig. 1B) and the latter a reduction in mitochondrial mass (Fig. 1C).

ROS production and GSH content

DCFH-DA fluorescence was significantly higher (Fig. 2A, P<0.05) and levels of GSH were significantly lower (Fig. 2B, P<0.05) among anorexic patients. These results confirmed an oxidative stress pattern in this group.

Mitochondrial complex I and III activity

As mitochondrial complexes I and III continuously generate ROS, they are particularly susceptible to oxidative damage. Therefore, we assessed the activity of both complexes in order to elucidate whether they were altered or not. Figure 3A shows the inhibition of mitochondrial complex I activity in anorexic patients (P<0.001), calculated as the rate of NADH oxidation in PMNs (expressed as % of control activity). The data suggest that complex I was the main target of the mitochondrial dysfunction in PMNs from the patients. No differences in complex III activity were detected between the anorexic and control groups (Fig. 3B). Human U937 leukocytes treated with rotenone or antimycin A were employed as controls and confirmed the inhibition of complex I and complex III respectively (P<0.001, data not shown).

Discussion

The present study highlights an impairment of mitochondrial function in PMNs from anorexic patients, expressed as a decrease in mitochondria O_2 consumption, $\Delta\Psi_m$ and GSH levels, and an increase in ROS production. We also demonstrate a reduction in mitochondrial mass in leukocytes from the same patients. Additionally, we propose complex I of the electron transport chain as a target of the ROS which are generated during anorexia. In line with this, we have previously demonstrated that complex I is more susceptible to oxidation than other mitochondrial complexes under oxidative stress conditions [16].

The mitochondrial electron transport chain is the principal site of ATP and ROS production in cells. In mammalian cells under normal conditions, mitochondrial complex I (CI) and mitochondrial complex III (CIII) are the main intracellular sources of the ROS generated by leaking electrons. In addition, ROS play several roles in cell and metabolic signalling [18–19]. Levels of ROS can increase dramatically during certain conditions, such as complex I dysfunction [10,16,20–21], resulting in oxidative stress and apoptosis [22]. In this context, an increase of ROS has previously been described in an animal model of anorexia – anx/anx mice [15] - which is in line with our observations of a decrease in O_2 consumption and $\Delta\Psi_m$ and an increase of ROS in human anorexic subjects. High ROS production has been related to the pathology of a high number of diseases, including atherosclerosis, cardiovascular disease, cancer and diabetes [13,15,17,23–24]. However, in addition to their status as oxidative molecules, ROS also act as metabolic signalling molecules [25]. The authors of the aforementioned study performed with the anx/anx mouse model hypothesized that a subclinical mitochondrial complex I deficiency increases ROS production and damages sensitive hypothalamic neurons, thereby inducing an impairment of appetite-regulating neuronal networks.

The present study highlights an increase in ROS production in the leukocytes of anorexic patients, which is relevant given that leukocytes are known to be highly sensitive to oxidative damage [26–27]. In fact, excessive ROS levels can be deleterious to cells, as they induce lipid peroxidation and apoptosis. However, these harmful effects of ROS can be counteracted by the organism's antioxidant system; antioxidants in general, and particularly GSH, play a key role in maintaining the viability of cells and protecting them from high levels of ROS/oxidative stress [28–30]. Malnutrition is usually accompanied by deficiency of vitamins and antioxidants; in fact, an undermined antioxidant status has been reported in AN [31], which supports the data of the present study. Furthermore, previous studies have shown that oxidative stress can accelerate hepatocyte injuries provoked during anorexia by increasing lipid peroxidation [32].

The increase in ROS production and decrease in GSH levels, mitochondrial O_2 consumption and $\Delta\Psi_m$ in our anorexic subjects point to an impairment of the electron transport chain that alters the function of mitochondria as a source of ATP. Moreover, we have witnessed a decrease of mitochondrial mass in these patients, which is relevant, as mitochondrial mass and morphology are important mediators of mitochondrial function [33–34]. A reduction in mitochondrial mass has been observed in different diseases, including diabetes [35,17], and hyperglycemia has been shown to induce mitochondrial fission, high ROS production and a reduction of ATP [36].

Importantly, while our anorexic patients exhibited lower mitochondrial mass than controls, they displayed a higher ROS production, indicating a pro-oxidant state despite the reduced amount of mitochondria. ROS production can disturb the GSH/GSSG ratio and redox state by reacting with thiol residues within redox-sensitive proteins. Our data show that AN leads to a decrease in GSH levels in leukocytes. In addition, we demonstrate that activity of complex I, but not of complex III, is impaired in anorexic patients, possibly due to high ROS production. In relation to this, different symptoms of anorexia have recently been linked to mitochondrial impairment in complex I in the previously mentioned study in a mouse model of anorexia (anx/anx mice), including poor feeding, neurodegeneration and muscle weakness [14–15].

Considered together, these findings confirm a state of oxidative stress in anorexic patients. PMNs are extremely sensitive under oxidative stress conditions in several diseases, including type 2 diabetes [10] and polycystic ovary syndrome [16]. In addition, oxidative stress can activate numerous inflammatory mediators, such as adhesion molecules, and proinflammatory cytokine expression (e.g. TNF-α, whose levels are enhanced in anorexia) [37] and immune signaling responses, including phospholipase activity, MAP kinase, and STAT and TLR signaling pathways [38]. In fact, TNF-α has been shown to mediate weight loss in experimental animal models through several mechanisms, including catabolic effects on energy storage tissue, suppression of food intake and lipoprotein lipase inhibition [37]. In light of this evidence, PMNs would seem to be one of the main types of inflammatory cells. Once activated, they release proinflammatory cytokines and ROS, which contribute to mitochondrial and endothelial dysfunction, reticulum stress, oxidative stress, inflammation and cardiovascular diseases (CVD) [10,16].

In summary, the present study demonstrates that oxidative stress is produced in the leukocytes of anorexic patients and that this stress is closely related to mitochondrial dysfunction. In fact, we show that mitochondrial complex I is inhibited in anorexic patients. Future research concerning mitochondrial dysfunction and oxidative stress should aim to determine the physiological mechanism involved in this effect and the physiological impact of anorexia.

Acknowledgments

We thank Isabel Soria for her work in the extraction of biological samples (University Hospital Dr Peset) and B Normanly for his editorial assistance (University of Valencia).

Author Contributions

Conceived and designed the experiments: AHM VMV LR. Performed the experiments: SR-L CB RF RC. Analyzed the data: MR VMV. Contributed reagents/materials/analysis tools: MR. Wrote the paper: VMV AHM. Supervision of the subjects in the study: VS-A MS LR-B LR.

References

1. Rojo L, Livianos L, Conesa L, García A, Domínguez A, et al. (2003) Epidemiology and risk factors of eating disorders. A two stage epidemiological study in a spanish population aged 12–18 years. Int J Eat Disord 34: 281–291.
2. Fairburn CG, Harrison PJ (2003) Eating disorders. Lancet 361: 407–416.
3. Ghaderi A (2003) Structural modeling analysis of prospective risk factors for eating disorder. Eating Behaviors 3: 387–396.
4. American Psychiatric Association (1994) Diagnostic and statistical manual of mental disorders. 4th ed. Washington DC: American Psychiatric Press.
5. Keel PK, Brown TA (2010) Update on Course and Outcome in Eating Disorders. Int J Eat Disord 43: 195–204.
6. Fisher M (2006) Treatment of eating disorders in children, adolescents, and young adults. Pediatr Rev 27: 5–16.
7. Neumärker KJ (1997) Mortality and sudden death in anorexia nervosa. Int J Eat Disord 21: 205–212.
8. Katzman DK (2005) Medical complications in adolescent with anorexia nervosa: a review of the literature. Int J Eat Disord 37: 552–559.
9. Victor VM, Rocha M, De la Fuente M (2004) Immune cells: free radicals and antioxidants in sepsis. Int Immunopharmacol 4: 327–347.
10. Hernandez-Mijares A, Rocha M, Apostolova N, Borras C, Jover A, et al. (2011) Mitochondrial complex I impairment in leukocytes from type 2 diabetic patients. Free Radic Biol Med 50: 1215–1221.
11. Murphy MP (2009) How mitochondria produce reactive oxygen species. Biochem J 417: 1–13.
12. James AM, Collins Y, Logan A, Murphy MP (2012) Mitochondrial oxidative stress and the metabolic syndrome. Trends Endocrinol Metab 23: 429–434.
13. Rovira-Llopis S, Rocha M, Falcon R, de Pablo C, Alvarez A, et al. (2013) Is Myeloperoxidase a Key Component in the ROS-Induced Vascular Damage Related to Nephropathy in Type 2 Diabetes? Antioxid Redox Signal 19: 1452–1458.
14. Luft R, Landau BR (1995) Mitochondrial medicine. J Intern Med 238: 405–421.
15. Lindfors C, Nilsson I, Garcia-Roves PM, Zuberi AR, Karimi M, et al. (2011) Hypothalamic mitochondrial dysfunction associated with anorexia in the anx/anx mouse. PNAS 108: 18108–18113.
16. Victor VM, Rocha M, Bañuls C, Sanchez-Serrano M, Sola E, et al. (2009) Mitochondrial complex I impairment in leukocytes from polycystic ovary syndrome patients with insulin resistance. J Clin Endocrinol Metab 94: 3505–3512.

17. Hernandez-Mijares A, Rocha M, Rovira-Llopis S, Bañuls C, Bellod L, et al. (2013) Human leukocyte/endothelial cell interactions and mitochondrial dysfunction in type 2 diabetic patients and their association with silent myocardial ischemia. Diabetes Care 36: 1695–1702.

18. Schagger H, de Coo R, Bauer MF, Hofmann S, Godinot C, et al. (2004) Significance of respirasomes for the assembly (stability of human respiratory complex I. J Biol Chem 2004; 279: 36349–36353.

19. Grad LI, Lemire BD (2006) Riboflavin enhances the assembly of mitochondrial cytochrome c oxidase in C elegans NADH-ubiquinone oxidoreductase mutants. Biochim Biophys Acta 1757: 115–122.

20. Ugalde C, Janssen RJ, van den Heuvel LP, Smeitink JA, Nijtmans LG (2004) Differences in assembly or stability of complex I and other mitochondrial OXPHOS complexes in inherited complex I deficiency. Hum Mol Genet 13: 659–667.

21. Victor VM, Rocha M, Bañuls C, Alvarez A, de Pablo C, et al. (2011) Induction of oxidative stress and human leukocyte/endothelial cell interactions in polycystic ovary syndrome patients with insulin resistance. J Clin Endocrinol Metab 96: 3115–3122.

22. Barrientos A, Moraes CT (1999) Titrating the effects of mitochondrial complex I impairment in the cell physiology. J Biol Chem 274: 16188–16197.

23. Esposito LA, Melov S, Panov A, Cottrell BA, Wallace DC (1999) Mitochondrial disease in mouse results in increased oxidative stress. Proc Natl Acad Sci U S A 96: 4820–4825.

24. Rocha M, Apostolova N, Herance JR, Rovira-Llopis S, Hernandez-Mijares A, et al. (2014) Perspectives and potential applications of mitochondria-targeted antioxidants in cardiometabolic diseases and type 2 diabetes. Med Res Rev 34: 160–189.

25. Diano S, Liu ZW, Jeong JK, Dietrich MO, Ruan HB, et al. (2011) Peroxisome proliferation-associated control of reactive oxygen species sets melanocortin tone and feeding in diet-induced obesity. Nat Med 17: 1121–1127.

26. De la Fuente M, Victor VM (2000) Antioxidants as modulators of immune function. Immunol Cell Biol 78: 49–54.

27. Sela S, Mazor R, Amsalam M, Yagil C, Yagil Y, et al. (2004) Primed polymorphonuclear leukocytes, oxidative stress, and inflammation antecede hypertension in the Sabra rat. Hypertension 44: 764–769.

28. Victor VM, Rocha M, Esplugues JV, De la Fuente M (2005) Role of free radicals in sepsis: antioxidant therapy. Curr Pharm Des 11: 3141–3158.

29. Yang YT, Whiteman M, Gieseg SP (2012) Intracellular glutathione protects human monocyte-derived macrophages from hypochlorite damage. Life Sci 90: 682–688.

30. Monsalve M, Borniquel S, Valle I, Lamas S (2007) Mitochondrial dysfunction in human pathologies. Front Biosci 12: 1131–1153.

31. Moyano D, Sierra C, Brandi N, Artuch R, Mira A, et al. (1999) Antioxidant status in anorexia nervosa. Int J Eat Disord 25: 99–103.

32. Tajiri K, Shimizu Y, Tsuneyama K, Sugiyama T (2006) A case report of oxidative stress in a patient with anorexia nervosa. Int J Eat Disord 39: 616–618.

33. Yoon Y (2005) Regulation of mitochondrial dynamics: another process modulated by Ca^{2+} signals? Sci STKE 2005: pe18.

34. Riva A, Tandler B, Loffredo F, Vazquez E, Hoppel C (2005) Structural differences in two biochemically defined populations of cardiac mitochondria. Am J Physiol Heart Circ Physiol 289: H868–H872.

35. Morino K, Petersen K, Dufour S (2005) Reduced mitochondrial density and increased IRS-1 serine phosphorylation in muscle of insulin-resistant offspring of type 2 diabetic parents. J Clin Invest 115: 3587–3593.

36. Yu T, Robotham JL, Yoon Y (2006) Increased production of reactive oxygen species in hyperglycemic conditions requires dynamic change of mitochondrial morphology. Proc Natl Acad Sci U S A 103: 2653–2658.

37. Tracey KJ, Morgello S, Koplin B, Fahey TJ 3rd, Fox J, et al. (1990) Metabolic effects of cachectin/tumor necrosis factor are modified by site of production. Cachectin/tumor necrosis factor-secreting tumor in skeletal muscle induces chronic cachexia, while implantation in brain induces predominantly acute anorexia. J Clin Invest 86: 2014–24.

38. Ivison SM1, Wang C, Himmel ME, Sheridan J, Delano J, et al. (2010). Oxidative stress enhances IL-8 and inhibits CCL20 production from intestinal epithelial cells in response to bacterial flagellin. Am J Physiol Gastrointest Liver Physiol 299: G733–741.

8

Silver-Zeolite Combined to Polyphenol-Rich Extracts of *Ascophyllum nodosum*: Potential Active Role in Prevention of Periodontal Diseases

Zohreh Tamanai-Shacoori[1]*, **Fatiha Chandad**[2], **Amélie Rébillard**[3], **Josiane Cillard**[3], **Martine Bonnaure-Mallet**[1,4]

1 Equipe de Microbiologie, EA 1254, Université Rennes 1, UEB, Rennes, France, **2** Groupe de Recherche en Ecologie Buccale, Faculté de médecine dentaire, Université Laval, Québec City, Québec, Canada, **3** Laboratoire Mouvement, Sport, Santé, EA 1274, Université Rennes 1, Université Rennes 2, UEB, Rennes, France, **4** Centre hospitalo-universitaire, Rennes, France

Abstract

The purpose of this study was to evaluate various biological effects of silver-zeolite and a polyphenol-rich extract of *A. nodosum* (ASCOP) to prevent and/or treat biofilm-related oral diseases. *Porphyromonas gingivalis* and *Streptococcus gordonii* contribute to the biofilm formation associated with chronic periodontitis. In this study, we evaluated *in vitro* antibacterial and anti-biofilm effects of silver-zeolite (Ag-zeolite) combined to ASCOP on *P. gingivalis* and *S. gordonii* growth and biofilm formation capacity. We also studied the anti-inflammatory and antioxidant capacities of ASCOP in cell culture models. While Ag-zeolite combined with ASCOP was ineffective against the growth of *S. gordonii*, it showed a strong bactericidal effect on *P. gingivalis* growth. Ag-zeolite combined with ASCOP was able to completely inhibit *S. gordonii* monospecies biofilm formation as well as to reduce the formation of a bi-species *S. gordonii/P. gingivalis* biofilm. ASCOP alone was ineffective towards the growth and/or biofilm formation of *S. gordonii* and *P. gingivalis* while it significantly reduced the secretion of inflammatory cytokines (TNFα and IL-6) by LPS-stimulated human like-macrophages. It also exhibited antioxidant properties and decreased LPS induced lipid peroxidation in gingival epithelial cells. These findings support promising use of these products in future preventive or therapeutic strategies against periodontal diseases.

Editor: Christophe Egles, Université de Technologie de Compiègne, France

Funding: Région Bretagne, Conseil Général du Finistère and OSEO Innovation. The funders had no role in study design, data collection and analysis, decision to publish, or preparation of the manuscript.

Competing Interests: The authors have declared that no competing interests exist.

* Email: zohreh.shacoori@univ-rennes1.fr

Introduction

Periodontal diseases (PD) are the most prevalent chronic infectious diseases worldwide [1]. These infections lead to progressive destruction of the tooth supporting tissues, bone resorption and tooth loss. Several studies have reported the potential link between PD and systemic diseases including diabetes, and cardiovascular disease. The pathogenesis of PD is associated with accumulation of an oral biofilm (also called dental plaque) and modulation of the host inflammatory response [2]. *Porphyromonas gingivalis,* a Gram-negative anaerobic bacterium [3,4], is one of the most important pathogens associated with the development of periodontitis. However, *P. gingivalis* requires others bacterial species called early-colonizers including *Streptococcus gordonii* [5], to form the subgingival biofilm. *P. gingivalis* and *S. gordonii* interact with gingival epithelial cells [6,7] and impair their functions [8]. In addition, *P. gingivalis* secretes a wide range of proteases and degrade various host proteins including collagen, fibronectin, immunoglobulins and cytokines [9]. The host immune reaction to these colonizing bacteria and their products, particularly lipopolysaccharides (LPS), induces the

secretion of a wide array of molecules, including cytokines, prostaglandins, proteolytic enzymes and oxidative stress products [1,10–12]. Thus, prevention of PD is focused on the development of strategies to inhibit both bacterial biofilm formation and to modulate the host inflammatory response.

Recently, marine algae have attracted the scientific interest as natural source of bioactive products possessing various biological properties. In fact, several studies have reported that extracts, rich in polysaccharides and polyphenols, from the marine brown alga *Ascophyllum nodosum*, possess various beneficial biological properties including anticoagulant and antithrombotic [13], antitumoral [14], antiviral [15], antioxidant [16,17] and potent anti-inflammatory effects [18].

On the other hand, ionic silver (Ag$^+$) has long been used for its broad-spectrum antimicrobial properties in different fields including dentistry [19], ocular infections and treatment of burns [20,21]. Advances in chemical technology allowed trapping Ag$^+$ within zeolite (a porous crystalline material of hydrated sodium aluminosilicate with a strong affinity for ionic heavy metals). This complex, called silver-zeolite (Ag-zeolite), has been applied to various materials as long-lasting antimicrobial disinfectant [22–25].

In the present study, we hypothesized that the biological properties of marine algae extracts combined to those of the complex silver-zeolite could have beneficial effects in the prevention of PD by inhibiting bacterial biofilm formation and modulating the host immune response. Our aims were then to investigate the effects of a polyphenol-rich extract from the algae *Ascophyllum nodosum* called ASCOP (for *Ascophyllum nodosum* polyphenols), combined or not with Ag-zeolite, on bacterial growth and biofilm formation of two oral bacterial species *S. gordonii* and *P. gingivalis*. The anti-inflammatory and antioxidant properties of the ASCOP were assessed in cell culture models.

Materials and Methods

Preparation of the complex Ag-zeolite

The complex Ag-zeolite was synthesized by an ion-exchange method [26]. Briefly, constant amounts of zeolite were suspended in 600 mL of demineralised water containing 2.60 g of silver nitrate ($AgNO_3$). The solution was stirred for 3 hours at 60°C to obtain a complex formed by zeolite loaded with ionic silver. After a vacuum filtration and three washes in distilled water, the Ag-zeolite complex was dried for 12 hours at 100°C. The obtained suspension was analysed by ICP MS (Inductive Coupled Plasma Mass Spectrometry) to determine the silver proportion in the complex Ag-zeolite. The final solution containing the active complex Ag-zeolite was formed by silver ($0.38 \ \mu g \ mL^{-1}$) and zeolite ($0.50 \ \mu g \ mL^{-1}$) and was distributed into aliquots and stored at $-80°C$ until use in experimental assays.

Preparation of polyphenol-rich extract of *Ascophyllum nodosum* (ASCOP)

The algae *A. nodosum* was harvested from the west coast of France. A polyphenol-rich extract from *A. nodosum* called ASCOP was prepared following the protocol described by Chandler and Dodds [27]. Briefly, ASCOP was obtained from *A. nodosum* by successive water extraction, alginate precipitation, filtration and final concentration by ultra-filtration procedures. Phenolics concentration was estimated by comparison to a calibration curve prepared with 0–50 μg gallic acid [27]. The final polyphenol-rich solution was lyophilized and stored at 4°C until use. ASCOP mixed with the Ag-zeolite was used in antibacterial and anti-biofilm assays. ASCOP was used alone in antioxidant and anti-inflammatory assays.

Bacterial culture

P. gingivalis ATCC 33277 and *S. gordonii DL1* were grown in brain-heart infusion broth (BHI) (DIFCO, France) and/or on blood Columbia agar plates (AES Chemunex, France) supplemented with hemin ($5 \ g \ mL^{-1}$) and menadione ($1 \ g \ mL^{-1}$) (Sigma Aldrich, France). *P. gingivalis* cultures were incubated under anaerobic conditions (N_2-H_2-CO_2 [80:10:10]) and *S. gordonii* was grown aerobically at 37°C.

Macrophage-like and gingival epithelial cell cultures

Cells from the human myeloid leukemia cell line U937 (ATCC CRL-1593.2) were grown in RPMI-1640 medium (Sigma-Aldrich). Cells from the human gingival epithelial carcinoma cell line Ca9-22 (Health Science Research Resources Bank, Osaka, Japan) were cultured in Dulbecco's Modified Eagle Medium (DMEM) (Lonza, France) at 37°C in humidified atmosphere of 5% CO_2. Both cell culture media were supplemented with 10% heat-inactivated fetal bovine serum (FBS, Lonza, France) and

antibiotics ($100 \ mg \ mL^{-1}$ penicillin/$50 \ mg \ mL^{-1}$ streptomycine) (Sigma Aldrich). Monocytic U937 cells were differentiated into macrophage-like cells using 16 nM phorbol-12-myristate-13-acetate (PMA) (Sigma Aldrich) in RPMI-1640 supplemented with 10% FBS for 48 hours. The adherent macrophage-like cells were washed and incubated for an additional 24 hours in fresh RPMI-1640-10% FBS medium. For all the experiments, a cellular count was carried out using a haemocytometer and the cells were suspended in RPMI supplemented with 1% FBS, seeded in six-well plates (1×10^6 cells/well/1 mL) and incubated at 37°C in a 5% CO2 atmosphere for 2 h prior to the ASCOP treatment and lipopolysaccharide (LPS) stimulations.

Antibacterial assay

The capacity of ASCOP mixed with Ag-zeolite to inhibit bacterial growth was assessed using a standard procedure according to the European norms prEN 1040 (AFNOR: NF EN 1040-1997) in chemical disinfectants and antiseptics section. Briefly, $1–5 \times 10^7$ cfu mL^{-1} of a fresh bacterial suspension (standard inoculum) was incubated in the presence of the tested product for 15 min at 15°C. For controls, the same experiments were carried out in the same conditions with sterile BHI but without the tested product. For bacterial viable count, samples (100 μL) of serial dilutions were plated onto blood Columbia agar plates and incubated at 37°C for 48 hours in aerobiosis for *S. gordonii*, and for 6 days, under anaerobic conditions for *P. gingivalis*. Each experiment was repeated three times and each colony count was repeated two times. The results were expressed as log_{10} values of the mean colony forming unit (cfu) count.

Anti-biofilm formation assay

The effect of the tested product on biofilm formation has been assessed using the Biofilm Ring Test method (BioFilm Control, Saint Beauzire, France) as described by the manufacturer. This assay is based on the immobilization of magnetic beads when they become embedded in bacterial aggregates. Briefly, bacterial inoculums (mono-specie and/or bi-species) of *P. gingivalis* and/or *S. gordonii* were prepared in BHI medium and adjusted to 10^7–10^8 cfu mL^{-1}. Bacteria (200 μl) were distributed in wells of polystyrene 96-well plates and mixed with 10 μL mL^{-1} of the toner solution (TON 005 containing magnetic beads, provided by the manufacturer) in the presence or absence of the test product. Controls without bacteria were also run in the assay to be sure that the tested product does not interfere with the beads. After 3 hours incubation at 37°C in an anaerobic atmosphere, plates were scanned before and after magnetization using the dedicated Scan Plate Reader (BioFilm Control, France) operated with the Biofilm Control Software (BioFilm Control, France). The biofilm formation was expressed as a Biofilm Formation Index (BFI) calculated by the software and based on attracted beads forming a black spot in the bottom of the wells and detected by the Scan Plate Reader. Calculated BFIs are inversely proportional to the biofilm formation density. A BFI value ≤ 2 corresponds to a densely formed biofilm whereas a BFI value ≥ 12 indicates the absence of biofilm formation. The results are expressed as the mean of BFI values of triplicate from three independent experiments.

Cytotoxicity assay

Eukaryotic cell viability was measured by MTT assay [3-(4, 5-dimethylthiazol-2-yl)-2, 5-diphenyl tetrazolium bromide (MTT; Sigma-Aldrich)]. The U937 macrophage-like cells (5×10^3 cells/ well), distributed in wells of 96-well plates, were exposed to increasing concentrations of ASCOP solution (0.10, 0.25 and 0.50 μg mL^{-1} in RPMI-1640 culture medium) with three wells for each concentration. After 24 hours incubation in the presence or absence of a bacterial stimuli (0.5 µg mL^{-1} *P. gingivalis* LPS (invivoGen, Toulouse, France), 10 µL of MTT (0.50 mg mL^{-1} final concentration) were added to each well. After 4 hours incubation at 37°C, the supernatant was removed and 100 µl of acidic (0.04 M HC) isopropanol were added to each well to solubilize the formazan crystals. After vigorous shaking, absorbance was measured using a microplate reader at 550 nm wavelength. A correction was carried out at 655 nm to exclude the cellular debris. The cellular percentage of viability was expressed according to the following formula: OD (optical density) of cells treated with ASCOP solution x 100/OD of untreated cells. The ASCOP concentrations showing less than 20% of cell mortality were selected as working concentrations for the subsequent experiments.

Anti-inflammatory activity

Macrophage-like cells U937 (5×10^6 cells/wells of six-well plates) were pre-incubated for 2 hours with non-toxic concentrations of ASCOP (0.10 µg mL^{-1}), and then stimulated for an additional 24 hours period with 0.5 µg mL^{-1} of *P. gingivalis* LPS. After the incubation period, the amounts of inflammatory cytokines TNFα and IL-6 were measured in the cell culture supernatants using commercial ELISA kits (R&D Systems, Minneapolis, MN) according to the manufacturer's protocol. Non LPS-stimulated and non ASCOP treated cells were used as negative controls. Cells stimulated with LPS but not treated with ASCOP also were used as positive controls of stimulation. Three independent experiments were conducted in triplicate and data are expressed as means ± SD.

Antioxidant activity of ASCOP

Free Radical scavenging activity. Superoxide anion (O2$^-$) was produced by the xanthine/xanthine oxidase system and hydroxyl radical (OH) was generated from decomposition of H_2O_2 by ferrous ions. Both reactions were carried out in the presence of a spin trap 5,5-dimethylpyrroline-N-oxide (DMPO). ASCOP solution was added at concentrations ranging respectively from 0.025 to 0.50 µg mL^{-1} for superoxide anion assay and 0.0025 to 0.05 µg mL^{-1} for hydroxyl radical assay. Electron Spin Resonance (ESR) spectra were recorded at room temperature using a Bruker ECS 106 spectrometer. The scavenging activity of ASCOP was evaluated by the decrease in the ESR signal expressed as arbitrary units. Scavenging activities were calibrated using the bovine erythrocyte superoxide dismutase (SOD, Sigma-Aldrich) as standard for superoxide anion, and benzoic acid as reference scavenging substance for hydroxyl radical. All ESR experiments were performed five times for each point and data are expressed as means ± SD.

Total Antioxidant Capacity. The Oxygen Radical Absorbance Capacity (ORAC) experiments were carried out according to Prior *et al*. [28]. ASCOP was used at a concentration of 0.10 µg mL^{-1}. A standard curve was performed using Trolox (6-hydroxy-2,5,7,8-tetramethylchroman-2-carboxylic acid) (Sigma Aldrich), a synthetic analogue of vitamin E, at concentrations ranging from 6.20 µM to 50 µM. Final values were expressed as micromole Trolox equivalents per gram. Trolox experiments were performed five times and the results are expressed as the mean ± SD of spectrophotometric absorbance.

Anti-lipoperoxidation activity

Ca9-22 gingival epithelial cells were seeded at 1×10^5 cells/well of 96-well plates in DMEM-10% FBS medium. After 24 hours incubation, cells were treated with ASCOP solution (10 µg mL^{-1}) for 1 hour before being stimulated with *P. gingivalis* LPS of (10 µg mL^{-1}) during 2 hours. Lipid peroxidation as a marker of oxidative stress was evaluated by measurement of 15 F$_2$ α-Isoprostanes (also called 8-Isoprostanes) released in the culture medium. F2 α-Isoprostanes were analyzed by LC-MS according to the protocol previously described [29]. Each experiment was performed in triplicate and repeated three times. Concentrations of isoprostanes (picogramme isoprostanes/mL) are expressed as means ± SD.

Statistical analysis

All data are expressed as means ± standard deviations of triplicates from at least three independent experiments. The significance of the results was assessed using the Student's *t*-test. An effect was considered statistically significant if its *p* value was lower than 0·05 (*p*<0.05 as significant) except in the case of antioxidant assay, it was lower than 0.01 (*p*<0.01 as significant).

Results

Antibacterial activities

After 60 min of exposure, the antibacterial activity of the tested products against *S. gordonii* and *P. gingivalis* were evaluated according to the European norms (Table 1). Ag-zeolite in the presence or absence of ASCOP showed strong bactericidal effect (*p*<0.05) by complete killing of *P. gingivalis*. In the same condition, silver alone at 0.38 µg mL^{-1} concentration revealed a weaker effect on the growth of *P. gingivalis* with 3 log reduction (*p*<0.05) (Table 1) compared to the starting inoculum. Both zeolite (0.50 µg mL^{-1}) and ASCOP (0.50 µg mL^{-1}), independently assessed, did not show significant effect on the growth of *P. gingivalis*.

For *S. gordonii*, none of the evaluated products showed any effect on the growth of this bacterial species. The number of bacteria (cfu mL^{-1}) remained similar to that of the non-treated control after 60 min of treatment with the tested products.

Anti-biofilm formation properties

The capacity of Ag-zeolite, combined or not to ASCOP, to inhibit biofilm formation by *S. gordonii in* monoculture or in coculture with *P. gingivalis*, was investigated. The BFI for *S. gordonii* monoculture biofilm or in combination with *P. gingivalis* (positive controls) were respectively 1.65±0.15 and 1.85±0.15. However, when bacteria were treated with Ag-zeolite combined to ASCOP, biofilm forming capacity of *S. gordonii* in monoculture or coculture with *P. gingivalis* was altered (Figures 1 and 2). Indeed, *S. gordonii* biofilm formation was completely inhibited in the presence of the complex Ag-zeolite combined to ASCOP (Figures 1A and 1B). The BFI reached 17.50±0.20 (*p*<0.05) in the case of *S. gordonii* monoculture biofilm and 6.42±0.10 (*p*<0.05) for the coculture *S. gordonii* + *P. gingivalis* biofilms (Figures 1A and 2A). The capacity of *S. gordonii* to form a biofilm was less affected by Ag-zeolite in the absence of ASCOP (BFI of 9.95±0.15) (*p*<0.05) (Figure 1A). Under the same conditions, a slight effect was observed on the biofilm formation of the coculture *S. gordonii* + *P. gingivalis* (BFI = 2.6±0.11) (*p*<0.05) (Figure 2A).

Anti-inflammatory activities of ASCOP

To investigate the effects of ASCOP on inflammatory cytokine (TNFα and IL-6) production, macrophage-like cells U937 were treated with ASCOP (0.10 µg mL^{-1} solution) before stimulation with LPS. Cytokine productions were measured in the cell culture medium by ELISA. As shown in Figure 3, ASCOP treatment caused significant decrease (*p*<0.05) of the secretion of TNFα

Table 1. Bacterial count (cfu mL^{-1}) of *S. gordonii* and *P. gingivalis* cultures after 60 min treatment with silver (Ag), ASCOP, zeolite, Ag-zeolite or Ag-zeolite+ASCOP.

Bacterium	Control	Ag	ASCOP	Zeolite	Ag-zeolite	Ag-zeolite+ASCOP
S. gordonii DL1	$2,16\times10^{7}\pm0,07$	$2,99\times10^{7}\pm0,12$	$2,91\times10^{7}\pm0,15$	$2,17\times10^{7}\pm0,17$	$2,70\times10^{7}\pm0,23$	$2,56\times10^{7}\pm0,25$
P. gingivalis ATCC33277	$2,33\times10^{7}\pm0,29$	$2,59\times10^{4*}\pm0,40$	$2,90\times10^{7}\pm0,45$	$1,23\times10^{7}\pm0,25$	0*	0*

Control: in absence of active products.
The values are means ±standard deviations for measurements obtained for three independent experiments (* $p < 0.05$; $n = 6$).

(Figure 3A) and IL-6 (Figure 3B) in LPS stimulated macrophage-like cells. The amounts of TNFα and IL-6 in the supernatant of treated cells were clearly less than those of the LPS stimulated control cells (94% and 84% of reduction respectively). ASCOP had no effects on unstimulated control cells (Figures 3A and B). To exclude the possibility that the decrease in cytokine amounts might have been caused by cytotoxic effects of ASCOP solution, we have evaluated the viability of the macrophage-like cells by an MTT assay. No cytotoxic effects were detected following treatments of

macrophages with increasing concentrations of ASCOP ranging from 0.10 to 0.50 μg mL^{-1}, and cell viability was ≥98% of the untreated controls in all experiments (data not shown).

Antioxidant activities of ASCOP

ASCOP at a concentration of 0.50 μg mL^{-1} decreased DMPO-OOH signal by 50%. The superoxide anion scavenging capacity of ASCOP was calculated to be equivalent to 207 UI SOD [30]. For hydroxyl radical, ASCOP at a concentration of 0.05 μg mL^{-1}

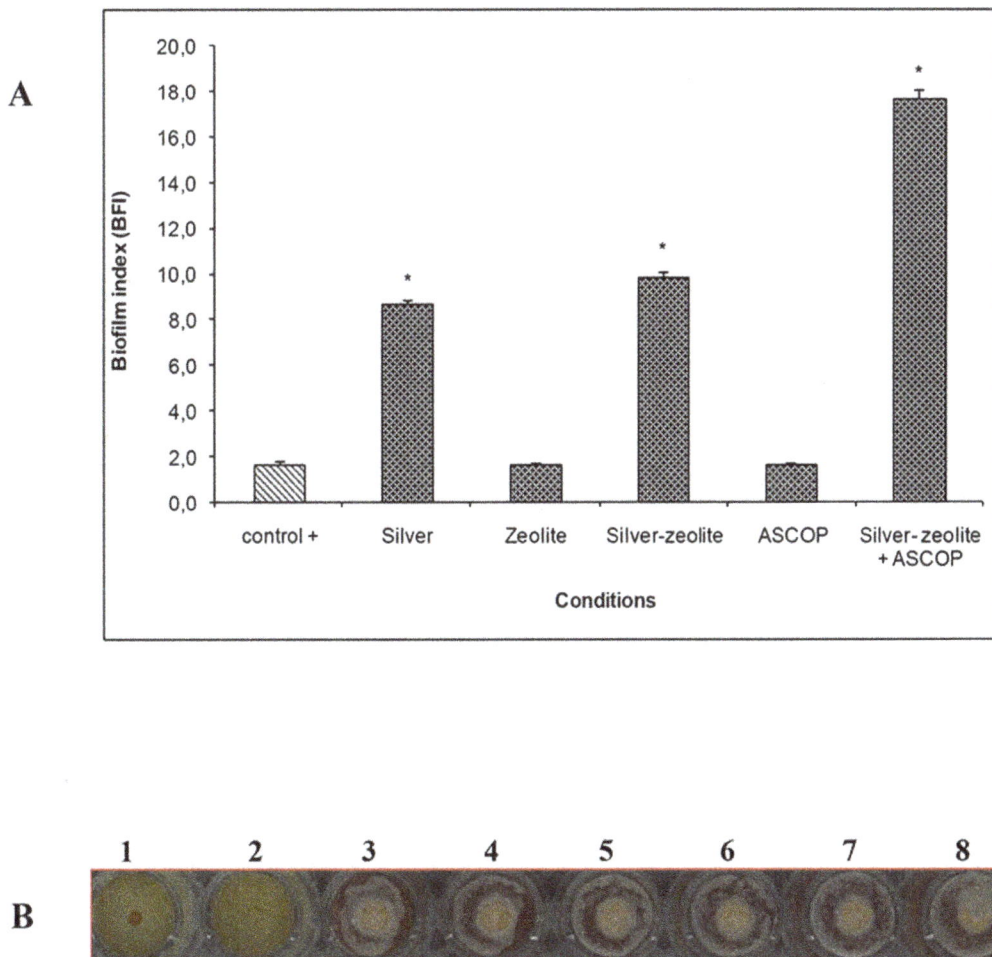

Figure 1. Biofilm formation of monoculture of *S. gordonii* treated with silver (Ag), ASCOP, zeolite, Ag-zeolite or Ag-zeolite+ASCOP.
A: BFI (biofilm formation index) values for monoculture of *S. gordonii* in absence or presence of silver (Ag); zeolite; Ag-zeolite; ASCOP or Ag-zeolite+ ASCOP. *Significantly different from control ($p<0.05$; n = 9). **B**: Biofilm formation of *S. gordonii* in the presence of Ag-zeolite combined to ASCOP. Well 1 (BHI, negative control), well 2 (positive control), wells 3 to 8 (replicate of *S. gordonii* in the presence of Ag-zeolite+ASCOP.

A

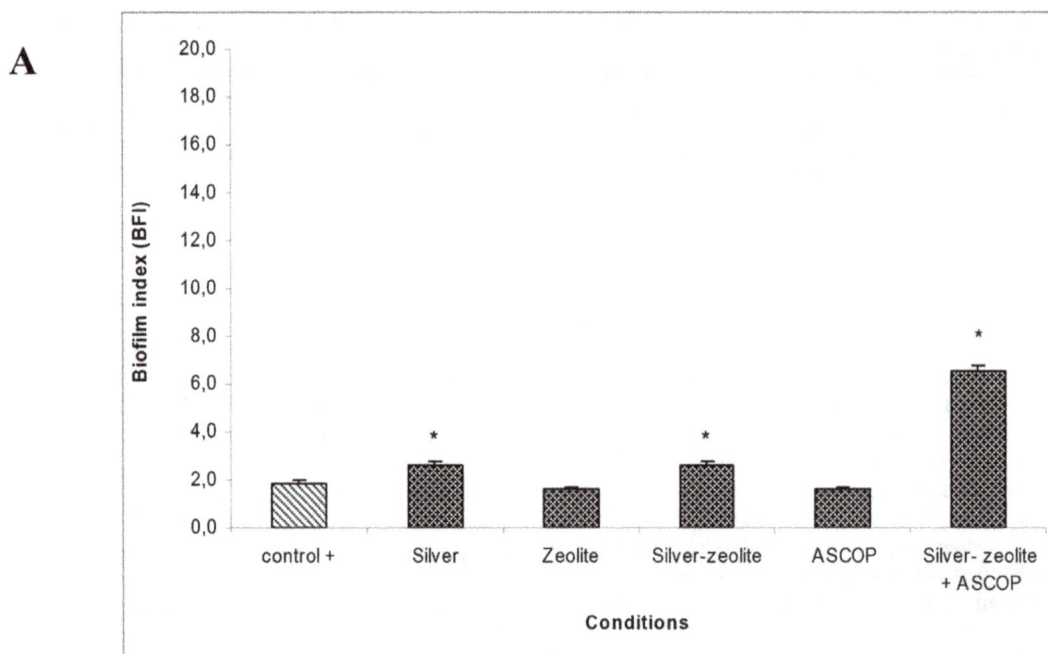

B

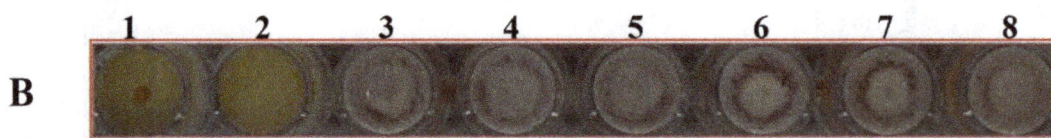

Figure 2. Biofilm formation of the coculture of *S. gordonii + P. gingivalis* **treated with silver (Ag), zeolite, Ag-zeolite, ASCOP or Ag-zeolite+ASCOP. A**: Biofilm formation of the coculture of *S. gordonii + P. gingivalis* treated with silver (Ag), zeolite, Ag-zeolite, ASCOP or Ag-zeolite+ ASCOP. *Significantly different from control ($p<0.05$; n=9). **B**: Biofilm formation of the coculture *S. gordonii + P. gingivalis* in the presence of Ag-zeolite combined to ASCOP. Well 1 (BHI, negative control), well 2 (positive control), wells 3 to 8 (replicate of the coculture *S. gordonii + P. gingivalis* in the presence of Ag-zeolite+ASCOP.

decreased DMPO-OH signal by 50%. Hydroxyl radical scavenging capacity of ASCOP was determined to be equivalent to 83 mg mL^{-1} of benzoic acid. It should be mentioned that in these experiments, the concentrations of ASCOP used to scavenge hydroxyl radical were 10 times lower than those used to scavenge superoxide anion. This is due to a higher reactivity of hydroxyl radical compared to superoxide anion.

The total antioxidant capacity (TAC) of ASCOP determined by ORAC assay was calculated to be 296 micromole Trolox equivalents per gram.

An inhibition of lipid peroxidation was observed in Ca9-22 epithelial cells treated with 0.10 μg mL^{-1} of ASCOP during 1 h before stimulation with *P. gingivalis* LPS as showed by the significant decrease of isoprostanes in culture medium ($p<0.01$) (Figure 4). No obvious effect of LPS (10 μg mL^{-1}) on the viability rate of Ca9-22 cells was observed after 4 h and 24 h of cell stimulation (data not shown).

Discussion

Over the past two decades, natural compounds with antibacterial, anti-inflammatory and/or anti-oxidant properties have received considerable attention as new therapeutic agents for the prevention and treatment of various infections. In this work, we investigated the biological properties of a polyphenol-rich extract from the marine algae *A. nodosum*, named ASCOP, combined with a complex of silver-zeolite named Ag-zeolite. To the best of our knowledge, no study has described before the bactericidal effect of algae extracts on oral pathogens. Nevertheless, bacteriostatical activities against positive and negative Gram bacteria have already been described for tannins extracted from the algae *Ecklonia kurome*, *E. cava* and *Fucus vesiculosus*, suggesting their potential use as natural preservatives in food industry or as antibacterial drugs [31,32]. In addition, algae extracts like phytochemical extracts have an advantage over synthetic antibacterial agents in that, pathogens are not frequently exposed to these

A

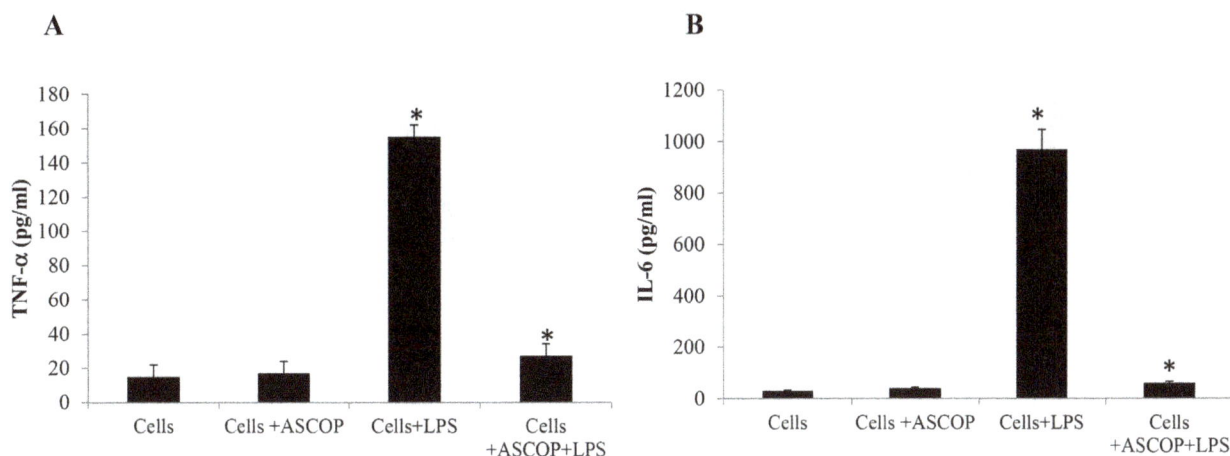

B

Figure 3. Cytokine measurement in cell culture medium of macrophage like cells U937. Levels of TNFα (**A**) and IL-6 (**B**) in culture supernatant of macrophage-like cells U937 stimulated with LPS (0.5 µg mL^{-1}) and treated or not with ASCOP (0.1 µg mL^{-1}). Values are expressed as means ± standard deviation of triplicates (* $p<0.05$).

natural compounds and should not develop resistance. On the other hand, the metallic silver, loaded onto several inorganic systems such as zeolites, was reported as efficient anti-microbial agents [33,34]. Indeed, the incorporation of silver into zeolite increases ions interaction with microorganism via a higher specific surface area. Lima *et al.* [35] reported that gold nanoparticles dispersed on zeolites are excellent biocide to rapidly eliminate *Escherichia coli* and *Salmonella typhi*. In our study, Ag-zeolite alone or in combination with ASCOP exhibited a high bactericidal activity against *P. gingivalis* while the viability of *S. gordonii* was not affected. This feature could be attributed to the nature of bacterial membrane of the Gram positive bacterium which seems to be more effective in the protection against any cytotoxic effects of these compounds. For ASCOP preparation, no antibacterial effect against *P. gingivalis* or *S.gordonii* was observed.

In addition, we show in this study, for the first time, that Ag-zeolite combined with ASCOP exhibits a marked synergistic effect in alteration of the biofilm forming capacity of *S. gordonii* alone or in coculture with *P. gingivalis*. This result becomes highly pertinent when we consider that the adherence of *P. gingivalis*, one of the late colonizers in the biofilm, depends on its capacity to adhere to the first colonizers including *Streptococcus spp.* [36]. Without affecting *S. gordonii* viability, addition of ASCOP to Ag-zeolite inhibited coculture *S. gordonii* + *P. gingivalis* biofilm formation while silver-zeolite alone did not reveal any specific anti-biofilm effect. This inhibitory effect is probably associated with a different interaction between ASCOP and Ag-zeolite conferring thus a new biological property.

Actually, there is no doubt that plaque bacteria are necessary to initiate the chronic inflammatory response in the periodontal tissues [37]. At the same time, there is strong evidence that

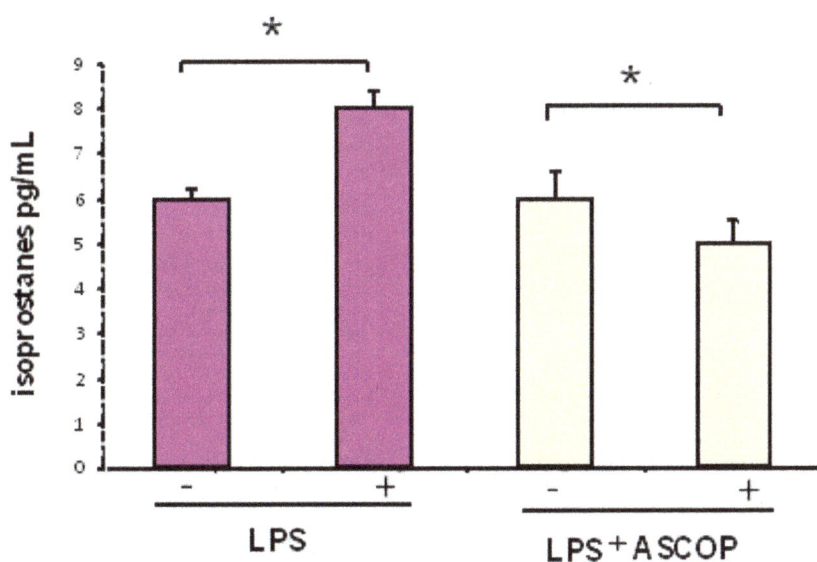

Figure 4. Isoprostanes release in culture media of epithelial gingival cells Ca9-22. Cells were treated with ASCOP (0.10 µg mL^{-1}) for 1 hour before been stimulated with LPS (10 µg mL^{-1}) during 2 hours. Data were expressed as means of pg isoprostanes per mL of culture medium for a minimum of three independent experiments (*: $p<0.01$).

destructive processes occurring as part of the host inflammatory response are responsible for the majority of soft-tissue breakdown leading to periodontal diseases. Chronic periodontitis occurs mainly as a result of activation of host-derived immune and inflammatory mechanisms. Cytokines are inflammatory mediators that play a major role in the pathogenesis of periodontal disease and tissue destruction [38,39]. There is a need to develop new and effective preventive and treatment approaches for periodontal diseases, based on recent advances in host modulation and inflammation resolution [40]. In the present study, we showed that ASCOP significantly decreases the production of two cytokines TNFα and IL-6 in a cell culture model of LPS stimulated macrophages. These results are in agreement with those of others. Studies of Dutot *et al.* [41] reported that a phlorotannin-rich natural extract from *A. nodosum* inhibits the release of pro-inflammatory cytokines. Another study from Bahar *et al.* [42] have also reported that extracts from *A. nodosum* seaweed have potential to suppress the pro-inflammatory response induced by the bacterial LPS in a pig colon model by suppressing LPS-induced pro-inflammatory cytokines IL-8, IL-6, and TNFα genes. Since cytokine release is associated with inflammation and destruction tooth-supporting tissue, these data suggest that ASCOP may contribute to reduction of host cell damage by decreasing secretion of inflammatory mediators [43,44]. Of note, the results in this study are obtained in a macrophage-like cell culture model using an established cell line. Further studies using primary human gingival cells should be performed to confirm this anti-inflammatory properties.

Our results also revealed that ASCOP exhibits antioxidant properties. Indeed ASCOP revealed a capacity to scavenge free radicals such as superoxide anion, hydroxyl radical and peroxyl radical. Free Radical scavenging activity of *A. nodosum* extracts have been previously reported by others [41]. O'Sullivan *et al.* [45] reported that among five different seaweed extracts, *Ascophyllum* showed the highest capacity to scavenge the free radical DPPH (2,2-diphenyl-1-picrylhydrazyl). Wang *et al.* [46] also showed a high correlation between total phenol content of *A. nodosum* and its high scavenging activity towards DPPH and peroxyl radical (ORAC). Recently, Abu *et al.* [17] showed that ascophyllan, a sulfated polysaccharide from *A. nodosum*, was more potent scavenger of superoxide anion than fucoidan. Nonetheless, ascophyllan and fucoidan showed similar scavenging activity towards hydroxyl radical.

In the present study, ASCOP inhibited oxidative stress by reducing lipid peroxidation induced by *P. gingivalis* LPS in gingival epithelial cells. In fact, bacteria produce a number of metabolites, which affect gingival tissue. One irritating agent, LPS is a major constituent of the outer membrane of Gram-negative bacteria and a critical determinant in initiation and progression of periodontal disease. It has been observed that LPS induces the production of reactive oxygen species (ROS) that could initiate lipid peroxidation [47]. Recent studies have demonstrated that epithelial cells also have a functionally active NADPH-oxidase complex for ROS production and oxidative stress responses [48]. Thus in our model, lipid peroxidation observed in LPS-stimulated epithelial gingival cells could involve the activation of NADPH oxidase by LPS leading to superoxide anion production and as a consequence to hydroxyl production. This later free radical is well known to oxidize polyunsaturated fatty acids in membranes. It has already been reported that application of the polyphenolic fraction of *Lonicera caerulea* fruit to LPS-treated human gingival fibroblasts significantly decreased ROS production, a marker of lipid peroxidation [49].

In summary, this study showed that ASCOP added to Ag-zeolite confers synergistic antibacterial and anti-biofilm properties to this complex and that ASCOP alone possess anti-oxidative and anti-inflammatory activities. Ag-zeolite and ASCOP act on oral bacteria and the host immune response, two etiological components involved in periodontitis. Their combination could be a promising compound in prevention and treatment of periodontal diseases. However, the perspectives of development of potential preventive or therapeutic product, containing ASCOP combined with Ag-zeolite, should be validated in *in vivo* models and should be more optimized in terms of galenic formulation and optimal concentrations presenting the minimal side effects on buccal cells and normal flora.

Acknowledgments

The authors would like to thank Yslab (Quimper, France), Algues&Mer (Ouessant, France), IRMAtech (Ploemeur, France) for providing ASCOP and Ag-zeolite, and the Pôle Mer Bretagne (Brest, France) for their scientific support.

We equally thank Hélène Sohli (EA 1254-Université Rennes 1); Brice Martin (EA 1274-Université Rennes 2); Dany Saligaut (EA 1274-Université Rennes 1) for their technical contributions and Céline Allaire (Université Rennes 1) for her editorial assistance.

Author Contributions

Conceived and designed the experiments: ZTS FC AR JC MBM. Performed the experiments: ZTS FC AR. Analyzed the data: ZTS FC JC. Contributed reagents/materials/analysis tools: ZTS FC AR JC MBM. Wrote the paper: ZTS FC JC MBM.

References

1. Petersen PE (2005) The burden of oral disease: challenges to improving oral health in the 21st century. Bull World Health Organ 83: 3.
2. Marsh PD (1992) Microbiological aspects of the chemical control of plaque and gingivitis. J Dent Res 71: 1431–1438.
3. Holt SC, Kesavalu L, Walker S, Genco CA (1999) Virulence factors of *Porphyromonas gingivalis*. Periodontol 2000 20: 168–238.
4. Socransky SS, Haffajee AD (2005) Periodontal microbial ecology. Periodontol 2000 38: 135–187.
5. Lamont RJ, Bevan CA, Gil S, Persson RE, Rosan B (1993) Involvement of *Porphyromonas gingivalis* fimbriae in adherence to *Streptococcus gordonii*. Oral Microbiol Immunol 8: 272–276.
6. Ximenez-Fyvie LA, Haffajee AD, Socransky SS (2000) Comparison of the microbiota of supra- and subgingival plaque in health and periodontitis. J Clin Periodontol 27: 648–657.
7. Lamont RJ, Jenkinson HF (2000) Subgingival colonization by *Porphyromonas gingivalis*. Oral Microbiol Immunol 15: 341–349.
8. Lamont RJ, Yilmaz O (2002) In or out: the invasiveness of oral bacteria. Periodontol 2000 30: 61–69.
9. Travis J, Potempa J (2000) Bacterial proteinases as targets for the development of second-generation antibiotics. Biochim Biophys Acta 1477: 35–50.
10. Fravalo P, Menard C, Bonnaure-Mallet M (1996) Effect of *Porphyromonas gingivalis* on epithelial cell MMP-9 type IV collagenase production. Infect Immun 64: 4940–4945.
11. Darveau RP, Belton CM, Reife RA, Lamont RJ (1998) Local chemokine paralysis, a novel pathogenic mechanism for *Porphyromonas gingivalis*. Infect Immun 66: 1660–1665.
12. Huang GT, Kim D, Lee JK, Kuramitsu HK, Haake SK (2001) Interleukin-8 and intercellular adhesion molecule 1 regulation in oral epithelial cells by selected periodontal bacteria: multiple effects of *Porphyromonas gingivalis* via antagonistic mechanisms. Infect Immun 69: 1364–1372.
13. Mourao PA (2004) Use of sulfated fucans as anticoagulant and antithrombotic agents: future perspectives. Curr Pharm Des 10: 967–981.
14. Choi EM, Kim AJ, Kim YO, Hwang JK (2005) Immunomodulating activity of arabinogalactan and fucoidan in vitro. J Med Food 8: 446–453.
15. Trinchero J, Ponce NM, Cordoba OL, Flores ML, Pampuro S, et al. (2009) Antiretroviral activity of fucoidans extracted from the brown seaweed *Adenocystis utricularis*. Phytother Res 23: 707–712.
16. Qi H, Zhang Q, Zhao T, Chen R, Zhang H, et al. (2005) Antioxidant activity of different sulfate content derivatives of polysaccharide extracted from *Ulva pertusa* (Chlorophyta) in vitro. Int J Biol Macromol 37: 195–199.

17. Abu R, Jiang Z, Ueno M, Okimura T, Yamaguchi K, et al. (2013) *In vitro* antioxidant activities of sulfated polysaccharide ascophyllan isolated from *Ascophyllum nodosum*. Int J Biol Macromol 59: 305–312.

18. Mizuno M, Nishitani Y, Hashimoto T, Kanazawa K (2009) Different suppressive effects of fucoidan and lentinan on IL-8 mRNA expression in in vitro gut inflammation. Biosci Biotechnol Biochem 73: 2324–2325.

19. Yoshida K, Tanagawa M, Atsuta M (1999) Characterization and inhibitory effect of antibacterial dental resin composites incorporating silver-supported materials. J Biomed Mater Res 47: 516–522.

20. Hartford CE, Ziffren SE (1972) The use of 0.5 percent silver nitrate in burns: results in 220 patients. J Trauma 12: 682–688.

21. Tokumaru T, Shimizu Y, Fox CL, Jr. (1974) Antiviral activities of silver sulfadiazine in ocular infection. Res Commun Chem Pathol Pharmacol 8: 151–158.

22. Takai K, Ohtsuka T, Senda Y, Nakao M, Yamamoto K, et al. (2002) Antibacterial properties of antimicrobial-finished textile products. Microbiol Immunol 46: 75–81.

23. De la Rosa-Gomez I, Olguin MT, Alcantara D (2008) Antibacterial behavior of silver-modified clinoptilolite-heulandite rich tuff on coliform microorganisms from wastewater in a column system. J Environ Manage 88: 853–863.

24. De Muynck W, De Belie N, Verstraete W (2010) Antimicrobial mortar surfaces for the improvement of hygienic conditions. J Appl Microbiol 108: 62–72.

25. Odabas ME, Cinar C, Akca G, Araz I, Ulusu T, et al. (2011) Short-term antimicrobial properties of mineral trioxide aggregate with incorporated silver-zeolite. Dent Traumatol 27: 189–194.

26. Inoue Y, Hoshino M, Takahashi H, Noguchi T, Murata T, et al. (2002) Bactericidal activity of Ag-zeolite mediated by reactive oxygen species under aerated conditions. J Inorg Biochem 92: 37–42.

27. Chandler SF, Dodds JH (1983) The effect of phosphate, nitrogen and sucrose on the production of phenolics and solasodine in callus cultures of *Solanum laciniatum*. Plant Cell Rep 2: 205–208.

28. Prior RL, Hoang H, Gu L, Wu X, Bacchiocca M, et al. (2003) Assays for hydrophilic and lipophilic antioxidant capacity (oxygen radical absorbance capacity (ORAC(FL))) of plasma and other biological and food samples. J Agric Food Chem 51: 3273–3279.

29. Youssef H, Groussard C, Pincemail J, Moussa E, Jacob C, et al. (2009) Exercise-induced oxidative stress in overweight adolescent girls: roles of basal insulin resistance and inflammation and oxygen overconsumption. Int J Obes (Lond) 33: 447–455.

30. McCord JM, Fridovich I (1969) Superoxide dismutase. An enzymic function for erythrocuprein (hemocuprein). J Biol Chem 244: 6049–6055.

31. Nagayama K, Iwamura Y, Shibata T, Hirayama I, Nakamura T (2002) Bactericidal activity of phlorotannins from the brown alga *Ecklonia kurome*. J Antimicrob Chemother 50: 889–893.

32. Sandsdalen E, Haug T, Stensvag K, Styrvold OB (2003) The antibacterial effect of a polyhydroxylated fucophlorethol from the marine brown alga, *Fucus vesiculosus*. World J Microbiol Biotechnol 19: 777–782.

33. Sabbani S, Gallego-Perez D, Nagy A, J W, Hansford D, et al. (2010) Synthesis of silver-zeolite films on micropatterned porous alumina and its application as an antimicrobial substrate. Micropor Mesopor Mater 135: 131–136.

34. Guerra R, Lima E, Viniegra M, Guzman G, Lara V (2012) Growth of *Escherichia coli* and *Salmonella typhi* inhibited by fractal silver nanoparticles supported on zeolites. Micropor Mesopor Mater 147: 267–273.

35. Lima E, Guerra R, Lara V, Guzman A (2013) Gold nanoparticles as efficient antimicrobial agents for *Escherichia coli* and *Salmonella typhi*. Chem Cent J 7: 11–17.

36. Kolenbrander PE, Palmer RJ, Jr., Periasamy S, Jakubovics NS (2010) Oral multispecies biofilm development and the key role of cell-cell distance. Nat Rev Microbiol 8: 471–480.

37. Kornman KS (1999) Host modulation as a therapeutic strategy in the treatment of periodontal disease. Clin Infect Dis 28: 520–526.

38. Kantarci A, Hasturk H, Van Dyke TE (2006) Host-mediated resolution of inflammation in periodontal diseases. Periodontol 2000 40: 144–163.

39. Dixon DR, Bainbridge BW, Darveau RP (2004) Modulation of the innate immune response within the periodontium. Periodontol 2000 35: 53–74.

40. Tonetti MS, Chapple IL, Working Group 3 of Seventh European Workshop on P (2011) Biological approaches to the development of novel periodontal therapies–consensus of the Seventh European Workshop on Periodontology. J Clin Periodontol 38 Suppl 11: 114–118.

41. Dutot M, Fagon R, Hemon M, Rat P (2012) Antioxidant, anti-inflammatory, and anti-senescence activities of a phlorotannin-rich natural extract from brown seaweed *Ascophyllum nodosum*. Appl Biochem Biotechnol 167: 2234–2240.

42. Bahar B, O'Doherty JV, Hayes M, Sweeney T (2012) Extracts of brown seaweeds can attenuate the bacterial lipopolysaccharide-induced pro-inflammatory response in the porcine colon ex vivo. J Anim Sci 90 Suppl 4: 46–48.

43. Okada H, Murakami S (1998) Cytokine expression in periodontal health and disease. Crit Rev Oral Biol Med 9: 248–266.

44. Holt SC, Ebersole JL (2005) *Porphyromonas gingivalis*, *Treponema denticola*, and *Tannerella forsythia*: the "red complex", a prototype polybacterial pathogenic consortium in periodontitis. Periodontol 2000 38: 72–122.

45. O'Sullivan AM, O'Callaghan YC, O'Grady MN, Queguineur B, Hanniffy D, et al. (2011) *In vitro* and cellular antioxidant activities of seaweed extracts prepared from five brown seaweeds harvested in spring from the west coast of Ireland. Food Chem 126 1064–1070.

46. Wang Q, Zhou X, Huang D (2009) Role for *Porphyromonas gingivalis* in the progression of atherosclerosis. Med Hypotheses 72: 71–73.

47. Nishio K, Horie M, Akazawa Y, Shichiri M, Iwahashi H, et al. (2013) Attenuation of lipopolysaccharide (LPS)-induced cytotoxicity by tocopherols and tocotrienols. Redox Biol 1: 97–103.

48. Cha B, Lim JW, Kim KH, Kim H (2010) HSP90beta interacts with Rac1 to activate NADPH oxidase in *Helicobacter pylori*-infected gastric epithelial cells. Int J Biochem Cell Biol 42: 1455–1461.

49. Zdarilova A, Rajnochova Svobodova A, Chytilova K, Simanek V, Ulrichova J (2010) Polyphenolic fraction of Lonicera caerulea L. fruits reduces oxidative stress and inflammatory markers induced by lipopolysaccharide in gingival fibroblasts. Food Chem Toxicol 48: 1555–1561.

9

Dimethyl Fumarate Protects Pancreatic Islet Cells and Non-Endocrine Tissue in L-Arginine-Induced Chronic Pancreatitis

Lourdes Robles, Nosratola D. Vaziri, Shiri Li, Yuichi Masuda, Chie Takasu, Mizuki Takasu, Kelly Vo, Seyed H. Farzaneh, Michael J. Stamos, Hirohito Ichii*

Departments of Surgery and Medicine, University of California Irvine, Irvine, CA, United States of America

Abstract

Background: Chronic pancreatitis (CP) is a progressive disorder resulting in the destruction and fibrosis of the pancreatic parenchyma which ultimately leads to impairment of the endocrine and exocrine functions. Dimethyl Fumarate (DMF) was recently approved by FDA for treatment of patients with multiple sclerosis. DMF's unique anti-oxidant and anti-inflammatory properties make it an interesting drug to test on other inflammatory conditions. This study was undertaken to determine the effects of DMF on islet cells and non-endocrine tissue in a rodent model of L-Arginine-induced CP.

Methods: Male Wistar rats fed daily DMF (25 mg/kg) or vehicle by oral gavage were given 5 IP injections of L-Arginine (250 mg/100 g×2, 1 hr apart). Rats were assessed with weights and intra-peritoneal glucose tolerance tests (IPGTT, 2 g/kg). Islets were isolated and assessed for islet mass and viability with flow cytometry. Non-endocrine tissue was assessed for histology, myeloperoxidase (MPO), and lipid peroxidation level (MDA). *In vitro* assessments included determination of heme oxygenase (HO-1) protein expression by Western blot.

Results: Weight gain was significantly reduced in untreated CP group at 6 weeks. IPGTT revealed significant impairment in untreated CP group and its restoration with DMF therapy (P <0.05). Untreated CP rats had pancreatic atrophy, severe acinar architectural damage, edema, and fatty infiltration as well as elevated MDA and MPO levels, which were significantly improved by DMF treatment. After islet isolation, the volume of non-endocrine tissue was significantly smaller in untreated CP group. Although islet counts were similar in the two groups, islet viability was significantly reduced in untreated CP group and improved with DMF treatment. *In vitro* incubation of human pancreatic tissue with DMF significantly increased HO-1 expression.

Conclusion: Administration of DMF attenuated L-Arginine-induced CP and islet function in rats. DMF treatment could be a possible strategy to improve clinical outcome in patients with CP.

Editor: Zoltan Rakonczay, University of Szeged, Hungary

Funding: This study was in part supported by grants from: NIH-NCRR UL1 TR000153, KL2 TR000147, and the Juvenile Diabetes Research Foundation International 17-2011-609. The funders had no role in the study design, data collection and analysis, decision to publish, or preparation of the manuscript.

Competing Interests: The authors have declared that no competing interests exist.

* Email: hichii@uci.edu

Introduction

Chronic pancreatitis (CP) is a progressive inflammatory disorder that results in the destruction and fibrosis of the pancreatic parenchyma and its endocrine and exocrine dysfunctions. Although CP can develop from repeated attacks of AP, this is not the only mechanism implicated. The specific pathogenesis is uncertain and has thus resulted in a lack of progress in developing specific therapies [1,2]. Data suggest that the incidence of CP continues to rise [3]. In structured questionnaires, patients with CP described themselves as living with a complex illness with a significant impact on their physical, social, and psychological wellbeing [4]. Likewise, financial problems are more frequent amongst patients with CP. In a United Kingdom series, 37% of CP patients were unemployed [5]. Moreover, the mortality rate appears to be higher in patient with long standing CP. At 5 years the survival rate is initially high at 97% however, this drops to between 45% and 63% at 20 years.

Currently, the main treatment for this debilitating disease is supportive care through nutrition and pain control. Dimethyl Fumarate (DMF) was recently approved by the Food and Drug Administration (FDA) for use in the treatment of patients with multiple sclerosis. The exact mechanism of action of DMF has yet to be clearly determined, however its unique antioxidant and inflammatory properties have been shown in experimental inflammatory conditions [6,7,8,9,10,11].

The aim of the present study was to test the hypothesis that DMF treatment would protect islets and non-endocrine cells from oxidative stress and inflammation caused by chronic pancreatitis.

Methods

Chronic pancreatitis

This study was carried out in strict accordance with the Guidelines for the Care and Use of Laboratory Animals of the National Institutes of Health. The protocol was approved by Institutional Animal Care and Use Committee of University of California, Irvine (Permit Number: 2012–3069). Animals were purchased from Charles River (Wilmington, MA). L-arginine and DMF were purchased from Sigma (St. Louis, MO). Male Wistar rats (250–300 g) were fed ad libitum on a standard diet with free access to water and maintained on a 12 h light/dark cycle. The rats were divided into four groups: Control (n = 3), DMF alone treated (n = 3), L-arginine + DMF-treated (n = 6), and L-arginine + vehicle- treated rats (n = 6).

All surgical procedures were performed under isoflurane anesthesia (1–5%) (Phoenix, St. Joseph, MO) adjusted to achieve no movement with paw prick testing. All efforts were made to minimize suffering. Experimental animals were given oral DMF (25 mg/kg) dissolved in methyl cellulose and fed via oral gavage 24 hours prior to initiating pancreatitis and daily thereafter until the animals were sacrificed. The dose of DMF was based on previously published studies [12] and preliminary studies done in our laboratory. The healthy control rats as well as the subgroup of rats with L-Arginine induced CP were given methyl cellulose vehicle (0.08%, 2.5–3 ml/rat). Weekly body weight assessments (Denver Instrument, Bohemia, NY) and change in body weight from baseline were calculated.

L-arginine

20% L-arginine was dissolved in normal saline and filtered through a syringe filter with pH adjusted to 7.0. The solution was administered to non-fasted rats in two intraperitoneal injections at a dose of 250 mg/100 g body weight, each injection separated by 1 hour. L-Arginine injections were given a total of 5 times three days apart (Days 1, 5, 9, 13, 17) and animals were sacrificed after 7 weeks (on day 54, 37 days after the last L-arginine injection) [13]. Animals, control and experimental, received Buprenorphine (Reckitt Benkiser, Richmond, VA) pain medication (0.01 mg/kg) IM twice a day for two days after each L-arginine injection. Animals had accesses to regular food and water and were not fasted prior to L-arginine injections. All efforts were made to minimize pain and suffering. Experimental animals continued to receive daily DMF via gavage along with a standard diet.

Intraperitoneal glucose tolerance Test

Biweekly 2 g/kg intraperitoneal glucose tolerance test (IPGTT) were performed after rats were fasted overnight. IPGTT assessments were conducted using a 45% glucose solution (Corning, Manassas, VA) diluted to a 20% solution using normal saline and given to fasted rats at a dose of 2 g/kg. Capillary blood glucose levels were obtained via tail prick using a standard glucometer (Contour, Bayer, Mishawaka, IN) prior to injection and at 10, 30, 60, 90, 120, and 150 minutes.

Histology

At the end of the study period, rats were sacrificed under isoflurane (Pirmal Critical Care, Bethleham, PA) anesthesia. Blood and tissue were obtained. Rat pancreases were weighed, measured and a small 0.2×0.2 cm section was cut from the pancreas tail for biochemical and histological assessments. Rat pancreas sections (5 μm thick) were fixed in 10% buffered formalin, embedded in paraffin blocks, and sectioned. The pancreas tissue was processed for hematoxylin-eosin (H&E) staining using standard techniques. Using Schmidt criteria, interstitial edema, leukocyte infiltration, acinar cell destruction, and total scores were evaluated individually by two pathologists blinded to the source of the histology sections they evaluated. Pancreatitis was scored using a quantitative grading system as described by Schmidt et al [14]. Classification (Table 1) is based on the presence of edema, leukocyte infiltration, acinar cell necrosis, and hemorrhage.

Pancreatic malondialdehyde content (MDA)

Pancreatic MDA was measured by thiobarbituric acid colorimetric method using MDA assay kit (Cayman Chemical Company, Ann Arbor, MI). Each pancreas tissue (100 mg) was placed in lysis buffer (RIPA, Thermo Scientific, Piscataway, NJ) and homogenized using a hand held Homogenizer (Power Gen, Fischer Scientific).

Samples were then centrifuged at 1200 RPM at 4°C. The absorbance of the supernatant was measured by spectrophotometry at 535 nm for MDA content, as MDA reacted with thiobarbituric acid and turned pink after a 1 hour boil. The MDA concentration was calculated from the standard curve and expressed as μM.

Pancreatic Myeloperoxidase (MPO) content

Pancreatic MPO was measured using a standard colorimetric ELISA kit (BioVision, Milpitas, CA). Each pancreatic tissue (100 mg) was placed in MPO assay buffer (Bio Vision) and homogenized using a hand held Homogenizer (Power Gen, Fischer Scientific). Samples were then centrifuged at 13,000 G at 4°C. Supernatant (50 μl) at a 1:100 dilution was added to the reaction mix and incubated for 30 minutes at 25°C. The absorbance of the supernatant was measured by spectrophotometry at 412 nM. The MPO concentration was calculated from the standard curve. MPO activity is reported as nmole/min/ml = mU/ml. One unit of MPO activity is defined as the amount of enzyme that hydrolyzes the substrate and generates taurine chloramine to consume 1.0 μmole of TNB per minute.

Islet isolation and assessment of endocrine function

After removing and weighing the pancreas, the pancreatic duct was cannulated and a small piece of plastic cannula was sutured into the pancreatic duct. Pancreatic islet isolation was carried out as described previously [15,16]. Briefly, the plastic tubing attached to the pancreatic duct was accessed and 20 mg Collagenase V (Sigma-Aldrich, St. Louis, Mo., USA) was infused into the pancreas. The pancreases of 4 rats per group were harvested, digested and islets were isolated by passing the tissue through a 500 μm mesh filter using Ficoll density solution. The islets were stained with dithizone and counted to estimate the islet equivalent (IEQ). Islet samples were transferred to 35 mm Petri dish with grid filled with1 mL of PBS and 10 drops of dithizone. The petri dish with islet sample was placed on inverted microscope to count. There is a scale in the left eye piece with each tick mark representing 25 μm when using the 4× objective. Islets of varying diameters are normalized to a number of Islet Equivalents of 150 μm diameter by mathematically compensating for their volumes. An islet with 150 um in diameter is counted as 1 IEQ [17,18].

Table 1. Quantitative grading score for pancreatitis.

Score	0	1	2	3
Interstitial edema	none	Interlobular	Lobule involved	Isolated island like acinar cells
Leukocyte infiltration	none	<20%	20–50%	>50%
Acinar cell necrosis	none	<5%	5–20%	>20%
Hemorrhage	none	<5%	5–20%	>20%

Assessment of islet viability

The cultured islets were dissociated into single cell suspensions using the previously described method [19]. Aliquots of 700 IEQ were re-suspended in 1 mL accutase (Innovative Cell Technologies, Inc, San Diego, CA) in a 15-mL tube, incubated at 37°C for 10 minutes, and then dispersed by gentle pipetting. Digestion was stopped with 1 mL cold newborn calf serum (NCS, HyClone labs, Logan, UT). Washed Cells were transferred into filtered flow cytometry (FACS) tubes (BD Falcon, Franklin Lakes, NJ) to remove undigested tissue. The cells were then stained with 100 ng/mL of tetramethylrhodamine ethyl ester (TMRE; Molecular Probes) for 30 min at 37°C in Phosphate Buffered Saline. TMRE selectively binds to mitochondrial membranes, allowing for detection of apoptosis. After washing, cells were stained with 7-aminoactinomycin D (7-AAD; Molecular Probes), which binds to DNA when cell membrane permeability is altered after cell death. Analysis was performed by flow cytometry (Accuri C6 cytometers, Ann Arbor, MI, BD Bioscience) Acurri (Accuri C6 software, San Jose, CA) software was used for analysis.

Assessment of alpha and beta ratio

The experiment was accomplished similarly to the above protocol prior to staining. Single cell suspensions were placed in 4% paraformaldehyde for 10 minutes at room temperature. After successive PBS (Corning, Manassas, VA) washes, the cells were stained with chicken polyclonal antibody to insulin (1:100; Abcam Inc., Cambridge, MA) and mouse monoclonal antibody to glucagon (1:100, Sigma, St. Louis, MO). Secondary antibodies were then applied, with goat anti-chicken (1: 200; Alexa Fluor 488 goat anti-chicken IgG, Life Technologies, Grand Island, NY) and

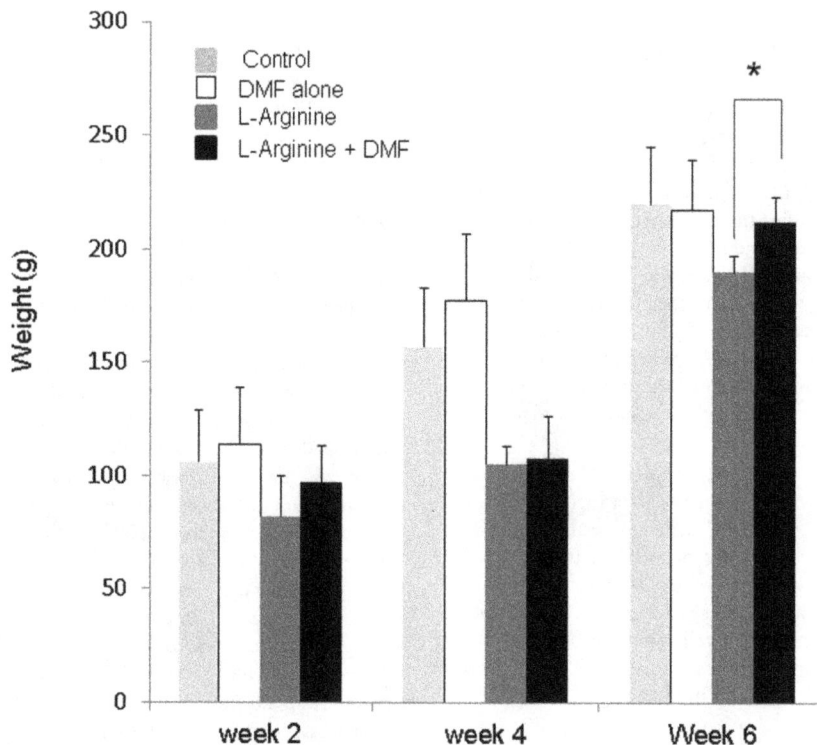

Body weight gain from baseline

Figure 1. Average change in body weight. Body weights were similar for all four experimental groups: control, DMF-alone, L-Arginine, and L-Arginine + DMF (n = 3, 3, 6, 6) at baseline and weeks 2, 4 and 6. There was a significant difference of the change in baseline weight at 6 weeks between L-Arginine and L-Arginine + DMF. * indicates a significant p<0.05 value. Data represent Mean ±S.D.

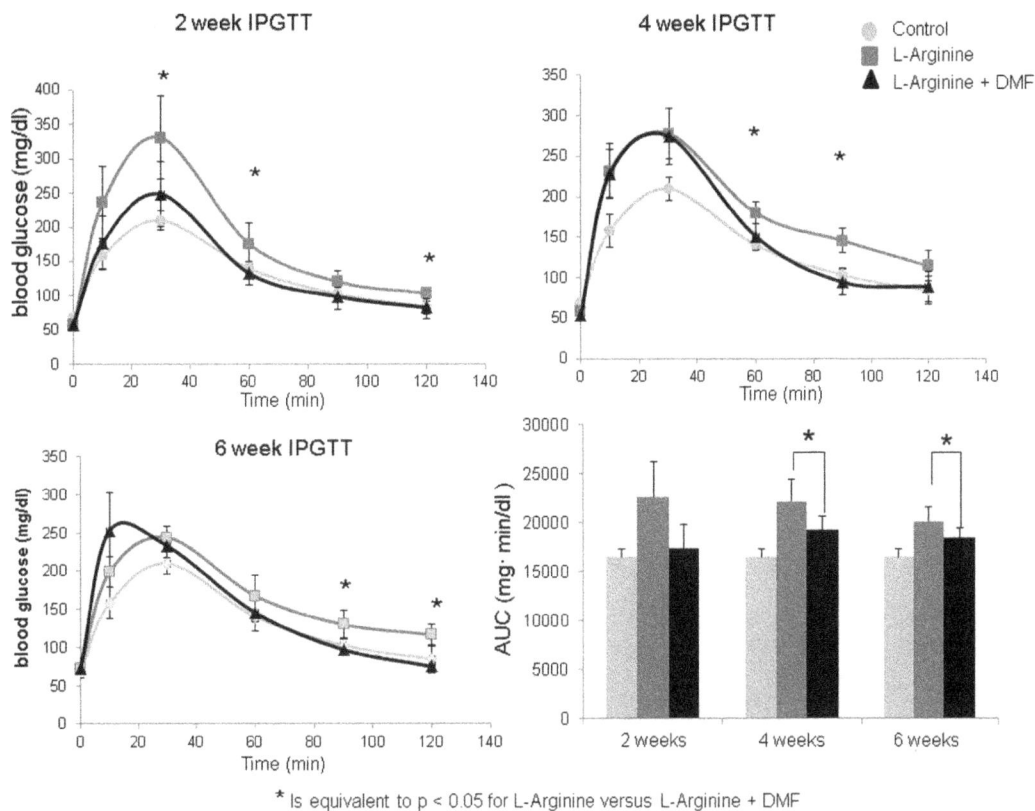

Figure 2. IPGTT at 2, 4, and 6 weeks. IPGTT conducted at 2 weeks reveals a significant change in the blood glucose level for L-Arginine (n = 6) and L-Arginine + DMF group (n = 6) at 30 and 60 minutes. At 4 weeks the differences between the two groups were seen at 60 and 90 minutes. Lastly, at 6 weeks there was a significant change between L-Arginine and L-Arginine + DMF group at 90 and 120 minutes. These differences indicate L-Arginine had a slower return to baseline glucose levels compared to the rats supplemented with DMF. An * indicates a significant differences with P<0.05. AUC was calculated. L-Arginine + DMF had a statistically lower blood glucose AUC compared to L-Arginine alone and results were similar to control rats for all weeks. * is equivalent to P<0.05 for L-Arginine versus L-Arginine + DMF.

goat anti-mouse (1: 200; Alexa Fluor 647 goat anti-chicken IgG, Life Technologies, Grand Island, NY). Omission of the primary antibody served as negative control. Analysis was performed by flow cytometry (Accuri C6 cytometers, Ann Arbor, MI, BD Bioscience) Acurri (Accuri C6 software, San Jose, CA) software was used for analysis.

In vitro human pancreatic tissue studies

In vitro studies were performed on human pancreatic tissue obtained from NIH/JDRF sponsored integrated islet distribution program (IIDP, https://iidp.coh.org/) or from collaborators. Institutional Review Board exemption was obtained at University of California Irvine. Our study does not involve any information including living individuals, identifiable and private information.

Human pancreatic tissues were obtained after removal of islet cells. Human non-endocrine pancreatic tissue was treated with DMF at preconditioned concentrations dissolved in dimethyl sulfoxide (Sigma, St. Louis, MO). Human pancreatic tissue was cultured in Roswell Park Memorial Institute (RPMI-1640) solution containing additionally 10% NCS and Penicillin 100 U/ml/ Streptomycin 50 μg/ml (Corning, Manassas, VA).

Human tissue was cultured with or without DMF. After a culture period of twenty four hours the tissue was homogenized (Power Gen 125, Fischer Scientific, Pittsburg, PA) with Lysis Buffer (RIPA, Thermo Scientific, Piscataway, NJ). Protein aliquots (45 μg) were mixed with sample buffer (Bio-Rad laboratories, Richmond, CA) boiled for 5 minutes and separated via 4–12%

BIS TRIS (2-[Bis(2-hydroxyethyl)amino]-2-(hydroxymethyl)-1, 3-propanediol) (Life Technologies, Carlsbad, CA). After transfer to nitrocellulose membranes (Biorad) the membranes were blocked with PBS/0.1%Tween containing 2% dry milk for 90 minutes at room temperature. The membranes were then probed with mouse monoclonal antibody to heme oxygenase (HO-1) (1:1000) and mouse monoclonal antibody to β-actin (1:1000) (Cell Signaling, Danvers, MA) followed by rabbit anti-mouse IgG (1:3000). The membranes were developed with an enhanced chemoluminescence detection kit (Bio-Rad) and exposed to X-ray film (Kodak, Rochester, NY). To evaluate the results of the western blot, the relative intensities of individual bands were determined with ImageQuant TL 7.0 (GE healthcare Life Sciences, Pittsburg, PA).

Statistical Analysis

Student's *t* test and one-way analysis of variance (ANOVA) were used in statistical analysis of the data using Excel for Windows software (Microsoft, Redmond, WA). P values equal to or less than 0.05 were considered significant. Data are expressed as mean ± SD.

Results

Effects of DMF on body weight in L-Arginine-induced CP

The average body weights for control, DMF alone treated, L-Arginine vehicle treated, and L-Arginine with DMF treated rats were similar at baseline and at three and six weeks during the

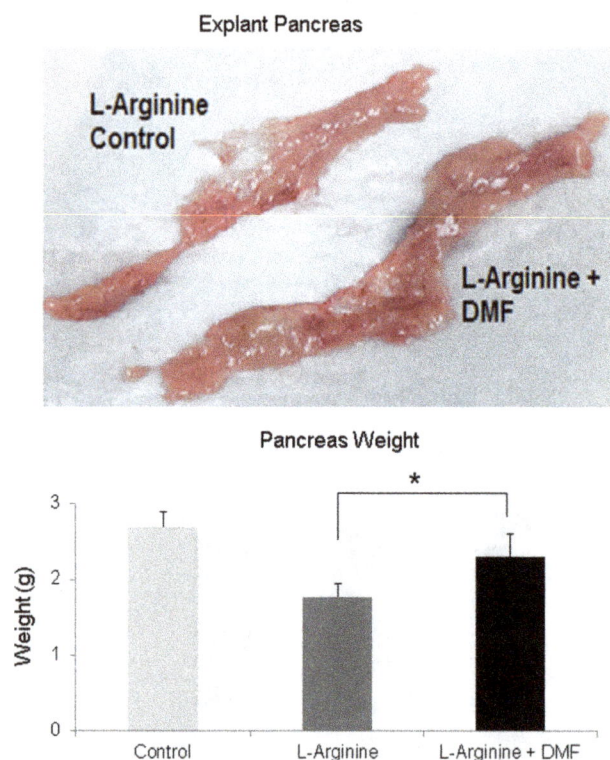

Figure 3. Explant pancreas weight. At explantation, pancreases from the control, L-Arginine and L-Arginine+ DMF rats were weighed at the end of 7 weeks. Results revealed a statistically larger pancreas weight (g) in the L-Arginine + DMF group. The image above shows an atrophic pancreas in the L-Arginine group compared to the L-Arginine + DMF group. The bar graphs demonstrated an average of 6 total L-Arginine rats and 6 L-Arginine + DMF rats. * indicates a significant $p < 0.05$ value. Data represent Mean ±S.D.

experiment. Compared to baseline the average weight gain in the L-Arginine + DMF treated group was similar to that found in the control and DMF alone treated rats. However, average weight gain was significantly reduced in the L-Arginine alone-treated group ($P < 0.05$) at 6 weeks (Figure 1).

Treatment with DMF improved glucose tolerance in rats with L-Arginine- induced CP

Intra-peritoneal glucose tolerance test performed at two, four, and six weeks revealed significant impairment in the untreated and significant improvement in the DMF-treated group at several time points (Figure 2). Moreover, the area under the curve (AUC) for the IPGTT revealed significantly improved glucose tolerance, as seen with lower blood glucoses, in the DMF treated rats (Figure 2).

Treatment with DMF improved pancreas pathology in rats with L-Arginine-induced CP

On explanation, following 7 weeks of L-Arginine induction, the pancreas of the L-Arginine alone treated rats was visibly atrophic and had a lower weight (g) compared to the L-Arginine + DMF treated rats ($p < 0.05$) (Figure 3). Pancreases of the DMF alone treated rats appeared grossly similar to the control rats' pancreas (Data not shown).

Administration of L-Arginine in rats caused significant histological changes in the pancreas including severe acinar architectural damage, edema, and fatty infiltration. Treatment with oral DMF resulted in significant ($p < 0.05$) reductions in acinar architectural damage, edema, and fatty infiltration (Figure 4&5). Moreover, the severity score determined by two pathologists who were blinded to the source of the histology sections, was significantly higher in the L-Arginine alone rats compared to the L-Arginine + DMF rats ($p < 0.05$) (Figure 5, Table 2). The severity scores in the normal and DMF alone treated rats were 0. Although, L-arginine has a mechanism of action that remains unclear there is evidence to support that L-arginine exerts its effects by producing oxidative stress and accumulation of nitric oxide *in vivo* [20]. DMF was extremely effective in protecting the treated rats against L-arginine induced chronic pancreatic changes most likely from the reduction in oxidative stress.

Improved biochemical parameters were seen in pancreatic tissue of rats treated with DMF

MPO catalyzes conversion of chloride and hydrogen peroxide to hypochlorite and is secreted actively by neutrophils during inflammatory conditions [21]. MPO was measured as a marker of inflammatory stress. MDA is a byproduct of lipid peroxidation and a marker of cellular damage and oxidative stress. Both the pancreatic MPO and MDA levels were significantly higher in the L-Arginine than in the control group and were significantly lower in the L-Arginine + DMF treated rats compared to the L-Arginine alone rats ($P < 0.05$)(Figure 6). The observed reduction of MPO and MDA levels demonstrates the efficacy of DMF in attenuating oxidative and inflammatory stress in this model.

Islets from each experimental group were isolated and compared. The pancreatic tissue volume (mainly acinar cells) was significantly larger in the L-Arginine + DMF group than in the L-Arginine alone group (Figure 7). The smaller non-endocrine pellet corresponds to the atrophy observed on the gross examination of pancreas in the L-Arginine alone group. Quantitatively, the number of islets was similar among all groups; however, the islets had improved viability on flow cytometry in the L-Arginine + DMF group compared to the L-Arginine alone group. The beta/alpha ratio appeared lower in the L-Arginine alone group but the difference did not reach statistical significance (Figure 7). The islets from the DMF treated rats were resistant to cell death and apoptosis *in vitro* which may account for the improved glucose tolerance in the rats *in vivo*.

HO-1 was upregulated in human pancreatic tissue treated with DMF in vitro

To explore the effect of DMF on expression of the pancreatic antioxidant enzyme HO-1, Western blot was performed 24 hours after incubation of pancreatic tissue with and without media containing DMF. Western blot revealed a significant increase in the HO-1 expression in DMF-treated human islets (Figure 8). Enhanced production of the key antioxidant enzyme in pancreatic tissue treated with DMF supports the hypothesis that DMF ameliorates oxidative stress through regulation of anti-oxidative enzymes.

Discussion

Due to the significant life changing processes that affect patients with CP, it is imperative that more effective treatments are explored. The results of this study revealed a pronounced difference in the pathology, histology, and pancreatic biochemical markers between the DMF treated animals and those given the vehicle alone. Our data indicates an overall improvement in the inflammatory and oxidative stress in the DMF treated animals as evidenced by the lowered levels of MDA and MPO. Although,

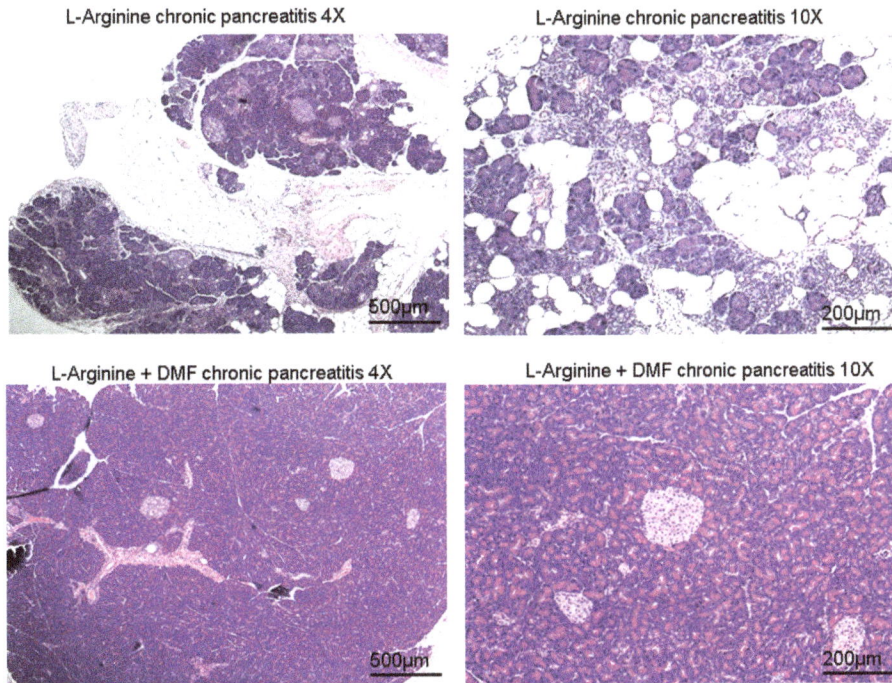

Figure 4. L-arginine induced chronic pancreatitis in a rodent model. Representative photomicrograph of an H&E stained section of pancreas after 7 weeks of chronic L-Arginine induction. L-Arginine + DMF treated rats had significantly reduced severity of destruction of acinar architecture, perilobular edema, and infiltration of fat.

fibrosis is a prominent feature of clinical chronic pancreatitis, we did not appreciate significant fibrosis in our model. Our findings were similar to the results achieved by Yamaguchi et al [13] in which the destroyed pancreas was replaced by fatty tissue instead.

Although this model does not fully resemble clinical CP, the use of L-arginine-induced CP in this study was effective in determining the effects of DMF on protection of islets and non-endocrine pancreatic tissue in experimental CP. Although our islets appeared

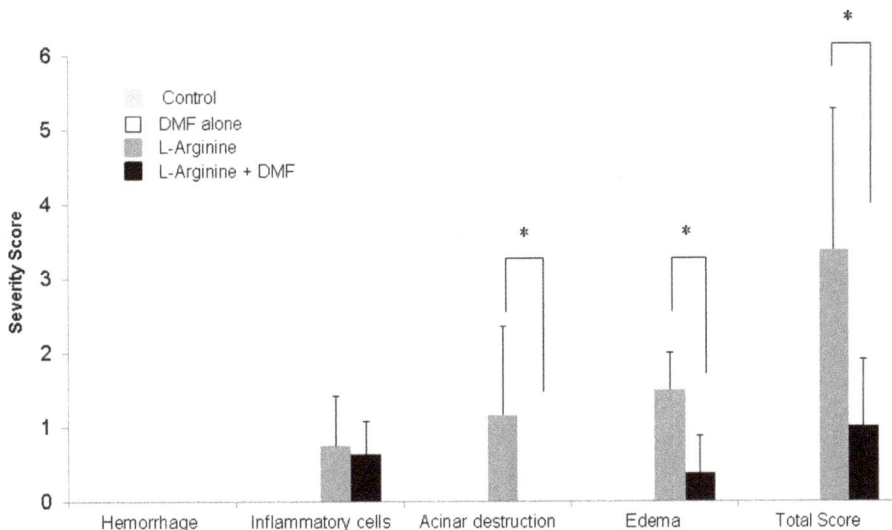

Figure 5. Quantitative chronic pancreatitis Score: hemorrhage, interstitial edema, leukocyte infiltration, acinar cell destruction, and average in total pancreatitis score. Histological pancreas slides were evaluated by two pathologists blinded to the source of the histology sections and given a score based on severity from 0–3 based on four criteria: hemorrhage, inflammatory cell infiltration, acinar destruction, and edema. The total score was also calculated. Based on quantitative scores for all four criteria there was a significantly higher severity score for L-arginine compared to L-arginine + DMF group. The severity scores in the normal and DMF alone treated rats were 0. (* indicates a significant $p < 0.05$ value for L-arginine versus L-Arginine + DMF).

Table 2. Chronic pancreatitis histology score.

Groups	Inflammatory Cells	Acinar destruction	Edema	Hemorrhage	Total score
Control	0	0	0	0	0
DMF alone	0	0	0	0	0
L-arginine	0.75±0.66	1.16±1.2	1.5±0.5	0	3.38±2.36
L-arginine + DMF	0.625±0.45	0	0.375±0.5	0	1±0.95

histologically normal and similar islet yield was obtained, islet cell viability was significantly impaired in vehicle-treated and improved with DMF administration.

It is postulated that the anti-oxidant effects of DMF gave the vulnerable islets the fortitude to withstand the stress of chronic L-Arginine-induced inflammation and the stress of tissue isolation. Given this finding, one would expect to see improved glucose tolerance tests as was observed. Enhanced glucose tolerance was observed by the DMF treatment. This observation suggest that by attenuating oxidative stress and fortifying the antioxidant capacity, DMF was effective in improve glucose homeostasis *in vivo*.

This phenomenon was also replicated in a study by Weaver et al. who established a CP model in a rat by daily L-Arginine injections for up to four weeks. After four weeks only single isolated acini remained within connective tissue however normal islets were seen histologically. Despite histologically normal islets, impairments in glucose homeostasis were seen in rats given chronic L-arginine injections, with significant changes seen on glucose tolerance tests between weeks two through four [22].

The endocrine pancreas develops as a highly organized microvascular network with elegant capillary fenestrations largely dependent on vascular endothelial growth factor (VEGF). Although, normal appearing islets were seen histologically in our study, severe destruction of neighboring acini were encountered and it is postulated that this highly organized capillary network was also disrupted. In an elegant study, Kostromina and associate showed that knockout mice of the signal transducer and activator transcription 3 (STAT-3), a transcription factor regulating VEGF, exhibited glucose intolerance and impaired insulin secretion *in vivo* but normal insulin secretion and equivalence in isolated islets *in vitro* [23].

Moreover, it has been established that beta cells are particularly vulnerable to oxidative stress. Endogenous antioxidant enzymes existing within host tissues primarily protect from excessive levels of reactive oxygen species. An important consideration would be the level of the host's antioxidant defenses within the cells. Islets are scattered throughout the whole pancreas and comprise only 1–2% of pancreatic tissue while acinar cells comprise 80–85% in the pancreas. It has been reported that the islets have very low level of

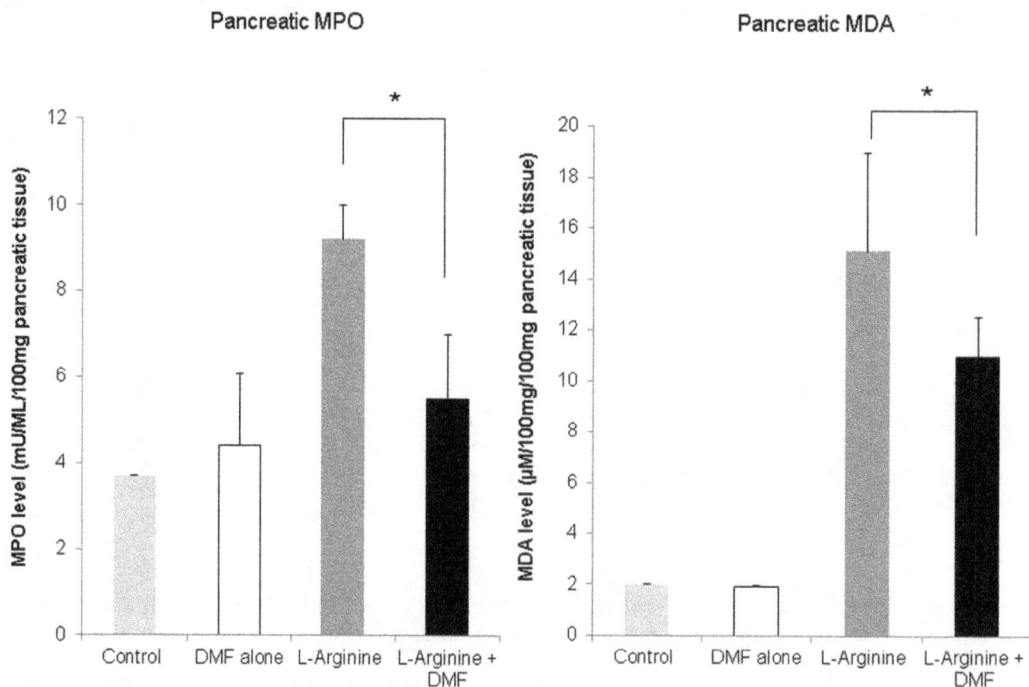

Figure 6. Effects of DMF on pancreatic MDA and MPO. MDA and MPO level in pancreatic tissue were determined after 7 weeks of chronic L-Arginine induction. There was a significant reduction of both pancreatic MDA and MPO levels in the L-Arginine + DMF treated rats (n = 3) compared to the L-Arginine alone treated rats (n = 3). There were no effects of DMF observed on MDA and MPO level under the condition of no L-Arginine induction. * indicates a significant p<0.05 value. Data represent Mean ±S.D.

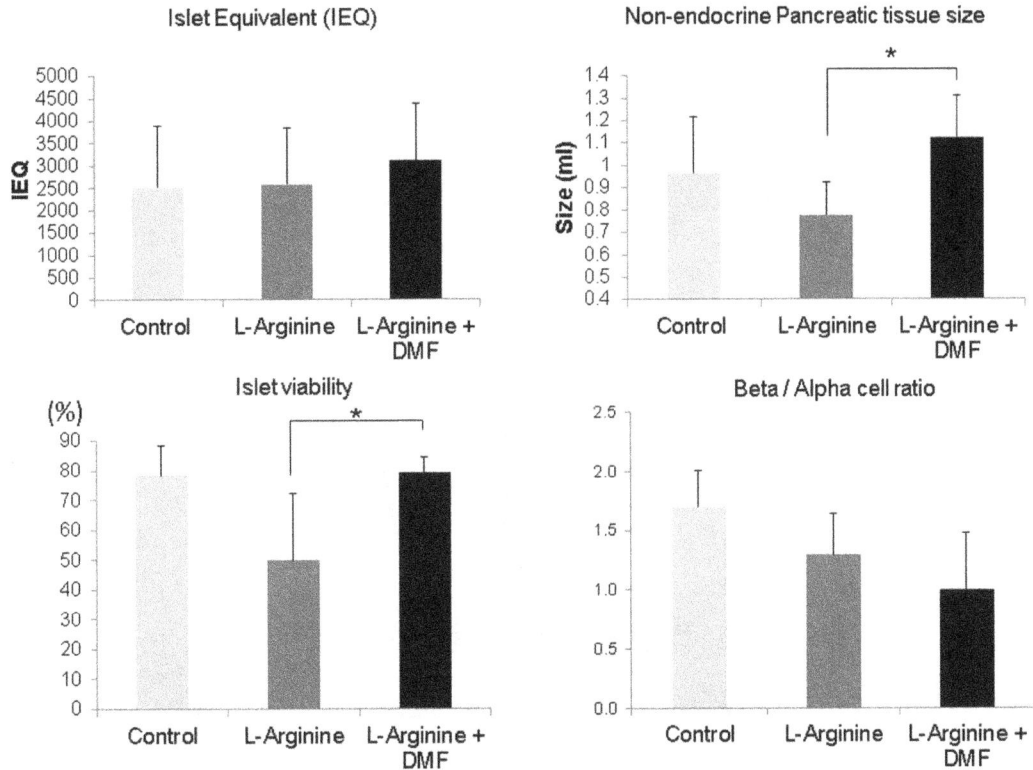

Figure 7. Endocrine and non-endocrine cells characteristics after isolation. After isolation of islets, the islet number was found to be similar between L-Arginine (n=6) and L-arginine + DMF group (n=6), however, the pancreatic tissue volume remaining after extraction of islets was significantly larger in the L-Arginine + DMF group compared to the L-Arginine alone group. Quantitatively, the islet number was similar among all groups. Islet viability in the L-Arginine + DMF group was significantly higher but beta/alpha ratio was similar. * indicates a significant p<0.05 value. Data represent Mean ±S.D.

intrinsic antioxidant enzyme expression and activity, including superoxide dismutase, catalase, and glutathione peroxidase [24]. However, the level of antioxidant enzyme expression in each type of human pancreatic endocrine and exocrine cells has yet to be reported. In previous experiments, (unpublished data) we have found beta cells to have a particularly low level of antioxidant enzymes compared to alpha cells. It is therefore, reasonable to deduce that improving the endogenous antioxidant capacity of the rats would enhance the viability of the islets exposed to chronic oxidant stress and improve glucose tolerance as was observed in this study.

Dimethyl Fumarate has a unique antioxidant and anti-inflammatory spectrum. Although the mechanism of DMF action remains unidentified, its low side effect profile has enabled its use and repurposing for over 20 years. Fumaric acid esters were first employed in the treatment of psoriasis under the trade name Fumaderm. This was based on the anti-proliferative effect of this compound on lymphocytes. Later reports found that DMF selectively up-regulated Th2 cytokines and suppressed a Th1 response [7,25,26]. Subsequent studies showed that DMF reduces expression of genes encoding pro-inflammatory cytokines and chemokines, and increases expression of anti-oxidant molecules [26,27] – effects likely to contribute to its antipsoriasis efficacy. These findings have led to increased interest in using DMF in treatment of other auto-immune or inflammatory diseases, including multiple sclerosis (MS). Recently, clinical trials demonstrated that in patients with multiple sclerosis, DMF (BG-12) significantly reduced the proportion of patients who had a relapse, the annualized relapse rate, the rate of disability progression, and

the number of lesions on MRI without significant adverse events [28]. These findings led to its FDA approval for first line oral therapy in MS patients on March 2013. Although clinically the exact mechanism of action of DMF has not been determined, DMF has been shown to induce expression of the potent endogenous antioxidant enzyme, HO-1 in experimental setting [29]. We were able to replicate these findings with *in vitro* assessments of HO-1 expression in DMF treated human tissue. HO-1 is a ubiquitously expressed antioxidant that is inducible in response to oxidative stress [30]. The upregulation of HO-1 in our experiment is a likely mechanism, among others, that lead to DMF's protective effects. Others have also implicated that DMF exerts its antioxidant effects as an Nrf2 activator. The pathway plays a critical role in the induction of genes that encode numerous antioxidants and detoxifying enzymes [31,32]. More likely, DMF has multiple mechanisms that afford its potent antioxidant efficacy.

In conclusion, long-term treatment with DMF was effective in ameliorating the histological lesions and biochemical abnormalities and improving beta cell function in our rodent model of L-Arginine-induced CP. Although, pain was not assessed in this study the authors wish to study experimental pain syndromes and DMF in future experiments given the wealth of knowledge that connects chronic pain with inflammation. Further research is needed to determine the efficacy of this drug for the treatment of CP in humans.

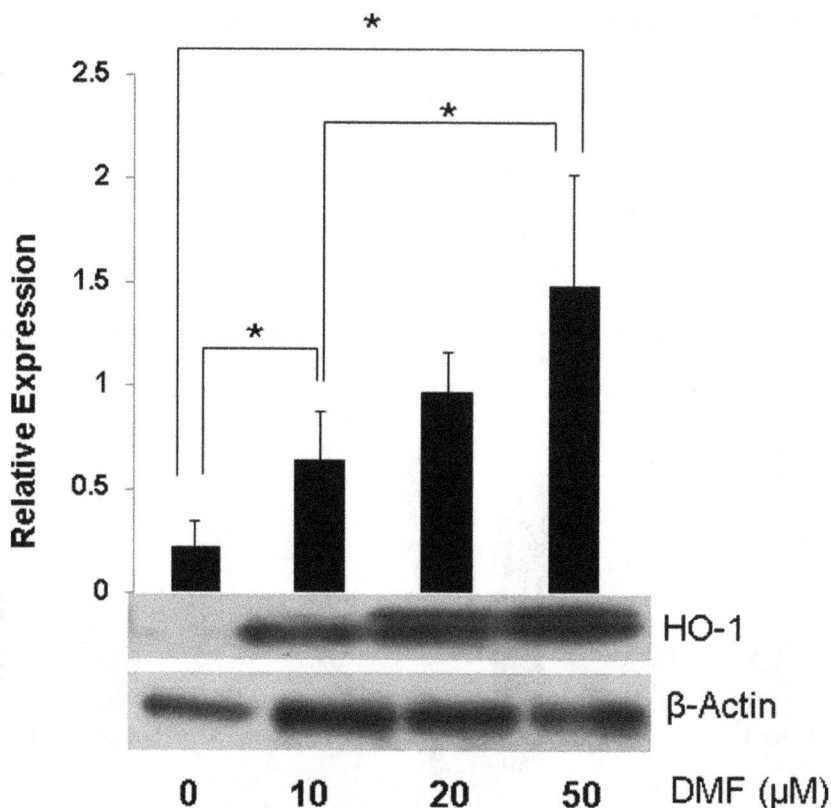

Figure 8. Effects of DMF on HO-1 expression in human pancreatic tissue. Representative western blots of HO-1. The bar graph summarizes the western blot data. DMF significantly enhanced protein expression of HO-1 in a dose dependent manner. Data are representative of four experiments using human islet preparations from independent donors and represent Mean ±S.D. * indicates a significant p<0.05 value.

Author Contributions

Conceived and designed the experiments: LR NV HI. Performed the experiments: LR SL YM CT MT KV. Analyzed the data: LR SL YM CT MT KV SF HI. Contributed reagents/materials/analysis tools: LR SL YM CT MT KV. Contributed to the writing of the manuscript: LR NV MS HI.

References

1. Braganza JM, Lee SH, McCloy RF, McMahon MJ (2011) Chronic pancreatitis. Lancet 377: 1184–1197.
2. Chen JM, Ferec C (2012) Genetics and pathogenesis of chronic pancreatitis: the 2012 update. Clin Res Hepatol Gastroenterol 36: 334–340.
3. Jupp J, Fine D, Johnson CD (2010) The epidemiology and socioeconomic impact of chronic pancreatitis. Best Pract Res Clin Gastroenterol 24: 219–231.
4. Fitzsimmons D, Kahl S, Butturini G, van Wyk M, Bornman P, et al. (2005) Symptoms and quality of life in chronic pancreatitis assessed by structured interview and the EORTC QLQ-C30 and QLQ-PAN26. Am J Gastroenterol 100: 918–926.
5. McEntee GP, Gillen P, Peel AL (1987) Alcohol induced pancreatitis: social and surgical aspects. Br J Surg 74: 402–404.
6. Ashrafian H, Czibik G, Bellahcene M, Aksentijevic D, Smith AC, et al. (2012) Fumarate is cardioprotective via activation of the Nrf2 antioxidant pathway. Cell Metab 15: 361–371.
7. Ghoreschi K, Bruck J, Kellerer C, Deng C, Peng H, et al. (2011) Fumarates improve psoriasis and multiple sclerosis by inducing type II dendritic cells. J Exp Med 208: 2291–2303.
8. Linker RA, Lee DH, Ryan S, van Dam AM, Conrad R, et al. (2011) Fumaric acid esters exert neuroprotective effects in neuroinflammation via activation of the Nrf2 antioxidant pathway. Brain 134: 678–692.
9. Meili-Butz S, Niermann T, Fasler-Kan E, Barbosa V, Butz N, et al. (2008) Dimethyl fumarate, a small molecule drug for psoriasis, inhibits Nuclear Factor-kappaB and reduces myocardial infarct size in rats. Eur J Pharmacol 586: 251–258.
10. Onai Y, Suzuki J, Kakuta T, Maejima Y, Haraguchi G, et al. (2004) Inhibition of IkappaB phosphorylation in cardiomyocytes attenuates myocardial ischemia/reperfusion injury. Cardiovasc Res 63: 51–59.
11. Scannevin RH, Chollate S, Jung MY, Shackett M, Patel H, et al. (2012) Fumarates promote cytoprotection of central nervous system cells against oxidative stress via the nuclear factor (erythroid-derived 2)-like 2 pathway. J Pharmacol Exp Ther 341: 274–284.
12. Oh CJ, Kim JY, Choi YK, Kim HJ, Jeong JY, et al. (2012) Dimethylfumarate attenuates renal fibrosis via NF-E2-related factor 2-mediated inhibition of transforming growth factor-beta/Smad signaling. Plos One 7: e45870.
13. Yamaguchi T, Kihara Y, Taguchi M, Nagashio Y, Tashiro M, et al. (2005) Persistent destruction of the basement membrane of the pancreatic duct contributes to progressive acinar atrophy in rats with experimentally induced pancreatitis. Pancreas 31: 365–372.
14. Schmidt J, Rattner DW, Lewandrowski K, Compton CC, Mandavilli U, et al. (1992) A better model of acute pancreatitis for evaluating therapy. Ann Surg 215: 44–56.
15. Gotoh M, Maki T, Kiyoizumi T, Satomi S, Monaco AP (1985) An improved method for isolation of mouse pancreatic islets. Transplantation 40: 437–438.
16. Shapiro AM, Hao E, Rajotte RV, Kneteman NM (1996) High yield of rodent islets with intraductal collagenase and stationary digestion–a comparison with standard technique. Cell Transplant 5: 631–638.
17. Ricordi C (1995) Methods in Cell Transplantation; Ricordi C, editor: R G Landes Co.
18. Ricordi C, Gray DW, Hering BJ, Kaufman DB, Warnock GL, et al. (1990) Islet isolation assessment in man and large animals. Acta Diabetol Lat 27: 185–195.
19. Ichii H, Inverardi L, Pileggi A, Molano RD, Cabrera O, et al. (2005) A novel method for the assessment of cellular composition and beta-cell viability in human islet preparations. Am J Transplant 5: 1635–1645.
20. Takacs T, Czako L, Morschl E, Laszlo F, Tiszlavicz L, et al. (2002) The role of nitric oxide in edema formation in L-arginine-induced acute pancreatitis. Pancreas 25: 277–282.
21. Lau HYB, Madhav (2012) Quantitating inflammation in a mouse model of acute pancreatitis. The Pancreapedia: Exocrine Pancreas Knowledge Base.

22. Weaver C, Bishop AE, Polak JM (1994) Pancreatic changes elicited by chronic administration of excess L-arginine. Exp Mol Pathol 60: 71–87.
23. Kostromina E, Gustavsson N, Wang X, Lim CY, Radda GK, et al. (2010) Glucose intolerance and impaired insulin secretion in pancreas-specific signal transducer and activator of transcription-3 knockout mice are associated with microvascular alterations in the pancreas. Endocrinology 151: 2050–2059.
24. Lenzen S, Drinkgern J, Tiedge M (1996) Low antioxidant enzyme gene expression in pancreatic islets compared with various other mouse tissues. Free Radic Biol Med 20: 463–466.
25. Mrowietz U, Asadullah K (2005) Dimethylfumarate for psoriasis: more than a dietary curiosity. Trends Mol Med 11: 43–48.
26. Stoof TJ, Flier J, Sampat S, Nieboer C, Tensen CP, et al. (2001) The antipsoriatic drug dimethylfumarate strongly suppresses chemokine production in human keratinocytes and peripheral blood mononuclear cells. Br J Dermatol 144: 1114–1120.

27. Seidel C, Bicker G (2002) Developmental expression of nitric oxide/cyclic GMP signaling pathways in the brain of the embryonic grasshopper. Brain Res Dev Brain Res 138: 71–79.
28. Gold R, Kappos L, Arnold DL, Bar-Or A, Giovannoni G, et al. (2012) Placebo-controlled phase 3 study of oral BG-12 for relapsing multiple sclerosis. The New England journal of medicine 367: 1098–1107.
29. Lehmann JC, Listopad JJ, Rentzsch CU, Igney FH, von Bonin A, et al. (2007) Dimethylfumarate induces immunosuppression via glutathione depletion and subsequent induction of heme oxygenase 1. J Invest Dermatol 127: 835–845.
30. Kikuchi G, Yoshida T, Noguchi M (2005) Heme oxygenase and heme degradation. Biochem Biophys Res Commun 338: 558–567.
31. Itoh K, Wakabayashi N, Katoh Y, Ishii T, Igarashi K, et al. (1999) Keap1 represses nuclear activation of antioxidant responsive elements by Nrf2 through binding to the amino-terminal Neh2 domain. Genes Dev 13: 76–86.
32. Li ZD, Ma QY, Wang CA (2006) Effect of resveratrol on pancreatic oxygen free radicals in rats with severe acute pancreatitis. World J Gastroenterol 12: 137–140.

10

Cardiovascular Disease-Related Parameters and Oxidative Stress in SHROB Rats, a Model for Metabolic Syndrome

Eunice Molinar-Toribio[1], Jara Pérez-Jiménez[1*¤], Sara Ramos-Romero[1,2], Laura Lluís[3], Vanessa Sánchez-Martos[3], Núria Taltavull[3], Marta Romeu[3], Manuel Pazos[4], Lucía Méndez[4], Aníbal Miranda[5,6], Marta Cascante[5,6], Isabel Medina[4], Josep Lluís Torres[1]

1 Institute of Advanced Chemistry of Catalonia (IQAC-CSIC), Barcelona, Spain, **2** Biomedical Research Networking Center in Bioengineering, Biomaterials, and Nanomedicine (CIBER-BBN), Zaragoza, Spain, **3** Unidad de Farmacología, Facultad de Medicina y Ciencias de la Salud, Universidad Rovira i Virgili, Reus, Spain, **4** Instituto de Investigaciones Marinas (IIM-CSIC), Vigo, Spain, **5** Department of Biochemistry and Molecular Biology, IBUB and unit associated with CSIC, Faculty of Biology, Universitat de Barcelona, Barcelona, Spain, **6** Institut d'Investigacions Biomèdiques August Pi i Sunyer (IDIBAPS), Barcelona, Spain

Abstract

SHROB rats have been suggested as a model for metabolic syndrome (MetS) as a situation prior to the onset of CVD or type-2 diabetes, but information on descriptive biochemical parameters for this model is limited. Here, we extensively evaluate parameters related to CVD and oxidative stress (OS) in SHROB rats. SHROB rats were monitored for 15 weeks and compared to a control group of Wistar rats. Body weight was recorded weekly. At the end of the study, parameters related to CVD and OS were evaluated in plasma, urine and different organs. SHROB rats presented statistically significant differences from Wistar rats in CVD risk factors: total cholesterol, LDL-cholesterol, triglycerides, apoA1, apoB100, abdominal fat, insulin, blood pressure, C-reactive protein, ICAM-1 and PAI-1. In adipose tissue, liver and brain, the endogenous antioxidant systems were activated, yet there was no significant oxidative damage to lipids (MDA) or proteins (carbonylation). We conclude that SHROB rats present significant alterations in parameters related to inflammation, endothelial dysfunction, thrombotic activity, insulin resistance and OS measured in plasma as well as enhanced redox defence systems in vital organs that will be useful as markers of MetS and CVD for nutrition interventions.

Editor: Christopher Torrens, University of Southampton, United Kingdom

Funding: This research was supported by the Spanish Ministries of Science and Innovation and of Economy and Competitiveness (Grants AGL2009-12374-C03-01, -02 and -03; AGL2013-49079-C2-1,2-R; respectively) and in part by the Generalitat de Catalunya regional authorities (2009SGR-1308). M.C. acknowledges ETHERPATHS (FP7-KBBE-222639) funded by the European Union and "ICREA Academia" award for excellence in research, funded by the ICREA Foundation of the Generalitat de Catalunya. The Panamanian Government (SENACYT/IFRHU) and the Spanish Ministry of Science and Innovation awarded graduate fellowships to E.M.-T. and L.M., respectively. The ISCIII and the Xunta de Galicia are also acknowledged for "Sara Borrell" and "Isidro Parga Pondal" postdoctoral contracts to J.P.-J. (CD09/00068) and M.P., respectively. The funders had no role in study design, data collection and analysis, decision to publish, or preparation of the manuscript.

Competing Interests: The authors have declared that no competing interests exist.

* Email: jara.perez@ictan.csic.es

¤ Current address: Department of Metabolism and Nutrition, Institute of Food Science, Technology and Nutrition (ICTAN-CSIC), Madrid, Spain

Introduction

The combination of CVD risk factors known as metabolic syndrome (MetS) is becoming a major public health problem which now affects 20%–30% of the adult population in developed countries [1]. The risk factors include abdominal obesity, hyperglycaemia, hypertension and/or hypertriglycerydaemia associated with a sedentary lifestyle [2]. The main underlying disorder in MetS appears to be insulin resistance, i.e., an impairment of insulin action within tissues (mainly muscle, liver and adipose tissues) that has been related to chronic low-level inflammation as well as oxidative stress (OS), as second-order underlying mechanisms for this pathological condition [3,4]. The factors defining MetS may lead to the onset of type-2 diabetes and CVD. This is the main reason why the study of the factors underlying MetS can be clinically useful.

There is wide interest in the development of strategies for the prevention of MetS, mainly via two different approaches: a)

pharmacology – based on the use of drugs such as certain statins or AMPK (5′ adenosine monophosphate-activated protein kinase) activating agents [5,6]; and b) nutrition–based on diet supplementation with functional compounds, e.g., proanthocyanidins [7] or iminosugars [8].

To test the efficacy of the different approaches, several animal models of MetS have been suggested, in which MetS is either induced by the diet [9,10] or results from some genetic alteration. Most of the genetically modified animals present mutations in the gene that codes for the leptin receptor [11], which impairs the capacity of leptin to regulate food intake and eventually leads to the development of insulin resistance. One such model is SHROB (spontaneously hypertensive obese) rats, also called Koletsky rats [12,13]. SHROB rats were generated by crossing a female spontaneously hypertensive rat (SHR), obtained by breeding high-blood-pressure Wistar-Kyoto rats, with a normotensive Sprague Dawley male, from which a single homozygous recessive trait appeared. That trait is a nonsense mutation in the leptin receptor, designated fa^k, which results in a premature stop codon in the extracellular domain of the leptin receptor that circumvents the process of transduction and thereby truncates all the leptin receptors [14,15]. SHROB rats, homozygous for this mutation, are therefore characterized by monogenetic obesity combined with a hypertensive background for which several phenotype aspects have been described, including hyperinsulinaemia, hyperlipidaemia and nephropathy [15]. SHROB rats are thus a model for MetS, in accordance with some of its currently accepted defining factors, i.e., insulin resistance, hypertension, increased plasma triglyceride levels and obesity [16]. It has also been suggested that in SHROB rats hyperinsulinaemia is not accompanied by hyperglycaemia, this model would be especially useful for the study of the prediabetic state [17], in contrast to other animal models (e.g. Zucker rats) which develop type-2 diabetes.

Despite its use as a model of MetS, a complete description of the SHROB rat phenotype, in relation to markers related to CVD and particularly OS, is lacking. Moreover, studies with SHROB rats have compared them with SHR, spontaneously hypertensive rats [15,18], a rat that is already mutated and in which several parameters are altered, and not with either of the original rat strains from which these rats were derived, i.e., Sprague-Dawley or Wistar Kyoto (WKY) rats.

The aim of this work is to complete a phenotypic description of SHROB rats using previously unexplored parameters related to CVD, and compare it with that of non-mutated WKY rats. We obtained new data of relevance for the use of SHROB rats in nutrition studies.

Materials and Methods

Materials and reagents

The A04 diet was from Harlan Iberica (Panlab S.L., Barcelona, Spain). Soybean oil, obtained from unrefined organic soy oil (first cold pressing), was from Clearspring Ltd. (London, UK).

Ketamine chlorhydrate was from Merial Laboratorios (Barcelona, Spain). Xylacine was from Quimica Farmaceutica (Barcelona, Spain). [2H4]-15-F2t-IsoP, 15-F_{2t}-IsoP and 15-F_{2t}-IsoP methyl ester were obtained from Cayman Chemical (Ann Arbor, MI, USA). 2,3,4,5,6-Pentafluorobenzyl (PFB) bromide, N,N-diisopropylethylamine (DIPE), acetonitrile, anhydrous sodium sulphate, heptane, phenylmethylsulphonyl fluoride (PMSF), dithiothreitol (DTT), iodoacetamide, ethylenediaminetetraacetic acid (EDTA), Tris-HCl, 3,3-cholaminopropyl-dimethylammonio-1-propanesulphonate (CHAPS), anhydrous magnesium chloride, bicinchoninic acid (BCA), 2,2′-Azobis(2-amidinopropane) dihydrochloride (AAPH), 6-hydroxy-2,5,7,8-tetramethylchroman-2-carboxylic acid (Trolox), fluorescein (sodium salt), acetone, phosphomolybdic acid, Bradford reagent, NADPH (β- Nicotinamide adenine dinucleotide 2′-phosphate reduced tetrasodium salt hydrate), glutathione reductase (GR from baker's yeast), L-glutathione reduced (GSH minimum 99%), t- tert-butyl hydroperoxide (t-BuOOH)) and L-glutathione oxidized (GSSG) were all obtained from Sigma-Aldrich (St. Louis, MO, USA). N,O-bis(trimethylsilyl)trifluoro-acetamide (BSTFA) was from Supelco (Bellefonte, PA, USA). Hydrochloric acid fuming 37%, ethanol absolute, ethyl acetate, methanol, chloroform, Na_2CO_3, $NaHCO_3$, EDTA Na^{2+}, o-phthalaldehyde (OPT), N-ethylmaleimide (NEM) and thiobarbituric acid were purchased from Merck KGaA (Darmstadt, Germany). Fluorescein-5-thiosemicarbazide (FTSC) was purchased from Invitrogen (Carlsbad, CA, USA). ProteoBlock protease inhibitor cocktail was purchased from Thermo Fisher Scientific Inc. (Rockford, IL, USA). Urea,

thiourea, SDS, glycine and glycerol were obtained from USB (Cleveland, OH, USA). Ammonium persulphate (APS), IPG buffer, pharmalyte 3-10; bromophenol blue and 1,2-bis(dimethyl-lamino)-ethane (TEMED) were purchased from GE Healthcare Bio-Sciences AB (Uppsala, Sweden). Acrylamide, bis (N,N′-methylene-bis-acrylamide) and the Bio-Rad protein assay were obtained from Bio-rad (Hercules, CA, USA). Drabkin Reagent and albumin were purchased from Química Clinica Aplicada (Tarragona, Spain). Na_2HPO_4, NaH_2PO_4, NaCl, epinefrine, KH_2PO_4, K_2HPO_4, trichloroacetic acid (TCA) and NaOH were purchased from Panreac Química (Barcelona, Spain). Water for the assay solutions was obtained using a Milli-Q water purification system from Millipore Corporation (Billerica, MA, USA).

Animals

Seven female, 11- to 14-week-old, spontaneously hypertensive obese rats (SHROB) (Charles River Laboratories, Wilmington, MA, USA) and seven female, 11-week-old WKY rats (control group) (Janvier, Le Genest-St-Isle, France) were used. They were kept away from male rats to minimize hormonal alterations.

Experimental design

The rats were kept in Macrolon cages ($n = 2$–3/cage, $425 \times 265 \times 180$ mm) under controlled conditions of stable humidity ($50 \pm 10\%$), and temperature ($22 \pm 2°C$) with a 12:12-h light/dark cycle. All the groups were fed a standard pelleted A04 diet, given water (Ribes, Barcelona, Spain) ad libitum and administered a weekly oral dose of 0.8 mL/kg of soybean oil for 13-weeks-fatty acid composition provided as **Table S1**. The additional dose of fat (weekly excess of 5–10% of fat intake) was intended to accelerate the appearance of alterations in CV risk factors and OS related parameters. At week 15, one week after the last intragastric dose of soybean oil and oral glucose tolerance test (OGTT)—see below—the rats were fasted overnight, anesthetized intraperitoneally with ketamine and xylacine (80 mg/kg and 10 mg/kg body weight respectively), and then killed by exsanguination. All the procedures follow the European Union guidelines for the care and management of laboratory animals and all efforts were made to minimize suffering. The pertinent permission for this specific study was obtained from the CSIC (Spanish Research Council) Subcommittee of Bioethical Issues (ref. AGL2009-12 374-C03-03).

Sample collection

For urine collection, at week 12 of the experiment, the rats were placed in metabolic cages and deprived of food for 18 h; the animals had previously been acclimated to the metabolic cages. At the end of the experimental period, after one week of recuperation since the final intragastric dose of soybean oil, blood was collected by cardiac puncture under anaesthesia. Plasma, serum and erythrocytes were collected. Tissue samples collected from heart, brain, liver, and kidney were washed with 0.9% NaCl solution and immediately frozen in liquid nitrogen. Abdominal fat was weighed and immediately frozen. All the samples were stored at $-80°C$ pending analysis. Before analysis, tissue samples were homogenized with sodium phosphate buffer and ultra-centrifuged.

Cardiovascular disease risk factors

Body weight was monitored weekly throughout the experiment.
Determination of plasma lipid profile. Total plasma cholesterol (CHOL), LDL-cholesterol (LDLc), HDL-cholesterol (HDLc) and triglycerides (TG) were measured by spectrophotometric methods using the corresponding kits from Spinreact

(Girona, Spain). ApoA1 and ApoB100 were measured using ELISA kits purchased from Cusabio Biotech (Hubei, China)

Determination of glycaemia. Blood glucose levels were measured by the enzyme electrode method using an Ascensia ELITE XL blood glucose meter from (Bayer Consumer Care (Basel, Switzerland). Plasma insulin was measured using ELISA kits from Millipore (Billerica, MA, USA). Homeostasis model assessments (HOMA) were calculated by applying the formula: fasting plasma glucose (mg/dL) times fasting insulin (mU/L) divided by 405 [19]. Glycated Hb was measured using a spectrophotometric kit from Spinreact. All these measurements were carried out at the end of the study.

An OGTT was conducted at week 14 of the experiment after 18 h of food deprivation. Rats were administered a glucose dose of 2 g/kg body weight by gastric probe using a 29% glucose solution. The glucose concentration was measured by the enzyme electrode method, using single drops of blood taken from the saphenous vein at 0, 15, 30, 45, 60, 90 and 120 min after glucose administration. The AUC for serum glucose was calculated over the 2 h period. This test was carried out 1 week after the last intragastric dose of soybean oil.

Blood pressure. Systolic and diastolic blood pressure were measured at week 13 of the experiment. In a quiet place, at an established time to reduce circadian rhythm interference, the rats were restrained in a rat pocket and maintained at 32°C. Systolic and diastolic blood pressure were measured three times by the tail-cuff method, using a non-invasive automatic blood pressure analyser (Panlab, Barcelona, Spain) as previously described [20]. Data are presented as the mean of three measurements.

Markers of endothelial function, inflammation and thrombotic activity. The corresponding ELISA kits from Cusabio Biotech (Hubei, China) were used to measure the following parameters in plasma: vascular cell adhesion molecule-1 (VCAM-1) and intercellular adhesion molecule-1 (ICAM-1) as markers of endothelial function; C-reactive protein (CRP) as an inflammation marker.; plasminogen activator inhibitor-1 (PAI-1) as a marker of thrombotic activity.

Endogenous antioxidant systems

Activity of superoxide dismutase (SOD) and catalase (CAT). SOD and CAT activities were measured using standard spectrophotometric methods [21,22] in the following samples: erithrocytes (0.23–1.84 μL and 0.5 μL, respectively), liver (167–417 μg and 1.25 mg, respectively), abdominal fat (1.6–4 μg and 12 mg, respectively), kidney (667–1667 μg and 10 mg, respectively), heart (333–833 μg and 5 mg, respectively) and brain (833–417 μg and 5 mg, respectively).

Glutathione system. Glutathione peroxidase (GPx) and glutathione reductase (GR) activities were measured by spectrophotometric methods [23,24]. Glutathione (GSH) and glutathione disulphide (GSSG) were determined using fluorometric methods [25].

GR and GPx analysis were measured in the following samples: erythrocytes (8–48 μL), liver (40–240 μg), abdominal fat (2–12 mg), kidney (80–480 μg), heart (80–480 μg) and brain (500–3000 μg). GSH and GSSG were measured in erythrocytes (149 μL), liver (75 μg), abdominal fat (372 μg), kidney (298 μg), heart (149 μg) and brain (372 μg). The standard curves used for the quantification of GSH and GSSG are provided as **Figures S1 and S2**.

In both cases, the activities of the enzymes were normalized to the amount of protein by the Bradford method [26] and to the amount of Hb in erythrocytes by the Drabkin method [27].

Oxidative stress

Determination of oxygen radical absorbance capacity. Total plasma antioxidant capacity was measured as the oxygen radical absorbance capacity (ORAC) [28], which measures the level of protection from the loss of intensity of the fluorescent molecules fluorescein, due to the action of peroxyl radicals generated from an azo-initiator. A standard curve for Trolox (reference compound for antioxidant capacity determination) was prepared in the range 12.5–100 μM.

Protein carbonylation. Protein concentrations in the homogenates were determined according to the method of Bradford [26], using a standard curve between 0.125 and 0.975 mg protein/mL standard. Preparation of homogenates from liver aliquots, determination of the protein concentration in the homogenates and protein separation by 10% SDS-PAGE proteins from 250 mg liver were fractionated according to hydrophobicity, into proteins soluble at low ionic strength, mostly water-soluble proteins, and proteins soluble at high ionic strength, mostly hydrophobic proteins. After homogenization, each liver fraction (300 μL) and plasma (25 μL) were independently incubated with 1 mM fluorescein-5-thiosemicarbazide (FTSC) in the dark as previously described [29,30]. After incubation, the proteins were precipitated with an equal volume of 20% TCA (v/v), centrifuged and finally, re-dissolved in urea buffer (7 M urea, 2 M thiourea, 2% CHAPS, 0.5% Pharmalyte 3–10, 0.5% IPG 3–10 buffer and 0.4% DTT). To evaluate the protein carbonyl levels, 30 μg of each sample were subjected to one-dimensional (1-DE) 10% SDS-PAGE [31] and run in a Mini-protean 3 cell (Bio-Rad). After electrophoresis, FTSC-tagged proteins were visualized by exposing the gel to a UV transilluminator Molecular Imager Gel Doc XR System (Bio-Rad) equipped with a 520 nm band-pass filter (520DF30 62 mm) and the scanned one-dimensional gels were analysed with the 1-D gel analysis software LabImage 1D from Kapelan Bio-Imaging Solutions (Halle, Germany). Finally, the scanned analysed gels were stained overnight with the Coomassie dye PhastGel Blue R-350 (GE Healthcare, Little Chalfont, UK) to visualize the total amount of protein in each sample. The global protein carbonylation level for each sample was quantified based on the overall optical volume of each lane in the FTSC-stained 1-D electrophoresis gel, whereas the oxidation level of a specific protein band was estimated by its optical intensity (peak height). Oxidized albumin (1 to 14 μg) was used as a positive control.

Oxidized LDL. Plasma oxidized LDL (LDL-ox) was determined with an ELISA kit from Cusabio Biotech, by measuring the absorbance at 450 nm on a PowerWave XS2 spectrophotometer from BioTec Instruments, Inc., (Winooski, VT, USA).

Malondialdehyde (MDA). MDA concentrations were measured in homogenized liver (80 μg of sample), kidney (80 μg), abdominal fat (80 μg), heart (10 μg) and brain (400 μg) with fluorescence detection [32]. The fluorescence at 515 nm excitation wavelength and 548 nm emission wavelength was determined on an LS50B spectrofluorimeter (Perkin Elmer, Alabama, USA).

Determination of isoprostane 15-F2t-IsoP. Urine 15-F2t-IsoP was determined by GC/negative ion chemical ionization/MS (GC-NICI-MS) following the method of Milne *et al.* [33]. Briefly, after addition of the deuterated internal standard [2H4]-15-F2t-IsoP to 250 μL of urine, the samples were subjected to solid phase extraction (SPE) purification, with a C18 Sep-Pak column and a silica Sep-Pak column (both from Waters Associates, Milford, MA, USA). The F2-Isoprostanes were derivatized to pentafluorobenzyl (PFB) esters and further purified by thin layer chromatography (TLC) using 15-F2t-IsoP methyl ester as the reference compound with an R_F value identical to the analyte. Finally, the pure derivatized analytes were converted to trimethylsilyl ether derivatives and analysed by GC-NICI-MS using a Shimadzu QP201 instrument (Tokyo, Japan), fitted with a DB1701 fused silica capillary column (15 m×0.25 mm i.d., 0.25 μM film thickness) from Agilent (J & W Scientific, Folsom, CA, USA). The 15-F2t-IsoP ion monitored was the carboxylate anion at m/z 569. Representative chromatograms used for the determination of 15-F2t-IsoP are provided as **Figure S3**. The final results are expressed in ng/mg creatinine. Creatinine levels from the urine samples were determined by a colorimetric method using a commercial kit from C-cromatest Linear Chemicals (Barcelona, Spain) by measuring absorbance at 510 nm on a SpectraMax M5 spectrophotometer (Molecular Devices, Sunnyvale, CA, USA).

Statistical analysis

The different analytical determinations in the biological samples were carried out in duplicate or triplicate, depending on the method. Results are expressed as the mean + SEM. The non-parametric Mann-Whitney U's test was applied to analyse the significant differences ($P<0.05$) between groups. The SPSS IBM19 package for Windows was used throughout.

The weight distribution between the groups of rats at each of the 15 time points was compared using the Wilcoxon Rank Sum test. Due to the large number of comparisons, a multi-test procedure that applies multiple comparisons as is known as the false discovery rate (FDR) [34] correction, with Simes' method [35] was used. With this procedure a comparison was considered statistically significant if the corresponding p-value was lower than or equal to the specific α-corrected value for the comparison. This analysis was performed using the statistical software STATA 12.0.

Results

Cardiovascular disease risk factors

The SHROB rats were already obese at week 16, with a body weight twice that of the WKY rats (483±9 g versus 221±4 g). Moreover, while the WKY rats maintained a constant body weight up to week 27, the SHROB rats showed an increase from 476.8±15.9 g at week 16 to 605.6±19.5 g at week 27. **Figure S4** shows the evolution of body weight of the SHROB and WKY rats during the study.

Abdominal fat at the end of the study, expressed as percentage of body weight was 50% higher in the SHROB than in the WKY rats (**Table 1**).

Plasma lipid profile. The SHROB rats presented significantly higher ($P<0.01$) levels of plasma total cholesterol, LDL-cholesterol, HDL-cholesterol and triglycerides than the WKY rats (**Table 1**). In particular, the SHROB rats showed a ninefold increase in total cholesterol and more than a tenfold increase in triglycerides, compared to the WKY rats. Plasma levels of both the anti-atherogenic ApoA1 and the pro-atherogenic Apo B100 were also significantly higher ($P<0.01$) in the SHROB rats than in the WKY rats (+33% and +62%, respectively).

Glycaemia. No significant differences were observed in fasting plasma glucose, OGTT or in glycated Hb between the SHROB and WKY rats. In contrast, plasma insulin was significantly higher ($P<0.01$) in the SHROB rats than in the WKY rats (1.0±0.3 nM versus 0.3±0.1 nM, respectively), and consequently, the HOMA index was also higher in the SHROB rats (**Table 1**).

Blood pressure. Both systolic and diastolic blood pressure were significantly higher ($P<0.001$) in the SHROB rats (193±12 mmHg and 135±5 mmHg, respectively) than in the WKY rats (121±2 mmHg and 106±2 mmHg) (**Table 1**).

Endothelial dysfunction. ICAM-1 and VCAM-1 were measured as markers of endothelial dysfunction; considered the earliest stage in the atherosclerosis process. ICAM-1 showed an 84% increase in plasma levels in the SHROB rats compared to the WKY rats ($P<0.001$). No significant differences were found in plasma VCAM-1 between the SHROB and WKY rats (**Table 1**).

Inflammation. Plasma C-reactive protein, determined as a marker of inflammation, was 65% higher in the SHROB rats than in the WKY rats ($P<0.001$) (**Table 1**).

Thrombotic activity. The SHROB rats presented significantly higher ($P<0.001$) plasma levels of PAI-1 than the WKY rats (6.4±0.3 μg/mL versus 11.6±0.5 μg/mL, respectively) (**Table 1**).

Endogenous antioxidant systems

Endogenous antioxidant systems were evaluated in erythrocytes, tissues and organs of the SHROB and WKY rats at the end of the study (**Table 2**).

SOD and CAT activity. The activity of the endogenous antioxidant enzymes was measured in erythrocytes, liver, abdominal fat, kidney and heart. No significant differences in SOD activity between SHROB and WKY rats were observed in any of the samples analysed. As regards CAT activity, brain was the only organ where significant differences ($P<0.01$) were found between the SHROB and WKY rats.

Glutathione system. The status of the glutathione system was evaluated by quantifying the two forms of glutathione (GSH and GSSG) to calculate the GSH/GSSG ratio; and by measuring the activity of the associated enzymes (GR, which regenerates reduced glutathione; and GPx, which catalyses the oxidation of GSH to GSSG). Higher concentrations of GSH in liver ($P<0.01$), abdominal fat ($P<0.05$) and brain ($P<0.01$) were found in the SHROB rats than the WKY rats. GSH/GSSG was significantly ($P<0.05$) higher in the adipose tissue of the SHROB rats. GPx activity was also higher in the abdominal fat tissue ($P<0.001$) and brain ($P<0.01$) of the SHROB rats. In contrast, higher concentration of GSSG were found in the heart of the SHROB rats than in the WKY rats ($P<0.01$) and the SHROB rats showed lower GPx activity in erythrocytes and in liver ($P<0.05$) and lower GR activity in liver ($P<0.05$).

Oxidative stress

Several biomarkers of OS were measured in blood, urine and different organs in the SHROB and WKY rats (**Table 3**). Plasma antioxidant capacity, as determined by ORAC assay, was significantly ($P<0.05$) higher in the SHROB than in the WKY rats. Lipid oxidation was evaluated by determining oxidized LDL in plasma, MDA in liver, kidney, abdominal fat, heart and brain, and 15-F$_{2t}$-IsoP in urine. Oxidized LDL in plasma was 50% higher in the SHROB rats than in the WKY rats, although this increase did not reach significance, due to the high interindividual variability of this parameter. Similarly, isoprostane 15-F$_{2t}$-IsoP in urine was non-significantly higher in the urine of SHROB rats. Creatinine was higher in SHROB rats than in WKY rats (68 mg/dL SEM 9 vs 58 mg/dL SEM 7); since 15-F$_{2t}$-IsoP is expressed per mg of creatinine, the higher values of this isoprostane in the SHROB rats is not an artefact resulting from increased creatinine values. In contrast, MDA in abdominal fat was significantly lower ($P<0.05$) in SHROB rats than in WKY rats and overall protein oxidation-measured as total carbonyls-was lower in the SHROB than in the WKY rats in both the low and high ionic strength fractions of liver proteins ($P<0.05$) as well as in plasma ($P=0.0571$).

Table 1. CVD risk factors evaluated in the plasma of SHROB and WKY rats (mean value and SEM)[1].

Category	Parameter	SHROB	SEM	WKY	SEM
Physical measurements	Abdominal fat (% bw)	6·7**	0·4	4·3	0·2
Plasma lipid profile	Total cholesterol (mM)	8·3**	1·2	3·3	0·2
	LDL-cholesterol (mM)	0·4*	0·1	0·1	0·004
	HDL-cholesterol (mM)	2·9*	0·2	1·9	0·1
	Total triglycerides (mM)	40·0**	0·0	5·6	1·1
	Apo A1 (mg/dL)	68·3*	1·9	51·4	5·0
	Apo B100 (mg/dL)	205·4*	18·7	126·8	5·3
Glycaemia	Glucose (mM)	3.4	0.1	3.5	0.1
	Insulin (nM)	1·0**	0·2·9	0·3	0·1
	HOMA index	15·6**	2·4	5·6	1·1
	OGTT (AUC)	5016·3	177·4	4494·0	122·8
	Glycated Hb (%)	6·8	0·4	6·4	0·4
Blood pressure	Systolic blood pressure (mmHg)	193·2**	12·5	121·0	2·2
	Diastolic blood pressure (mmHg)	134·8**	5·2	106·5	1·7
Endothelial dysfunction	VCAM-1 (µg/mL)	2·7	0·3	3·4	0·6
	ICAM-1 (ng/mL)	1·0**	0·1	0·5	0·03
Inflammation	C reactive protein (pg/mL)	285·9**	22·0	172·8	14·4
Thrombotic activity	PAI-1 (µg/mL)	11·6**	0·5	6·4	0·3

[1]SHROB, Spontaneously Hypertensive Obese; WKY, Wistar Kyoto; OGTT, oral glucose tolerance test; VCAM-1, vascular cell adhesion molecule-1; ICAM-1, intercellular adhesion molecule-1; PAI-1, plasminogen activator inhibitor-1.
Statistically significant differences between the samples are indicated by * ($P<0.05$), ** ($P<0.01$) and *** ($P<0.001$).

Discussion

SHROB rats represent a particularly interesting animal model for MetS, a situation prior to the onset of type-2 diabetes or CVD, in which the different metabolic alterations may be addressed without the use of drugs. The aim of the present study was to contribute to the description of this animal model, by examining parameters related to cardiovascular function, inflammation and oxidative stress not previously reported.

Total cholesterol, triglycerides, fasting glucose, insulin, glycated haemoglobin and blood pressure, have been examined before in SHROB rats [15,17] and in the related SHRSP (stroke-prone spontaneously hypertensive rat) model, after supplementation with soybean oil [36]. Our results concord with previous reports except for glycaemia; some authors found hyperglycaemia [15,37,38] while others reported normoglycaemia, [17,39], as we do. Anti-atherogenic ApoA1 and pro-atherogenic Apo B100 are now included in the lipid profile. Certain markers of endothelial dysfunction (ICAM-1 and VCAM-1), inflammation (C-reactive protein) and thrombotic activity (PAI-1) are also reported here for the first time.

The SHROB rats exhibited significant alterations in abdominal fat, plasma lipid profile (total cholesterol, LDL-cholesterol, HDL-cholesterol, triglycerides, apoA1, apoB100), insulin, blood pressure, ICAM-1, C-reactive protein and PAI-1 (**Table 1**). In many of these parameters (lipid profile, markers of endothelial dysfunction, inflammation and thrombotic activity), the values in the SHROB rats were at least 50% higher than in the WKY rats. Impairment of endothelial function in SHROB rats has previously been related to alterations in the nitric oxide pathway and the presence of visceral prostaglandins derived from perivisceral adipose tissue [36,37] All these results are consistent with high

circulating fat, visceral fat accumulation and the state of low-level inflammation that precedes insulin resistance [40]. Inflammation appears to be the link between obesity and the development of insulin resistance in MetS [41]. The mutation (fa^k) in the leptin receptor of SHROB rats that impairs the ability of leptin to regulate fat intake would explain these effects with a direct relation to an excess of fat.

Since OS is a complex process, where there are different interactions between endogenous antioxidants systems, progress of oxidation in biomolecules and levels of circulating exogenous antioxidants [42], we decided to measure markers corresponding to each one of these components of OS. The picture that emerges from our results is of a marked difference between systemic OS (as measured via the endogenous antioxidant system in erythrocytes and oxidized LDL in plasma) and OS in organs (as measured via the endogenous antioxidant system in tissues and organs, and via final lipid and protein oxidation products in organs and in urine). Both SOD and GPx activities in erythrocytes were significantly reduced in the SHROB rats, and this attenuation of the endogenous defence system was concomitant with a 50% increase in LDL oxidation. This is consistent with the preceding observations related to CVD biomarkers, since OS, particularly low SOD activity, has been shown to be present in subjects with MetS who also show high C-reactive protein levels [4]. However, this systemic OS was not immediately translated to the different organs, since the levels of MDA in liver and kidney and of 15-F$_{2t}$-IsoP in urine were not significantly modified in the SHROB rats. Indeed, compared to the WKY rats, the SHROB strain presented a significant increase in GSH in liver, abdominal fat and brain as well as a significant decrease in overall protein carbonylation and lipid oxidation in abdominal fat. We found that, in SHROB rats, OS may present later than other reported organ disturbances such

Table 2. Endogenous antioxidant systems in SHROB and WKY rats (mean value and SEM)[1].

Organ	Parameter	SHROB	SEM	WKY	SEM
Erythrocytes	SOD (U/g Hb)	768·0	224·0	1444·0	161·0
	CAT (mmol/min/g Hb)	51·9	4·1	41·5	13·1
	GR (U/g Hb)	0·9	0·1	0·9	0·1
	GPx (U/g Hb)	51·5*	10·3	101·5	14·4
Liver	SOD (U/g mg prot)	8·3	0·5	8·7	0·6
	CAT (µmol/min/mg prot)	70·8	9·8	81·1	10·9
	GR (mU/mg prot)	66·7*	3·1	88·8	8·3
	GPx (mU/mg prot)	245·4*	31·0	383·8	37·1
	GSH (nmol/mg prot)	61·2**	9·6	29·9	2·6
	GSSG (nmol/mg prot)	133·7	12·1	61·2	9·6
	GSH/GSSG	0·5*	0·1	0·5	0·1
Abdominal fat	SOD (U/g mg prot)	4·2	0·7	6·5	1·4
	CAT (µmol/min/mg prot)	27·8	4·9	28·3	2·5
	GR (mU/mg prot)	31·2	7·3	28·3	2·1
	GPx (mU/mg prot)	38·7**	2·6	15·8	4·0
	GSH (nmol/mg prot)	110·4*	24·9	41·7	6·4
	GSSG (nmol/mg prot)	49·8	4·8	47·7	3·0
	GSH/GSSG	2·2*	0·5	0·9	0·1
Kidney	SOD (U/g mg prot)	2·2	0·3	2·8	0·4
	CAT (µmol/min/mg prot)	24·1	3·1	33·5	7·6
	GR (mU/mg prot)	47·1	11·72	41·64	3·93
	GPx (mU/mg prot)	57·2	9·07	48·0	3·82
	GSH (nmol/mg prot)	33·4	7·4	36·7	3·7
	GSSG (nmol/mg prot)	0·5	0·1	0·6	0·1
	GSH/GSSG	71·0	18·1	64·5	8·6
Heart	SOD (U/g mg prot)	6·0	0·5	5·6	0·7
	CAT (µmol/min/mg prot)	15·1	0·6	13·4	1·1
	GR (mU/mg prot)	23·6	1·4	27·4	2·3
	GPx (mU/mg prot)	146·6	9·9	159·6	9·0
	GSH (nmol/mg prot)	21·5	2·8	18·1	2·1
	GSSG (nmol/mg prot)	6·4**	0·6	4·5	0·3
	GSH/GSSG	3·4	0·5	4·0	0·5
Brain	SOD (U/g mg prot)	8·0	0·2	7·4	1·5
	CAT (µmol/min/mg prot)	6·4**	0·9	2·2	0·7
	GR (mU/mg prot)	67·4	7·3	49·8	3·7
	GPx (mU/mg prot)	49·0**	5·3	30·9	1·5
	GSH (nmol/mg prot)	87·2**	16·5	24·2	7·3
	GSSG (nmol/mg prot)	5·2	0·4	3·0	1·0
	GSH/GSSG	16·8	3·4	8·0	3·5

[1]SHROB, Spontaneously Hypertensive Obese; WKY, Wistar Kyoto; SOD, superoxide dismutase; CAT, catalase; GR, glutathione reductase; GPx, glutathione peroxidase; GSH, glutathione; GSSG, glutathione disulphide; Hb, haemoglobin.
Statistically significant differences between the samples are indicated by * ($P<0.05$), ** ($P<0.01$) and *** ($P<0.001$).

as increased renal macrophage infiltration [43]. Also, it should be noted that even if total protein carbonylation in SHROB rats is shown to be lower than in WKY rats, we recently reported that key proteins involved in redox homeostasis, such as aldehyde dehydrogenase mitochondrial, protein disulphide-isomerase A3 or protein disulphide-isomerase, suffer higher oxidation in SHROB rats than in WKY rats [44]. Finally, the higher plasma antioxidant capacity in the SHROB rats, concordant with the lower protein carbonylation found in SHROB plasma may be the result of the activation of defence mechanisms that are not observed to have been overwhelmed in most organs. The observed differences between the different markers of OS, corresponding to different stages and elements of this process, emphasize the need to carry

Table 3. Oxidative stress biomarkers in SHROB and WKY rats (mean value and SEM)[1].

Organ	Parameter	SHROB	SEM	WKY	SEM
Plasma	ORAC (μmol Trolox/mL)	44·8[*]	3·2	30·3	3·6
	LDL-ox (ng/mL)	154·6	21·4	109·0	10·2
	Overall protein oxidation (FTSC intensity)	78·9	12·0	136·0	2·4
Liver	MDA (nmol/mg prot)	9·9	0·8	8·1	1·0
	Overall low ionic strength protein oxidation (FTSC intensity)	51·3[*]	2·7	74·7	0·7
	Overall high ionic strength protein oxidation (FTSC intensity)	81·4[*]	6·9	295·7	23·6
Abdominal fat	MDA (nmol/mg prot)	5·6[*]	1·2	16·0	3·1
Kidney	MDA (nmol/mg prot)	0·7	0·1	0·8	0·1
Heart	MDA (nmol/mg prot)	4·8	0·8	4·3	0·9
Brain	MDA (nmol/mg prot)	28·7	10·0	18·2	1·2
Urine	15-F_{2t}-IsoP (ng/mg creatinine)	2·9	0·2	1·9	0·1

[1]SHROB, Spontaneously Hypertensive Obese; WKY, Wistar Kyoto; ORAC, oxygen radical absorbance capacity; MDA, malondialdehyde.
Statistically significant differences between the samples are indicated by * ($P<0.05$), ** ($P<0.01$) and *** ($P<0.001$).

out this kind of integrated evaluations of OS in *in vivo* studies on metabolic syndrome.

The results presented here provide an updated picture of CVD-related markers in SHROB rats. In blood, the animals show elevated levels of markers related to inflammation, endothelial dysfunction, thrombotic activity, insulin resistance and oxidative stress (C-reactive protein, total cholesterol, LDL-cholesterol, triglycerides, apoA1, apoB100, abdominal fat, blood pressure, ICAM-1 and PAI-1, insulin and oxidized LDL). In other organs (abdominal fat, liver and brain) the glutathione system is activated and oxidative stress remains low, according to the observed concentrations of final lipid and protein oxidation products. All these observations are consistent with a pre-diabetic obese status of SHROB rats with a high risk of developing CVD that may be used to evaluate the effects of nutritional interventions on the metabolic alterations present in MetS.

Supporting Information

Figure S1 Standard curve used to quantify GSH (gluta-thione).

Figure S2 Standard curve used to quantify GSSG (glutathione disulphide).

References

1. Grundy SM (2008) Metabolic syndrome pandemic. Arterioscl Thormb Vasc Biol 28: 629–36.
2. Eckel RH, Alberti KGMM, Grundy SM, Zimmet PZ (2010) The metabolic syndrome. The Lancet 375: 2010, 181–83.
3. Festa A, D'Agostino R, Howard G, Mykkännen L, Tracy RP, et al. (2000) Chronic subclinical inflammation as part of the insulin resistance syndrome: The insulin resistance atherosclerosis study (IRAS). Circulation 102: 42–47.
4. Armutcu F, Ataymen M, Atmaca H, Gurel A (2008) Oxidative stress markers, C-reactive protein and heat shock protein 70 levels in subjects with metabolic syndrome. Clin Chem Lab Med 46: 785–90.
5. Güçlü F, Özmen B, Hekimsoy Z, Kirmaz C (2004) Effects of a statin group drug, pravastatin, on the insulin resistance in patients with metabolic syndrome. Biomed Pharmacother 58: 614–18.
6. Zhang BB, Zhou G, Li C (2009) AMPK: An emerging drug target for diabetes and metabolic syndrome. Cell Metabolism 9: 407–16.

Figure S3 Representative chromatogram of endogenous 15-F_{2t}-IsoP in rat urine. A) The m/z 573 ion current chromatogram represents the [$^2H_4$]-15-F_{2t}-IsoP internal standard; the signal used to quantify 15-F_{2t}-IsoP. B) The m/z 569 ion current chromatogram represents endogenous 15-F_{2t}-IsoP. The injection volume was 1 μL.

Figure S4 Evolution of the body weight of SHROB and WKY rats from week 13 to week 27 of life.

Table S1 Fatty acid composition of the soybean oil provided weekly. Values are given as mean ± SD.

Acknowledgments

We thank Lorena Barros and Mª Jesus Gonzalez for technical support, as well as María José Bleda Hernández for support with the statistical analysis. Language revision by Christopher Evans is appreciated.

Author Contributions

Conceived and designed the experiments: IM JLT. Performed the experiments: EMT JPJ LL VSM NT MR MP LM AM. Analyzed the data: EMT JPJ SRR MC JLT. Wrote the paper: EMT JPJ SRR.

7. Castell-Auvi A, Cedó L, Pallarés V, Blay MT, Pinent M, et al. (2012) Procyanidins modify insulinemia by affecting insulin production and degradation. J Nutr Biochem 23: 1565–72.
8. Kimura T, Nakagawa K, Kubota H, Kojima Y, Goto Y, et al. (2007) Food-grade mulberry powder enriched with 1-deoxynojirimycin suppresses the elevation of postprandial blood glucose in humans. J Agric Food Chem 55: 5869–5874.
9. Hariri N, Thibault L (2010) High-fat diet-induced obesity in animal models. Nutr Res Rev 23: 270–99.
10. Poudyal H, Panchal S, Brown L (2010) Comparison of purple carrot juice and β-carotene in a high-carbohydrate, high-fat diet-fed rat model of the metabolic syndrome. Br J Nutr 104: 1322–32.
11. Chua SC, Chung WK, Wu-Peng XS, Zhang Y, Liu SM, et al. (1996) Phenotypes of mouse diabetes and rat fatty due to mutations in the OB (leptin) receptor. Sci 271: 994–96.
12. Koletsky S (1973) Obese spontaneously hypertensive rats: a model for study of atherosclerosis. Exp Molec Pathol 19: 53–60.

13. Koletsky S (1975) Animal model of human disease: hypertension, obesity, type 4 hyperlipidemia, vascular disease. Am J Pathol 81: 463–66.

14. Takaya K, Ogawa Y, Hiraoka J, Hosoda K, Yamori Y, et al. (1996) Nonsense mutation of leptin receptor in the obese spontaneously hypertensive Koletsky rat. Nature Genetics 14: 130–31.

15. Ernsberger P, Koletsky RJ, Friedman JE (1999) Molecular pathology in the obese spontaneous hypertensive Koletsky rats: a model of syndrome X. Annals New York Acad Sci 892: 315–18.

16. Alberti KGMM, Eckel RH, Grundy SM, Zimmet PZ, Cleeman JI, et al. (2009) Harmonizing the metabolic syndrome: A joint interim statement of the international diabetes federation task force on epidemiology and prevention; National heart, lung, and blood institute; American heart association; World heart federation; International atherosclerosis society; And international association for the study of obesity. Circul 120: 1640–45.

17. Ernsberger P, Koletsky RJ (2012) The glucose tolerance test as a laboratory toll with clinical implications. In Glucose Tolerance [S Chackrewarthy, editor] InTech 2012.

18. Ishizuka T, Ernsberger P, Liu S (1998) Phenotypic nonsequences of a nonsense mutation in the leptin receptor gene (fa^k) in obese spontaneously hypertensive Koletsky rats (SHROB). J Nutr 128: 2299–2306.

19. Matthews D, Hosker J, Rudenski A, Naylor BA, Treacher DF, et al. (1985) Homeostasis model assessment: insulin resistance and B-cell function from fasting plasma glucose and insulin concentrations in man. Diabetologia 28: 412–9.

20. Buñag RD (1973) Validation in awake rats of a tail-cuff method for measuring systolic pressure. J Appl Physiol 34: 279–82.

21. Cohen G, Dembiec D, Marcus J (1970) Measurement of catalase activity in tissue extracts. Anal Biochem 34: 30–38.

22. Misra HP, Fridovich I (1972) The role of superoxide anion in the autoxidation of epinephrine and a simple assay for superoxide dismutase. J Biol Chem 247: 3170–3175.

23. Goldberg DM, Spooner RJ (1983) Glutathione reductase. In Methods of enzymatic analysis, 3rd ed, pp. 258–265 [HU . Bergmeyer, editor] Weinheim: Verlag Chemie 1983.

24. Wheeler CR, Salzman JA, Elsayed NM, Omaye ST, Korte DW (1990) Automated assays for superoxide dismutase, catalase, glutathione peroxidase, and glutathione reductase activity. Anal Biochem 184: 193–199.

25. Hissin PJ, Hilf R (1976) A fluorometric method for determination of oxidized and reduced glutathione in tissues. Anal Biochem 74: 214–26.

26. Bradford MM (1976) A rapid and sensitive method for the quantitation of microgram quantities of protein utilizing the principle of protein-dye binding. Anal Biochem 72: 248–254.

27. Drabkin D, Austin J (1935) Spectrophotometric studies. II. Preparations from washed blood cells; nitric oxide hemoglobin and sulfhemoglobin. J Biol Chem 112: 51–65.

28. Cao G, Booth SL, Sadowski JA, Prior RL (1998) Increases in human plasma antioxidant capacity after consumption of controlled diets high in fruit and vegetables. Am J Clin Nutr 68: 1081–1087.

29. Chaudhuri AR, de Waal EM, Pierce A, Van Remmen H, Ward WF, et al. (2006) A detection of protein carbonyls in aging liver tissue: A fluorescence-based proteomic approach. Mech Ageing Dev 127: 849–861.

30. Méndez L, Pazos M, Gallardo JM, Torres JL, Pérez-Jiménez J, et al. (2013) Reduced protein oxidation in Wistar rats supplemented with marine omega-3 PUFAs. Free Radical Biol Med 55: 8–20.

31. Laemmli UK (1970) Cleavage of structural proteins during the assembly of the head of bacteriophage T4. Nature 227: 680–685.

32. Buege JA, Aust SD (1978) Microsomal lipid peroxidation. Methods Enzymol 52: 302–10.

33. Milne GL, Sánchez CS, Musiek ES, Morrow DJ (2007) Quantification of F2-isoprostanes as a biomarker of oxidative stress. Nature Protocols 2: 221–226.

34. Benjamini Y, Hochberg Y (1995) Controlling the false discovery rate: A practical and powerful approach to multiple testing. J R Stat Soc C-Appl 57: 283–90.

35. Simes RJ (1986). An improved bonferroni procedure for multiple tests of significance. Biometrika 73: 751–54.

36. Papazzo A, Conlan XA, Lexis L, Lewandowski PA (2011) Differential effects of dietary canola and soybean oil intake on oxidative stress in stroke-prone spontaneously hypertensive rats. Lipids Health Dis 10: 98.

37. Mendizábal Y, Llorens S, Nava E (2011) Reactivity of the aortic and mesenteric arteries from the obese spontaneously hypertensive rat: effect of glitazones. Am J Physiol Heart Circ Physiol 301:H1319–30.

38. Mendizábal Y, Llorens S, Nava E (2013) Vasoactive effects of prostaglandins from the perivascular fat of mesenteric resistance arteries in WKY and SHROB rats. Life Sci 93: 1023–32.

39. Fellman L, Nascimento AR, Tibiriça E, Bousquet P (2012) Murine models for pharmacological studies on the metaoblic syndrome. Pharmacol Therapeut 137: 331–40.

40. Samuel VT & Shulman GI (2012) Mechanisms for insulin resistance: common threads and missing links. Cell 148: 852–871.

41. Chawla A, Nguyen KD, Goh YPS (2011) Macrophage-.mediated inflammation in metabolic disease. Nat Rev Inmunol 11: 738–49.

42. Maritim AC, Sanders RA, Watkins JB (2003) Diabetes, oxidative stress, and antioxidants: A review. J Biochem Molec Toxicol 17: 24–38.

43. Imig JD, Walsh KA, Khan MA, Nagasawa T, Cherian-Shaw M, et al. (2012) Soluble epoxide hydrolase inhibition and peroxisome proliferator activated receptor γ agonist improve vascular function and decrease renal injury in hypertensive obese rats. Exp Biol Med 237: 1402–12.

44. Méndez L, Pazos M, Giralt M, Nogués MR, Pérez-Jiménez J, et al. (2014) Targets of protein carbonylation in Koletsky Spontaneously Hypertensive Obese Rats and healthy Wistar counterparts: a potential role on metabolic disorders. J Proteom 106: 246–59.

11

Quantitative Analyses of Schizophrenia-Associated Metabolites in Serum: Serum D-Lactate Levels Are Negatively Correlated with Gamma-Glutamylcysteine in Medicated Schizophrenia Patients

Takeshi Fukushima[1]*, Hideaki Iizuka[1], Ayaka Yokota[1], Takehiro Suzuki[1], Chihiro Ohno[1], Yumiko Kono[1], Minami Nishikiori[1], Ayaka Seki[1], Hideaki Ichiba[1], Yoshinori Watanabe[2], Seiji Hongo[2], Mamoru Utsunomiya[3], Masaki Nakatani[3], Kiyomi Sadamoto[4], Takashi Yoshio[5]

1 Department of Analytical Chemistry, Faculty of Pharmaceutical Sciences, Toho University, Funabashi-shi, Chiba, Japan, 2 Nanko Clinic of Psychiatry, Himorogi group, Medical Corporation JISENKAI, Shirakawa-shi, Fukushima, Japan, 3 Public Interest Incorporated Foundation, Sumiyoshi-kaiseikai Sumiyoshi hospital, Koufu-shi, Yamanashi, Japan, 4 Department of Clinical Pharmacy, Yokohama College of Pharmacy, Yokohama-shi, Kanagawa, Japan, 5 Department of Clinical Pharmacy, Faculty of Pharmaceutical Sciences, Toho University, Funabashi-shi, Chiba, Japan

Abstract

The serum levels of several metabolites are significantly altered in schizophrenia patients. In this study, we performed a targeted analysis of 34 candidate metabolites in schizophrenia patients ($n = 25$) and compared them with those in age- and gender-matched healthy subjects ($n = 27$). Orthogonal partial least square-discriminant analysis revealed that complete separation between controls and patients was achieved based on these metabolites. We found that the levels of γ-glutamylcysteine (γ-GluCys), linoleic acid, arachidonic acid, D-serine, 3-hydroxybutyrate, glutathione (GSH), 5-hydroxytryptamine, threonine, and tyrosine were significantly lower, while D-lactate, tryptophan, kynurenine, and glutamate levels were significantly higher in schizophrenia patients compared to controls. Using receiver operating characteristics (ROC) curve analysis, the sensitivity, specificity, and the area under curve of γ-GluCys, a precursor of GSH, and D-lactate, a terminal metabolite of methylglyoxal, were 88.00%, 81.48%, and 0.8874, and 88.00%, 77.78%, and 0.8415, respectively. In addition, serum levels of D-lactate were negatively correlated with γ-GluCys levels in patients, but not in controls. The present results suggest that oxidative stress-induced damage may be involved in the pathogenesis of schizophrenia.

Editor: James D. Clelland, The Nathan Kline Institute, United States of America

Funding: This research was financially supported by the Japan Society for the Promotion of Science, Grant-in-Aid for Scientific Research (C) Grant Numbers 23617027 and 25460224, and the Faculty of Pharmaceutical sciences, Toho University. The funders had no role in study design, data collection and analysis, decision to publish, or preparation of the manuscript.

Competing Interests: The authors have declared that no competing interests exist.

* Email: t-fukushima@phar.toho-u.ac.jp

Introduction

Schizophrenia is a severe psychiatric disease that affects approximately 1% of the world's population; it is comprised of positive and negative symptoms and cognitive deficits, with an onset during adolescence [1]. Optimal treatment thus requires early detection and suitable medication, which in turn require highly trained psychiatrists. Recently, metabonomic studies have revealed significant alterations in endogenous metabolites, including amino acids, polyunsaturated fatty acids (PUFAs), myo-inositol, and citrate, in the serum of schizophrenia patients [2–4]. These alterations reflect the impairment of systemic metabolism in peripheral tissues, and indicate that schizophrenia should be regarded as not only a dysfunction of the central nervous system (CNS), but also as a disorder of systemic metabolism. In previous studies, however, the discriminatory power of metabonomics was found to be heavily dependent on the capacity of the instruments used for analysis; consequently, several different metabolites have

been proposed as crucial factors in the pathogenesis of schizophrenia.

In the present study, we focused on metabolites that have previously been suggested to be associated with schizophrenia. For example, the glutamate hypothesis of schizophrenia etiology suggests that endogenous D-serine is a crucial factor related to the hypofunction of the N-methyl-D-aspartate (NMDA) receptor [5–7]. Oxidative stress is also associated with schizophrenia [8], and a low level of the antioxidant glutathione (GSH) has been reported in schizophrenia patients [9]. Thus, we selected 34 target metabolites, many of which have been implicated in schizophrenia, and performed quantitative analyses of their levels in serum from schizophrenia patients. Subsequently, we applied a multivariate analysis between controls and the patients, and a correlation matrix approach to determine whether there was any association between these metabolites.

Methods

1. Participants

Table 1 lists the demographic features of the patients and controls that participated in this study. Twenty-five schizophrenia patients (11 men and 14 women) were clinically diagnosed by experienced doctors according to International Classification of Diseases (ICD)-10 criteria and recruited from Sumiyoshi Hospital (Koufu-shi) and the Nanko Clinic of Psychiatry (Shirakawa-shi), both located in Japan; the mean ± SD age of patients was 28.2±4.4 years. All were medicated outpatients, treated with olanzapine (60%; $n = 15$), aripiprazole (40%, $n = 10$), risperidone long acting injection (16%, $n = 4$), levomepromazine (8%; $n = 2$), blonanserin (8%; $n = 2$), paliperidone (8%; $n = 2$), quetiapine (4%; $n = 1$), fluphenazine (4%; $n = 1$), risperidone (4%; $n = 1$), or sulpiride (4%; $n = 1$). Eleven patients (44%) had taken more than 2 kinds of antipsychotics. Age-matched healthy human volunteers ($n = 27$), including 12 men and 15 women with a mean ± SD age of 26.5±5.6 years, comprised the control group.

Ethics statement: Written informed consent was obtained from all subjects prior to participation, and the protocol was approved by the ethics committee in the Faculty of Pharmaceutical Sciences, Toho University (approval number 23-1, 24-6). The capacities of all patients to provide consent were established by psychiatrists with more than 10 years' experience. In this study, there were no surrogate consent procedures required.

2. Blood sampling

Five milliliters of blood was drawn from the arm vein of participants at 11:00 AM–12:00 PM before lunch to avoid the effect of food intake wherever possible, and collected in Venoject-II AUTOSEP tubes (Terumo Corporation; Tokyo, Japan); samples were allowed to stand for 30 min at room temperature, consistent with a previous procedure for serum D-serine analysis [6,10]. Tubes were then centrifuged at 1200×g for 15 min. The serum obtained was divided into aliquots of 100 μL each in screw-capped vials, which were stored at –80°C.

3. Determination of targeted metabolites in serum

A total of 34 target metabolites were examined: L-tryptophan (Trp), L-kynurenine (Kyn), kynurenic acid (KYNA), 5-hydroxy-tryptamine (5-HT), D-serine (D-Ser), D-lactate, L-lactate, 3-hydroxybutyrate (3-HB), GSH, γ-glutamylcysteine (GluCys), cysteine (Cys), cysteinylglycine (CysGly), L-amino acids (His, Arg, Gln, Ser, Asn, Glu, Gly, Pro, Thr, Ala, Leu, Ile, Val, Phe,

Lys, and Tyr), fatty acids [linoleic acid (LA), arachidonic acid (AA), oleic acid, linolenic acid, and palmitoleic acid], and glucose. The serum levels of these metabolites were determined by using high-performance liquid chromatography (HPLC) methods. An HPLC with fluorescence detection method was used for quantification of L-amino acids [11–13], thiol compounds [14], D- and L-Ser [6,15], D- and L-lactate [16], 3-HB [17,18], fatty acids [19], and KYNA [20,21].

Serum Trp and Kyn levels were determined using an HPLC with mass spectrometric detection method as described previously [22], and 5-HT levels were determined using HPLC-electrochemical detection [23]. Glucose levels were determined using a commercial kit (Wako; Osaka, Japan). These methods have already been validated at the serum level for each metabolite.

4. Statistical analyses

The non-parametric Mann-Whitney U-test (2-tailed) was performed for statistical analysis of metabolite concentrations, with $p<0.05$ considered significant. The Spearman rank correlation test was performed to determine statistical correlations between variables.

For multivariate analysis, the collected data were imported to SIMCA 13.0.3 software (Umetrics; Umea, Sweden), and an orthogonal partial least square-discrimination analysis (OPLS-DA) was carried out. The statistics, R^2 (cumulative) and Q^2 (cumulative), were calculated by OPLS-DA. R^2 and Q^2 represent explanatory variable estimating the goodness of fit of the model and predictor, which is the 7-fold cross-validated predictive ability, respectively. The statics range (minimum–maximum) is 0–1. Receiver operating characteristics (ROC) curve tests for metabolites were performed using GraphPad Prism 6 (GraphPad Software, Inc.; La Jolla, CA, USA).

Results

1. Subject characteristics

For the purpose of early detection of schizophrenia, young patients, aged 21–35 years, were enrolled in the present study. In addition, age- and gender-matched healthy subjects were enrolled as controls. As shown in Table 1, no significant difference in sex ratio or age was observed between controls and patients ($p = 0.807$ and $p = 0.251$, respectively).

Table 1. Characteristics of subjects.

	Controls		Patients		p value
Number of subjects	27		25		
Gender (male/female)	12/15		11/14		0.8065
Age (year)	26.5±5.6	(18–37)	28.2±4.4	(21–35)	0.251
Onset age (year)			21.4±4.9	(15–30)	
Duration of illness (month)			84.5±57.8	(1–240)	
Chlorpromazine equivalent (mg)			605±345	(150–1455)	
Diabetes mellitus (Y/N)	0/27		0/25		
Smoker/nonsmoker	1/26		10/15		<0.001
BMI (kg/m²)	21.4±2.8	(17.4–27.8)	24±4.1	(14.4–31.2)	0.014

The comparison between 2 groups was performed using the χ^2 test for gender difference and smoking, and the Student's t-test for age and body mass index (BMI).

2. Discrimination of controls and patients

A total of 34 serum metabolites were quantified from controls and from schizophrenia patients. A multivariate analysis, OPLS-DA, was then carried out, and the results are shown in Fig. 1a. Clear separation between controls and patients was achieved with an R^2 (cumulative) and a Q^2 (cumulative) of 0.8606 and 0.7203, respectively. For Q^2, a predictor calculated by cross-validation, a value above 0.4 indicates that the OPLS-DA model is reliable; these results showed that patients could be discriminated from controls using these serum metabolite levels. Among the 34 compounds tested, 12 had a variable importance in the projection (VIP; an indicator of discriminatory power) value above 1.0; these were γ-GluCys, LA, D-lactate, Trp, AA, Kyn, D-Ser, Glu, 3-HB, L-lactate, Gly, and GSH (Fig. 1b). The relatively large VIP values of γ-GluCys (2.26), LA (1.98), and D-lactate (1.70) showed that these metabolites were the main contributors to the patient-group separation in this study.

3. Comparison of serum levels between controls and patients

The serum level results are categorized into 5 separate tables (Tables S1, S2, S3, S4, and S5). The metabolites for which serum levels differed between controls and schizophrenia patients are listed in Table 2. With regard to serum amino acids, the levels of Glu ($p = 0.0145$), D-Ser ($p = 0.00163$), Tyr ($p = 0.0469$), and Thr ($p = 0.0286$) were significantly altered between patients and controls. Serum levels of D-lactate ($p = 2.43 \times 10^{-5}$) and 3-HB

($p = 0.00438$) were significantly different between the patient and control groups. The analysis of thiol compounds and fatty acids, respectively, revealed that levels of GSH ($p = 0.0344$), γ-GluCys ($p = 1.75 \times 10^{-6}$), LA ($p = 1.61 \times 10^{-5}$), and AA ($p = 0.00149$) were significantly altered in patients. With regard to Trp metabolites, serum levels of Trp ($p = 0.00101$), Kyn ($p = 0.00568$), and 5-HT ($p = 0.0131$), but not KYNA ($p = 0.6145$), were significantly altered.

In summary, the serum levels of 9 compounds, γ-GlyCys, LA, AA, D-Ser, 3-HB, GSH, 5-HT, Thr, and Tyr, were significantly decreased, whereas those of 4 compounds, D-lactate, Trp, Kyn, and Glu, were significantly increased in patients compared to controls.

When a Bonferroni correction was applied, levels of 4 metabolites (γ-GluCys, LA, D-lactate, and Trp) were still significantly different between control and patient groups, while the following metabolites were present at similar levels in both groups: AA, Kyn, D-Ser, Glu, 3-HB, GSH, 5-HT, Thr, and Tyr (Table 2).

Similar to a previous study [10], there was a higher number of smokers among enrolled schizophrenia patients than controls (Table 1). There were no significant differences in the serum levels of metabolites between smokers and non-smokers with the exception of γ-GluCys ($p = 0.035$) (Table S6). Regarding γ-GluCys, however, significant differences between control and patient groups were observed in both non-smoking ($p = 5.71E-07$) and smoking patients ($p = 0.0152$, Bonferroni test).

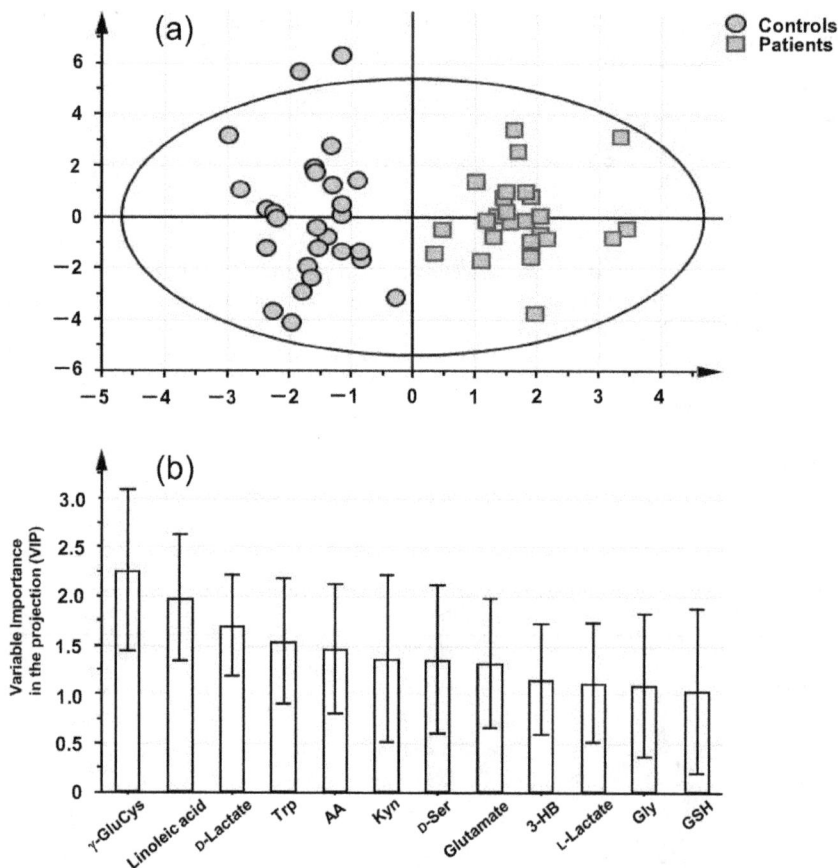

Figure 1. Score plot derived from orthogonal partial least square-discriminant analysis (OPLS-DA) based on the serum levels of 34 targeted metabolites in the subjects (a), and variable importance in the projection (VIP) data of the compounds with VIP values above 1.0 (b).

Table 2. Serum levels of metabolites (µmol/L) that were differentially expressed between controls and schizophrenia patients.

Compound	Levels in serum		p value*
	Controls (n=27)	Schizophrenia patients (n=25)	
γ–Glutamylcysteine	3.05±0.11	2.07±0.12	1.746E-06[a]
Linoleic acid	264±17.0	159±12.0	1.610E-05[a]
D-Lactate	7.26±0.481	13.1±1.42	2.426E-05[a]
L-Tryptophan	81.3±3.36	101±4.48	0.001011[a]
Arachidonic acid	55.4±4.48	38.5±2.18	0.001485
L-Kynurenine	1.74±0.121	2.35±0.162	0.005676
D-Serine	1.88±0.07	1.57±0.07	0.00163
Glutamate	35.5±3.20	71.3±12.3	0.0145
3-Hydroxybutyrate	46.5±10.1	17.6±3.84	0.004378
Glutathione	3.67±0.241	3.03±0.149	0.03437
5-Hydroxytryptamine	0.85±0.077	0.61±0.096	0.01308
Threonine	126±7.44	111±10.3	0.0286
Tyrosine	65.1±2.55	57.2±3.33	0.0469

Only p values below 0.05 are included in this table.
*Non-parametric Mann-Whitney U-test.
[a]Significantly different following Bonferroni correction (<0.05/34).

4. ROC curve analysis

The ROC curves of serum levels of γ-GluCys, LA, and D-lactate, which displayed relatively large VIP values, are shown in Fig. 2. The AUC values for these metabolites were 0.8874, 0.8489, and 0.8415, respectively. The sensitivity and specificity at the cut-off points for γ-GluCys, LA, and D-lactate were 88.00 and 81.48%, 80.00 and 77.78%, and 88.00 and 77.78%, respectively.

5. Correlations of the serum levels in controls and patients

Among the 13 compounds that discriminated the control and patient groups (Table 2), a negative correlation between D-lactate and γ-GluCys levels was observed ($p = 0.00533$, $r = -0.5400$) in patients (Fig. 3b), but not in controls (Fig. 3a). A positive correlation between γ-GluCys and GSH was observed in controls ($r = 0.652$, $p = 0.000229$) (Fig. 3c), but not in patients ($r = 0.044$, $p = 0.8351$) (Fig. 3d).

Serum Tyr and 5-HT levels in patients were significantly correlated with daily chlorpromazine (CP) equivalents, and the levels of D-Ser, Glu, 3-HB, AA, and LA were positively correlated with duration of illness (Table 3).

Discussion

Our data revealed that analysis of 34 serum metabolites was sufficient to discriminate between controls and schizophrenia patients by OPLS-DA (Fig. 1 (a)), and that the decreased levels of γ-GluCys and increased levels of D-lactate were the major contributors to this discrimination (Fig. 1 (b)). To the best of our knowledge, there have been no reports to date showing that serum levels of γ-GluCys or D-lactate are altered in schizophrenia patients. By analyses of ROC curves (Fig. 2), the serum levels of these metabolites revealed sufficient AUC values (0.8874 and 0.8415) to discriminate patients from controls. The sensitivity and selectivity values were also satisfactory (Fig. 2).

Oxidative stress may be involved in the pathogenesis of schizophrenia [8,24]. On the other hand, carbonyl stress, such as the glycation and inactivation of proteins by the dicarbonyl compound methylglyoxal (MGO), is involved in diabetic complications [25,26]. In the glyoxalase pathway, glyoxalase I converts MGO to S-lactoylglutathione, and subsequently, S-lactoylglutathione is converted to D-lactate by glyoxalase II [25] (Fig. S1). Increased D-lactate levels have been found in diabetes mellitus, likely due to enhanced MGO production [25]. Indeed, we previously reported a significant increase in the serum D-lactate level in diabetic patients [16]. Recently, it was reported that carbonyl stress was enhanced in a subpopulation of schizophrenia patients due to a decline in glyoxalase I activity [27]. Therefore, a reduction in glyoxalase I activity would be expected to lead to a lower serum D-lactate level. However, our current data show that the serum D-lactate level was significantly increased in patients. Although further experiments are required, we suggest that increased activity of glyoxalase II in patients may underlie the increased D-lactate level.

Another finding in the present study is that the serum γ-GluCys level was remarkably reduced in schizophrenia patients. γ-GluCys is a precursor of an endogenous antioxidant, GSH, and is produced from Glu and Cys by glutamatecysteine ligase (GCL; Fig. S2). GCL activity is a rate-limiting enzyme for GSH synthesis, and genetic polymorphisms in GCL significantly modulate schizophrenia risk [28,29]. As shown in Table 2, the low GSH level observed in patients is consistent with previous reports [9,30]. However, to the best of our knowledge, we are the first to report a decreased level of the GSH precursor γ-GluCys in the sera of schizophrenia patients. In addition, the level of Glu, which is a precursor of γ-GluCys, was significantly increased in patients (Table 2), suggesting that GCL activity might also be attenuated. The significant decrease in the GSH level of patients indicates that anti-oxidant defenses against reactive oxygen species (ROS) and reactive nitrogen species (RNS) may be compromised in schizophrenia. Interestingly, a significant negative correlation between D-lactate and γ-GluCys was observed specifically in the patients' sera (Fig. 3b). Since S-lactoylglutathione is metabolized by glyoxalase II to release D-lactate and GSH (Fig. S2), elevated

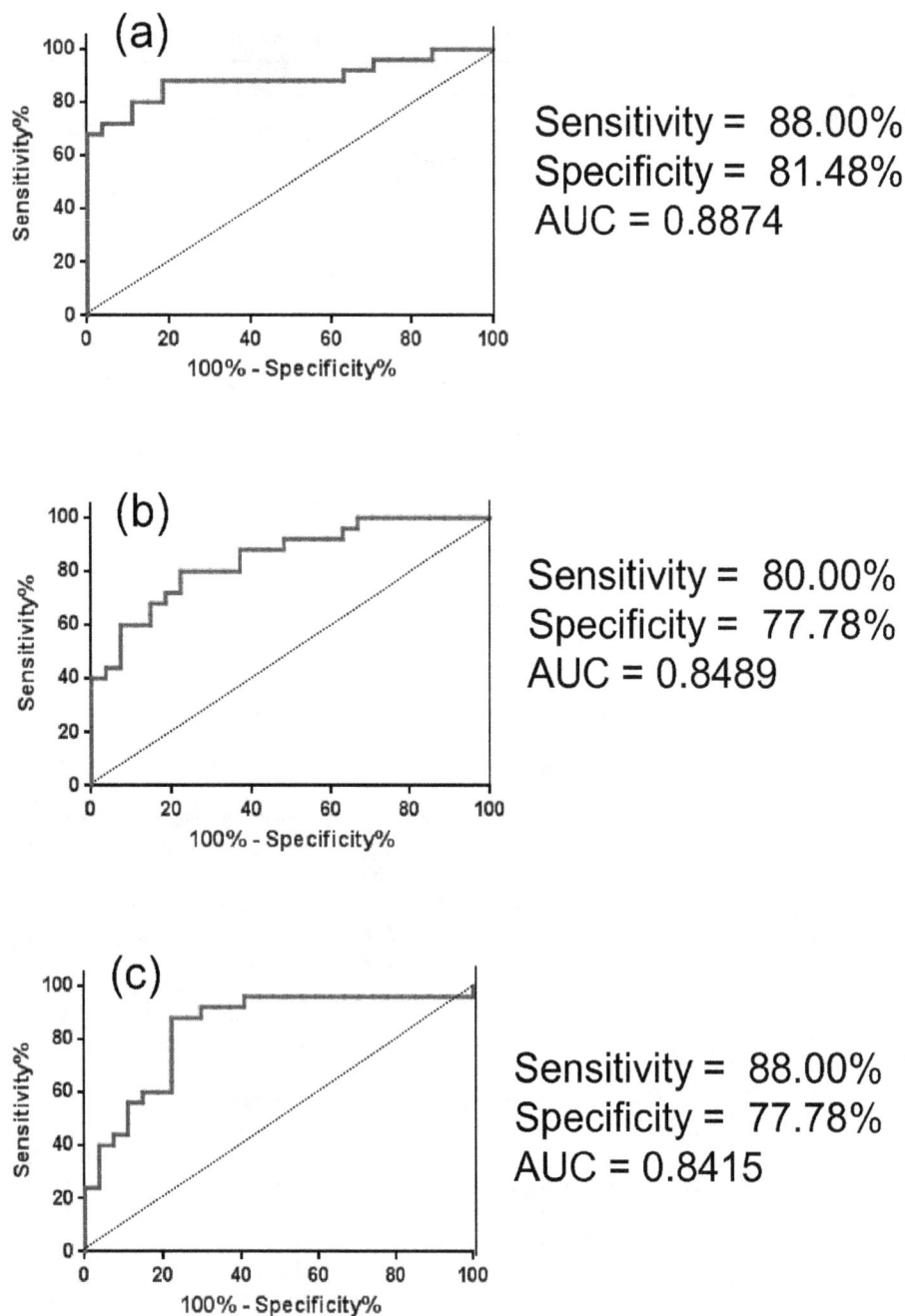

Sensitivity = 88.00%
Specificity = 81.48%
AUC = 0.8874

Sensitivity = 80.00%
Specificity = 77.78%
AUC = 0.8489

Sensitivity = 88.00%
Specificity = 77.78%
AUC = 0.8415

Figure 2. Receiver operating characteristic (ROC) curve analyses of γ-GluCys (a), lenoleic acid (b), and D-lactate (c).

GSH levels would be expected in patient serum; however, we observed low serum GSH levels in patients (Table 2). In addition, a positive correlation between serum γ-GluCys and GSH levels was observed specifically in controls (Fig. 3c and d). Taken together, these data suggest that reduced GSH levels in schizophrenia patients may be due to the rapid consumption of GSH during its anti-ROS or -RNS activities.

Recently, an increased 3-HB level was observed in serum from schizophrenia patients in a metabonomics study [2]. Conversely, Cai et al. (2012) reported a decreased 3-HB level in the serum of patients. As shown in Table 2, we found that 3-HB levels were reduced in patient serum. As a ketone body, 3-HB is produced from acetoacetate, which in turn is derived from fatty acids (Fig.

S3). 3-HB levels increase as a result of fasting and in diabetic subjects due to limited utilization of glucose; under these conditions, there is instead enhanced utilization of ketone bodies for energy production. A recent report showed that 3-HB-dependent increases in transcription of the oxidative stress resistance factors FOXO3A and MT2 constitute an anti-oxidant pathway [31]. Thus, depletion of endogenous 3-HB in patients may induce oxidative stress, which is implicated in schizophrenia etiology [8].

Regarding PUFAs, we found that serum AA and LA levels were significantly decreased in patients (Table 2). These results are consistent with previous reports of low PUFA levels in schizophrenia patients [32]. LA is initially obtained from the daily diet,

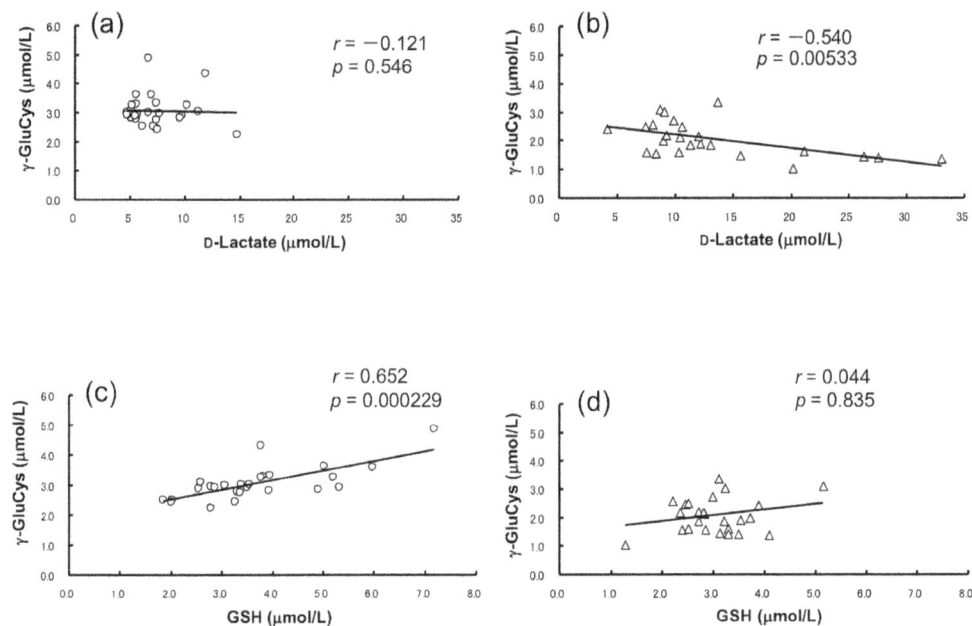

Figure 3. Correlation plots of D-lactate and γ-GluCys serum levels in controls (a) and in patients with schizophrenia (b), and between GSH and γ-GluCys in controls (c) and in patients with schizophrenia (d).

and is then converted to AA by elongase and desaturase (Fig. S3). Considering these facts, it is likely that the reduction in PUFA levels in schizophrenia patients is caused by their excess oxidative stress. In addition, it has been reported that increased tissue expression of fatty acid binding protein (FABP) is closely associated with the etiology of schizophrenia [33], and both LA and AA are bound by FABP7 [33,34]. Therefore, FABP7-dependent seques-tering of circulating PUFAs in biological fluids might also contribute to reduced serum PUFA levels in patients.

In the present study, we examined Trp and its metabolites, Kyn, KYNA, and 5-HT, since the associated metabolic pathways produce several neuroactive substances [35,36]. Our data revealed that serum Trp and Kyn levels were significantly increased in patients (Table 2). Trp is metabolized to Kyn by tryptophan 2,3-dioxygenase or indoleamine 2,3-dioxygenase in the Kyn pathway, and to 5-HT by tryptophan hydroxylase (TH) and aromatic amino acid decarboxylase (AAD) in the serotonin pathway (Fig. S4) [37,38]. Since only medicated patients were enrolled in the present study, our present results regarding serum Trp levels are consistent with the report of Xuan et al. [4], who found increased Trp levels in the serum of medicated patients. By contrast, the 5-HT level was significantly decreased in patients compared to controls

(Table 2). Therefore, activities of TH or AAD might also be decreased in patients. 5-HT is further metabolized to melatonin, which possesses anti-oxidant activity [36,39]. We speculate that the decreased level of 5-HT will lead to lower melatonin levels, and thus compromised antioxidant defenses, in patients.

Conversely, the serum KYNA level was not altered significantly between controls and patients ($p = 0.6145$), although increased KYNA levels in the post-mortem brain tissue [40] or cerebrospinal fluids [41] from schizophrenia patients have been reported. KYNA acts as an endogenous antagonist of the glycine site of the NMDA receptor. However, we found no alteration in the serum KYNA levels of patients, indicating that increased KYNA levels might occur only in the CNS. By contrast, we did observe a significant decrease in serum levels of D-serine, a co-agonist of the glycine site of the NMDA receptor [5,42] (Table 2), which is consistent with previous reports [6,10]. Genetic studies of schizophrenia show that the susceptibility gene G72 plays a role in regulation of D-amino acid oxidase (DAO), an enzyme that is upregulated in schizophrenia [43,44]. Thus, high-level expression of DAO in several tissues, including the brain, liver, and kidney, may underlie the observed decreased serum D-serine level in patients.

Table 3. Correlations between serum levels of metabolites and CP equivalent (mg) or duration of illness (months).

	Tyr	5-HT			
CP equivalent	$r = -0.488$	$r = 0.397$			
(mg)	($p = 0.0133$)	($p = 0.0491$)			
	D-Ser	**Glu**	**3-HB**	**Arachidonic acid**	**Linoleic acid**
Duration of illness	$r = 0.478$	$r = 0.397$	$r = 0.540$	$r = 0.630$	$r = 0.415$
(months)	($p = 0.0157$)	($p = 0.0491$)	($p = 0.0064$)	($p = 0.0007$)	($p = 0.0390$)

In this study, we were only able to include medicated patients, as recruitment of drug-naïve patients was not possible. Therefore, we cannot exclude the potential effects of medication in the interpretation of our results. Serum Tyr and 5-HT levels were significantly correlated with daily CP, and the levels of both metabolites were significantly lower in patients. The negative correlation between the serum Tyr level and CP equivalent is likely due to a medication-induced effect. Tyr is produced from Phe by phenylalanine hydroxylase (PH), and is then converted to catecholamines (e.g., dopamine and noradrenaline) by several enzymes such as tyrosine hydrolase and dopa decarboxylase. Since the serum level of Phe was not altered (Table S1), the involvement of decreased activity of PH or enhanced enzyme activities of catecholamines biosynthesis might occur in patients.

By contrast, the serum 5-HT level was positively correlated with CP equivalents. 5-HT is sensitive to oxidation; thus, elevated ROS or RNS in patients could lead to non-enzymatic decomposition of 5-HT in vivo. The second generation antipsychotics (SGA) aripiprazole and quetiapine have indirect anti-oxidative effects via induction of the anti-oxidative enzyme, superoxide dismutase [45]. Thus, the positive correlation between 5-HT levels and CP equivalents may be due to the SGA-dependent suppression of 5-HT oxidation.

The serum levels of D-Ser, Glu, 3-HB, AA, and LA exhibited a significant positive correlation with duration of illness (Table 3). Since the serum Glu level is reportedly increased even in drug-naïve patients [46], the effect of medication on the Glu level might be negligible. Calcia et al. [10] reported that plasma D-Ser levels were lower in non-medicated than in medicated patients. Consistent with this, D-Ser levels were higher in patients with a longer history of recorded illness, suggesting that sustained medication use may increase D-Ser levels. Indeed, we observed that SGAs possess DAO-inhibitory activity in vitro (data not shown). Furthermore, the anti-oxidant effects of SGAs [45] may explain why prolonged treatment of patients restores the levels of 3-HB, AA, and LA, as each of these metabolites are sensitive to oxidative stress.

There are nonetheless limitations to the current study. In the present study, blood samples were not collected from subjects in the early morning in a fasting state. Therefore, future studies should be performed under this condition to exclude the possibility that feeding is a confounding variable. Next, we only studied relatively young patients (≤ 35 years old), and we therefore cannot extrapolate our findings to a broader patient range. In addition, all patients were medicated, and it is therefore important to gather information from drug-naïve patients in future studies.

Conclusion

The present finding that the serum levels of 13 metabolites may be differentially regulated in schizophrenia patients extends our knowledge of the pathophysiology of the disease. Building upon this study, future investigations could identify which metabolites are suitable biomarkers for the early detection and prognosis of schizophrenia and its associated treatment regimens.

Supporting Information

Figure S1   D-Lactate-associated biosynthetic and metabolic pathways. Rectangles denote the quantified compound, and bold red rectangles denote metabolites that were differentially altered in patients compared to controls. Red upward or downward arrows indicate that the level increased or decreased, respectively.

Figure S2   Relevant biosynthetic and metabolic pathways associated with GSH. Rectangles denote quantified compounds, and bold red rectangles denote the metabolites that were differentially altered in the serum of patients versus controls. Red upward or downward arrows indicate that the level increased or decreased, respectively.

Figure S3   Relevant biosynthetic and metabolic pathway of PUFAs. Rectangles denotes the compounds that were quantified, and bold red rectangles denote the metabolites that differed between patients and controls. Red downward arrow means that the level decreased.

Figure S4   Relevant metabolic pathway of Trp. Rectangle denotes compounds quantified and bold red rectangle denotes the compounds whose levels were altered in patients compared to healthy controls. Red upward or downward arrows indicate that the level increased or decreased, respectively.

Table S1   Serum levels of amino acids (including D-serine) in controls and patients with schizophrenia.

Table S2   Serum levels of glucose, D-lactate, L-lactate, and 3-hydroxybutyrate (3-HB) in controls and patients with schizophrenia.

Table S3   Serum levels of thiol compounds in controls and patients with schizophrenia.

Table S4   Serum levels of unsaturated fatty acids in controls and patients with schizophrenia.

Table S5   Serum levels of Trp and its metabolites in controls and patients with schizophrenia.

Table S6   Serum levels of metabolites (μmol/L) in smoking and non-smoking schizophrenia patients.

Acknowledgments

The authors thank emeritus Prof. C. Nishimura, Toho University, for his kind and helpful advice on the statistical analyses, Drs. H. Yamada and S. Iwasa, Toho University, for their valuable discussions during this research, Mr. H. Ohashi, Mr. K. Suzuki, Miss M. Koshikawa, and Miss M. Kume, Toho University, for their technical assistance, and Mr. T. Takaku of the Himorogi group for his kind management of blood sampling from patients. The authors also thank all the participants who provided blood samples.

Author Contributions

Conceived and designed the experiments: TF H. Iizuka H. Ichiba TY. Performed the experiments: H. Iizuka AY TS CO YK M. Nishikiori AS TF. Analyzed the data: H. Iizuka H. Ichiba TF. Contributed reagents/materials/analysis tools: H. Iizuka AY TS CO YK M. Nishikiori AS TF. Wrote the paper: H. Iizuka H. Ichiba TF. Collected blood sample and the clinical data: YW SH MU M. Nakatani KS TY.

References

1. Freedman R (2003) Schizophrenia. N Engl J Med 349: 1738–1749.
2. Yang J, Chen T, Sun L, Zhao Z, Qi X, et al. (2013) Potential metabolite markers of schizophrenia. Mol Psychiatry 18: 67–78.
3. Cai H-L, Li H-D, Yan X-Z, Sun B, Zhang Q, et al. (2012) Metabolomic analysis of biochemical changes in the plasma and urine of first-episode neuroleptic-naive schizophrenia patients after treatment with risperidone. J Proteome Res 11: 4338–4350.
4. Xuan J, Pan G, Qiu Y, Yang L, Su M, et al. (2011) Metabolomic profiling to identify potential serum biomarkers for schizophrenia and risperidone action. J Proteome Res 10: 5433–5443.
5. Schell M, Brady R, Molliver M, Snyder S (1997) D-Serine as a neuromodulator: Regional and developmental localizations in rat brain glia resemble NMDA receptors. J Neurosci 17: 1604–1615.
6. Hashimoto K, Fukushima T, Shimizu E, Komatsu N, Watanabe H, et al. (2003) Decreased serum levels of D-serine in patients with schizophrenia: evidence in support of the N-methyl-D-aspartate receptor hypofunction hypothesis of schizophrenia. Arch Gen Psychiatry 60: 572–576.
7. Hashimoto K, Shimizu E, Iyo M (2005) Dysfunction of glia-neuron communication in pathophysiology of schizophrenia. Curr Psychiatry Rev 1: 151–163.
8. Bitanihirwe BKY, Woo T-UW (2011) Oxidative stress in schizophrenia: An integrated approach. Neurosci Biobehav Rev 35: 878–893.
9. Raffa M, Mechri A, Ben Othman L, Fendri C, Gaha L, et al. (2009) Decreased glutathione levels and antioxidant enzyme activities in untreated and treated schizophrenic patients. Prog Neuro-Psychopharmacol Biol Psychiatry 33: 1178–1183.
10. Calcia Marilia A, Madeira C, Alheira Flavio V, Silva Thuany CS, Tannos Filippe M, et al. (2012) Plasma levels of D-serine in Brazilian individuals with schizophrenia. Schizophr Res 142: 83–87.
11. Tomiya M, Fukushima T, Kawai J, Aoyama C, Mitsuhashi S, et al. (2006) Alterations of plasma and cerebrospinal fluid glutamate levels in rats treated with the N-methyl-D-aspartate receptor antagonist, ketamine. Biomed Chromatogr 20: 628–633.
12. Tomiya M, Fukushima T, Watanabe H, Fukami G, Fujisaki M, et al. (2007) Alterations in serum amino acid concentrations in male and female schizophrenic patients. Clin Chim Acta 380: 186–190.
13. Aoyama C, Santa T, Tsunoda M, Fukushima T, Kitada C, et al. (2004) A fully automated amino acid analyzer using NBD-F as a fluorescent derivatization reagent. Biomed Chromatogr 18: 630–636.
14. Isokawa M, Funatsu T, Tsunoda M (2013) Fast and simultaneous analysis of biothiols by high-performance liquid chromatography with fluorescence detection under hydrophilic interaction chromatography conditions. Analyst (Cambridge, U K) 138: 3802–3808.
15. Fukushima T, Kawai J, Imai K, Toyo'oka T (2004) Simultaneous determination of D- and L-serine in rat brain microdialysis sample using a column-switching HPLC with fluorimetric detection. Biomed Chromatogr 18: 813–819.
16. Hasegawa H, Fukushima T, Lee J-A, Tsukamoto K, Moriya K, et al. (2003) Determination of serum D-lactic and L-lactic acids in normal subjects and diabetic patients by column-switching HPLC with pre-column fluorescence derivatization. Anal Bioanal Chem 377: 886–891.
17. Tsai Y, Liao T, Lee J (2003) Identification of L-3-hydroxybutyrate as an original ketone body in rat serum by column-switching high-performance liquid chromatography and fluorescence derivatization. Anal Biochem 319: 34–41.
18. Hsu WY, Kuo CY, Fukushima T, Imai K, Chen CM, et al. (2011) Enantioselective determination of 3-hydroxybutyrate in the tissues of normal and streptozotocin-induced diabetic rats of different ages. J Chromatogr B 879: 3331–3336.
19. Prados P, Fukushima T, Santa T, Homma H, Tsunoda M, et al. (1997) 4-N,N-Dimethylaminosulfonyl-7-N-(2-aminoethyl)amino-benzofurazan as a new pre-column fluorescence derivatization reagent for carboxylic acids (fatty acids and drugs containing a carboxyl moiety) in liquid chromatography. Anal Chim Acta 344: 227–232.
20. Fukushima T, Mitsuhashi S, Tomiya M, Iyo M, Hashimoto K, et al. (2007) Determination of kynurenic acid in human serum and its correlation with the concentration of certain amino acids. Clin Chim Acta 377: 174–178.
21. Mitsuhashi S, Fukushima T, Kawai J, Tomiya M, Santa T, et al. (2006) Improved method for the determination of kynurenic acid in rat plasma by column-switching HPLC with post-column fluorescence detection. Anal Chim Acta 562: 36–43.
22. Ohashi H, Iizuka H, Yoshihara S, Otani H, Kume M, et al. (2013) Determination of l-tryptophan and l-kynurenine in human serum by using LC-MS after derivatization with (R)-DBD-PyNCS. Int J Tryptophan Res 6: 9–14.
23. Hubbard KE, Wells A, Owens TS, Tagen M, Fraga CH, et al. (2010) Determination of dopamine, serotonin, and their metabolites in pediatric cerebrospinal fluid by isocratic high performance liquid chromatography coupled with electrochemical detection. Biomed Chromatogr 24: 626–631.
24. Yao JK, Keshavan MS (2011) Antioxidants, redox signaling, and pathophysiology in schizophrenia: An integrative view. Antioxid Redox Signaling 15: 2011–2035.
25. Thornalley PJ (1994) Methylglyoxal, glyoxalases and the development of diabetic complications. Amino Acids 6: 15–23.
26. Kalapos M (1999) Methylglyoxal in living organisms - Chemistry, biochemistry, toxicology and biological implications. Toxicol Lett 110: 145–175.
27. Arai M, Yuzawa H, Nohara I, Ohnishi T, Obata N, et al. (2010) Enchanced carbonyl stress in a subpopulation of schizophrenia. Arch Gen Psychiatry 67: 589–597.
28. Gysin R (2007) Impaired glutathione synthesis in schizophrenia: convergent genetic and functional evidence. Proc Natl Acad Sci U S A 104: 16621–16626.
29. Nichenarnetla SN, Ellison I, Calcagnotto A, Lazarus P, Muscat JE, et al. (2008) Functional significance of the GAG trinucleotide-repeat polymorphism in the gene for the catalytic subunit of gamma-glutamylcysteine ligase. Free Radical Biol Med 45: 645–650.
30. Gawryluk JW, Wang J-F, Andreazza AC, Shao L, Young LT (2011) Decreased levels of glutathione, the major brain antioxidant, in post-mortem prefrontal cortex from patients with psychiatric disorders. Int J Neuropsychopharmacol 14: 123–130.
31. Shimazu T, Hirschey MD, Newman J, He W, Shirakawa K, et al. (2013) Suppression of oxidative stress by β-hydroxybutyrate, an endogenous histone deacetylase inhibitor. Science (Washington, DC, U S) 339: 211–214.
32. Ramos-Loyo J, Medina-Hernandez V, Estarron-Espinosa M, Canales-Aguirre A, Gomez-Pinedo U, et al. (2013) Sex differences in lipid peroxidation and fatty acid levels in recent onset schizophrenia. Prog Neuro-Psychopharmacol Biol Psychiatry 44: 154–161.
33. Maekawa M, Owada Y, Yoshikawa T (2011) Role of polyunsaturated fatty acids and fatty acid binding protein in the pathogenesis of schizophrenia. Curr Pharm Des 17: 168–175.
34. Iwayama Y, Hattori E, Maekawa M, Yamada K, Toyota T, et al. (2010) Association analyses between brain-expressed fatty-acid binding protein (FABP) genes and schizophrenia and bipolar disorder. Am J Med Genet, Part B 153B: 484–493.
35. Myint AM (2012) Kynurenines: from the perspective of major psychiatric disorders. FEBS J 279: 1375–1385.
36. Yao JK, Dougherty GG Jr, Reddy RD, Keshavan MS, Montrose DM, et al. (2010) Altered interactions of tryptophan metabolites in first-episode neuroleptic-naive patients with schizophrenia. Mol Psychiatry 15: 938–953.
37. Moroni F (1999) Tryptophan metabolism and brain function: focus on kynurenine and other indole metabolites. Eur J Pharmacol 375: 87–100.
38. Batabyal D, Yeh S-R (2007) Human tryptophan dioxygenase: A comparison to indoleamine 2,3-dioxygenase. J Am Chem Soc 129: 15690–15701.
39. Reiter RJ, Tan DX, Jou MJ, Korkmaz A, Manchester LC, et al. (2008) Biogenic amines in the reduction of oxidative stress: Melatonin and its metabolites. Neuroendocrinol Lett 29: 391–398.
40. Schwarcz R, Rassoulpour A, Wu HQ, Medoff D, Tamminga CA, et al. (2001) Increased cortical kynurenate content in schizophrenia. Biol Psychiatry 50: 521–530.
41. Erhardt S, Blennow K, Nordin C, Skogh E, Lindstrom LH, et al. (2001) Kynurenic acid levels are elevated in the cerebrospinal fluid of patients with schizophrenia. Neurosci Lett 313: 96–98.
42. Schell M, Molliver M, Snyder S (1995) D-Serine, an endogenous synaptic modulator - localization to astrocytes and glutamate-stimulated release. Proc Natl Acad Sci USA 92: 3948–3952.
43. Chumakov I, Blumenfeld M, Guerassimenko O, Cavarec L, Palicio M, et al. (2002) Genetic and physiological data implicating the new human gene G72 and the gene for D-amino acid oxidase in schizophrenia. Proc Natl Acad Sci USA 99: 13675–13680.
44. Madeira C, Freitas ME, Vargas-Lopes C, Wolosker H, Panizzutti R (2008) Increased brain D-amino acid oxidase (DAAO) activity in schizophrenia. Schizophr Res 101: 76–83.
45. Miljevic C, Nikolic-Kokic A, Nikolic M, Niketic V, Spasic MB, et al. (2013) Effect of atypical antipsychotics on antioxidant enzyme activities in human erythrocytes (in vitro study). Hum Psychopharmacol Clin Exp 28: 1–6.
46. Tortorella A, Monteleone P, Fabrazzo M, Viggiano A, De Luca L, et al. (2001) Plasma concentrations of amino acids in chronic schizophrenics treated with clozapine. Neuropsychobiol 44: 167–171.

12

Methotrexate-Related Response on Human Peripheral Blood Mononuclear Cells May Be Modulated by the Ala16Val-SOD2 Gene Polymorphism

Fernanda Barbisan[2], Jéssica de Rosso Motta[1], Alexis Trott[4], Verônica Azzolin[2],
Eduardo Bortoluzzi Dornelles[3], Matheus Marcon[1], Thaís Doeler Algarve[3],
Marta Maria Medeiros Frescura Duarte[1], Clarice Pinheiro Mostardeiro[1], Taís Cristina Unfer[1],
Karen Lilian Schott[3], Ivana Beatrice Mânica da Cruz[1,2,3]*

1 Biogenomic Laboratory, Federal University of Santa Maria, Santa Maria, RS, Brazil, 2 Pharmacology Graduate Program, Federal University of Santa Maria, Santa Maria, RS, Brazil, 3 Biochemical Toxicology Graduate Program, Federal University of Santa Maria, Santa Maria, RS, Brazil, 4 Laboratory of Molecular Biology, University of Western Santa Catarina, UNOESC, Chapecó, SC, Brazil

Abstract

Methotrexate (MTX) is a folic acid antagonist used in high doses as an anti-cancer treatment and in low doses for the treatment of some autoimmune diseases. MTX use has been linked to oxidative imbalance, which may cause multi-organ toxicities that can be attenuated by antioxidant supplementation. Despite the oxidative effect of MTX, the influence of antioxidant gene polymorphisms on MTX toxicity is not well studied. Therefore, we analyzed here whether a genetic imbalance of the manganese-dependent superoxide dismutase (SOD2) gene could have some impact on the MTX cytotoxic response. An *in vitro* study using human peripheral blood mononuclear cells (PBMCs) obtained from carriers with different Ala16Val-SOD2 genotypes (AA, VV and AV) was carried out, and the effect on cell viability and proliferation was analyzed, as well as the effect on oxidative, inflammatory and apoptotic markers. AA-PBMCs that present higher SOD2 efficiencies were more resistance to high MTX doses (10 and 100 µM) than were the VV and AV genotypes. Both lipoperoxidation and ROS levels increased significantly in PBMCs exposed to MTX independent of Ala16Val-SOD2 genotypes, whereas increased protein carbonylation was observed only in PBMCs from V allele carriers. The AA-PBMCs exposed to MTX showed decreasing SOD2 activity, but a concomitant up regulation of the SOD2 gene was observed. A significant increase in glutathione peroxidase (GPX) levels was observed in all PBMCs exposed to MTX. However, this effect was more intense in AA-PBMCs. Caspase-8 and -3 levels were increased in cells exposed to MTX, but the modulation of these genes, as well as that of the Bax and Bcl-2 genes involved in the apoptosis pathway, presented a modulation that was dependent on the SOD2 genotype. MTX at a concentration of 10 µM also increased inflammatory cytokines (IL-1β, IL-6, TNFα and Igγ) and decreased the level of IL-10 anti-inflammatory cytokine, independent of SOD2 genetic background. The results suggest that potential pharmacogenetic effect on the cytotoxic response to MTX due differential redox status of cells carriers different SOD2 genotypes.

Editor: Jian Jian Li, University of California Davis, United States of America

Funding: This study was funded by CNPq – Conselho Nacional do Desenvolvimento Científico e Tecnológico, CAPES – Coordenação de Aperfeiçoamento de Pessoal de Nível Superior, and FAPERGS – Fundação de Amparo a Pesquisa do Rio Grande do Sul. All funders are no-profit Brazilian Governmental Agencies. The funders had no role in study design, data collection and analysis, decision to publish, or preparation of the manuscript.

Competing Interests: The authors have declared that no competing interests exist.

* Email: ibmcruz@hotmail.com

Introduction

Methotrexate (MTX) is a drug that has been used since the 1950 s to treat a broad number of morbidities such as cancer and autoimmune diseases. The basis for its therapeutic efficacy is the inhibition of dihydrofolate reductase (DHFR), a key enzyme in folic acid (FA) metabolism [1]. At low concentrations, MTX has anti-inflammatory and/or immunosuppressive effects [2] related to the induction of lymphocyte apoptosis through oxidative stress and increasing caspase-3 levels [3,4]. For this reason, it is the first-line therapy for the treatment of moderate to severe psoriasis and psoriatic arthritis all over the world [5].

In contrast, the continued use of MTX has being associated with oxidative imbalance, which may cause multi-organ toxicities, including hepato-, neuro-, lung- and nephrotoxicity and testicular damage [6–9]. Investigations suggest that oxidative stress caused by MTX involves decreasing in some antioxidant enzymes as glutathione peroxidase, glutathione reductase, catalase and super-oxide dismutase, increasing of lipoperoxidation and reactive oxygen species (ROS) levels, as well as apoptosis induction [4,10].

Despite the fact that the clinical response to MTX and its adverse effects exhibit marked interpatient variability indicating pharmacogenetic effects [11], the influence of antioxidant gene polymorphisms on MTX efficacy and toxicity is not well studied.

Human beings present genetic polymorphisms in antioxidant enzymes, which have an impact on cell oxidative metabolism and are associated with the risk of chronic diseases, such as the Ala16Val polymorphism in manganese-dependent superoxide dismutase (MnSOD or SOD2) [12]. This single nucleotide polymorphism (SNP) (rs4880) occurs in the target sequence of the SOD2 enzyme, where a valine to alanine substitution causes a SOD2 conformational change from beta-sheet to alpha helix, compromising the ability to neutralize O_2- radicals. The α-helix SOD2 protein form produced by the A allele is related to a 30–40% increase in enzyme activity, whereas the V allele is related to reduced SOD2 enzyme efficiency [13].

Previous investigations have suggested that the AA genotype increases the susceptibility to develop some cancer types such as breast and prostate cancer, whereas other studies have associated the V allele with a higher risk of developing metabolic diseases such as obesity and hypercholesterolemia [14,15]. In addition, the toxicogenetic and pharmacogenetic effects of the Ala16Val-SOD2 polymorphism were described to include the *in vitro* influence on the toxic response of human lymphocytes exposed to UV radiation [16] and methylmercury [17]. The differential response of peripheral blood mononuclear cells (PBMCs) to a clomiphene citrate, a gynecological drug with antioxidant activity, was also reported [18]. The investigation performed by Montano et al. [19] also described that the Ala16Val-SOD2 polymorphism could trigger PBMCs to produce different levels of proinflammatory cytokines when exposed to culture medium richest in glucose and/or insulin. In this case, the V allele presented higher levels of proinflammatory cytokines than did the A allele.

Therefore, we analyzed here whether the Ala16Val-SOD2 polymorphism could have some impact on the MTX cytotoxic response via an *in vitro* study using human peripheral blood mononuclear cells (PBMCs) from carriers of different Ala16Val-SOD2 genotypes.

Therefore, we analyzed the MTX effect at different concentrations on PBMCs viability and proliferation with different SOD2 genotypes. In addition, effect on redox metabolism, inflammatory and apoptosis pathway by MTX exposition was also investigated from evaluation of the levels of ROS, lipoperoxidation, protein carbonylation, genotoxicity, antioxidant enzymes activities, cytokines production and caspases (CASP) levels. Modulation of gene expression of antioxidant enzymes and some molecules involved with apoptosis pathway by MTX exposition was also determined.

Materials and Methods

General experimental design

An *in vitro* analysis was performed using human peripheral mononuclear cells (PBMCs) obtained from carriers of different SOD2 genotypes. The present research study was approved by the Ethics Committee of the UFSM (no 23081.015838/2011-10), and all blood cell donors signed a consent form.

Reagents

MTX, thiazolyl blue tetrazolium bromide, 2′,7′-dichlorofluor-escin diacetate, silver nitrate, and xanthine were obtained from Sigma-Aldrich (St. Louis, MO, USA). The Quant-iT TM Picogreen® dsDNA Assay Kit was obtained from Life-Technologies (Carlsbad, CA, USA). Reagents for cell culture including RPMI 1640 Medium, fetal bovine serum, penicillin/streptomycin

and amphotericin were obtained from Sigma-Aldrich Reagents for molecular biology were as follows: Phusion Blood Direct PCR Kit (Thermo Scientific, Waltham, MA, USA), Trizol®, Dnase, SYBR® Green Master Mixes (Life-Technologies). The iScript cDNA synthesis kit was obtained from Bio-Rad (Berkeley, CA, USA). Caspase and cytokine immunoassays were performed using Quantikine® Colorimetric kits (R&D Systems, Minneapolis, MN, USA). The equipment used for ARMS-PCR (genotyping) and Q-PCR were Thermocycler (MaxygenII-Axygen, Union City, CA-USA) and StepOne Plus (Applied Biosystems, Foster City, CA, USA) instruments. Fluorimetric readings were obtained using a SpectraMax M2/M2e Multi-mode Plate Reader (Molecular Devices Corporation, Sunnyvale, CA, USA).

The effects of SOD2 genotype on cell viability, apoptosis induction, oxidative metabolism imbalance, genotoxicity and inflammatory cytokine levels were analyzed. To perform the experiments, we first collected blood samples and genotyped the Ala16Val-SOD2 gene single nucleotide polymorphism (SNP) of 120 healthy adult subjects. The SOD2 genotypes frequencies (AA = 22.8%, VV = 27.6% and AV = 48.7%) were in Hardy-Weinberg equilibrium that was calculated by chi-square goodness-of-fit statistical test. Further, some subjects with similar lifestyle profiles were invited to donate blood again and these samples were used to perform the *in vitro* assays. From this second blood donation, the PBMCs (1×10^5 cells) were obtained and cultured in controlled conditions with and without MTX exposure (0, 0.1, 1, 10, and 100 µM). There are few studies involving MTX effects on PBMCs cells. Therefore we used a broad concentration range based in a previous investigation performed by Sakuma et al [20]. The cell viability was determined, and the effect of MTX on apoptosis, oxidative stress and inflammatory metabolism was evaluated and compared among all treatments. Apoptosis pathway induction by MTX was evaluated by quantifying caspase-8 and -3 levels. Caspase-8 is an apoptosis initiator molecule, which activates caspase-3, and represents a key point in the transmission of the proteolytic signal. The gene expression levels of these CASP were also determined. Because MTX oxidative stress could be related to mitochondrial damage that triggers apoptosis, we also analyzed the effect of MTX treatments on Bcl-2 and BAX gene modulation. These genes belong to the Bcl-2 family of gene proteins that is also involved in the apoptosis pathway. The effect of MTX on PBMC oxidative metabolism was evaluated by quantifying ROS, lipoperoxidation, protein carbonylation and genotoxicity levels. The levels of antioxidant enzymes [SOD1, SOD2, catalase (CAT), and glutathione peroxidase, (GPX)] were also determined, as were the effects of MTX on the gene expression of these enzymes. Because PBMCs produce important inflammatory cytokines modulated by MTX [21], the levels of interleukin-1 beta (IL-1β), interleukin-6 (IL-6), tumor necrosis factor alpha (TNFα), interferon gamma (IFNγ) and the anti-inflammatory cytokine interleukin-10 (IL-10) were measured and compared among PBMCs with different Ala16Val-SOD2 genotypes that had been exposed to MTX. The caspase-1 level was also determined because this intracellular cysteine protease is required for processing the IL-1 precursor into the mature and active form that can then be secreted from the cell [1]. All experiments were performed in triplicate, and the assays used to perform these analyses are described below.

Ala16Val-SOD2 SNP genotyping

To obtain PBMCs, the blood samples were first collected by venipuncture from 120 healthy adult subjects (26.4 ± 7.3 years old) living in a Brazilian region (Rio Grande do Sul) without a history of diseases that are treated with MTX, non-smokers, not obese, no use of chronic medication or vitamin supplements, no previous cardiovascular medical history or hypertensive disorder, and no metabolic diseases or other morbidity that could affect the results. The Ala16Val-SOD2 genotyping was determined by polymerase chain reaction using a direct total blood cell sample and Tetra-Primer ARMS-PCR assay as described by Ruiz-Sanz et al. [22] with slight modifications. Briefly, two primer pairs were used to amplify and determined the genotype of a DNA fragment containing the Ala16Val SNP in the human SOD2 sequence. The 3'-end of the allele-specific primers is underlined. Underlined lowercase bases indicate the introduced mismatches. The PCR reaction was carried out in a total volume of 40 μL containing 20–40 ng of genomic DNA as the template, 0.5 μM of each primer, 100 μM of each dNTP, 1.25 mM of MgCl2, PCR buffer (20 mM Tris-HCl (pH 8.4), 50 mM KCl), 5% dimethyl sulfoxide (DMSO), and 1.25 Units of DNA polymerase. The PCR amplification was carried out with an initial denaturation at 94°C for 7 min, followed by 35 cycles of 60 s of denaturation at 94°C, 20 seconds of annealing at 60°C, and 30 s of extension at 72°C, and an additional 7 minutes of extension at 72°C at the end of the final cycle. A 20-μL aliquot of the PCR products was mixed with 6 μL of loading buffer and resolved by electrophoresis in a 1.5% agarose gel. This procedure resulted in three bands in heterozygotes (514, 366, and 189 bp) and two bands in homozygotes (Val/Val resulting in bands of 514 and 189 bp, and Ala/Ala resulting in bands of 514 and 366 bp) (Figure 1).

PBMCs *in vitro* culture

From the subjects genotyped, a sub-group of 6–8 subjects per genotype with the Ala16Val-SOD2 genotype were invited to donate blood again in order to perform cell culture and *in vitro* assays involving MTX exposure as previously described in Montano et al. [19]. The 20 mL blood samples were collected by venipuncture using heparinized vials and then transferred to tubes with Ficoll histopaque (1:1). The tubes were centrifuged for 30 min at 252×g and PBMCs were positioned in the interfase, PBMCs were centrifuged again (10 minutes at 2000 rpm) and transferred to culture medium containing 1 ml RPMI 1640 (GIBCO) with 10% fetal calf serum (FCS) and 1% penicillin/streptomycin. Culture tubes for each subject were prepared at a final concentration of 1×10^6 cells/mL. The PBMC cultures were incubated at 37°C and 5% CO_2 for 24 h before performing the experiments.

Viability and Cell proliferation assays

Based on previous reports that low dose MTX exerts anti-inflammatory and immunosuppressive effects that induce apoptosis and oxidative stress [3], we exposed PBMCs from carriers of different Ala16Val-SOD2 genotypes to different MTX concentrations (0.1–100 μM). The effect of genotype on cell viability was analyzed after 24 hs of exposure and the effect on cell proliferation was assessed after 72 hs of exposure. Cell viability after 24 h of MTX exposition and cell proliferation after 72 h of MTX exposition was analyzed by the MTT (3-[4,5dimethylthiazol-2-yl]-2,5-diphenyltetrazolic bromide) reduction assay as described by

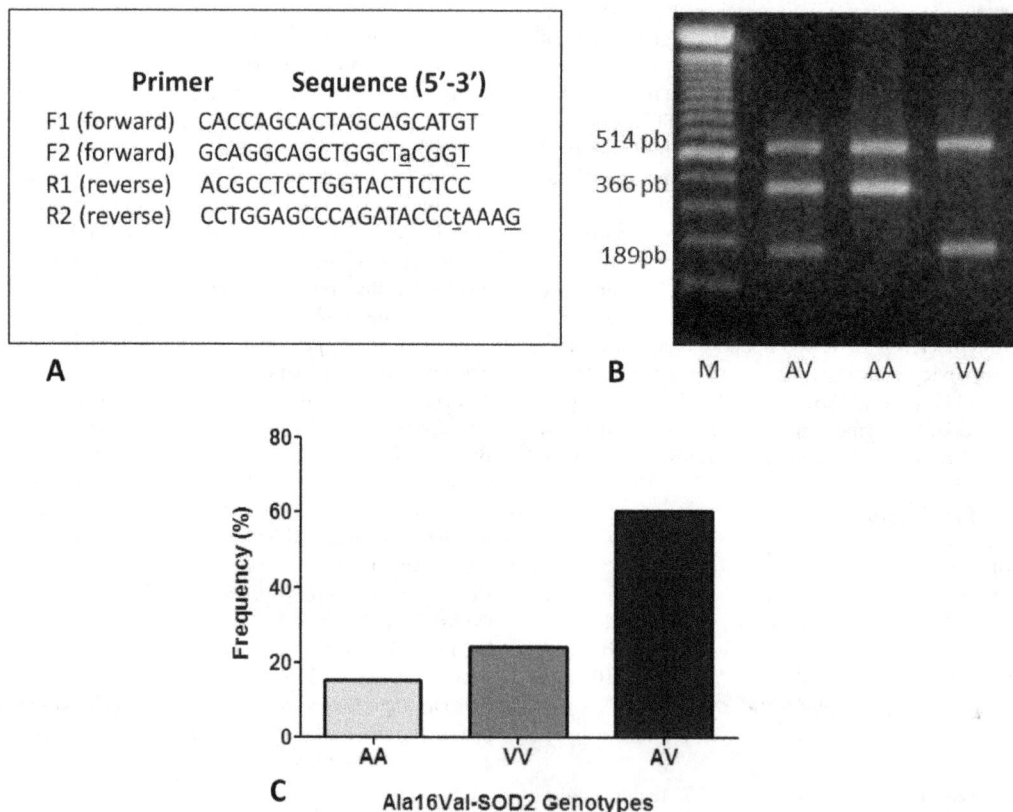

Primer	Sequence (5'-3')
F1 (forward)	CACCAGCACTAGCAGCATGT
F2 (forward)	GCAGGCAGCTGGCTaCGGT
R1 (reverse)	ACGCCTCCTGGTACTTCTCC
R2 (reverse)	CCTGGAGCCCAGATACCCtAAAG

A

514 pb
366 pb
189pb

B   M   AV   AA   VV

C   Ala16Val-SOD2 Genotypes

Figure 1. Ala16Val-SOD2 genotyping. (A) primers used to perform tetra-primer ARMS-PCR assay; (B) Gel electrophoresis showing different fragments used to identify the SOD2 genotypes; (C) Genotypic frequency distribution of AA, VV and AV genotypes in the 120 adult health samples subject that donate blood sample to perform the PBMCs *in vitro* assays.

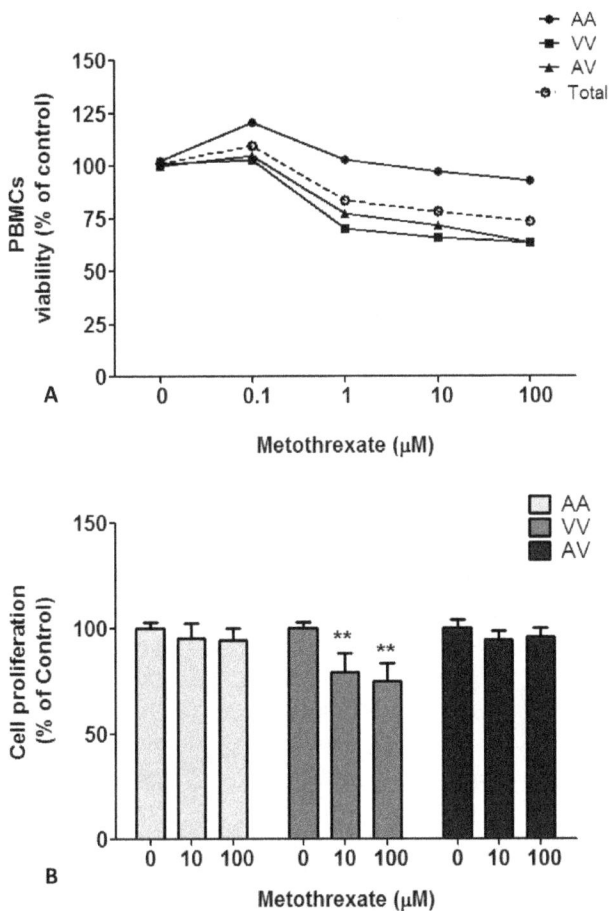

Figure 2. MTX effect on PBMCs carrier's different Ala16Val-SOD2 genotypes. (A) cell viability at different MTX concentrations evaluated after 24 h of MTX exposition; (B) cell proliferation at different MTX concentrations evaluated after 72 h of MTX exposition. **$p<0.01$ was determined by two-way analysis of variance followed by Bonferroni *post hoc* test. Viability and cell proliferation were evaluated by MTT assay.

Mosmann [23]. Briefly, treated cells were incubated for 4 h with MTT reagent. After the formazan salt was dissolved, the absorbance was measured at 570 nm. The cells were photographed before the addition of DMSO in order to observe the formazan crystals. The MTT assay was performed using a 96-well plate in three independent replications. The Trypan blue dye exclusion assay was also performed to confirm the MTX effect on PBMCs viability [24]. The results were expressed as a percentage of the untreated control values.

2'–7'-dichlorofluorescein diacetate (DCFDA) ROS production assay

The effect of 24 h of MTX exposure on the oxidative metabolism of PBMCs from carriers of different Ala16Val-SOD2 genotypes was evaluated for different oxidant and antioxidant variables. The ROS level was determined using the non-fluorescent cell permeating compound 2'–7'-dichlorofluorescein diacetate (DCFDA) assay. In this technique, the DCFDA is hydrolyzed by intracellular esterases to DCFH, which is trapped within the cell. This non-fluorescent molecule is then oxidized to fluorescent dichlorofluorescein (DCF) by cellular oxidants. After the designated treatment time, the cells were treated with DCFDA

(10 µM) for 60 minutes at 37°C. In the assay, 1×10^5 cells from each sample were used to measured ROS levels [18]. The fluorescence was measured at an excitation of 488 nm and an emission of 525 nm, and the results were expressed as picomoles/mL of 2',7'-dichlorofluorescein (DCF) production from 2',7'-dichlorofluorescin in reaction with ROS molecules present in the samples.

Spectrophotometric assays

Oxidative stress indicators were measured in PBMCs samples. Thiobarbituric acid reactive substances (TBARS) were measured according to the modified method of Jentzsch et al. [25]. The carbonylation of serum proteins was determined by the Levine method with modifications [31]. Whole blood catalase (CAT) activity was determined by the method of Aebi [26] by measuring the rate of decomposition of H_2O_2 at 240 nm. Whole blood superoxide dismutase (SOD) activity was measured as described by McCord & Fridovich [27]. The Glutathione peroxidase activity was measured as Glutathione Peroxidase (GPX) as described by Flohe e Gunzler with modifications [28].

DNA comet genotoxicity assay

The alkaline comet assay was performed as described by Singh et al. [29] in accordance with the general guidelines for use of the comet assay [30]. One hundred cells (50 cells from each of the two replicate slides) were selected and analyzed. Cells were visually scored according to tail length and received scores from 0 (no migration) to 4 (maximal migration). Therefore, the damage index for cells ranged from 0 (all cells with no migration) to 400 (all cells with maximal migration). The slides were analyzed under blind conditions by at least two different individuals.

Caspase and cytokine immunoassays

The analyses of CASP- 8, -3, and -1 and cytokines IL-1β, IL-6, TNFα, IgY, IL-10 were performed using the Quantikine Human Caspase Immunoassay to measure CASP in the cell culture supernatants, according to the manufacturer's instructions. Briefly, all reagents and working standards were prepared and the excess microplate strips were removed. The assay diluent RD1W was added (50 mL) to each well. Further, 100 mL of standard control for our sample was added per well, after which the well was covered with the adhesive strip and incubated for 1.5 h at room temperature. Each well was aspirated and washed twice for a total of three washes. The antiserum of each molecule analyzed here was added to each well and covered with a new adhesive strip and incubated for 30 min at room temperature. The aspiration/wash step was repeated, and the caspase-1 conjugate (100 mL) was added to each well and incubated for 30 min at room temperature. The aspiration/wash step was repeated and 200 mL of substrate solution was added to each well and incubated for 20 min at room temperature. Finally, the 50 mL stop solution was added to each well and the optical density was determined within 30 min using a microplate reader set to 450 nm.

mRNA expression analysis by quantitative QT-PCR assay

The expression levels of eight genes were measured by QT-PCR assay in PBMCs from carriers of different Ala16Val-SOD2 genotypes exposed to MTX: four genes belong to oxidative metabolism [superoxide dismutase genes (SOD1, SOD2), catalase (CAT) and glutathione peroxidase (GPX)]. The gene expression of some proteins involved in the apoptosis cascade, initiator caspase-8 (CASP 8) and effector caspase-3 (CASP 3) were also evaluated, as

Table 1. Comparison of oxidative metabolism variables of peripheral blood mononuclear cells (PBMCs) carrier's different Ala16Val-SOD2 genotypes exposed to Methotrexate.

Variables	MTX (µM)	Ala16Val-SOD2 Genotypes		
		AA	**VV**	**AV**
		Mean ± sd	Mean ± sd	Mean ± sd
TBARS (mmol MDA/mg protein)	0	3.210±0.014[a]	3.805±0.020[a]	3.390±0.031[a]
	10	5.165±0.274[b]	5.307±0.08[b]	6.290±0.215[b]
	100	5.008±0.301[b]	4.948±0.176[b]	6.000±0,412[b]
Protein carbonylation (mmol/mg protein)	0	0.226±0.023[a]	0.201±0.023[a]	0.195±0.024[a]
	10	0.267±0.022[a]	0.292±0.030[b]	0.339±0.079[b]
	100	0.213±0.015[a]	0.329±0.035[c]	0.306±0.04[b]
ROS (DCF picomoles/mL)	0	3104±177[a]	2680±199[a]	2855±330[a]
	10	3704±193[a]	2829±132[a]	2693±261[a]
	100	5632±191[b]	7311±269[b]	4999±509[b]
SOD1 (UMnOD/mg protein)	0	0.747±0.09[a]	0. 610±0.04[a]	0.654±0.04[a]
	10	0.507±0.05[b]	0.423±0.05[b]	0.456±0.06[b]
	100	0.498±0.06[b]	0.411±0.04[b]	0.432±0.05[b]
SOD2 (UMnOD/mg protein)	0	2.170±0.190[a]	0.728±0.05a[a]	1.050±0.160[a]
	10	1.577±0.125[b]	0.756±0.05[a]	0.870±0.270[a]
	100	1.170±0.04[b]	0.580±0.01[b]	0.960±0.110[a]
Catalase (K/mg protein)	0	0.050±0.004[a]	0.043±0.008[a]	0.033±0.008[a]
	10	0.024±0.003[b]	0.037±0.002[b]	0.041±0.006[a]
	100	0.027±0.003[b]	0.041±0.018[a]	0.039±0004[a]
GPX (U/mL)	0	4.01±0.82[a]	11.04±2.02[a]	11.75±3.04[a]
	10	12.96±2.02[b]	16.73±3.04[b]	46.86±4.03[b]
	100	20.53±3.50[c]	22.23±3.06[c]	36.39±3.02[c]

MTX = methotrexate; sd = standard deviation; Different letters (a, b, c) indicate significant differences among each MTX treatment determined by analysis of variance followed by Tukey's post hoc test at p<0.05.

was the pro-apoptotic Bcl-2-associated X protein (BAX) gene, which has been shown to be involved in p53-mediated apoptosis.

Total RNA was isolated using TRIzol reagent. RNA yields were measured using a Nanodrop 2000 spectrophotometer. First strand cDNA was synthesized from total RNA (2 µg) using a First Strand cDNA Synthesis Kit and oligo dT primers. Q-PCR was performed in a 10 µl reaction that contained 0.5 µl of the cDNA and 1×KAPA SYBR® FAST Universal qPCR Master Mix (Kapa Biosystems, Woburn, MA, USA) using the following PCR parameters: 95°C for 3 min followed by 40 cycles of 95°C for 10 s, 60°C for 30 s followed by a melt curve of 65°C to 95°C in 0.5°C increments for 5 s. The expression level of beta-actin was used as an internal control. The relative expression was calculated using the comparative Ct and was expressed as the fold expression compared to the control. The specific primer pairs of antioxidant gene enzymes are presented used in this study were: SOD1 Forward GCACACTGGTGGTCCATGAA and Reverse ACAC-CACAAGCCAAACGACTT; SOD2 Forward- 5′GCCCTGG-AACCTCACATCAA3′ and Reverse- GGTACTTCTCCTCG-GTGACGTT; CAT = Forward- GATAGCCTT CGACCCA-AGCA and Reverse- ATGGCGGTGAGTGTCAGGAT; GPX = Forward- GGTTTTCATCTATGAGGGTGTTTCC and Reverse-GCCTTGGT CTGGCAGAGACT; BAX = Forward- CCCTT-TTCTACTTTGCCAGCAA and Reverse- CCCGGAGGAAGTC-CAATGT; Bcl-2 = Forward- GAGGATT GTGGCCTTCTTT-GAGT; Reverse- AGTCATCCACAGGGCGATGT; CASP3 =

Forward- TTTGAGCCTGAGCAGAGACATG and Reverse-TACCAGT GCGTATGGAGAAATGG; CASP 8 = Forward- AG-GAGCTGCTCTTCCGAATT and Reverse- CCCTGCCTG-GTGTCTGAAGT.

Statistical analysis

All analyses were carried out using the Graph Pad Prism 5 software, and the results were expressed as the mean ± standard deviation (SD). The comparison of all PBMC samples from different Ala16Val-SOD2 donors treated with and without MTX was performed using the two-way analysis of variance followed by a *post hoc* Tukey's test. All p values were two-tailed. The alpha value was set to <0.05 to determine statistical relevance.

Results

The MTX exposure caused significant cytotoxicity from 1 µM concentration in human PBMCs. However, this effect was significantly influenced by the Ala16Val-SOD2 SNP (Figure 2A). PBMCs from carriers with the V allele (VV and AV) exhibited decreased viability when exposed to MTX at 1, 10 and 100 µM concentrations, whereas AA-PBMC viability was not affected by these treatments. These results were confirmed by trypan assay.

Based on these results, a second analysis was performed to evaluate the prolonged MTX effect at 10 and 100 µM concentrations on PBMC proliferation. Again, the cell response was influenced by the Ala16Val-SOD2 SNP. As seen in Figure 2B, MTX did not influence the cell proliferation of PBMCs from A-carriers (AA and AV). The VV-PBMCs treated with MTX showed significant decreases in proliferation rate when compared to the untreated control group. However, the influence on VV-cell proliferation was similar at the 10 and 100 μM MTX concentrations.

The influence of MTX on PBMC oxidative metabolism after 24 h of exposure was then analyzed, and the results are presented in Table 1. Lipoperoxidation as well as ROS levels increased significantly in PBMCs exposed to MTX independent of Ala16Val-SOD2 genotype. However, the effect on lipoperoxidation was not dependent on MTX concentration (10 and 100 μM), whereas the increase in ROS levels only occurred at the higher MTX dose tested here (100 μM). On the other hand, protein carbonylation was not affected in AA-PBMCs, whereas AV and VV PBMCs presented an increase in this oxidative parameter. However, the effect of MTX on protein carbonylation was dose-dependent only in VV-PBMCs.

The effects of MTX on antioxidant enzyme activity and gene expression were evaluated. However, considering the results obtained in the analysis of antioxidant activity, the effect on gene expression was evaluated only in cells exposed to 10 μM MTX (Table 1, Figure 3). SOD1 was strongly affected by MTX exposure, resulting in decreased enzyme activity and gene expression independent of the Ala16Val-SOD2 genotype.

In contrast, the SOD2 activity and the gene expression were influenced by the Ala16Val-SOD2 SNP. The AA-PBMCs exposed to MTX showed decreasing SOD2 activity. However, SOD2 gene expression significantly was upregulated in the cells exposed to MTX. The VV-PMCs presented a decrease in SOD2 activity only when exposed to the higher MTX concentration (100 μM). Unlike the AA-PBMCs, these cells presented SOD2 gene down regulation when compared to the control group. Despite the fact that AV-PBMCs also presented SOD2 gene down regulation, the SOD2 activity was maintained in cells treated with MTX.

Catalase activity decreased only in AA-PBMCs cells exposed to MTX. However, these cells did not demonstrate any effect on catalase gene expression. The PBMCs from carriers of the A allele (AA and AV) did not show a decrease in catalase levels, but the effect on catalase gene expression was evident. Whereas, VV-PBMCs exposed to MTX exhibited downregulated catalase gene expression, heterozygous cells demonstrated catalase upregulation.

After 24 hs of MTX exposure, PBMCs presented high levels of GPX enzyme when exposed to MTX drug, independent of genetic background. The GPX gene was strongly upregulated in cells treated with MTX when compared to untreated control cells.

The potential genotoxic effect in survival cells exposed to MTX at 10 μM concentration was evaluated. The results presented in Figure 4 show no statistically significant differences in terms of DNA damage in PBMCs obtained from carriers of different Ala16Val-SOD2 genotypes.

The cytokines involved in inflammatory response were also determined in PBMCs from carriers of different Ala16Val-SOD2 genotypes exposed to MTX. The results described in Table 2 show that 24 h of 10 μM MTX exposure significantly increase levels of inflammatory cytokines (IL-1β, IL-6, TNFα and Igγ) and significantly decrease IL-10, an anti-inflammatory cytokine. These results were similar in all PBMCs independent of Ala16Val-SOD2 genotype.

The effect of MTX on PBMC apoptosis was evaluated by determining CASP-3 and -8 gene and protein levels. The results presented in Figure 5 show increased CASP-1, -3 and -8 levels in cells exposed to 10 μM MTX. This result was independent of the Ala16Val-SOD2 SNP. However, the gene expression analysis showed significant differences among PBMCs with different genotypes. VV-PBMCs exposed to MTX presented the down regulation of both CASP genes (-8 and -3) when compared to the control group. In contrast, casp-8 was upregulated in AA-PBMCs. The heterozygous genotype showed an intermediary pattern of casp gene expression, where casp-8 was downregulated similar to

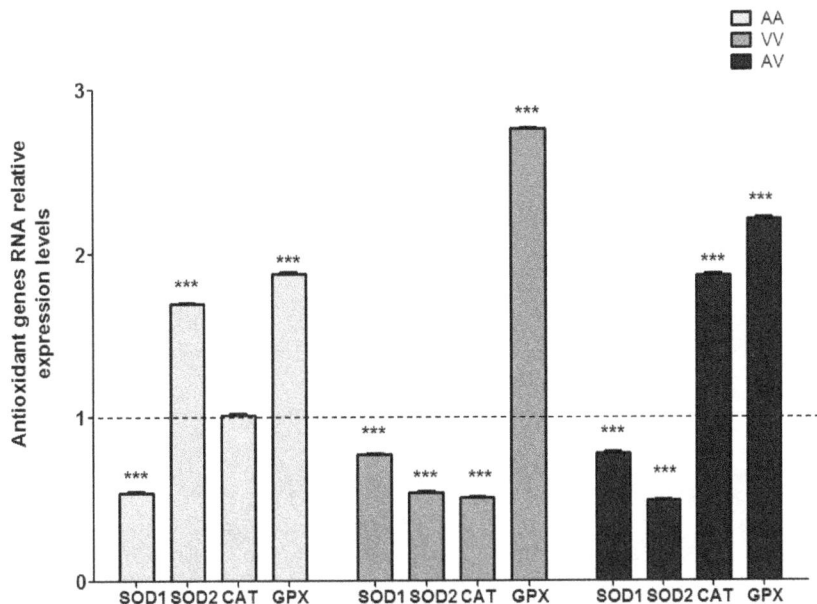

Figure 3. MTX (10 μM) effect on antioxidant SOD1, SOD2, CAT and GPX genes expression. The dashed line on the value 1 indicate that each untreated control group of PBMCs carrier's different Ala16Val-SOD2 genotypes was used as reference to calculated the relative mRNA expression of the antioxidant enzymes. **p≤0.01 and *** p≤0.001 were determined by two-way analysis of variance followed by Bonferroni *post hoc* test.

ALKALINE DNA COMET DAMAGE LEVELS

A No damage   Damage 1   Damage 2   Damage 3   Damage 4

B

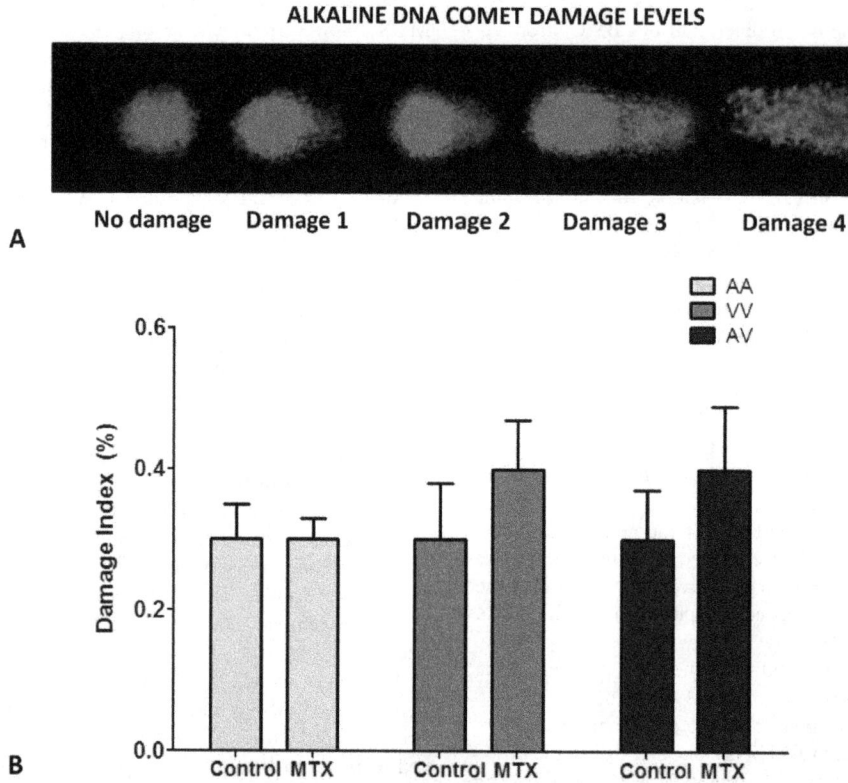

Figure 4. DNA damage to MTX exposition in PBMCs from subjects with different Ala16Val-SOD2 genotypes. (A) alkaline DNA comet assay showing nucleus without damage, and the nucleus with different damage levels; (B) Index damage of cells no-exposed and exposed to MTX 10 μM. No significant differences were observed between treatments.

the VV genotype and casp-3 was upregulated similar to the AA genotype.

The effect of MTX on BAX and Bcl-2 gene expression was also evaluated, and the results showed an imbalance between these genes that was influenced by the SOD2 genetic background

(Figure 6). The BAX gene was down regulated only in AV-PBMCs, whereas the BAX gene was upregulated in homozygous genotypes. The Bcl-2 gene was strongly upregulated in AA and AV-PBMCs and slightly upregulated in VV-PBMCs. Considering that the BAX/Bcl-2 balance defines the proapoptotic and

Table 2. Comparison of cytokines involved in immune response of peripheral blood mononuclear cells (PBMCs) carrier's different Ala16Val-SOD2 genotypes exposed to Methotrexate.

Variables	MTX (μM)	Ala16Val-SOD2 Genotypes		
		AA	VV	AV
		Mean ± sd	Mean ± sd	Mean ± sd
Interleukin 1β (pg/mL)	0	46.3±5.9[a]	51.7±2.0[a]	44.6±3.7[a]
	10	210.3±16.6[b]	346.1±12.6[b]	321.1±6.9[b]
Interleukin 6 (pg/mL)	0	58.0±5.9[a]	56.3±7.8[a]	60.7±4.1[a]
	10	251.9±43.1[b]	472.8±108[b]	433.3±8.6[b]
TNFα (pg/mL)	0	86.0±4.3[a]	86.3±7.6[a]	88.6±2.14[a]
	10	278.7±57.5[b]	494.9±7[b]	449.3±60.9[b]
Igγ (pg/mL)	0	103.2±9.4[a]	100.7±7.6[a]	108.6±6.8[a]
	10	351.2±68.1[b]	668.2±25.9[b]	589.7±9.4[b]
Interleukin 10 (pg/mL)	0	86.7±4.7[a]	90±4.2[a]	90.0±6.1[a]
	10	68.3±16.3[b]	54.6±9.6[b]	46.9±2.4[b]

MTX = methotrexate; sd = standard deviation; Different letters (a, b, c) indicate significant differences among each MTX treatment determined by analysis of variance followed by Tukey's post hoc test at p<0.05.

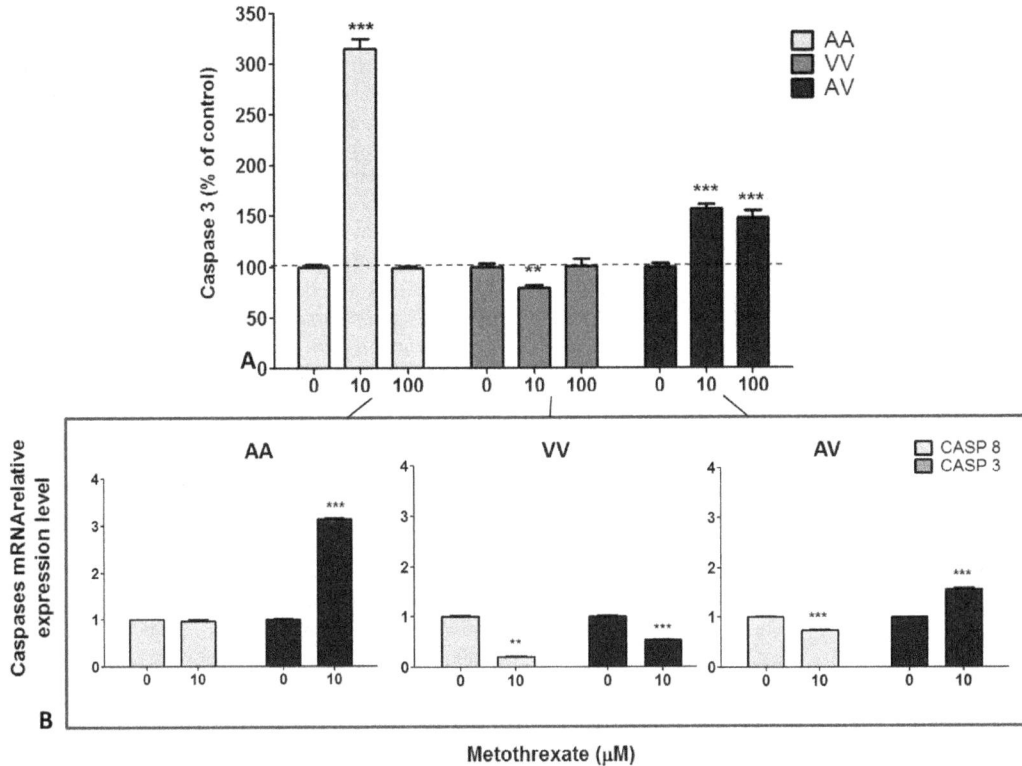

Figure 5. MTX (10 μM) effect on (A) CASP 8 and 3 protein levels determined by immunoassay tests and (B) respective gene expression in PBMCs carriers different Ala16Val-SOD2 genotypes. The dashed line on the value 1 indicate that each untreated control group of PBMCs carrier's different Ala16Val-SOD2 genotypes was used as reference to calculated the relative mRNA expression of the antioxidant enzymes. $**p \leq 0.01$ and $***$ $p \leq 0.001$ were determined by two-way analysis of variance followed by Bonferroni *post hoc* test.

antiapoptotic cell state, we also calculated the BAX/Bcl-2 ratio. The results showed an antiapoptotic ratio in AA and AV-PBMCs and a proapoptotic ratio in VV-PBMCs after 24 h of 10 μM MTX exposure.

Discussion

The present study, confirmed that the cytotoxic effect of MTX, a commonly used anti-inflammatory, antiproliferative, and immunosuppressive drug, on human PBMCs involves an acute imbalance of cell oxidative and inflammatory metabolism and triggers apoptosis [14,10,11,25]. However, our results showed that this effect was directly influenced by genetic background related to oxidative metabolism, specifically by the Ala16Val-SOD2 SNP.

The PBMCs obtained from healthy adult carriers of different Ala16Val-SOD2 genotypes showed a differential response to MTX in terms of cell viability and proliferation. Whereas AA showed some resistance to the immunosuppressive effect caused by MTX, presenting similar viability and cell proliferation levels than untreated cells, VV was more susceptible and presented reduced viability and cell proliferation. On the other hand, the heterozygous genotype (AV) showed an intermediary response to MTX exposure, observed as decreased cell viability as observed in VV-PBMCs and the maintenance of cell proliferation as observed in AA-PBMCs.

These results suggest that the SOD2 balance could play some pharmacogenetic or toxicogenetic role in the cellular MTX response. A robust number of studies have described that MTX at high concentrations causes oxidative stress in some types of cells. This observation was noted in the *in vitro* investigation performed

by Chibbers et al. [31] which showed that MTX alone or in combination with Cu (II) was able to inhibit scavengers of ROS and exhibit pro-oxidant action. The oxidative imbalance in the Jurkat T lymphocytic line exposed *in vitro* to MTX was also described and related to apoptosis events [25]. Another investigation showed that MTX-induced oxidative stress in liver mitochondria caused a significant increase in mitochondrial lipid peroxidation, protein carbonyl content, superoxide radical ($O_2^{-\bullet}$) generation and also affected the mitochondrial thiol profile [32]. MTX concentrations ≥ 10 μM also cause reduced antioxidant enzyme levels including superoxide dismutase, catalase and glutathione levels.

In the present study, the effect of MTX on AA-PBMC viability and cell proliferation was less intense than that observed in V allele carriers, indicating that MTX toxicity could be influenced by oxidative metabolism involving SOD2 modulation. This suggestion was confirmed by the analysis of potential causal mechanisms associated with the differential MTX response of PBMC carriers with different Ala16Val-SOD2 genotypes. The results showed that some variables presented a similar response to MTX independent of genetic background, including the increase of lipoperoxidation, inflammatory cytokines and apoptotic CASPs (-8 and -3) and GPX activity and gene expression, and the decrease in SOD1 activity and gene expression and IL-10, an anti-inflammatory cytokine.

However, in contrast to that observed in cytokine modulation some oxidative and apoptotic markers were differentially modulated in the PBMCs from carriers with different Ala16Val-SOD2 genotypes.

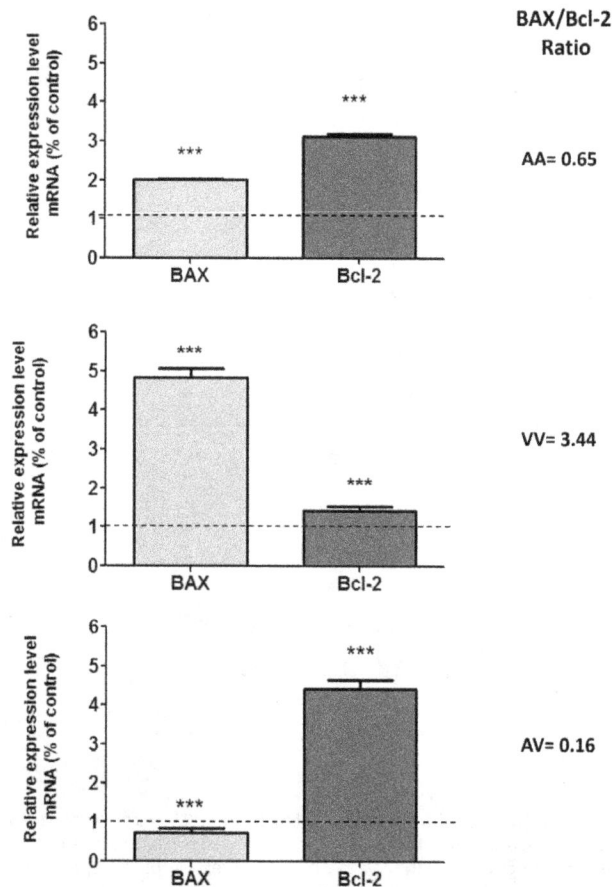

Figure 6. MTX (10 μM) effect on BAX and Bcl-2 gene expression of PBMCs carriers different Ala16Val-SOD2 genotypes. The dashed line on the value 1 indicate that each untreated control group of PBMCs carrier's different Ala16Val-SOD2 genotypes was used as reference to calculated the relative mRNA expression of the antioxidant enzymes. **$p \le 0.01$ and *** $p \le 0.001$ were determined by two-way analysis of variance followed by Bonferroni *post hoc* test. The ratio between expressions of BAX/Bcl-2 was also calculated. Values ≥ 1 indicate proapoptotic tendency and $<$ indicate antiapoptotic tendency.

Considering the oxidative metabolism, we observed that AA-PBMCs did not show an increase in protein carbonylation, as occurred in the VV and AV genotypes. These cells also showed a decrease in SOD2 activity although we also observed the up regulation of this gene and an important increase in GPX enzyme levels and gene expression. The AA cells treated with MTX showed an approximately four-fold increase in GPX enzyme levels when compared to the untreated control group. Despite the fact that the VV and AV cells also presented increased GPX activity when treated with MTX, this effect was not as intense. The AA-PBMCs exposed to MTX also presented a decrease in catalase activity despite the fact that the gene expression of this enzyme maintained levels similar to those observed in the control group.

The AA genotype has been associated with high efficiency to dismutate $O_2^{-\bullet}$ ions in hydrogen peroxide (H_2O_2) [12], and this property could be responsible for decreasing the oxidative stress caused by high levels of MTX and the subsequent decrease in apoptosis events observed in PBMCs from V allele carriers. In addition to the greater efficiency of AA-PBMCs in the dismutation of superoxide into hydrogen peroxide, these cells presented a significant increase in GPX levels when exposed to MTX, which

probably offered some protection against toxic effects caused by hydrogen peroxide produced by superoxide dismutation.

The relevance of the AA genotype's efficiency in controlling $O_2^{-\bullet}$ and H_2O_2 levels in the cells exposed to MTX could have a consequence as a superior control mechanism for protein carbonylation production. Both $O_2^{-\bullet}$ and H_2O_2 are capable of altering proteins chemically, thereby influencing their function. The main protein modifications originating from such an increase in oxidative stress comprise direct oxidation, namely that of amino acids with a thiol group such as cysteine, oxidative glycation, and carbonylation. In this context, it is remarkable that oxidative protein carbonylation, apparently the most frequent type of protein modification in response to oxidative stress, is thought to be irreversible and destined only to induce protein degradation in a nonspecific manner [33].

Therefore, events that prevent the production of high levels of protein carbonylation, including SOD2 efficiency and increased GPX activity and gene expression observed in AA-PBMCs exposed to MTX could explain why this genotype has protective effects against apoptosis events caused by MTX exposure.

On the other hand, VV cells exposed to MTX presented higher lipoperoxidation, protein carbonylation and ROS levels than untreated cells (Table 1). These results indicated increase in H_2O_2 levels triggered by MTX. However, opposite effects on main enzymes that catalyze H_2O_2 were also observed, since VV cells exposed to MTX showed lower CAT activity and higher GPX activity. These differences appear to be triggered by differential mRNA regulation of these enzymes (down regulation of CAT and upregulation of GPX genes). Considering the role of H_2O_2 in different signaling cellular cascades, this molecule is under sophisticated fine control of several antioxidant enzymatic molecules. However, despite CAT to be frequently used by cells to rapidly catalysis of H_2O_2 into less reactive gaseous oxygen and water molecules, the predominant scavengers of H_2O_2 in normal mammalian cells are likely other molecules as GPX and peroxiredoxins [34]. Our results suggest that in the presence of prooxidant molecules as MTX, the control of H_2O_2 production is directly influenced by efficiency of SOD2 enzyme. This suggestion can be partially corroborated by a previous study performed by Paludo et al. [35] suggested that Ala16Val-SOD2 SNP actively participates in the regulation of cellular redox environment involving H_2O_2 catalysis However the nature of the differential regulation of enzymes involving in H_2O_2 catalysis need to be clarified from complementary studies using antagonist and agonist molecules of SOD2 enzyme.

The heterozygous genotype (AV) showed an intermediary response to MTX exposition when compared to homozygous genotypes (AA and VV) or, sometimes the response was similar to AA genotype or to VV genotype.

The lesser effect of MTX on AA-PBMCs can also be observed when the expression of BAX and Bcl-2 genes was analyzed. In many systems, members of the bcl-2 family modulate apoptosis, with the BAX/Bcl-2 ratio serving as a rheostat with which to determine the susceptibility to apoptosis. Bcl-2 protein is able to repress a number of apoptotic death programs. Therefore, Bcl-2 is specifically considered an important anti-apoptotic protein and is, therefore, classified as an oncogene. In contrast, overexpressed BAX accelerates apoptotic death [36]. In healthy cells, BAX protein is largely found in the cytosol. However, upon initiation of apoptotic signaling, Bax undergoes a conformational shift and becomes organelle membrane-associated, in particular with the mitochondrial membrane. The main BAX effect involves the induction of opening of the mitochondrial voltage-dependent anion channel that results in the release of pro-apoptotic factors from the mitochondria, leading to the activation of CASPs [37].

The results showed differential Bax/Bcl-2 ratio gene expression in PBMCs from carriers of different Ala16Val-SOD2 genotypes exposed to MTX. Whereas the BAX/Bcl-2 ratio was below one in AA- and AV-PBMCs indicating a tendency to antiapoptotic events, VV-PBMCs showed a higher Bax/Bcl-2 ratio indicating the maintenance of cellular apoptosis. Therefore, these results confirmed the influence of Ala16Val-SOD2 on PBMC susceptibility to MTX exposure.

Another important result described here was the massive effect of MTX at the 10 μM concentration on human PBMC inflammatory cytokine levels. As previously mentioned, cells treated with MTX showed higher levels of IL-1β, IL-6, TNFα and Igγ. A reduction of IL-10, an anti-inflammatory cytokine, was also observed in cells exposed to MTX. Some of the results on the MTX inflammatory effect of PBMCs exposed to high levels of this drug have being described in previous studies performed in experimental models. For example, nephrotoxicity in rats induced by high doses of MTX increase the TNFα cytokine levels [38]. Rats with hepatorenal oxidative injury induced by high doses of MTX also showed increasing TNFα and IL-1β levels when compared to the untreated control group [39]. The number of studies analyzing the effect of MTX on IL-6 and Igγ is much lower [24,40]. Therefore, to the best of our knowledge, the study of the concomitant effect of MTX on IL-1β, CASP 1, IL-6, TNFα, Igγ and IL-10 has not been previously published in the literature.

The clinical relevance of the data presented here could be related to the lower cytotoxic effect observed in AA-PBMCs exposed to MTX. This effect could be desirable in cancer patients undergoing chemotherapy using MTX. For example, neurocognitive sequelae associated with oxidative stress have been described in pediatric lymphoblastic leukemia patients treated with MTX [38], as have hepatotoxic and nephrotoxic effects [10,11,12].

However, the immunosuppressive activities of MTX have been studied in the context of cell proliferation and recruitment, and an inverse effect of MTX at low concentrations on some inflammatory cytokines is well established. Low MTX doses are able to reduce some important cytokines as TNFα that are elevated in autoimmune diseases such as rheumatoid arthritis [41]. Taking into account the results described here and published in the literature, we can suggest that MTX presents an important dose-dependent modulation of immune cytokines in PBMCs. This effect does not seem to be directly influenced by oxidative metabolism involving SOD2 activity because the results found here were independent of the Ala16Val-SOD2 SNP.

In conclusion, despite the methodological limitations related to *in vitro* experimental studies including the limited number of subjects used to obtain PBMCs with different SOD2 genotypes, the results described here suggest that the differential modulation of the cell's $O_2^{-\bullet}$ and H_2O_2 balance is genetically determined by SOD2 gene variation, which could influence the MTX cytotoxic effect.

These results are in consonance with previous studies describing the toxicogenetic and pharmacogenetic effects of the Ala16Val-SOD2 SNP on PBMCs exposed to xenobiotic molecules [21,22]. Another important effect observed in this study was the MTX effect on cytokines involved in the inflammatory response, but this result seems to not be influenced by SOD2 metabolism.

Author Contributions

Conceived and designed the experiments: FB AT IBMC. Performed the experiments: JRM VA MM MMMFD TDA CPM TCU KLS. Analyzed the data: FB EBD IBMC. Contributed reagents/materials/analysis tools: MMMFD IBMC AT. Contributed to the writing of the manuscript: FB IBMC AT.

References

1. Khan ZA, Tripathi R, Mishra B (2012) Methotrexate: a detailed review on drug delivery and clinical aspects. Expert Opin Drug Deliv 9: 51–56.

2. Herman S, Zurgil N, Deutsch M (2005) Low dose methotrexate induces apoptosis with reactive oxygen species involvement in T lymphocytic cell lines to a greater extent than in monocytic lines. Inflamm Res 54: 273–280.

3. Elango T, Dayalan H, Gnanaraj P, Malligarjunan H, Subramanian S (2013) Impact of methotrexate on oxidative stress and apoptosismarkers in psoriatic patients (2013). Clin Exp Med [Epub ahead of print].

4. Kozub P, Simaljakova M (2011) Systemic therapy of psoriasis:methotrexate (2011). Bratisl Lek Listy 112: 390-344.

5. Tobias H, Auerbach R (1973) Hepatotoxicity of long-term methotrexate therapy for psoriasis. Arch Intern Med 132: 391–396.

6. Vardi N, Parlakpinar H, Ates B, Cetin A, Otlu A (2009) Antiapoptotic and antioxidant effects of beta-carotene against methotrexate-induced testicular injury. Fertil Steril 92: 2028–2033.

7. D'Andrea N, Triolo L, Margagnoni G, Aratari A, Sanguinetti CM (2010) Methotrexate-induced pneumonitis in Crohn's disease. Case report and review of the literature Multidiscip Respir 31: 312–319.

8. Brock S, Jennings HR (2004) Fatal acute encephalomyelitis after a single dose of intrathecal_h. Pharmacoth 24: 673–676.

9. Ali N, Rashid S, Nafees S, Hasan SK (2014) Beneficial effects of Chrysin against Methotrexate-induced hepatotoxicity via attenuation of oxidative stress and apoptosis. Mol Cell Biochem. 385: 215–23.

10. Malik F, Ranganathan P (2013) Methotrexate pharmacogenetics in rheumatoid arthritis: a status report. Pharmacogen 14: 305–314.

11. Bresciani G, Cruz IB, de Paz JA, Cuevas MJ, González-Gallego J (2013) The MnSOD Ala16Val SNP: relevance to human diseases and interaction with environmental factors. Free Radic Res 47: 781–792.

12. Sutton A, Khoury H, Prip-Buus C, Cepanec C, Pessayre D, et al. (2003) The Ala16Val_geneticdimorphism modulates the import of human manganese superoxide dismutase into rat liver mitochondria. Pharmacog 13: 145–157.

13. Shimoda-Matsubayashi S, Matsumine H, Kobayashi T, Nakagawa-Hattori Y, Shimizu Y, et al. (1996) Structural dimorphism in the mitochondrial targeting sequence in the human manganese superoxide dismutase gene. A predictive evidence for conformational change to influence mitochondrial transport and a study of allelic association in Parkinson's disease. Biochem. Biophys. Res. Commun., 226 (1996): 561–565.

14. Duarte MM, Moresco RN, Duarte T, Santi A, Bagatini MD, et al. (2010) Oxidative stress in hypercholesterolemia and its association with Ala16Val superoxide dismutase gene polymorphism. Clin Biochem 43: 18–23.

15. Montano MA1, Barrio Lera JP, Gottlieb MG, Schwanke CH, da Rocha MI, et al. (2009) Association between manganese superoxide dismutase (MnSOD) gene polymorphism and elderly obesity. Mol Cell Biochem 328: 33–40.

16. Dos Santos Montagner GF, Sagrillo M, Machado MM, Almeida RC, Mostardeiro CP, et al. (2010) Toxicological effects of ultraviolet radiation on lymphocyte cells with different manganese superoxide dismutase Ala16Val polymorphism genotypes. Toxicol In Vitro 24: 1410–1416.

17. Algarve TD, Barbisan F, Ribeiro EE, Duarte MM, Mânica CMF, et al. (2013) In vitro effects of Ala16Val manganese superoxide dismutase gene polymorphism on human white blood cells exposed to methylmercury. Genet Mol Res 12: 5134–5144.

18. Costa F, Dornelles E, Mânica-Cattani MF, Algarve TD, Souza Filho OC, et al. (2012) Influence of Val16Ala SOD2 polymorphism on the in-vitro effect of clomiphene citrate in oxidative metabolism. Reprod Biomed 24: 474–481.

19. Montano MA, da Cruz IB, Duarte MM, Krewer C da C, da Rocha MI et al. (2012) Inflammatory cytokines in vitro production are associated with Ala16Val superoxide dismutase gene polymorphism of peripheral blood mononuclear cells. Cytok 60: 30–33.

20. Sakuma S, Kato Y, Nishigaki F, Magari K, Miyata S, et al. (2001) Effects of FK506 and other immunosuppressive anti-rheumatic agents on T cell activation mediated IL-6 and IgM production in vitro. Int Immunopharmacol 1: 749–57.

21. Olsen NJ, Spurlock CF, Aune TM (2014) Methotrexate induces production of IL-1 and IL-6 in the monocytic cell line U937. Arthritis Res Ther 16: 17–25.

22. Ruiz-Sanz JI, Aurrekoetxea I, Matorras R, Ruiz-Larrea MB (2011) Ala16Val SOD2 polymorphism is associated with higher pregnancy rates in in vitro fertilization cycles. Fertil Steril 95: 1601–1605.

23. Mosmann T (1983) Rapid colorimetric assay for cellular growth and survival: application to proliferation and cytotoxicity assays. J Immunol Methods 65: 55–63.

24. Burrow ME, Weldon CB, Tang Y, Navar GL, Krajewski S, et al. (1998) Differences in susceptibility to tumour necrosis factor alpha-induced apoptosis among MCF-7 breast cancer cell variants. Cancer Res 58: 4940–4946.

25. Jentzsch AM, Bachmann H, Fürst P, Biesalski HK (1983) Improved analysis of malondialdehyde in human body fluids. Free Radic Biol Med 20: 251–256.

26. Aebi H Catalase invitro (1984) Methods Enzymol 105: 121–126.

27. McCord JM, Fridovich I (1988) Superoxide dismutase: the first twenty years. Free Radic Biol Med 5: 363–369.

28. Flohe' L, Gunzler WA (1984) Glutathione peroxidase and reductase in vitro. Methods Enzymol 105: 114–121].

29. Singh N, McCoy M, Tice R, Schneider E (1988) A simple technique for quantitation of low levels of DNA damage in individual cells. Exp Cell Re 175: 184–191.

30. Hartmann A, Agurell E, Beevers C, Brendler-Schwaab S, Burlinson B, et al. (2003) Recommendations for conducting the in vivo alkaline Comet assay. International Comet Assay Workshop 4th. Mutagenesis 18: 45–55.

31. Chibber S, Hassan I, Farhan M, Naseem I (2011) In vitro pro-oxidant action of Methotrexate in presence of white light. J Photochem Photobiol B 104: 387–393.

32. Tabassum H, Parvez S, Pasha ST, Banerjee BD, Raisuddin S (2010) Protective effect of lipoic acid against methotrexate-induced oxidative stress in liver mitochondria. Food Chem Toxicol 48: 1973–1979.

33. Dalle-Donne I, Aldini G, Carini M, Colombo R, Rossi R, et al. (2006) Protein carbonylation, cellular dysfunction, and disease progression. J Cell Mol Med 10: 389–406.

34. Nicholls P (2012) Classical catalase: ancient and modern. Arch Biochem Biophys. 525: 95–101.

35. Paludo FJ, Simões-Pires A, Alho CS, Gelain DP, Moreira JC (2013) Participation of 47C>T SNP (Ala-9Val polymorphism) of the SOD2 gene in the intracellular environment of human peripheral blood mononuclear cells with and without lipopolysaccharides. Mol Cell Biochem.372: 127–35.

36. Oltvai Z, Milliman C, Korsmeyer SJ (1993) Bcl-2 heterodimerizes in vivo with a conversed homolog, Bax, that accelerates programmed cell death. Cell 74: 609–619.

37. Weng C, Li Y, Xu D, Shi Y, Tang H (2005) Specific cleavage of Mcl-1 by caspase-3 in tumor necrosis factor-related apoptosis-inducing ligand (TRAIL)-induced apoptosis in Jurkat leukemia T cells. J. Biol. Chem 280: 10491–10500.

38. Ibrahim MA, El-Sheikh AA, Khalaf HM, Abdelrahman AM (2014) Protective effect of peroxisome proliferator activator receptor (PPAR)-α and -γ ligands against methotrexate-induced nephrotoxicity. Immunopharmacol Immunotoxicol 36: 130–137.

39. Shandala T, Shen Ng Y, Hopwood B, Yip YC, Foster BK, et al. (2012) The role of osteocyte apoptosis in cancer chemotherapy induced bone loss. J Cell Physiol 227: 2889–2897.

40. Caron JE, Krull KR, Hockenberry M, Jain N, Kaemingk K, et al. (2009) Oxidative stress and executive function in children receiving chemotherapy for acute lymphoblastic leukemia. Pediatr Blood Cancer 53: 551–556.

41. Ma X, Xu S (2013) TNF inhibitor therapy for rheumatoid arthritis. Biomed Rep 1: 177–184.

13

Treatment of FANCA Cells with Resveratrol and N-Acetylcysteine

**Marta Columbaro[1]⬥, Silvia Ravera[2]⬥, Cristina Capanni[3], Isabella Panfoli[2], Paola Cuccarolo[4],
Giorgia Stroppiana[5], Paolo Degan[4]⬥, Enrico Cappelli[6]*⬥**

1 SC Laboratory of Musculoskeletal Cell Biology, IOR, Bologna, Italy, 2 DIFAR-Biochemistry Lab., University of Genova, Genova, Italy, 3 CNR-National Research Council of Italy, Institute of Molecular Genetics, Unit of Bologna-IOR, Bologna, Italy, 4 S. C. Mutagenesis, IRCCS AOU San Martino – IST (Istituto Nazionale per la Ricerca sul Cancro), Genova, Italy, 5 Centro di Diagnostica Genetica e Biochimica delle Malattie Metaboliche, Istituto Giannina Gaslini, Genova, Italy, 6 Hematology Unit, Istituto Giannina Gaslini, Genova, Italy

Abstract

Fanconi anemia (FA) is a genetic disorder characterised by chromosome instability, cytokine ipersensibility, bone marrow failure and abnormal haematopoiesis associated with acute myelogenous leukemia. Recent reports are contributing to characterize the peculiar FA metabolism. Central to these considerations appears that cells from complementation group A (FANCA) display an altered red-ox metabolism. Consequently the possibility to improve FA phenotypical conditions with antioxidants is considered. We have characterized from the structural and biochemical point of view the response of FANCA lymphocytes to N-acetyl-cysteine (NAC) and resveratrol (RV). Surprisingly both NAC and RV failed to revert all the characteristic of FA phenotype and moreover their effects are not super imposable. Our data suggest that we must be aware of the biological effects coming from antioxidant treatment.

Editor: Mauro Salvi, University of Padova, Italy

Funding: The authors have no funding or support to report.

Competing Interests: The authors have declared that no competing interests exist.

* Email: enricocappelli@ospedale-gaslini.ge.it

⬥ These authors contributed equally to this work.

Introduction

Fanconi anemia (FA) is a genetic disorder characterised by chromosome instability and cytokine hypersensitivity. Bone marrow failure and abnormal haematopoiesis are associated with high frequency to clonal hematopoietic stem cells (HSC) expansion, acute myelogeneous leukemia via a mechanism involving genomic instability and inflammation [1].

We recently reported [2,3] different structural abnormalities in FANCA cells underlying an impaired mitochondrial functionality affecting the energy metabolism. A defective respiration at the mitochondrial oxidative phosphorylation complex I is associated with a reduced ATP production and altered ATP/AMP ratio. These defects are consistently associated with impaired oxygen metabolism [4]. Therefore the possibility to improve FA patients physiological state with antioxidants as therapy adjuvants appears promising.

N-acetyl-cysteine (NAC) is a sulphydryl-group providing compound which acts as a precursor of reduced glutathione (GSH) and as direct scavenger of reactive oxygen species (ROS). Intracellular reduced GSH is often depleted as a consequence of increased oxidative stress and inflammation. Hence NAC can regulate the red-ox status in the cells interfering with several signalling pathways. NAC is widely used in clinical treatment [5] as support in treatment of diseases related to oxidative stress. Actually almost 250 studies with NAC are enlisted in the Clinical Trials governmental registry (www.clinicaltrials.gov).

Resveratrol (RV) is a naturally-occurring polyphenol mainly found in grapes. A growing body of literature has demonstrated the beneficial effects of RV on age-related metabolic deterioration and its protective role in metabolic diseases. RV exerts its potent anticarcinogenic effect by inducing apoptosis and inhibiting tumor promoter-induced cell transformation [6]. RV protects against the deregulation of energy homeostasis, up-regulates eNOS and many cellular anti-oxidant enzymes, down regulates TNFα and NF-κB expression and inhibits NADPH oxidases [7]. Moreover, crystallographic studies showed that RV (and other related polyphenols) directly inhibits the rotary mechanism of mitochondrial F_oF_1-ATP synthase (ATP synthase) by binding to a site in γ-subunit and hence its ATP synthetic activity [8]. More than 70 clinical trials with RV are actually listed in the National Institutes of Health website.

In FA, the use of NAC and RV has already been proposed. Treatment with NAC, in association with Lipoic Acid (LA) [9] increased cellular viability as well as GSH and ATP contents, and reduced spontaneous and DEB-induced chromosomal instability in lymphocyte from FA patients. The protective abilities of NAC, RV and tempol were compared in the FANCD2 murine model [10]. NAC and RV partially corrected the abnormal cell cycle state of the HSP cells and helped maintaining them in a quiescent state. In turn tempol substantially delayed tumor onset apparently without a beneficial effect on hematopoiesis. Finally an antioxidant dietary formulate containing lysine, proline, ascorbic acid and green tea extracts, was successfully reported to inhibit in vitro and in vivo FANCA-associated head and neck squamous cell carcinoma [11].

Notwithstanding the potential interest concerning these results the still crucial and open question is that we do not know yet which molecular mechanisms and metabolic pathways are relevant in the FA pathological phenotype. Here we evaluate the biological effects of RV and NAC, two most promising antioxidants which act with different biochemical mechanisms.

Materials & Methods

Ethics statement

Study approval was obtained from the Ethics Committee at the Gaslini Hospital, Genova, Italy (protocol N° J5002 date: 24/9/2010). Informed written consent was obtained from the adult subjects and from parents, on the behalf of their children, involved in the study. All clinical investigations were conducted according to the principles expressed in the Declaration of Helsinki.

Cell culture and treatments

FANCA primary fibroblast cell lines, isogenic FANCA primary fibroblasts corrected with S11FAIN [12] retrovirus and wild type (wt) cells were grown as monolayer at 37°C in RPMI supplemented with 10% fetal calf serum and antibiotics. All the cell lines between the 5th and 15th passage, were grown with the same density and conditions. During treatment we didn't observe significant changes in the cellular viability. FANCA and wt lymphoblast cell lines were grown at 37°C in RPMI supplemented with 10% fetal calf serum and antibiotics. Primary lymphocytes were isolated using Ficoll-Paque Plus and grown at 37°C in RPMI supplemented with 10% fetal calf serum, antibiotics and phytohemagglutinin (20 μg/ml). N-acetyl-cysteine (500 μM), resveratrol (10 μM) were added to the cells once a day for five days. One hour after the last treatment, cells were used for protein extracts or fixed for electron microscopy experiments. FANCA corrected cells always behaved alike wt [3].

Oxygen consumption measurements

To measure oxygen consumption, an amperometric electrode (Unisense-Microrespiration, Unisense A/S, Denmark) was used. Experiments were performed in a closed chamber at 25°C. For each experiment 500.000 cells were permeabilized with 0.03 mg/ml digitonin for 1 minute, centrifuged for 9 minutes at 1000 rpm and resuspended in: 137 mM NaCl, 0.7 mM NaH_2PO_4, 5 mM KCl and 25 mM Tris HCl pH 7.4. The same medium was used in the oximetric experiments. To stimulate the pathway composed by the respiratory complexes I, III and IV, 10 mM pyruvate and 5 mM malate was added to the sample, while to stimulate the pathway II, III and IV 20 mM succinate was used as respiratory substrate. To confirm that the oxygen consumption was really due to oxidative phosphorylation (OXPHOS) machinery, 0.1 mM rotenone or 0.2 mM antimycin A were used as inhibitors for the first and second pathway, respectively [13].

Electron transfer from Complex I to Complex III

The electron transfer between Complex I to Complex III was studied spectrophotometrically, following the reduction of cytochrome c at 550 nm. The extinction molar coefficient used for reduced cytochrome c was 1 mM^{-1} cm^{-1}. For each assay, 50 μg of total proteins was used. The assay medium containing; 100 mM Tris-HCl pH 7,4 and 0,03% cytochrome c. The reaction was started with the addition of 0,7 mM NADH [3]. If the electron transport between Complex I and Complex III is conserved, the electrons pass from NADH to Complex I, then to Complex III via coenzyme Q, and finally to cytochrome c.

Adenylate kinase (AK) assay

AK activity was assayed spectrophotometrically, following NADH oxidation at 340 nm [14]. ATP and GTP in the assay mixture are needed to assay the ATP-AMP phosphotransferase activity (AK1 + AK2) or the GTP-AMP phosphotransferase activity (mitochondrial AK3), respectively. Results are reported for the activity of the enzyme (U/mg) per sample.

ATP and AMP quantification

ATP and AMP were measured according to the enzyme coupling method of Bergmeyer et al. [15]. For ATP assay, medium contained 20 μg of sample, 50 mM Tris- HCl pH 8.0, 1 mM NADP, 10 mM $MgCl2$, and 5 mM glucose in 1 ml final volume. Samples were analyzed spectrophotometrically before and after the addition of 4 μg of purified hexokinase/glucose-6-phosphate dehydrogenase (Boehringer). The rise in absorbance at 340 nm, due to NADPH formation, was proportional to the ATP concentration. For AMP assay, the medium contained 20 μg of sample, 50 mM Tris-HCl pH 8.0, 1 mM NADH, 10 mM $MgCl2$, and 10 mM phosphoenolpyruvate (PEP), 2 mM ATP in 1 ml final volume. Samples were analyzed spectrophotometrically before and after the addition of 4 μg of purified pyruvate kinase/lactate dehydrogenase (Boehringer). The rise in absorbance at 340 nm, due to NADH oxidation, was proportional to the AMP concentration. For all biochemical experiments, protein concentrations were determined using the Bradford method.

Electron microscopy

Lymphocyte pellets from healthy donor and FANCA patients (subjected or not to antioxidant treatments) were fixed with 2.5% glutaraldehyde 0.1 M cacodylate buffer pH 7.6 for 1 h at room temperature. After post-fixation with 1% $OsO4$ in cacodylate buffer for 1 h, pellets were dehydrated in an ethanol series and embedded in Epon resin. Ultrathin sections stained with uranylacetate and lead citrate were observed with a Jeol Jem-1011 transmission electron microscope. Two hundred mitochondria were examined for each sample.

Cytometry

ROS were quantified by cytometry with 2′,7′-dichlorodihydrofluorescein diacetate (H2DCFH-DA). This dye is a cell-permeable, nonfluorescent molecule, which is very sensitive to intracellular redox change. When $H_2DCFH-DA$ enters into the cell it is cleaved by intracellular esterases into 2′,7′-dichlorodihydrofluorescein (H_2DCF) which, in presence of H_2O_2, oxidize to the fluorescent molecule dichlorofluorescein (DCF). Fluorescence from this probe is measured by flow cytometry, as the dye is excited by the 488-nm laser. $H_2DCFH-DA$ has a good specificity for H_2O_2, and it has been shown that the fluorescence of the product DCF appears to be mediated mainly by H_2O_2. Cytometry measures were performed on a Cyan ADP cytometer (Beckman Coulter, Mountain View, CA, USA) equipped with three laser lamps.Ten thousand cells per sample were analyzed, and the results are reported as the percentage of cells, relative to the relevant control, that display a fluorescence shift.

Statistical analysis

Data were analyzed by one-way ANOVA and unpaired two-tail Student's t test using instat software (GraphPad Software, Inc., La Jolla, CA, USA). Data are expressed as mean ± standard deviation (SD) from 3 to 5 independent determinations performed in duplicate. In the figures SD are shown as error bars. An error probability with P<0.05 was selected as significant.

Results

1 – Cytometric ROS quantification

An enhanced oxidative stress appears the common denominator of the many altered functions in FANCA cells. In fact, we reported [2,3] an enhanced ROS production in FANCA cells associated with a scarce NADH utilization or availability at the mitochondrial respiratory Complex I. NAC and RV, although with different mechanisms as discussed below, provide significant reduction in intracellular ROS production. When FANCA cells were treated with NAC or RV a significant decrease (p<0,01) in intracellular ROS production was measured (Table 1). The large differences reported among the samples analysed might be attributed to the different functional characteristics of the mutant FANCA proteins produced. In this context, the structure-function relationships in mutant FANCA proteins (in the various patients) are however as yet not fully available to-date and cannot be properly discussed at this time. Castella et al. [19] reported cytoplasmic expression of mutated FANCA protein without functional correlation between genotype and phenotype. Moreover, this work evaluated the effect of FANCA mutated protein only in the perspective of the DNA repair activity without considering other possible functions for FANCA protein. Indeed, these putative functions may be the cause of the high variability observed.

2 – Biochemical Parameters

2.1 - Oxygen consumption. As described by Ravera et al. [3], FANCA cells display defective respiration trough the pathway composed by Complex I, III and IV. In our experimental setting, FANCA and wild type (wt) primary fibroblasts were treated with 500 µM NAC or 10 µM RV for 5 days. In these conditions the ability of FANCA cells to respire from the Complex I, III and IV pathway were fully restored (Fig. 1A) after NAC and only partially after RV treatment.

Moreover RV reduced the ability of wt cells to respire both in the presence of pyruvate/malate and with succinate, as respiring substrates. This effect may be explained considering that RV is an inhibitor of the activity of ATP synthase [16,17]. Namely, being oxygen consumption coupled to ATP synthesis, when ATP synthase is inhibited, the electron transport chain activity also slows down, and so does oxygen consumption. In conclusion, even though the effects of NAC and RV follow different pathways, the net results is a reduction of ROS generated at the level of Complex I. Genetic complementation by FANCA gene corrects the respiratory defect. The same results were obtained in lymphoblast cell lines from the same patients (data not shown).

2.2 - Complex I to Complex III electron transfer. Defective respiration in FANCA cells is due to defect in electron transfer from Complex I to Complex III and is associated with reduced ATP production and altered ATP/AMP ratio [3]. However, as shown above, the treatment of FANCA cells with NAC restores their ability to respire through Complex I and, accordingly, electron transfer efficiency between Complex I and III is restored in FANCA at level comparable to wt cells. By contrast, RV only partially recovered the FANCA cells electron transfer efficiency. Also, in line with the results for oxygen consumption, it reduced the electron transfer ability in wt cells (Fig. 1B). The difference among the effect of NAC and RV likely depends on their different target. In fact, being a precursor of GSH NAC is really an antioxidant molecule able to decrease the damage due to ROS production consequent to impaired functioning of Complex I. By contrast, RV acts by inhibiting the activity of ATP synthase, thus reducing the speed of electron transport chain, i.e. of Complex I. This causes a lower production of ROS thus allowing cell scavengers systems to work.

2.3 - Intracellular ATP and AMP quantification. In FANCA the ATP/AMP ratio is very low with respect to the control (Fig. 1C) in agreement with what can be expected from the impairment of Complexes I-III electron transport. By contrast,

Table 1. Cytometric quantification of the ROS reduction (%) in FANCA cells after treatment with NAC and RV.

Samples	ROS reduction (%)	
	+ NAC	+ RV
FANCA 1	32.67	31.28
FANCA 2	42.11	30.37
FANCA 3	27.70	37.03
FANCA 4	41.24	60.94
FANCA 5	41.40	28.71
FANCA 6	46.33	47.10
FANCA 7	35.85	64.18
FANCA 8	39.67	44.29
FANCA 9	44.81	57.17
FANCA 10	16.59	46.84
FANCA 11	59.26	n.d.
FANCA 12	45.50	43.94
FANCA 13	26.65	36.58
FANCA 14	77.84	16.31

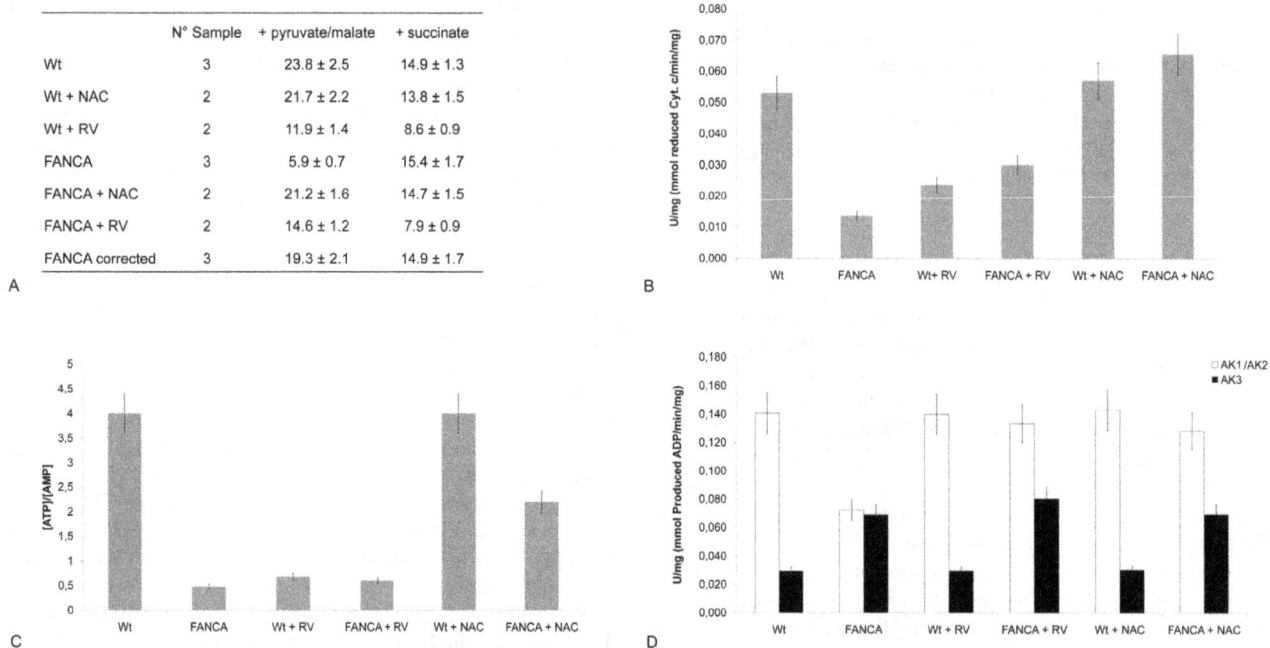

	N° Sample	+ pyruvate/malate	+ succinate
Wt	3	23.8 ± 2.5	14.9 ± 1.3
Wt + NAC	2	21.7 ± 2.2	13.8 ± 1.5
Wt + RV	2	11.9 ± 1.4	8.6 ± 0.9
FANCA	3	5.9 ± 0.7	15.4 ± 1.7
FANCA + NAC	2	21.2 ± 1.6	14.7 ± 1.5
FANCA + RV	2	14.6 ± 1.2	7.9 ± 0.9
FANCA corrected	3	19.3 ± 2.1	14.9 ± 1.7

Figure 1. Biochemical parameters in FANCA and wild-type (wt) cells untreated or treated with 500 μm nac or 10 μm rv for 5 days. A. Table reports values for oxygen consumption (μM O_2/min/mg) in FANCA and wild type (wt) primary fibroblasts treated NAC or RV after induction with pyruvate/malate (Complexes I, III and IV), or succinate (Complexes II+III+IV). B. Assay of the electron transfer from Complex I to Complex III on wt and FANCA samples. Electron transfer between Complex I and III was measured following the reduction of cytochrome c at 550 nm after the addition of 0.7 mM NADH, the substrate of Complex I. Data are reported as μmol reduced Cytochrome c/min/mg. C. Figure shows the ratio among ATP and AMP concentration in wt and FANCA samples. D. Histogram reports a comparison of the ATP-AMP phosphotransferase activity (AK1+AK2 white columns) and GTP-AMP phosphotransferase (AK3, black columns) activity on wt and FANCA samples. The activity is expressed as μmol of ADP produced/min/mg. Data are expressed as mean ± SD. Each panel is representative of at least five experiments.

after NAC treatment, the ATP level in FANCA cells was restored and the AMP concentration decreases, although it remained higher than in wt, allowing to reach a good ATP/AMP ratio (Fig. 1C). In the case of RV treatment only a partial recovery of ATP was seen in FANCA and a strong reduction in wt cells was observed. This is likely related to the inhibitor effect of RV on ATP synthase, considering that ATP synthase is the principal source of ATP production for the cell.

2.4 - Adenylate Kinase (AK) activity. Adenylate Kinase (AK) activities were also investigated. These enzymes catalyse the interconversion of adenine nucleotides and contributing to the regulation of the cellular energy homeostasis. In particular, we assayed the ATP-AMP phosphotransferase isoforms (AK1 and AK2), which catalyze the interconversion of ADP to ATP+AMP and the GTP-AMP phosphotransferase isoform, typical of the mitochondrial matrix, which utilizes GTP as donor for the phosphate group to AMP [3]. In FANCA cells ATP-AMP phosphotransferase activity was impaired while GTP-AMP phosphotransferase activity was increased (Fig. 1D). Both NAC and RV treatment restored FANCA ATP-AMP phosphotransferase activity, to a level similar to wt cells. By contrast, as already observed [3], the GTP-AMP phosphotransferase activity was higher in FANCA cells with respect to controls. Thus FANCA cells appear to preferably use GTP, from Krebs cycle, as alternative source of energy. This could be explained considering that in FANCA cells the electron transport among Complex I and III is impaired. Consequently ATP synthesis from oxidative phosphorylation is lower with respect to control. Interestingly, RV and NAC treatments do not restore the GTP-AMP phospho-transferase activity to the control level, suggesting that energetic

metabolism restoration by the antioxidant treatment in FANCA cells is not complete.

3 – Electron Microscopy

By ultrastructural analysis (Fig. 2A), we observed striking mitochondrial changes in FANCA lymphocytes after NAC, RV or NAC plus RV treatments compared to untreated FANCA lymphocytes Indeed in NAC treated FANCA1 lymphocytes many mitochondria (30%) were greatly enlarged with disrupted cristae and rarefaction of matrix density (Fig. 2b) rather than the swollen shape mitochondrial observed in untreated FANCA1 lymphocytes (Fig. 2a). On the contrary, NAC treatment did not cause detectable changes in mitochondrial structure in FANCA2 lymphocytes (Fig. 2d) compared to untreated FANCA2 cells (Fig. 2c). In fact, before and after NAC treatment, most of the mitochondria appeared swollen with matrix rarefaction and altered cristae. Surprisingly, in RV treated FANCA3 lymphocytes a significant recovery in the mitochondria organization (40%) consisting in elongated, small or rod –like shape mitochondria with dense matrix and normal distribution of cristae (Fig. 2f), was seen compared to untreated FANCA3 lymphocytes characterized by altered swollen mitochondria with fewer cristae (80%) (Fig. 2e). In untreated FANCA4 lymphocytes most mitochondria had normal morphology, but 30% of them showed highly condensed matrix with swollen internal cristae (Fig. 2g), which are indicative of mitoptosis, a kind of dead mitochondria [18]. After NAC treatment the number of mitochondria in mitoptosis decreases and the cells shown normal mitochondrial structure (Fig. 2h). However, the number of apoptotic cells increased with about 30% of cells in apoptosis (data not shown). After RV treatments, we

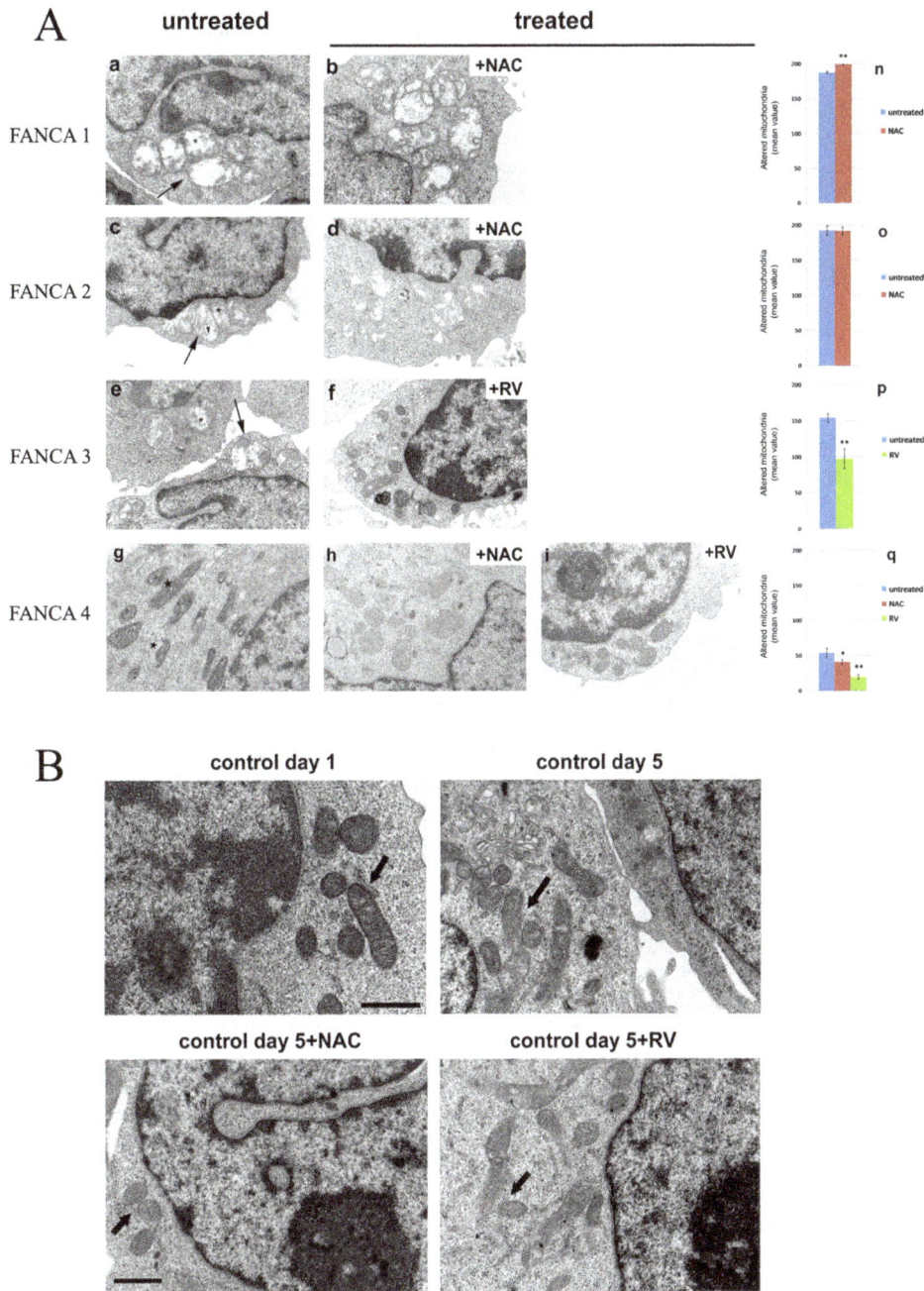

Figure 2. Morphological changes of mitochondria in FANCA lymphocytes and healthy controls. A. Representative transmission electron microscopy images of morphologically altered mitochondria from untreated (a,c,e,g) and treated FANCA (b,d,f,h,i) with different antioxidants. Mitochondria of untreated lymphocytes from FANCA patients 1, 2, 3 (a,c,e) appeared swollen (black arrows) with increased size, disrupted cristae (black asterisks) and rarefacted matrix (black arrowheads). On the contrary, mitochondria in untreated lymphocytes from FANCA4 patient were small, oval and round with dark matrix and swollen internal cristae (black stars). (b) Mitochondria of FA1 lymphocytes showed worsened alteration such as more enlarged shape (white arrow) after NAC treatment. (d) Mitochondria of FANCA2 lymphocytes appeared indistinguishable from untreated (b) in overall aspect, after NAC treatment (white arrowheads). (f) Mitochondria of FANCA3 and FANCA4 lymphocytes showed a striking rescue after NAC or RV treatments (white asterisks). (Scale bars, 1 μm) **B.** Representative micrographs of morphologically normal mitochondria (arrowheads) in control lymphocytes at day 1 and day 5 before and after NAC or RV treatments. (Scale bars 1μm).

observed an increased of percentage of ameliorated mitochondria (20%) with dense matrix and regularly distributed cristae (Fig. 2i). Small, electron-dense granules were occasionally seen in untreated and treated FANCA4 lymphocytes.

Fig. 2B shows representative micrographs of morphologically normal mitochondria from control lymphocytes at day 1 and day 5 before and after NAC or RV treatments.

Discussion

FANCA cells display an altered red-ox metabolism [4]. The possibility to improve this altered physiological conditions with the employment of antioxidants has been consequently forwarded/proposed. Here we evaluated the biological effects of two antioxidants featuring different biochemical mechanisms. While from the point of view of the biochemistry and the energy metabolism NAC treatment appears advantageous, the here reported results concerning cellular morphology suggests attention especially in the view to employ NAC as therapeutic in FA. On the contrary RV induces only a partial recovery of the biochemical parameters, but great improvement in cellular morphology.

Our data suggest that we must be aware of possible pitfalls of the employment of antioxidants as therapeutics. While short time exposure (from few hours to 2 days) to NAC appears beneficial in FA [9,20], upon mere observation of the biochemical parameters, the effect of NAC appears positive for the FANCA cells. However when we extend our observation to the cellular ultrastructure, some cellular defects don't improve and negative effects are seen, such as worsening of mitochondrial structure. A possible explanation for this could paradoxically be the recovery of electron transport chain functioning by NAC. The pro-oxidant FA phenotype cells is characterized by alterations in the electron transport efficiency in the inner mitochondrial membrane with loss of efficiency of electron transfer from Complex I to Complex III which can in fact be restored by administration of exogenous Coenzyme Q [3]. NAC decreases ROS production and normalizes mitochondrial respiration. Therefore it is expected that in FA cells with increased ROS production, oxygen consumption will increase in the presence of NAC (Fig. 1A). The ability of NAC to restore Complex I activity is however inherently linked to an increase in ROS production and therefore in worsening of the already existent structural damage typical of FACA cells. This is also suggestive of the existence of a primary damage to mitochondrial membranes in the FANCA phenotype. The sole increase in GSH reductive potential in FANCA cells appears insufficient to restore a fully functional phenotype. NAC was already reported [21] to be only partially effective in limiting GSH depletion, particularly when employed in drugs targeted to mitochondria. While the negative phenotypic outcomes from the chronic NAC treatment in FANCA cells were almost unexpected its possible detrimental effects are already known. The forced increase in intracellular GSH was indeed reported to induce a paradoxical triggering of mitochondrial oxidative stress [22]. After either pharmacologic (NAC supplementation) or genetic (glutamate cysteine ligase overexpression) maneuvers an initially more reducing GSH redox potential or reductive stress was promptly followed by a pathogenic mitochondrial oxidation. The GSH-mediated reductive stress culminated with pro-oxidative consequences in mitochondria contrary to the common belief that NAC functions solely as an antioxidant.

The various lymphocytes here analysed do show various types of mitochondrial alterations. It has been reported that no apparent correlation exists between the genotypic defect and the phenotypic expression [19]. However it also holds true that no molecular function or metabolic regulation other than DNA repair has been exploited to date.

The different response to NAC observed in the analysed samples may be correlated to the different genetic background. It appears clear, however, that the effect of NAC on the overall cell population examined is null or negative. In FANCA1 NAC treatment (fig. 2b) result in mitochondria with greatly enlarged, disrupted cristae and rarefaction in matrix density where in FANCA2 (fig. 2d) no detectable changes are seen in mitochondrial structure; in FANCA4 (fig. 2h) we observe a normal mitochondrial structure and a decrease in the number of mitochondria in mitoptoses but with a concomitant increase in the number of apoptotic cells. It appears peculiar that the level of the apoptotic cells in the NAC treated sample equals the level of mitoptotic cells in the untreated. It has been reported that ROS produced by the respiratory chain inside mitochondria could also induce mitochondrial fission as the initial step of mitoptosis [23]. The same degeneration in the mitochondrial reticulum here reported has been described by us in FA fibroblasts [2].

RV treatment partially restored the FANCA biochemical activity but resulted in significant recovery of a normal structure. It may appear surprising that in the presence of RV mitochondrial functions like ATP production and oxygen uptake are increased in FANCA cells (and decreased in wild type cells, as expected). To explain this apparent contradiction the cited defective phenotype of Complex I in FANCA cells [3], as well as the results from Gledhill et al. [8] should be taken into consideration. These Authors, by structural analysis of ATPase crystallized in the presence of RV demonstrated that it binds the inside surface of F_1 npreventing both the synthetic and hydrolytic activities of ATPase [8]. In this respect, RV cannot be considered a mere ROS scavenger, rather its action is exerted also through mild control of the ATP synthase activity. Being an inhibitor of ATP synthase [8], RV slows down the electron transport chain activity and NADH utilization by Complex I which has the result to lower free radical production. It can be hypothesized that in these conditions aerobic respiration is more efficient and more directed to ATP production increasing O_2 utilization finalized to H_2O and not to ROS production. RV alone inhibits ATP synthase and decreases electron transport chain activity producing less free radicals. In fact, when the ATP synthase is inhibited also the electron transport chain activity slows, and consequently the oxygen consumption decreases with a kind of indirect scavenging.

RV was shown to reduce mitochondrial respiration, and Complex IV activity and to extend lifespan. In fact diminished mitochondrial OXPHOS is associated with lower ROS production and reduced longevity. A beneficial effect of RV in tumors may derive in part by its preventing mitochondrial ATP synthesis, thereby inducing apoptosis. RV was shown to decrease tumor cell viability, an effect that can be reverted by overexpression of Bcl-2 [24]. However, RV may exert other effects, also in dependence of the model used. For example, treatment of the whole animal (mice) in vivo with RV causes induction of OXPHOS genes, an effect likely related to activation of the protein deacetylase, SIRT1 [25].

We have also tested a combination of NAC and RV. Unfortunately, the double treatment did not restore the correct OXPHOS activity in FANCA-cells, nor the electron transport from Complex I to Complex III (data not shown). We may explain these results considering the single contribution from each compound: NAC restores the functionality of Complex I, while RV reduces mitochondrial respiration, and ATP synthesis, by reversibly inhibiting ATP synthase. In the FANCA case, the combination of the two has the effect of both blocking mitochondrial respiration and improving the functioning of Complex I: this would cause a backlog of electrons, augmenting ROS production and increasing oxidative damage to the mitochondrial inner membranes. Literature reports that a mild uncoupling between electron transport chain and ATP synthase induces a H^+ leak and increases ROS production.

Ultrastructural analysis also showed that the combined treatment of NAC plus RV did not improve mitochondrial alterations (data not shown). Instead, concomitant treatment with RV and NAC worsened the mitochondrial phenotype (data not shown). In this case ATP synthase blockade by RV on one hand and promotion of electron transfer by NAC on the other produce an increase in oxidative damage.

In conclusion, both NAC and RV failed to revert the biochemical and structural phenotype FANCA phenotype. Moreover, their effects are not super imposable. Even though the NAC treatment did restore the OXPHOS functionality in FA cells, the phenotype did not improve; by contrast RV exerted a better effect on FA cell phenotype, although it was not able to revert all the characteristic of the mutant cells. Therefore, an antioxidant therapy is likely to be beneficial in several pathological conditions; however an evaluation of the effects of the single antioxidant employed should be carefully scrutinized to avoid possible detrimental consequences. Our knowledge of the proper use and the effects of any single antioxidant, and for their combined use as well, is as yet quite limited.

Acknowledgments

The samples were obtained from the "Cell Line and DNA Biobank from Patients affected by Genetic Diseases" (G. Gaslini Institute) - Telethon Genetic Biobank Network (Project No. GTB07001). AIRFA, ERG spa, Cambiaso & Risso, Rimorchiatori Riuniti, Saar Depositi Oleari Portuali, UC Sampdoria are aknowledged for supporting the activity of the Clinical & Experimental Hematology Unit of G. Gaslini Institute.

Author Contributions

Conceived and designed the experiments: MC SR GS PC CC IP EC PD. Performed the experiments: MC SR GS PC CC. Analyzed the data: PD EC IP. Contributed reagents/materials/analysis tools: IP CC EC PD. Contributed to the writing of the manuscript: EC PD.

References

1. Li X, Yang Y, Yuan J, Hong P, Freie B et al. (2004) Continuous in vivo infusion of interferon-gamma (IFN-gamma) preferentially reduces myeloid progenitor numbers and enhances engraftment of syngeneic wild-type cells in Fancc-/- mice. Blood 104: 1204–1209.
2. Capanni C, Bruschi M, Columbaro M, Cuccarolo P, Ravera S et al. (2013) Changes in vimentin, lamin A/C and mitofilin induce aberrant cell organization in fibroblasts from Fanconi anemia complementation group A (FA-A) patients. Biochimie 95: 1838–47.
3. Ravera S, Vaccaro D, Cuccarolo P, Columbaro M, Capanni C et al. (2013) Mitochondrial respiratory chain Complex I defects in Fanconi anemia complementation group A. Biochimie 95: 1828–1837.
4. Cappelli E, Ravera S, Vaccaro D, Cuccarolo P, Bartolucci M et al. (2013) Mitochondrial respiratory complex I defects in Fanconi anemia. Trends Mol Med 19: 513–514.
5. Dodd S, Dean O, Copolov DL, Malhi GS, Berk M (2008) N-acetylcysteine for antioxidant therapy: pharmacology and clinical utility. Expert Opinion on Biological Therapy 8: 1955–1962.
6. Dong Z (2003) Molecular mechanism of the chemopreventive effect of resveratrol. Mutat Res. 523–524: 145–50.
7. Csiszar A (2011) Anti-inflammatory effects of resveratrol: possible role in prevention of age-related cardiovascular disease. Ann N Y AcadSci 1215: 117–22.
8. Gledhill JR, Montgomery MG, Leslie AG, Walker JE (2007) Mechanism of inhibition of bovine F1-ATPase by resveratrol and related polyphenols. Proc Natl Acad Sci U S A. 104: 13632–7.
9. Ponte F, Sousa R, Fernandes AP, Gonçalves C, Barbot J et al. (2012) Improvement of genetic stability in lymphocytes from Fanconi anemia patients through the combined effect of α-lipoic acid and N-acetylcysteine. Orphanet J Rare Dis 16: 7–28.
10. Zhang QS, Marquez-Loza L, Sheehan AM, Watanabe-Smith K, Eaton L et al. (2014) Evaluation of resveratrol and N-acetylcysteine for cancer chemoprevention in a Fanconi anemia murine model. Pediatr Blood Cancer. 61: 740–742.
11. Roomi MW, Kalinovsky T, Roomi NW, Niedzwiecki A, Rath M (2012) In vitro and in vivo inhibition of human Fanconi anemia-associated head and neck squamous cell carcinoma by a novel nutrient mixture. Int J Oncol. 41: 1996–2004.
12. Hanenberg H, Batish SD, Pollok KE, Vieten L, Verlander PC et al. (2002) Phenotypic correction of primary Fanconi anemia T cells with retroviral vectors as a diagnostic tool. Exp Hematol. 30: 410–20.
13. Ravera S, Panfoli I, Calzia D, Aluigi MG, Bianchini P et al. (2009) Evidence for aerobic ATP synthesis in isolated myelin vesicles. Int J Biochem Cell Biol.41: 1581–1591.
14. Ravera S, Calzia D, Bianchini P, Diaspro A, Panfoli I (2007) Confocal laser scanning microscopy of retinal rod outer segment intact disks: new labeling technique. J Biomed Opt.12: 050501.
15. Bergmeyer HU, Grassl M, Walter HE (1983) Methods of Enzymatic Analysis, Verlag-Chemie, Weinheim,p. 249.
16. Hong SM, Pedersen PL (2008) ATP Synthase and the Actions of Inhibitors Utilized To Study Its Roles in Human Health, Disease, and Other Scientific Areas. Microbiol Mol Biol Rev 72: 590–641.
17. Zheng J, Ramirez VD (2000) Inhibition of mitochondrial proton F0F1-ATPase/ATP synthase by polyphenolic phytochemicals. Br. J. Pharmacol 130: 1115–1123.
18. Jangamreddy JR, Los MJ (2012) Mitoptosis, a novel mitochondrial death mechanism leading predominantly to activation of autophagy. Hepat Mon. 12(8):e6159.
19. Castella M, Pujol R, Callén E, Trujillo JP, Casado JA et al. (2011) Origin, functional role, and clinical impact of Fanconi anemia FANCA mutations. Blood 117: 3759–69.
20. Kumari U, Ya Jun W, Huat Bay B, Lyakhovich A (2014) Evidence of mitochondrial dysfunction and impaired ROS detoxifying machinery in Fanconi Anemia cells. Oncogene 33: 165–172.
21. Cuccarolo P, Viaggi S, Degan P (2012) New insights into redox response modulation in Fanconi's anemia cells by hydrogen peroxide and glutathione depletors. FEBS J. 279: 2479–94.
22. Zhang H, Limphong P, Pieper J, Liu Q, Rodesch CK et al. (2012) Glutathione-dependent reductive stress triggers mitochondrial oxidation and cytotoxicity. FASEB J. 26: 1442–51.
23. Pletjushkina OY, Lyamzaev KG, Popova EN, Nepryakhina OK, Ivanova OY et al. (2006) Effect of oxidative stress on dynamics of mitochondrial reticulum. BiochimBiophysActa. 1757: 518–24.
24. Low IC, Chen ZX, Pervaiz S. (2010) Bcl-2 modulates resveratrol-induced ROS production by regulating mitochondrial respiration in tumor cells. Antioxid. Redox Signal. 13, 807–819.
25. Lagouge M, Argmann C, Gerhart-Hines Z, Meziane H, Lerin C et al. (2006) Resveratrol Improves Mitochondrial Function and Protects against Metabolic Disease by Activating SIRT1 and PGC-1α. Cell, 127, 1109–1122.

14

Azelnidipine Inhibits Cultured Rat Aortic Smooth Muscle Cell Death Induced by Cyclic Mechanical Stretch

Jing Zhao, Kentaro Ozawa, Yoji Kyotani, Kosuke Nagayama, Satoyasu Ito, Akira T. Komatsubara, Yuichi Tsuji, Masanori Yoshizumi*

Department of Pharmacology, Nara Medical University School of Medicine, Kashihara, Nara, Japan

Abstract

Acute aortic dissection is the most common life-threatening vascular disease, with sudden onset of severe pain and a high fatality rate. Clarifying the detailed mechanism for aortic dissection is of great significance for establishing effective pharmacotherapy for this high mortality disease. In the present study, we evaluated the influence of biomechanical stretch, which mimics an acute rise in blood pressure using an experimental apparatus of stretching loads in vitro, on rat aortic smooth muscle cell (RASMC) death. Then, we examined the effects of azelnidipine and mitogen-activated protein kinase inhibitors on mechanical stretch-induced RASMC death. The major findings of the present study are as follows: (1) cyclic mechanical stretch on RASMC caused cell death in a time-dependent manner up to 4 h; (2) cyclic mechanical stretch on RASMC induced c-Jun N-terminal kinase (JNK) and p38 activation with peaks at 10 min; (3) azelnidipine inhibited RASMC death in a concentration-dependent manner as well as inhibited JNK and p38 activation by mechanical stretch; and (4) SP600125 (a JNK inhibitor) and SB203580 (a p38 inhibitor) protected against stretch-induced RASMC death; (5) Antioxidants, diphenylene iodonium and tempol failed to inhibit stretch-induced RASMC death. On the basis of the above findings, we propose a possible mechanism where an acute rise in blood pressure increases biomechanical stress on the arterial walls, which induces RASMC death, and thus, may lead to aortic dissection. Azelnidipine may be used as a pharmacotherapeutic agent for prevention of aortic dissection independent of its blood pressure lowering effect.

Editor: Hiromi Yanagisawa, UT-Southwestern Med Ctr, United States of America

Funding: The study was supported by JSPS KAKENHI Grants, number 23590306 and 26460345, to MY. (http://www.e-rad.go.jp/index.html). The funders had no role in study design, data collection and analysis, decision to publish, or preparation of the manuscript.

Competing Interests: The authors have declared that no competing interests exist.

* Email: yoshizu@naramed-u.ac.jp

Introduction

With the rapid progress of population aging in most developed countries, the number of patients with atherosclerosis has remarkably increased; this is becoming an extremely serious problem requiring urgent attention [1,2]. Among cardiovascular diseases, acute aortic dissection presents with sudden onset of severe pain and a high fatality rate [3,4]. It has been reported that various endovascular techniques with minimally invasive characteristics have been applied extensively to elderly patients and have proven to be effective in acute aortic dissection treatment. However, most successful cases to date have been restricted to surgical operations, and there is little evidence relating to effective drug treatment or pharmacotherapy.

It is well recognized that aortic dissection occurs when a small tear generated in the inner aortic wall extends along the wall of the aorta and causes blood to flow between the layers of the tunica media and adventitia of the aorta, forcing the layers apart. Despite the pathophysiological interpretation, the detailed mechanism for aortic dissection still remains unclear. Various efforts have been recently made to clarify the possible reasons for aortic dissection. Collins et al. reported that progressive loss of smooth muscle cells is observed in the specimens of acute aortic dissection character-

ized by aortic medial degeneration [5]. Wernig et al. and Chen et al. confirmed that mechanical stretch can induce apoptosis in vascular smooth muscle cells (VSMCs) [6,7]. Hipper and Isenberg found that cyclic mechanical strain reduced DNA synthesis in VSMCs [8]. Along with these findings, we hypothesized that acute mechanical stretching force, which mimics an acute rise in blood pressure, may cause rat aortic smooth muscle cell (RASMC) death including apoptosis, thus leading to the occurrence of aortic dissection.

Azelnidipine has been approved for the treatment of patients with hypertension and is extensively used in developed countries [9–11]. Many researchers considered that the effects of azelnidipine can be attributed primarily to its protection of cardio-renal functions by means of lowering blood pressure. Kondo et al. and Fujimoto et al. reported that azelnidipine had protective effects on renal injury induced by angiotensin II infusion through improvement in renal microcirculation [12,13]. In addition, it was reported that azelnidipine imparted antihypertensive effects and prevented cardiac hypertrophy in the Spontaneously Hypertensive Rat [14] and improved contractile dysfunction in stunned myocardium in dogs [15]. However, most of these studies have only emphasized the protective effects of azelnidipine on cardio-renal functions through lowering of blood pressure, and there have been almost no findings on the pathophysiological mechanism by which azelnidipine protects against progression of acute aortic dissection. Based on the findings mentioned above, we hypothesized that azelnidipine, in addition to its blood pressure lowering effect, may inhibit VSMC death (including apoptosis) and thereby reduce the occurrence of aortic dissection.

In the present study, we used an experimental apparatus of stretching loads in vitro that can simulate sudden increases of blood pressure and observed RASMC death induced by biomechanical stretch. Furthermore, we investigated whether azelnidipine inhibited stretch-induced VSMC death. The effect of azelnidipine on changes in intracellular signaling by biomechanical stretch was also examined to provide a possible mechanism by which azelnidipine may be used as a pharmacotherapeutic agent for the prevention of aortic dissection independent of its blood pressure lowering effect.

Materials and Methods

Cell culture and mechanical stretch

The study design was approved by an ethics review board of guidelines for the use of laboratory animals of Nara Medical University (No. 11011) and this study conducted in accordance with the guide for the Care and Use of Laboratory Animals as adopted and promulgated by the United States National Institutes of Health.

RASMCs were isolated from the thoracic aorta of 8-week-old male Sprague–Dawley rats by enzymatic digestion, as previously described [16]. Cells were grown in Dulbecco's modified Eagle's medium (DMEM, Sigma-Aldrich, St Louis, MO) supplemented with 10% fetal bovine serum (FBS, HyClone, Logan, UT), penicillin (100 U/mL, Invitrogen, Carlsbad, CA), and streptomy-

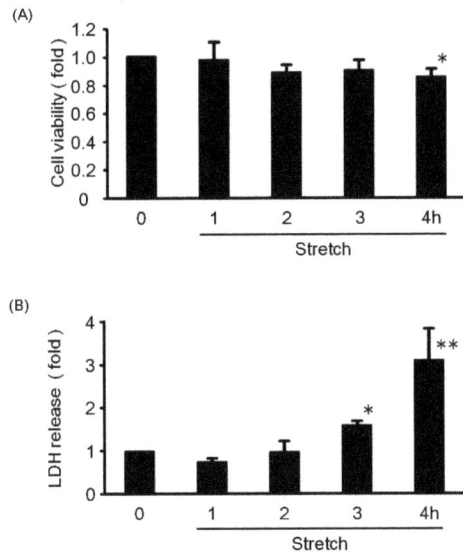

Figure 1. Time course for the effects of cyclic mechanical stretch (15% elongation) on cell viability (A) and cell death (B) in RASMCs up to 4 h. The cells cultured under standard conditions were exposed to cyclic mechanical stretch by 15% elongation for various time periods (from 1 to 4 h) and then incubated for 24 h. Cell viability and cell death were evaluated by MTT assay and the release of lactate dehydrogenase (LDH), respectively. Colorimetric analysis of each value was normalized by arbitrarily setting the absorbance value of the control cells (Ctrl.) to 1. Each value represents the mean ± standard deviatin (S.D.) (n = 4). The asterisks represent significant differences compared with the control value (*P<0.05).

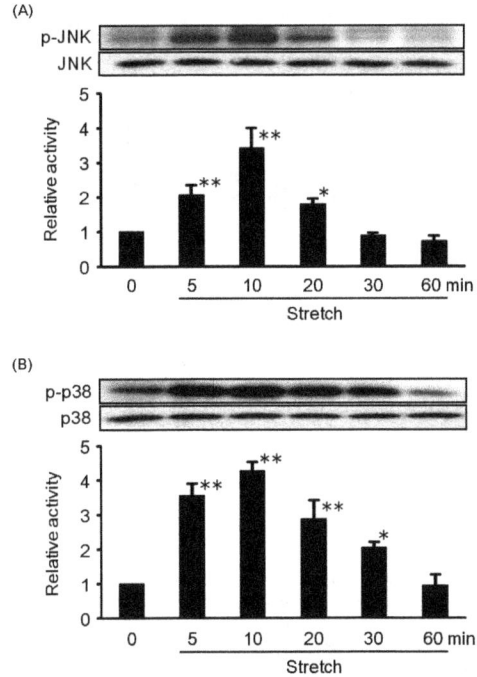

Figure 2. Time course for the effects of cyclic mechanical stretch (15% elongation) on the activation of JNK (A) and p38 (B) in RASMCs. The cells cultured under standard conditions were exposed to cyclic mechanical stretch by 15% elongation for various time periods (from 5 min to 60 min). The phosphorylation of JNK (A) and p38 (B) were measured as described under Materials and Methods. Densitometric analysis of each value was normalized by arbitrarily setting the densitometric value of the control cells (Ctrl.) to 1. Each value represents the mean ± S.D. (n = 3). The asterisks represent significant differences compared with the control value (*P<0.05, **P< 0.01).

cin (100 μg/mL, Invitrogen) at 37°C under 5% CO_2 in a humidified incubator. RASMCs were used for experiments between the third and sixth passages. The cells were cultured in collagen I-coated (70 μg/cm^2) silicon chambers (STREX Inc, Osaka, Japan). When the cell confluency in culture was estimated to be 70–80%, the medium was replaced with unsupplemented DMEM. The cells were further cultured for 24 h and then subjected to cyclic mechanical stretch (60 cycles/min, 15% elongation) for a given time period using the computer-controlled mechanical Strain Unit (STREX Inc, Osaka, Japan). After cyclic stretch, the medium was replaced with DMEM-containing 0.1% FBS. For western blot analysis, a portion of the RASMCs were lysed immediately after stretch stimulation and lysate proteins were collected in the manner described earlier [17]. In addition, a portion of the RASMCs were further incubated for 24 h to detect cell viability by MTT assay and cell death by the release of lactate dehydrogenase (LDH). In some experiments, RASMCs were pre-incubated with azelnidipine and mitogen-activated protein (MAP) kinase inhibitors (SP600125 or SB203580) 20 min prior to stimulation with cyclic mechanical stretch. Azelnidipine (CS905), SP600125, and SB203580 are abbreviated as CS, SP, and SB in figures. Band intensities were quantified by densitometry of the immunoblots using NIH Image J software. The values of phospho-MAP kinase have been normalized to total MAP kinase measurements and then expressed as the ratio of normalized values to protein in the control group as 1 (n = 3 per group).

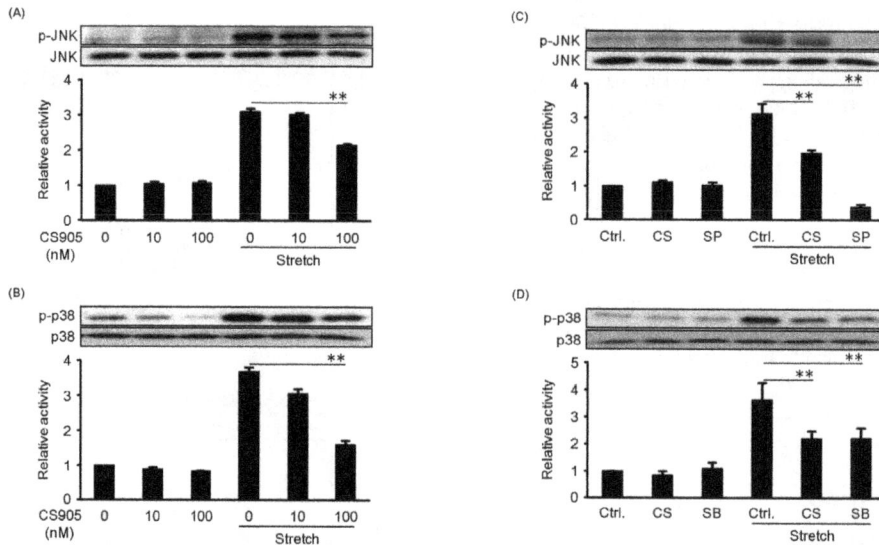

Figure 3. Effects of different concentrations of azelnidipine on the activation of JNK (A) and p38 (B) induced by cyclic mechanical stretch in RASMCs; and the comparison of the effects of azelnidipine and MAP kinase inhibitors on the activation of JNK (C) and p38 (D) induced by cyclic mechanical stretch in RASMCs. The cells were pre-incubated by CS905 (10 nM, 100 nM), SP600125 (20 μM), and SB203580 (20 μM) for 20 min prior to exposing to cyclic mechanical stretch by 15% elongation for 10 min. The phosphorylation of JNK and p38 were measured as described under *Materials and Methods*. Azelnidipine (CS905), SP600125, and SB203580 are abbreviated as CS, SP, and SB. Densitometric analysis of each value was normalized by arbitrarily setting the densitometric value of the control cells (Ctrl.) to 1. Each value represents the mean ± S.D. (n = 3). The asterisks represent significant differences compared with the stretched control value (*$P<0.05$, **$P<0.01$).

Materials

Materials were purchased from Wako (Kyoto) or Nacalai Tesque (Kyoto) unless stated otherwise. Azelnidipine (CS905) was from Daiichi Sankyo, Inc (Osaka). The antibodies used for western blot analyses were as follows: anti-phospho-SAPK/JNK (Thr183/Tyr185) antibody and anti-phospho-p38 MAP kinase (Thr180/Tyr182) antibody were purchased from Cell Signaling Technology, while ECL and ECL plus systems were purchased from GE Healthcare. Collagen I was purchased from Nippon Meat Packers, Inc. (Osaka). All chemical compounds were dissolved in dimethyl sulfoxide (DMSO) at final concentration less than 1% except for special notification.

Statistical analysis

All experimental values were expressed as mean ± standard deviation. Analysis of variance along with subsequent Student's *t*-test was used to determine significant differences in multiple comparisons. A *P* value<0.05 was considered to be significant.

Results

Effects of cyclic mechanical stretch on cell viability in RASMCs

The effect of cyclic mechanical stretch on the viability of RASMCs was firstly examined by measuring MTT reduction and LDH released. Figures 1A and 1B show the viability and death rate (reflected by LDH released to the medium) of RASMCs subjected to cyclic mechanical stretch by 15% elongation for various time periods, respectively. It was observed that viability was reduced with an increase in stretch time; the viability of RASMCs stimulated for 4 h decreased by 14% as compared with those of untreated cells. In the meantime, the death rate of RASMCs increased nearly three-fold with increase in stretch time from 1 h up to 4 h. These results suggest that cyclic mechanical stretch induced cell death in RASMCs.

Cyclic mechanical stretch induced the activation of MAP kinases in RASMCs

The effects of cyclic mechanical stretch on the activation of JNK and p38 (members of MAP kinases family proteins) were assessed by western blot analysis (Figure 2). RASMCs were exposed to cyclic mechanical stretch with a 15% elongation for different periods of time, and the phosphorylation of JNK (A) and p38 (B) was measured. As shown in Figures 2A and 2B, both JNK and p38 in RASMCs were activated by cyclic mechanical stretch. For both JNK and p38, the extent of activation increased with increase in stretch time, reaching a peak at 10 min and then gradually decreasing to basal level with further increasing stretch time up to 60 min. These findings imply that the activation of JNK and p38 seemed to be involved in was well as influence RASMCs death. The results obtained here are in agreement with those reported earlier in the literature [18,19].

In order to clarify the possible mechanisms of how cyclic mechanical stretch influences cell death, the following two experiments were undertaken.

Azelnidipine inhibited cyclic mechanical stretch-induced JNK and p38 MAP kinase activation in RASMCs

The effects of azelnidipine on cyclic mechanical stretch-induced activation of JNK and p38 in RASMCs were firstly examined and the results are shown in Figures 3A and 3B, respectively. In Figures 3C and 3D, we compared the effects of azelnidipine and MAP kinase inhibitors on cyclic mechanical stretch-induced activation of JNK and p38 in RASMCs, respectively. It was obvious that JNK and p38 MAP kinase activation were significantly attenuated by azelnidipine in a dose-dependent manner. Both JNK and p38 activation induced by cyclic mechanical stretch were inhibited by their respective inhibitors (SP600125 and SB203580), implying that the inhibition of JNK and p38 activation could be beneficial to suppressing mechanical stretch-induced RASMC death.

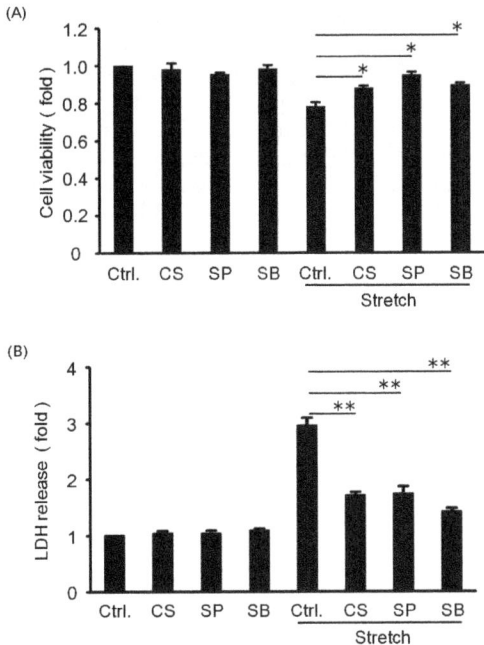

(A)

(B)

Figure 4. Comparison of the cell viability (A) and LDH release (B) induced by cyclic mechanical stretch in RASMCs with or without azelnidipine or MAP kinase inhibitors. The cells were pre-incubated by CS905 (100 nM), SP600125 (20 μM), and SB203580 (20 μM) for 20 min prior to exposing to cyclic mechanical stretch by 15% elongation for 4 h and then incubated for 24 h. Cell viability and cell death were evaluated by MTT assay and the release of lactate dehydrogenase (LDH), respectively. Azelnidipine (CS905), SP600125, and SB203580 are abbreviated as CS, SP, and SB. Colorimetric analysis of each value was normalized by arbitrarily setting the absorbance value of the control cells (Ctrl.) to 1. Each value represents the mean ± S.D. (n = 4). The asterisks represent significant differences compared with the stretched control value (*$P < 0.05$, **$P < 0.01$).

Cyclic mechanical stretch-induced cell death was inhibited by azelnidipine and MAP kinase inhibitors in RASMCs

Figure 4A compares the relative cell viability for RASMCs in culture media with or without azelnidipine or MAP kinase inhibitors. It was found that azelnidipine, SP600125, and SB203580 all significantly increased the viability of RASMCs. Figure 4B compares the LDH released from the RASMCs into the culture media with or without azelnidipine or MAP kinase inhibitors. Compared with the positive control, azelnidipine, SP600125, and SB203580 significantly reduced the death rate of RASMCs. These results indicate that azelnidipine and MAP kinase inhibitors potentially inhibit RASMC death induced by cyclic mechanical stretch.

Effects of antioxidants, diphenylene iodonium (DPI) and tempol on cyclic mechanical stretch-induced cell death

It has been reported that azelnidipine has the effects of anti-inflammation and antioxidant in mouse aneurysmal models [20,21]. Therefore, we next examined the effects of antioxidants, DPI and tempol on cyclic mechanical stretch-induced RASMC death. As shown in Figure 5, pretreatment with both DPI and tempol failed to inhibit mechanical stretch-induced RASMCs death, suggesting that oxidative stress may not be involved in RASMC death induced by cyclic mechanical stretch.

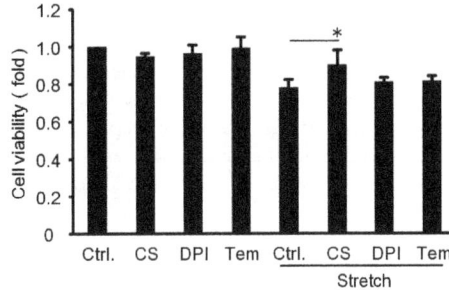

Figure 5. Effects of antioxidants on cyclic mechanical stretch-induced RASMC death. The cells were pre-incubated by CS905 (100 nM), diphenylene iodonium (5 μM), and tempol (1 μM) for 20 min prior to exposing to cyclic mechanical stretch by 15% elongation for 4 h and then incubated for 24 h. Cell viability was evaluated by MTT assay. Azelnidipine (CS905), diphenylene iodonium, and tempol are abbreviated as CS, DPI, and Tem. Colorimetric analysis of each value was normalized by arbitrarily setting the absorbance value of the control cells (Ctrl.) to 1. Each value represents the mean ± S.D. (n = 4). The asterisks represent significant differences compared with the stretched control value (*$P < 0.05$, **$P < 0.01$).

Discussion

The major findings of the present study are as follows: (1) cyclic mechanical stretch of RASMC caused cell death in a time-dependent manner up to 4 h; (2) cyclic mechanical stretch of RASMCs induced JNK and p38 activation with peaks at 10 min; (3) azelnidipine, a calcium channel blocker, inhibited the activation of JNK and p38 by cyclic mechanical stretch in a concentration-dependent manner; and (4) azelnidipine and JNK or p38 inhibitors protected against stretch-induced RASMC death; (5) Antioxidants, DPI and tempol failed to inhibit stretch-induced RASMC death.

In this work, we recall the assumption that acute biomechanical stretch applied to cultured VSMCs in vitro simulating a sudden increase in blood pressure resulted in VSMC death that led to aortic dissection. As shown in Figure 1A, we found that cyclic mechanical stretch caused cell death of RASMCs in a time-dependent manner. The cell fate also can be supported by the fact that LDH release from the cells was increased (Fig. 1B). This implies that RASMC death induced by rapidly developed biomechanical stretch is one of the likely reasons for aortic dissection. Some other researchers have also reported that stretching loads induce smooth muscle cell death, which is consistent with the present study [6,7,22,23]. On the other hand, it has been reported that cyclic mechanical stretch of cells results in cell proliferation [23,24]. Such a phenomenon was also observed as we applied mechanical stretch to RASMCs in vitro for 24 h using a stretching apparatus (data not shown here). In our experimental conditions, cell death occurred after stretch stimulation for 4 h and subsequently surviving cells entered into a proliferation cycle, showing a gradual increase in cell numbers that might be higher than that of the control at the end of 24 h as a result of growth and division. From the above findings, we concluded that mechanical stretch led to both cell death and cell proliferation. It appeared that the extent and duration of mechanical stretch decided what would happen to those SMCs in vitro. Our experimental results indicated that acute mechanical stretch primarily contributed to SMC death.

Azelnidipine is a calcium channel antagonist (blocker) that has been applied extensively to the treatment of patients with hypertension all over the world. In the present study, we found that azelnidipine inhibited RASMC death induced by cyclic mechanical stretch (Fig. 4A). Under the present conditions, the protective effects of azelnidipine on RASMCs seemed to be different from its antihypertensive effects, because the cyclic mechanical stretch was applied. It has been reported that azelnidipine exhibited a suppressing effect on aneurysm development in mouse models of aortic aneurysms, which was thought to be independent of its antihypertensive action [20,21]. Those researchers considered that azelnidipine suppressed the progression of aortic aneurysm through both anti-inflammatory [20] and antioxidant mechanisms [21]. Although the exact mechanisms are unresolved, our findings suggest that the preventive effects of azelnidipine against aortic aneurysm should be associated with its inhibitory effect of RASMCs death induced by cyclic mechanical stretch, apart from its antihypertensive effect. Such an assumption needs to be further confirmed by examining the fate of SMCs using an in vivo model of acute aortic dissection and may be a topic for future research. In addition, attention should also be paid to other calcium channel blockers in future with the aim of comparing their effects on stretch-induced RASMC death.

Among MAP kinases, JNK and p38 were recognized to be related to cell death or apoptosis [25–27]. Our experimental data demonstrated that JNK and p38 in RASMCs were activated by cyclic mechanical stretch (Fig. 2). Cheng et al. also reported that JNK activation was involved in mechanical stretch-induced VSMC death [7]. Yoshimura et al. found that JNK played a significant role in the formation and development of aortic aneurysm [28]. Similarly, some researchers reported that mechanical stretch led to p38 activation [18], which is in agreement with our results. Actually, we found that cyclic mechanical stretch-induced RASMC death was suppressed when the activity of JNK and p38 was inhibited by their inhibitors (Fig. 4). These findings indicated that JNK and p38 activation is likely to be associated with cyclic mechanical stretch-induced RASMC death. Since azelnidipine inhibited both JNK and p38 activation by cyclic mechanical stretch, it can be assumed that azelnidipine prevented cyclic mechanical stretch-induced RASMC death through inhibition of JNK and p38 activation in RASMCs.

We have reported in the previous study that p38 and JNK are oxidative stress sensitive [29]. Ohyama et al. also reported that azelnidipine has an effect of antioxidant in mouse aneurysmal models [21]. Therefore, it is conceivable that azelnidipine inhibited cyclic mechanical stretch-induced cell death through inhibiting JNK and p38 activation via its anti-oxidative mechanisms. In order to clarify this point, we performed additional experiments of cyclic mechanical stretch-induced RASMC death using antioxidants, diphenylene iodonium and tempol. As shown in Fig. 5, pretreatment with these anti-oxidants did not affected the relative cell viability of RASMCs, suggesting that the inhibiting effects of azelnidipine on stretch-induced cell death could not be attributed to its anti-oxidative effect.

In conclusion, azelnidipine inhibited RASMC death induced by acute cyclic mechanical stretch (originating from a simulated increase in blood pressure in vitro). JNK and p38 in RASMCs were activated by cyclic mechanical stretch; however, the activation was inhibited by azelnidipine. Similar to azelnidipine, pharmacological inhibition of JNK and p38 activation by mechanical stretch suppressed cyclic mechanical stretch-induced RASMC death. It is expected that the mechanism of acute aortic dissection will be clarified from further study of the fate of VSMCs by acute cyclic mechanical stretch. Azelnidipine may be an alternative candidate for prevention of acute aortic dissection independent of its blood pressure lowering effect.

Acknowledgments

We are grateful to Sankyo, Co., Ltd. (Tokyo, Japan) for supplying azelnidipine. We would also like to thank Professor Eiichi Taira in the Department of Pharmacology, Iwate Medical University School of Medicine for the help on the silicon chamber coating in this research.

Author Contributions

Conceived and designed the experiments: MY. Performed the experiments: JZ YK KN SI. Analyzed the data: JZ MY. Contributed reagents/materials/analysis tools: KO MY. Contributed to the writing of the manuscript: JZ MY. Interpreted results of experiments: JZ KO YK KN SI ATK YT MY.

References

1. Wang JC, Bennett M (2012) Aging and atherosclerosis: mechanisms, functional consequences, and potential therapeutics for cellular senescence. Circ Res 111: 245–259.
2. Costopoulos C, Liew TV (2008) Bennett M. Ageing and atherosclerosis: Mechanisms and therapeutic options. Biochem Pharmacol 75: 1251–1261.
3. Guilmet D, Bachet J, Goudot B, Dreyfus G, Martinelli GL (1993) Aortic dissection: anatomic types and surgical approaches. J. Cardiovasc Surg 34: 23–32.
4. Fares A (2013) Winter cardiovascular diseases phenomenon N Am J Med Sci 5: 266–279.
5. Collins MJ, Dev V, Strauss BH, Fedak PW, Butany J (2007) Variation in the histopathological features of patients with ascending aortic aneurysms: a study of 111 surgically excised cases. Clin Pathol. 61: 519–523.
6. Wernig F, Mayr M, Xu Q (2003) Mechanical stretch-induced apoptosis in smooth muscle cells is mediated by beta1-integrin signaling pathways. Hypertension 41: 903–911.
7. Cheng WP, Wang BW, Chen SC, Chang H, Shyu KG (2012) Mechanical stretch induces the apoptosis regulator PUMA in vascular smooth muscle cells. Cardiovasc Res 93: 181–189.
8. Hipper A, Isenberg G (2000) Cyclic mechanical strain decreases the DNA synthesis of vascular smooth muscle cells. Pflugers Arch 440: 19–27.
9. Eguchi K, Tomizawa H, Ishikawa J, Hoshide S, Fukuda T, et al. (2007) Effects of new calcium channel blocker, azelnidipine, and amlodipine on baroreflex sensitivity and ambulatory blood pressure. J Cardiovasc Pharmacol 49: 394–400.
10. Oizumi K, Nishino H, Koike H, Sada T, Miyamoto M, et al. (1989) Antihypertensive effects of CS-905, a novel dihydropyridine Ca++ channel blocker. Jpn J Pharmacol 51: 57–64.
11. Zhao X, Wu F, Jia S, Qu P, Li H, et al. (2010) Azelnidipine and amlodipine: a comparison of their effects and safety in a randomized double-blinded clinical trial in Chinese essential hypertensive patients. Clin Exp Hypertens 32: 372–376.
12. Kondo N, Kiyomoto H, Yamamoto T, Miyatake A, Sun GP, et al. (2006) Effects of calcium channel blockade on angiotensin II-induced peritubular ischemia in rats. J Pharmacol Exp Ther 316: 1047–1052.
13. Fujimoto S, Satoh M, Nagasu H, Horike H, Sasaki T, et al. (2009) Azelnidipine exerts renoprotective effects by improvement of renal microcirculation in angiotensin II infusion rats. Nephrol Dial Transplant 24: 3651–3658.
14. Oizumi K, Nishino H, Miyake S, Shiga H, Sada T, et al. (1990) Hemodynamic changes following long-term administration of CS-905, a novel dihydropyridine calcium blocker, in conscious SHR. Jpn J Pharmacol 54: 1–6.
15. Satoh K, Yamamoto A, Hoshi K, Ichihara K (1998) Effects of azelnidipine, a dihydropyridine calcium antagonist, on myocardial stunning in dogs. Jpn J Pharmacol 76: 369–376.
16. Yoshizumi M, Abe J, Haendeler J, Huang Q, Berk BC (2000) Src and Cas mediate JNK activation but not ERK1/2 and p38 kinases by reactive oxygen species. J Biol Chem 275: 11706–11712.
17. Nakayama H, Zhao J, Ei-Fakhrany A, Isosaki M, Satoh H, et al. (2009) Neuroprotective effects of pramipexole against tunicamycin-induced cell death in PC12 cells. Clin Exp Pharmacol Physiol 36: 1183–1185.
18. Cornelissen J, Armstrong J, Holt CM (2004) Mechanical stretch induces phosphorylation of p38-MAPK and apoptosis in human saphenous vein. Arterioscler Thromb Vasc Biol 24: 451–456.
19. Hamada K, Takuwa N, Yokoyama K, Takuwa Y (1998) Stretch activates Jun N-terminal kinase/stress-activated protein kinase in vascular smooth muscle cells through mechanisms involving autocrine ATP stimulation of purinoceptors. J Biol Chem 273: 6334–6340.
20. Kurobe H, Matsuoka Y, Hirata Y, Sugasawa N, Maxfield MW, et al. (2013) Azelnidipine suppresses the progression of aortic aneurysm in wild mice model through anti-inflammatory effects. J Thorac Cardiovasc Surg 146: 1501–1508.

21. Ohyama T, Sato K, Kishimoto K, Yamazaki Y, Horiguchi N, et al. (2012) Azelnidipine is a calcium blocker that attenuates liver fibrosis and may increase antioxidant defence. Br J Pharmacol 165: 1173–1187.

22. Su BY, Shontz KM, Flavahan NA, Nowicki PT (2006) The effect of phenotype on mechanical stretch-induced vascular smooth muscle cell apoptosis. J Vasc Res 43: 229–237.

23. Song Jt, Hu B, Qu Hy, Bi Cl, Huang Xz, et al. (2012) Mechanical stretch modulates microRNA 21 expression, participating in proliferation and apoptosis in cultured human aortic smooth muscle cells. PLoS One 7: e47657.

24. Chahine MN, Dibrov E, Blackwood DP, Pierce GN (2012) Oxidized LDL enhances stretch-induced smooth muscle cell proliferation through alterations in nuclear protein import. Can J Physiol Pharmacol 90: 1559–1568.

25. Iryo Y, Matsuoka M, Wispriyono B, Sugiura T, Igisu H (2000) Involvement of the extracellular signal-regulated protein kinase (ERK) pathway in the induction of apoptosis by cadmium chloride in CCRF-CEM cells. Biochem Pharmacol 60: 1875–1882.

26. Huh JE, Kang KS, Chae C, Kim HM, Ahn KS, et al. (2004) Roles of p38 and JNK mitogen-activated protein kinase pathways during cantharidin-induced apoptosis in U937 cells. Biochem Pharmacol 67: 1811–1818.

27. Kim BC, Kim HG, Lee SA, Lim S, Park EH, et al. (2005) Genipin-induced apoptosis in hepatoma cells is mediated by reactive oxygen species/c-Jun NH2-terminal kinase-dependent activation of mitochondrial pathway. Biochem Pharmacol 70: 1398–1407.

28. Yoshimura K, Aoki H, Ikeda Y, Furutani A, Hamano K, et al. (2006) Regression of abdominal aortic aneurysm by inhibition of c-Jun N-terminal kinase in mice. Ann N Y Acad Sci 1085: 74–81.

29. Kyaw M, Yoshizumi M, Tsuchiya K, Kirima K, Tamaki T. (2001) Antioxidants inhibit JNK and p38 MAPK activation but not ERK 1/2 activation by angiotensin II in rat aortic smooth muscle cells. Hypertens Res. 24: 251–261.

15

Arsenic Trioxide and Resveratrol Show Synergistic Anti-Leukemia Activity and Neutralized Cardiotoxicity

Yuhua Fan[1]◐, Meng Chen[2]◐, Jia Meng[3], Lei Yu[1], Yingfeng Tu[4], Lin Wan[5], Kun Fang[1], Wenliang Zhu[6]*

1 College of Pharmacy, Harbin Medical University-Daqing, Daqing, China, 2 Department of Respiratory Medicine, the Fourth Hospital of Harbin Medical University, Harbin, China, 3 Department of Geriatrics, the Second Affiliated Hospital of Harbin Medical University, Harbin, China, 4 Department of Cardiology, the Fourth Hospital of Harbin Medical University, Harbin, China, 5 Radiology Department and Key Laboratory of Molecular Imaging, the Fourth Hospital of Harbin Medical University, Harbin, China, 6 Institute of Clinical Pharmacology, the Second Affiliated Hospital of Harbin Medical University, Harbin, China

Abstract

Cardiotoxicity is an aggravating side effect of many clinical antineoplastic agents such as arsenic trioxide (As_2O_3), which is the first-line treatment for acute promyelocytic leukemia (APL). Clinically, drug combination strategies are widely applied for complex disease management. Here, an optimized, cardiac-friendly therapeutic strategy for APL was investigated using a combination of As_2O_3 and genistein or resveratrol. Potential combinations were explored with respect to their effects on mitochondrial membrane potential, reactive oxygen species, superoxide dismutase activity, autophagy, and apoptosis in both NB4 cells and neonatal rat left ventricular myocytes. All experiments consistently suggested that 5 µM resveratrol remarkably alleviates As_2O_3-induced cardiotoxicity. To achieve an equivalent effect, a 10-fold dosage of genistein was required, thus highlighting the dose advantage of resveratrol, as poor bioavailability is a common concern for its clinical application. Co-administration of resveratrol substantially amplified the anticancer effect of As_2O_3 in NB4 cells. Furthermore, resveratrol exacerbated oxidative stress, mitochondrial damage, and apoptosis, thereby reflecting its full range of synergism with As_2O_3. Addition of 5 µM resveratrol to the single drug formula of As_2O_3 also further increased the expression of LC3, a marker of cellular autophagy activity, indicating an involvement of autophagy-mediated tumor cell death in the synergistic action. Our results suggest a possible application of an As_2O_3 and resveratrol combination to treat APL in order to achieve superior therapeutics effects and prevent cardiotoxicity.

Editor: Pierre Bobé, INSERM-Université Paris-Sud, France

Funding: This work was supported by National Natural Science Foundation of China (No. 31301136) and Foundation of Health Department of Heilongjiang Province of China (No. 2011-233). The funders had no role in study design, data collection and analysis, decision to publish, or preparation of the manuscript.

Competing Interests: The authors have declared that no competing interests exist.

* Email: wenzwl@yeah.net

◐ These authors contributed equally to this work.

Introduction

Due to its substantial anticancer effect, arsenic trioxide (As_2O_3) has been recommended as the front-line agent for treatment of acute promyelocytic leukemia (APL), particularly for cases of relapsed or refractory APL [1–3]. Although generally considered a relatively safe therapeutic strategy [4], numerous clinical reports have indicated that chronic exposure to a therapeutic dose of As_2O_3 could damage cardiac structure and functions and evoke severe cardiac side effects such as ventricular arrhythmia, even resulting in sudden cardiac death in certain cases [5–8]. This issue may become increasingly relevant due to the significantly extended survival time of APL patients, and therefore increased likelihood of long-term exposure to As_2O_3 resulting in cardiovascular disease. Thus, prophylactic treatment is urgently required for managing the consequent cardiotoxicity in clinical applications of As_2O_3.

A better understanding of the potential mechanism by which As_2O_3 induces its cardiotoxicity will undoubtedly be of value for developing specific and effective preventive measures. Recently, many experimental observations have revealed that mitochondrial microstructural changes and dysfunctions might play crucial roles in As_2O_3-mediated cardiotoxicity via inducing excessive production of reactive oxygen species (ROS), and the subsequent increase

in cell apoptosis [9–12]. Indeed, enrichment of mitochondriain cardiomyocytes enhanced their susceptibility to oxidative damage compared to other cells [13]. Accordingly, a prophylactic strategy was proposed that is based on maintaining mitochondrial function to guard against As_2O_3-induced oxidative stress [14]. This suggests that natural, strong antioxidants might be ideal drug candidates. Recently, such antioxidants have been investigated as rational cardioprotectants against the cardiotoxicity induced by As_2O_3, including the flavonoid genistein (Gen) as well resveratrol (Rev), a stilbene that is enriched in red wine [15,16]. These investigations have pointed to the use of a combination treatment of Gen or Rev (Gen/Rev) and As_2O_3 as a novel therapeutic strategy for APL to prevent cardiotoxicity. Nonetheless, many important issues have yet to be considered. First, the exact mechanism regarding the cardioprotective effect of Gen/Rev against As_2O_3 remains elusive. Second, due to poor bioavailability of polyphenolic compounds, a reasonable and feasible choice of drugs is necessary [17]. Third, the potential antitumor effects of the use of Gen/Rev and As_2O_3 in combination in APL are unknown. Finally, although previous studies have validated the anticancer effect of Gen and Rev independently [18,19], it is still unknown whether they can be effective at suppressing the proliferation of APL cancer cells and assist As_2O_3. This is a particularly important line of evidence that is required to determine whether the proposed new method is superior to the currently widely applied As_2O_3 monotherapy strategy.

Therefore, in this study, the ability of these two natural antioxidants, Gen and Rev, to reverse As_2O_3-induced oxidative stress injuries and simultaneously enhance the anticancer effect of As_2O_3 was investigated *in vitro* in neonatal rat left ventricular myocytes (NRLVMs) and NB4 cells, respectively. Our experiments focused on drug-induced alterations of mitochondria-derived ROS generation and the secondarily triggered cell apoptosis. Due to an intrinsic functional relationship between the mediators implicated in regulating oxidative stress and autophagy [20], we also measured the protein expression of LC3, a marker of cellular autophagy activity. We designed these experiments with the aim of providing mechanism-based answers to the open questions related to the potential of Gen/Rev plus As_2O_3 combinatorial therapy for APL.

Materials and Methods

Reagents and drugs

Gen and Rev were provided by Xi'an QingYue Biotechnology Co. Ltd. (China) and Sigma Chemical Co. (St. Louis, MO, USA), respectively. As_2O_3 was acquired from Harbin YI-DA Pharmaceutical Limited Company. The 3-(4,5-dimethylthiazol-2-yl)-2,5-diphenyl-tetrazolium bromide (MTT), cell-penetrating lipophilic cationic fluorochrome JC-1 (5,5′,6,6′-tetrachloro-1,1′,3,3′-tetraethylbenzimidazole-carbocyanine iodine), the Total Superoxide Dismutase Assay Kit with 2-(4-iodophenyl)- 3-(4-nitrophenyl)-5-(2,4-disulfophenyl)-2H-tetrazolium, monosodium salt (WST-1), and Annexin V-FITC Apoptosis Detection Kit were bought from Beyotime Institute of Biotechnology (China) and stored at $-20°C$ in the dark. The 2′,7′-dichlorofluorescein diacetate (DCFH-DA) was provided by Molecular Probes (Eugene, OR, USA). The TUNEL detection kit was purchased from Roche (Cell Death Detection Kit; Roche Biochemicals; Mannheim, Germany). LC3A/B monoclonal antibody was purchased from Cell Signaling Technology, Inc. (Danvers, MA, USA).

Culture of NB4 cells and NRLVMs

Human promyelocytic leukemia NB4 cell line, established in 1991 from a patient suffering from APL having the t(15;17) translocation, was a kind gift from Dr. M. Lanotte (INSERM Unit301, St Louis Hospital, Paris, France) [21]. NB4 cells were collected, washed two times in RPMI1640, counted and resuspended at 500,000 cells/ml in RPMI1640 with 10% fetal bovine serum (FBS). After 24 h cultivation, the cells were sedimented by centrifugation ($1500 \times g$ for 5 min). NRLVMs were isolated from neonatal rat hearts of 1- to 2-day-old Sprague-Dawley rats. Briefly, the rats were immersed in 75% alcohol and decapitated, and the hearts were then quickly removed and seeded in cold Dulbecco's modified Eagle medium (DMEM). These hearts were cut into small pieces with scissors and digested with 0.25% trypsin solution. The isolated cardiomyocytes were placed in DMEM with 10% FBS and centrifuged, and pellets were resuspended and cultured for 90 min at 37°C. Cardiomyocyte-enriched suspensions were removed from the culture flask and placed in fresh medium. The use of animals complied with the Guide for the Care and Use of Laboratory Animals published by the US National Institutes of Health (NIH Publication, No. 85–23, revised 1996) and the study protocol was pre-approved by the Experimental Animal Ethics Committee of the Harbin Medical University, China (Animal Experimental Ethical Inspection

Protocol, No. 2009104). NRLVMs were pretreated with Rev (5 µM) or Gen (50 µM) for 1 h and then co-incubated with As_2O_3 (5 µM) [22] for another 24 h. The procedure was the same for NB4 cells, except that a concentration of 2 µM As_2O_3 was used [23].

Measurement of ROS production

Measurement of intracellular ROS production was based on the oxidation of DCFH-DA to fluorescent 2′,7′-dichlorofluorescin (DCF). Cells were cultured for 12 h followed by incubation with Rev (5 µM) or Gen (50 µM) for 1 h, and then co-incubation with As_2O_3, or were incubated with As_2O_3 alone for 12 h. A concentration of 5 µM and 2 µM of As_2O_3 was used for NRLVMs and NB4 cells, respectively. The cells were then further incubated with 10 µM DCFH-DA at 37°C for 30 min, and then washed twice with serum-free medium and stored in FBS-free medium. Cellular DCF fluorescence intensities were detected by confocal microscopy with excitation and emission spectra of 488 nm and 525 nm, respectively.

Measurement of intracellular GSH

NB4 cells or NRLVMs were seeded in 6-well plate. After the cells grew into 90% confluence, they were treated with Rev+As_2O_3 or Rev at the indicated concentration. After 24 hours of Rev+As_2O_3 or Rev exposure, the cells were trypsinized, harvested and centrifuged at $1000 \times g$, for 3 min. Cell pellets were removed to 1.5 mL eppendorf tubes, cleaned twice with cold PBS and resuspended in ice-cold metaphosphoric acid (MPA). After homogenization, the solution was centrifuged at $10,000 \times g$ at 4°C for 10 min and then the supernatant was applied to measure levels of GSH according to the manufacturer's instructions (Bioxytech-GSH 400, OxisResearch, Portland, OR, USA). The assay was carried out in eppendorf tubes and transferred to flat-bottom 96-well plates for absorbance measurement at 400 nm. The pellet from the centrifugation was dissolved in 100 µL of 0.1 M NaOH and the protein concentration was determined by the Bio-Rad microprotein assay in 96-well plate using bovine serum albumin as the standard. The GSH level was expressed as nmol GSH/mg cellular protein.

Measurement of mitochondrial membrane potential (MMP)

JC-1 was applied to explore the effects of Gen and Rev on mitochondrial function by measuring MMP in As_2O_3-treated cardiomyocytes and NB4 cells. Cells were placed in a 6-well plate and cultured for 12 h at 37°C and then incubated with Rev (5 µM) or Gen (50 µM) for 1 h prior to co-treatment with As_2O_3, or were incubated with As_2O_3 alone for another 12 h. A concentration of 5 µM and 2 µM of As_2O_3 was used for NRLVMs and NB4 cells, respectively. Red emission of the dye represents normal MMP and green fluorescence indicates mitochondria with depolarized MMP. MMP was measured using a confocal laser-scanning microscope (Fluoview-FV300; Olympus, Tokyo, Japan).

Determination of superoxide dismutase (SOD) activity

The activity of the anti-oxidant enzyme SOD in NRLVMs and NB4 cells was detected by using a Total Superoxide Dismutase Assay Kit with WST-1 according to the manufacturer's protocol. Briefly, cells were exposed to Rev (5 µM) or Gen (50 µM) for 1 h following treatment with As_2O_3 for another 24 h. A concentration of 5 µM and 2 µM of As_2O_3 was used for NRLVMs and NB4 cells, respectively. Then, the cell suspension was centrifuged ($800 \times g$, 10 min, 4°C), and the cell pellets were ultrasonicated for

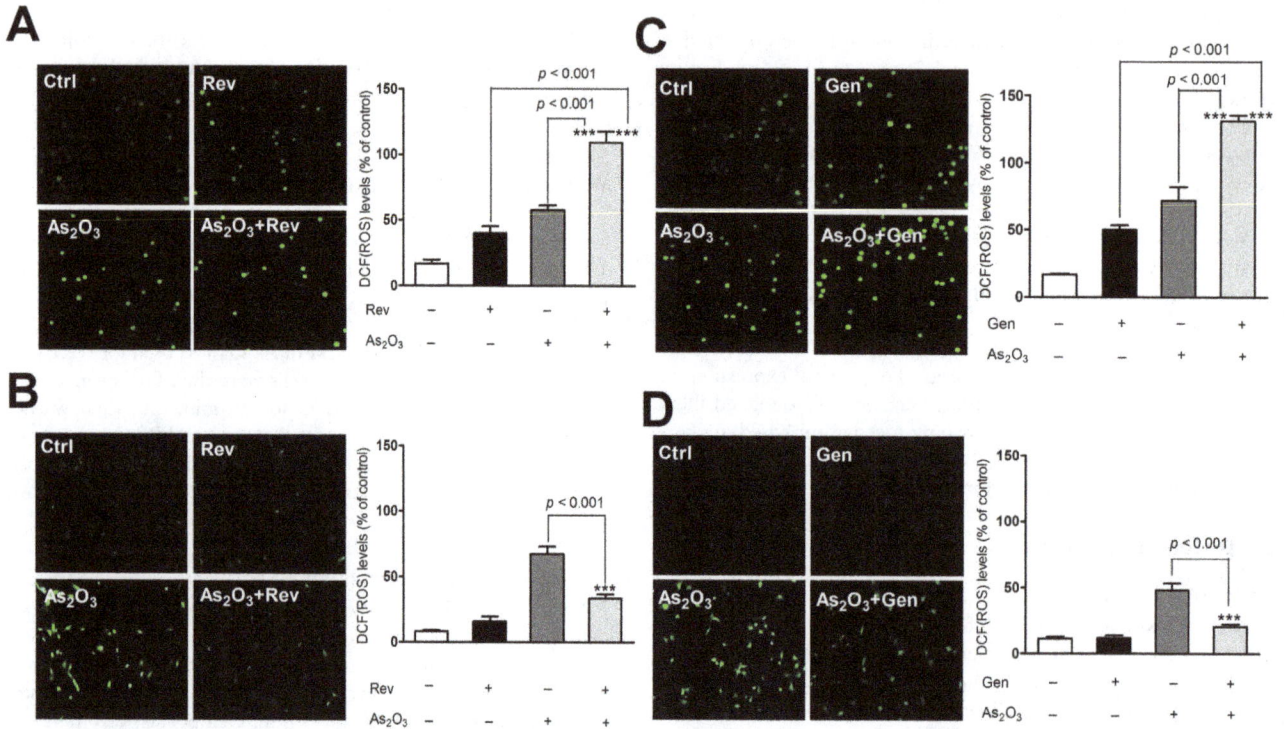

Figure 1. Effect of Gen/Rev on As$_2$O$_3$-induced oxidative stress in NB4 cells and NRLVMs (n = 6). Co-treatment of 5 µM Rev or 50 µM Gen further increased ROS production in NB4 cells compared to As$_2$O$_3$ alone (A, C) but reduced the ROS level in NRLVMs (B, D). ***$p < 0.001$, As$_2$O$_3$+Rev versus As$_2$O$_3$ or Rev; ***$p < 0.001$, As$_2$O$_3$+Gen versus As$_2$O$_3$ or Gen.

15 min (every 15 s with 5-min intervals) at 4°C in cell lysate buffer [RIPA buffer, 50 mM Tris, pH 7.4, 150 mM NaCl, 1% Triton X-100, 1% sodium deoxycholate, 0.1% sodium dodecyl sulfate (SDS), sodium orthovanadate, sodium fluoride, ethylenediamine tetraacetic acid, and leupeptin]. After the cell-lysed buffer was centrifuged at 2000×g for 15 min, the supernatant was removed. Supernatants, enzyme-working solutions, and WST-1 were

prepared and added to a 96-well plate. The mixtures were incubated at 37°C for 20 min, and the absorbance was finally determined at 450 nm using a microplate reader.

Protein extraction and immunoblotting analysis

Protein samples were isolated from NRLVMs and NB4 cells. NRLVMs and NB4 cells were seeded in 6-well plate at 37°C in

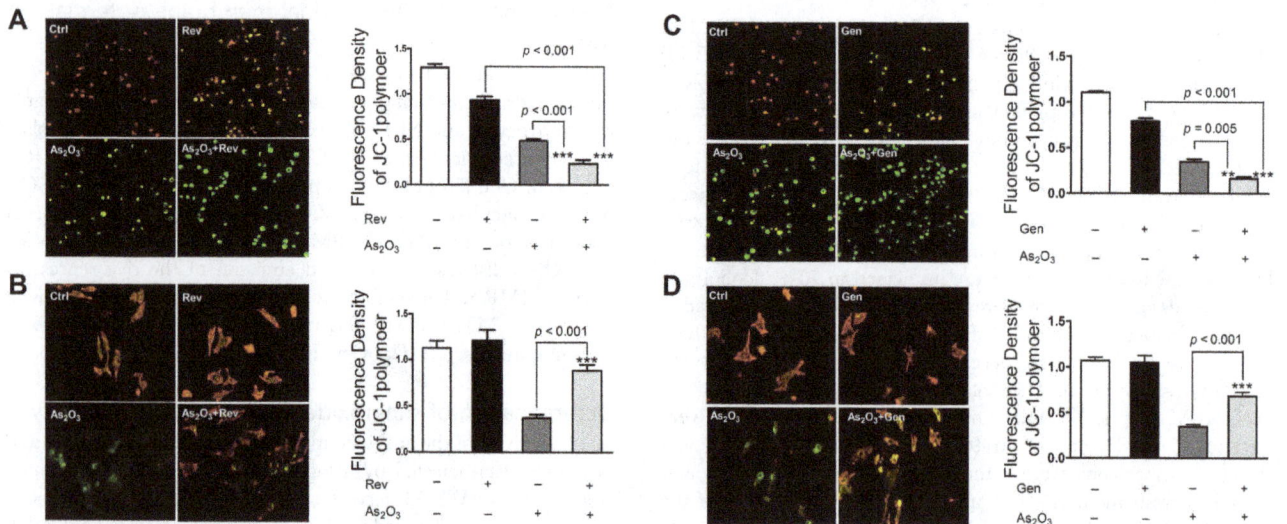

Figure 2. Effect of co-treatment of As$_2$O$_3$ and Rev/Gen on MMP of NB4 cells and NRLVMs (n = 6). Co-treatment of 5 µM Rev or 50 µM Gen further decreased the MMP in NB4 cells compared to As$_2$O$_3$ alone (A, C) but restored MMP in NRLVMs (B, D). ***$p < 0.001$, As$_2$O$_3$+Rev versus As$_2$O$_3$ or Rev; ***$p < 0.001$, As$_2$O$_3$+Gen versus Gen; **$p = 0.005$, ***$p < 0.001$, As$_2$O$_3$+Gen versus As$_2$O$_3$.

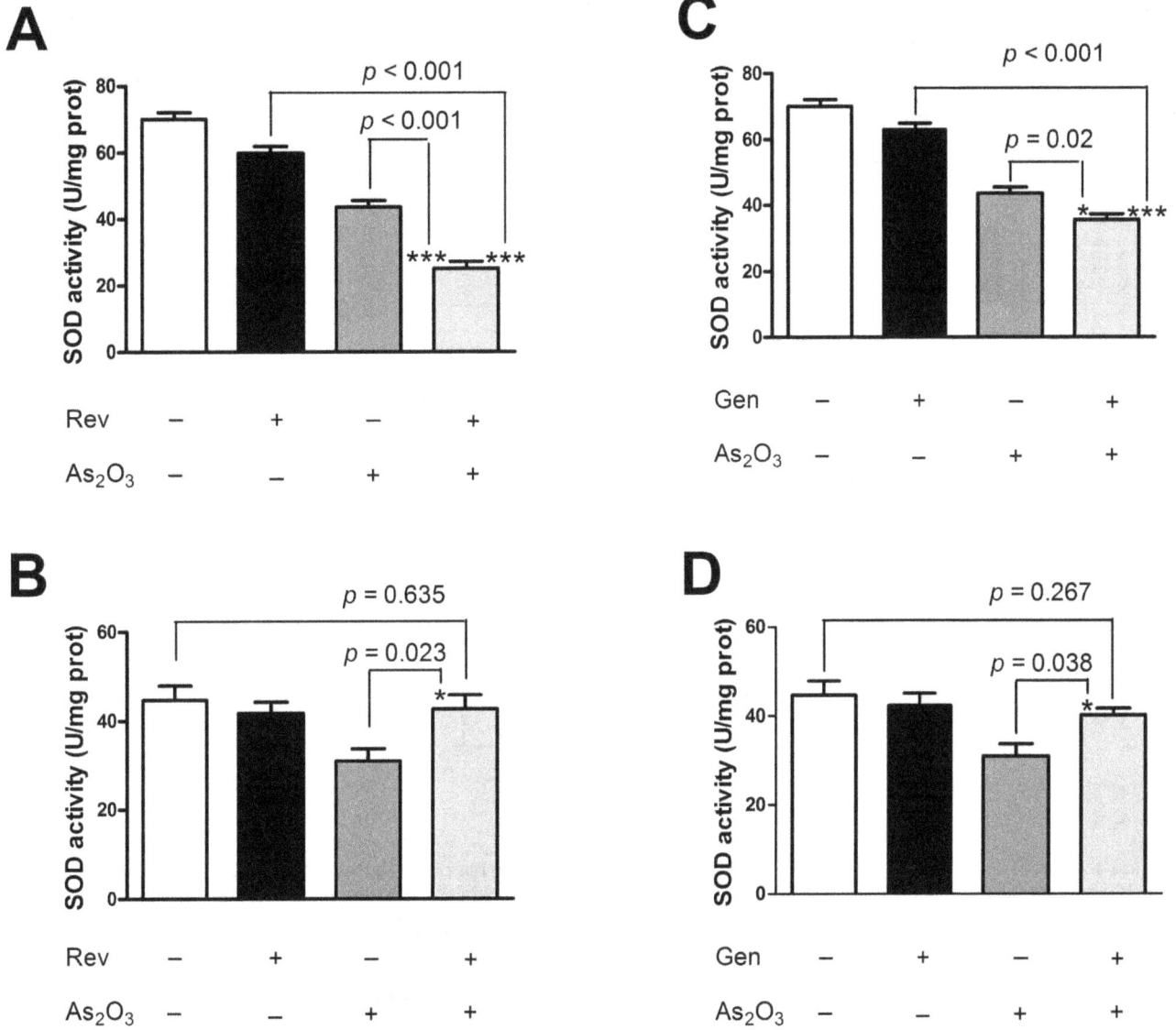

Figure 3. Effect of Gen/Rev on As_2O_3-induced SOD activity in NB4 cells and NRLVMs (n = 6). Co-treatment of 5 µM Rev or 50 µM Gen further decreased the SOD activity in NB4 cells compared to As_2O_3 alone (A, C) but restored it in NRLVMs (B, D). ***$p<0.001$, As_2O_3+Rev versus Rev; *$p = 0.023$, ***$p<0.001$, As_2O_3+Rev versus As_2O_3; ***$p<0.001$, As_2O_3+Gen versus Gen; *$p = 0.02$, **$p = 0.038$, As_2O_3+Gen versus As_2O_3.

5% CO_2. After treatment with different types of drugs, the two types of cells were collected from 6-well plate, then the cell suspension was centrifuged ($800 \times g$, 10 min, 4°C), and the cell pellets were ultrasonicated for 15 min (every 15 s with 5 min intervals) at 4°C in cell lysate buffer (RIPA buffer, 50 mM Tris pH 7.4, 150 mM NaCl, 1% Triton X-100, 1% sodium deoxycholate, 0.1% SDS, sodium orthovanadate, sodium fluoride, EDTA and leupeptin). After cells-lysed buffer was centrifuged at $1000 \times g$ for 15 min, the supernatant protein samples were kept for the following experiments. The isolated protein samples were subjected to 15% SDS-polyacrylamide gel electrophoresis, blotted to a nitrocellulose membrane, and then blocked with 5% non-fat milk for 120 min. Next, the membranes were probed with LC3A/B in phosphate-buffered saline (PBS) containing 1% BSA and incubated overnight at 4°C. Thereafter, membranes were washed three times with PBS for 30 min and incubated with secondary antibody (Alexa Fluor; Molecular Probes; Eugene, OR, USA) for 1 h. The

bands were acquired using an imaging system (LI-COR Biosciences; Lincoln, NE, USA), and quantified with Odyssey v3.0 software by measuring the band intensity [area×optical density (OD)] in each group using β-actin (anti-β-actin antibody) as an internal control for normalization.

Measurement of cell viability

The cell viability was measured with an MTT reduction assay using a previously described method [24]. Briefly, cells were seeded in serum-free DMEM for 24 h, followed by administration with the indicated concentrations of agents at each time point. After incubation, the cells were quickly washed twice with cold PBS and added to MTT solution (final concentration, 5 mg/mL) for 4 h at 37°C. Then, the supernatant was removed and formazan crystals were dissolved with dimethylsulfoxide (150 µL) for 10 min. The absorbance was measured at 490 nm. Notably, the effect of Rev and As_2O_3 on the cell viability of NB4 cells was

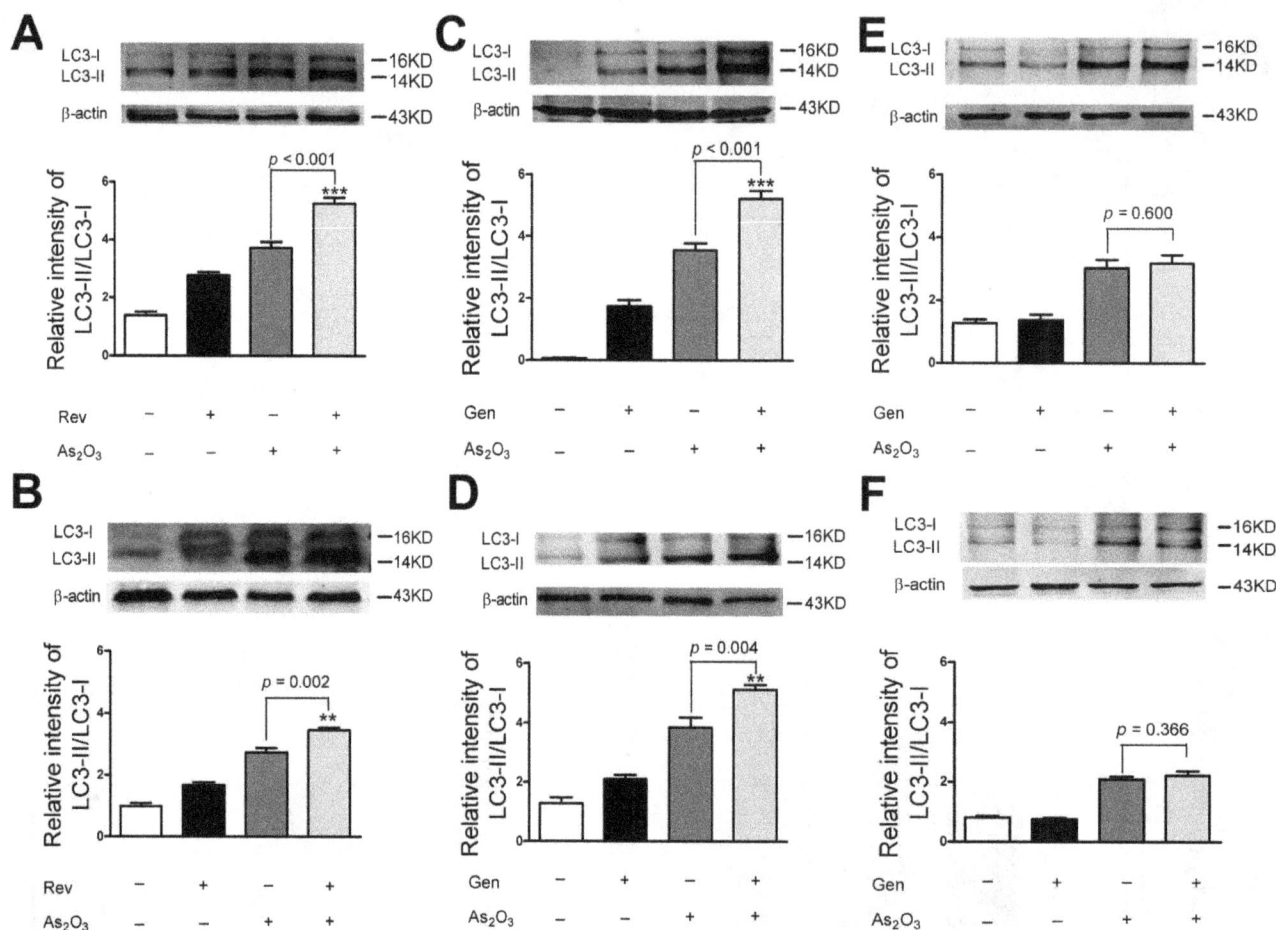

Figure 4. Effect of co-treatment of As$_2$O$_3$ and Gen/Rev on LC3 expression in NB4 cells and NRLVMs (n = 3). Co-treatment of 5 µM Rev or 50 µM Gen further increased the expression ratio of LC3 II/LC3 I in NB4 cells (A, C) and NRLVMs (B, D) compared to As$_2$O$_3$ alone. **$p = 0.002$, ***$p < 0.001$, As$_2$O$_3$+Rev versus As$_2$O$_3$; **$p = 0.004$, **$p < 0.005$, As$_2$O$_3$+Gen versus As$_2$O$_3$. No significant difference was found in the expression ratio of LC3 II/LC3 I in NB4 cells (E) and NRLVMs (F) with co-treatment of 5 µM Gen compared to As$_2$O$_3$ alone.

quantitatively assessed by calculating combination index (CI) as described before [25].

TUNEL assay

The cells were treated as described above. DNA fragmentation of the cells was then determined using the TUNEL assay. Briefly, air-dried slides were fixed with 4% paraformaldehyde for 30 min at room temperature, washed three times with PBS, and then permeabilized with 1% Triton X-100 for 4 min at 4°C. Subsequently, a TdT-labeled nucleotide mix was added to each slide and incubated at 37°C for 60 min in the dark. Slides were washed twice with PBS and then counterstained with 10 mg/mL 4,6-diamidino-2-phenylindole (DAPI) for 5 min at 37°C.

Flow cytometric analysis of cell apoptosis

The extent of apoptosis was detected by using annexinV-FITC apoptosis detection kit as described in the manufacturer's instructions [26]. After NB4 cells or NRLVMs had been treated with Rev+As$_2$O$_3$ or Rev for 24 h, cells were harvested, and carefully washed with PBS for three times. After centrifugation at $1000 \times g$ for 5 min, the cell pellets were resuspended in 195 µL annexin V binding buffer and gently mixed by adding another 5 µL annexin V binding buffer. The suspension was then incubated in the dark for 10 min at room temperature. Thereafter,

the supernatant was removed by centrifugation at $1000 \times g$ for 5 min. After 190 µL of annexin V binding buffer and 10 µL of propidiumiodide (50 mg/mL) were added, the fluorescence of these cells were analyzed by flow cytometry using the FloMax software. The fraction of cell population in different quadrants was analyzed using quadrant statistics. The lower left quadrant indicated normal cells; lower right quadrant represented early apoptotic cells and in the upper right quadrant was late apoptotic cells. The upper left quadrant was necrotic cells.

Statistical analysis

Data are presented as the mean ± SEM. The significance of differences between groups was assessed using one-way ANOVA followed by Dunnett's test. Two-tailed $p < 0.05$ was considered to be a statistically significant difference.

Results

Co-treatment of Gen/Rev further increased As$_2$O$_3$-induced oxidative stress in NB4 cells but relieved oxidative stress in NRLVMs

Consistent with previous studies [27–29], the individual compounds, Rev, Gen, and As$_2$O$_3$, substantially induced endogenous production of ROS in NB4 cells (Figure 1A and C).

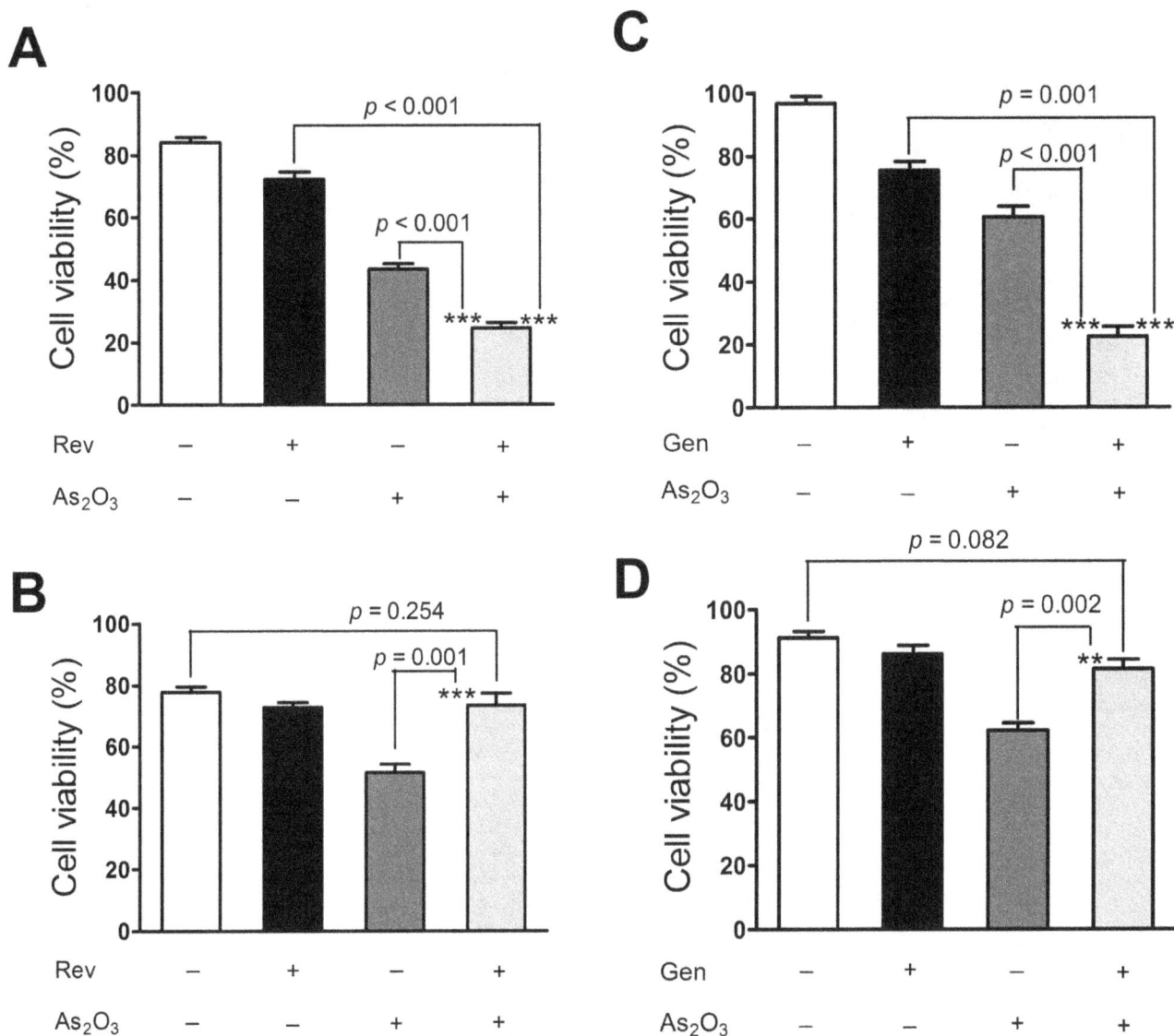

Figure 5. Effect of Gen/Rev on As$_2$O$_3$-induced cell viability of NB4 cells and NRLVMs (n = 6). Co-treatment of 5 µM Rev or 50 µM Gen further decreased the cell viability of NB4 cells (A, C) but reversed the cell viability of NRLVMs (B, D). ***p<0.001, As$_2$O$_3$+Rev versus Rev or As$_2$O$_3$; ***p<0.001, As$_2$O$_3$+Gen versus Gen; **p = 0.002, ***p<0.001, As$_2$O$_3$+Gen versus As$_2$O$_3$.

Mitochondrial malfunction, in conjunction with other factors such as increased metabolic activity and oncogenic stimulation, contributed to the heightened redox status of cancer cells, whereas excessive ROS generation inevitably aggravated tumor cell damage [30]. Significant alteration of MMP clearly indicated drug-induced damage to the mitochondria, the main intrinsic source of ROS, in NB4 cells (Figure 2A and C). Combination of As$_2$O$_3$ and Gen/Rev led to a more dramatic release of ROS from dysfunctional mitochondria than single drug treatment. Combined application of As$_2$O$_3$ and Gen/Rev also caused a remarkable decline in SOD activity (Figure 3A and C). As SOD is one of the main endogenous free radical scavenging enzymes, this finding suggests the continuous accumulation of ROS. Simultaneously reduced GSH level further exacerbated the injuries by excessive cellular oxidative stress (Figure S1A). In contrast to these phenomena observed in NB4 cells, the drug combination treatment in NRLVMs showed neutralized effects on ROS generation, MMP, GSH level, and SOD activity rather than

synergistic effects (Figures 1–3 and S1B). Both Rev (5 µM) and Gen (50 µM) obviously mitigated the As$_2$O$_3$-induced increase of ROS and mitochondrial injury in cardiomyocytes, demonstrating cytoprotection against the cardiotoxicity caused by As$_2$O$_3$. In addition, successful reversal of SOD activity to basal levels suggested the restored ability of cardiomyocytes to scavenge ROS.

Gen/Rev enhanced As$_2$O$_3$-induced autophagy in NB4 cells and NRLVMs

Increased release of ROS is one of the main endogenous factors for enhancement of cell autophagy [31]. Accordingly, As$_2$O$_3$ obviously increased the expression ratio of LC3 II/LC3 I in NB4 cells following the excessive generation of ROS (Figure 1A and 4A). Our result was in line with a previous study by Qian et al., in which another autophagy marker, Beclin-1, was confirmed to be up-regulated by As$_2$O$_3$ in leukemia cells [32]. Co-treatment with Rev substantially enhanced the effect of As$_2$O$_3$ on autophagy in NB4 cells (Figure 4A). However, to achieve the same effect with

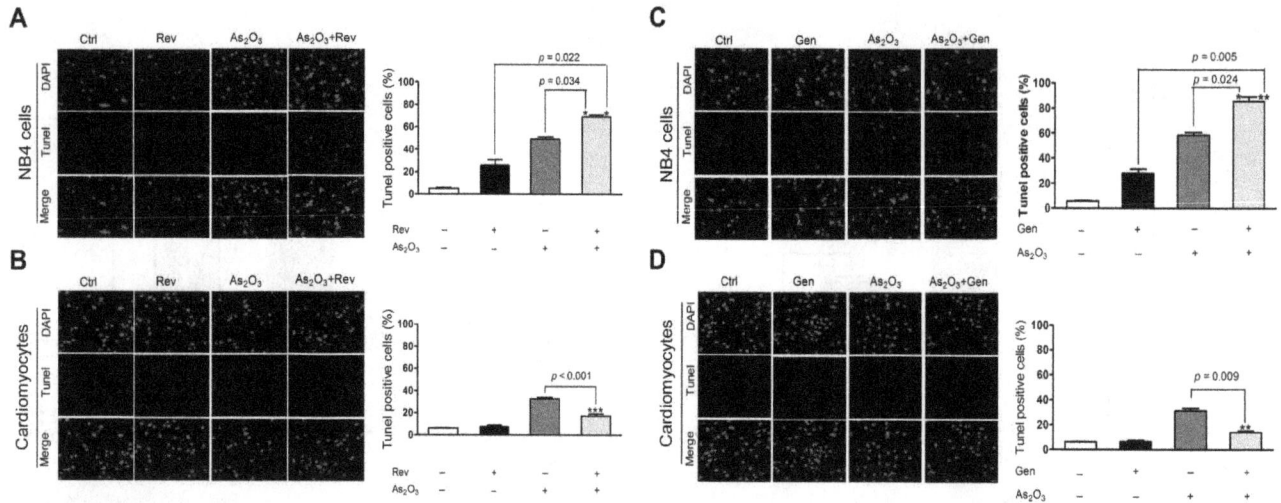

Figure 6. Effect of Gen/Rev on As$_2$O$_3$-induced apoptosis of NB4 cells and NRLVMs as determined by a TUNEL assay (n=6). Co-treatment of 5 μM Rev or 50 μM Gen further aggravated the As$_2$O$_3$-induced apoptosis of NB4 cells (A, C) but reversed that of NRLVMs (B, D). ***$p <$ 0.001, As$_2$O$_3$+Rev versus Rev; ***$p =$ 0.001, ***$p < 0.001$, As$_2$O$_3$+Rev versus As$_2$O$_3$; ***$p =$ 0.001, As$_2$O$_3$+Gen versus Gen; **$p =$ 0.002, ***$p < 0.001$, As$_2$O$_3$+ Gen versus As$_2$O$_3$.

Gen, a ten-fold concentration was required (Figure 4C and E). We further confirmed that the autophagy induced by As$_2$O$_3$ was also enhanced by co-treatment with Gen/Rev in NRLVMs (Figure 4B and D). This result is consistent with the cardioprotection that Rev provides via activation of autophagy [33]. As observed in NB4 cells, an equal concentration of Gen failed to enhance autophagy, implying a dosage advantage of Rev relative to Gen (Figure 4F).

Gen/Rev promoted As$_2$O$_3$-induced apoptosis in NB4 cells but protected against apoptosis in NRLVMs

MTT and TUNEL assays consistently verified that only 2 μM As$_2$O$_3$ was sufficient to substantially induce cell apoptosis of NB4 cells (Figure 5A and 6A), in line with its good therapeutic effect for APL [3]. However, this apoptosis-promoting activity might also contribute to marked cardiac toxicity [16]. Our results indicated that As$_2$O$_3$ substantially decreased the cell viability of NRLVMs and induced cardiomyocyte apoptosis (Figure 5B and 6B). However, addition of Gen/Rev changed the picture. On the one hand, Rev or Gen further exacerbated the apoptotic damage caused by As$_2$O$_3$ in NB4 cells (Figure 5C and 6C), whereas no obvious damage to cell viability and apoptosis was observed in these co-treated cardiomyocytes (Figure 5D and 6D). Additionally, the results of MTT-based CI calculation indicated that Rev act synergistically with As$_2$O$_3$ on inducing cell apoptosis of NB4 cells (Figure S2). This finding was further confirmed by the result of flow cytometry (Figure S3A). Co-administration of 2 μM As$_2$O$_3$ and 5 μM Rev dramatically increased the proportions of early apoptotic cells (27.16%) and late apoptotic cells (34.82%), compared with those of the control NB4 cells (early apoptotic cells, 0.87%; late apoptotic cells, 0.73%). However, 5 μM Rev obviously alleviated As$_2$O$_3$-induced apoptosis in NRLVMs by substantially reducing early apoptotic cells from 20.37% to 12.17% and late apoptotic cells from 7.71% to 1.55% (Figure S3B). The above findings were consistent with the results obtained with respect to ROS generation and LC3 expression in NB4 cells and NRLVMs (Figures 1–4).

Discussion

The outstanding benefit of As$_2$O$_3$ treatment for APL is due to its ability to specifically initiate the degradation of PML/RAR alpha, a core driving oncoprotein of APL [34]. Non-specific actions of As$_2$O$_3$, such as increasing ROS production, also greatly contribute to the mechanism by which APL can be cured with As$_2$O$_3$ [35]. However, as with many drugs, there is another side to these beneficial effects. The excessively amplified ROS generation flux induced by As$_2$O$_3$ inevitably leads to above-threshold toxicity levels in normal cells. Cardiomyocytes are likely to bear the brunt of this toxicity due to enrichment of mitochondria and their particular susceptibility to oxidative stress injury [13]. This has been validated experimentally [9–12] and confirmed by a plethora of clinical drug toxicity event reports [5–8]. In this study, combinations of As$_2$O$_3$ and the natural antioxidants Gen/Rev were investigated *in vitro* for the first time to explore their potential for treating APL without inducing cardiotoxicity.

Because of its multiple phenolic hydroxyl groups, the natural product Rev shows strong cytoprotective capacity against ROS generated by different inducers in non-tumor cells [36], which was confirmed in the present study. Rev successfully reversed the As$_2$O$_3$-induced ROS outbreak in NRLVMs. An equivalent effect was achieved with another natural antioxidant, Gen, but at a ten-fold concentration. Interestingly, we found that Rev and Gen played the role of accomplice to As$_2$O$_3$ in NB4 cells by exacerbating intracellular oxidative stress instead of adversary by extinguishing the ROS outbreak. Tumor cells employ a different mechanism to that of non-tumor cells for regulating mitochondrial functions [37,38], which eventually leads to disparate effectsof the same drug in tumor cells relative to non-tumor cells. Accordingly, in this study, we validated that both Rev and Gen could exacerbate As$_2$O$_3$-induced mitochondrial damage in the NB4 cells, but mitigated the mitochondrial injury caused by As$_2$O$_3$ in cardiomyocytes, in agreement with previous studies [28,29,37,38]. In addition, our experiments demonstrated that Gen/Rev further reduced SOD activity and deteriorated the intracellular ROS environment of NB4 cells by shifting the balance between ROS scavenging factors and ROS release factors. Ultimately, Gen/Rev might accelerate the As$_2$O$_3$-mediated degradation of PML/RARA oncoprotein via maintaining a high level of intracellular ROS, as proposed by Jeanne et al. [35]. This potential mechanism is reasonable to explain the synergistic proapoptotic effect observed by the combination of As_2O_3 and Gen/Rev.

While significantly relieving the oxidative injury caused by As_2O_3, 5 μM Rev was still able to enhance the autophagic flux of NRLVMs, indicating ROS-independent activation of autophagy. This role is likely the main contributor to Rev's myocardial protection, as revealed in previous studies [39,40]. Although there is currently no consensus as to whether activation or inhibition intervention of autophagy in APL is recommended [41], a study by Qian et al. strongly demonstrated that obvious enhancement of autophagy was indeed associated with the As_2O_3-mediated cell death of leukemia cells [32]. The results of our study further verified this finding, as autophagic cell death was implicated in the mechanisms by which As_2O_3 counteracts cell proliferation and promotes apoptosis of NB4 cells; Gen/Rev strengthened its pro-apoptotic effect via further elevating the level of autophagy.

In conclusion, we presented here *in vitro* evidence for synergistic antileukemic action of As_2O_3 and Rev from multiple aspects including oxidative stress, autophagy, and apoptosis. Meanwhile, the cardioprotective potential of Rev was also validated against As_2O_3-induced cardiomyocytes injury. Compared with Gen, the lower effective concentration of Rev indicates its potential as a rational drug candidate for APL treatment in combination with As_2O_3. Our findings provide a novel therapeutic possibility for APL with enhanced efficiency and reduced toxicity. Further functional experiments *in vivo* are required to validate our findings.

References

1. Soignet SL, Maslak P, Wang ZG, Jhanwar S, Calleja E, et al. (1998) Complete remission after treatment of acute promyelocytic leukemia with arsenic trioxide. N Engl J Med 339: 1341–1348.
2. Fox E, Razzouk BI, Widemann BC, Xiao S, O'Brien M, et al. (2008) Phase 1 trial and pharmacokinetic study of arsenic trioxide in children and adolescents with refractory or relapsed acute leukemia, including acute promyelocytic leukemia or lymphoma. Blood 111: 566–573.
3. Mathews V, Chendamarai E, George B, Viswabandya A, Srivastava A (2011) Treatment of acute promyelocytic leukemia with single-agent arsenic trioxide. Mediterr J Hematol Infect Dis 3: e2011056.
4. Barbey JT, Pezzullo JC, Soignet SL (2003) Effect of arsenic trioxide on QT interval in patients with advanced malignancies. J Clin Oncol 21: 3609–3615.
5. Drolet B, Simard C, Roden DM (2004) Unusual effects of a QT-prolonging drug, arsenic trioxide, on cardiac potassium currents. Circulation 109: 26–29.
6. Mumford JL, Wu K, Xia Y, Kwok R, Yang Z, et al. (2007) Chronic Arsenic Exposure and Cardiac Repolarization Abnormalities with QT Interval Prolongation in a Population-based Study. Environ Health Perspect 115: 690–694.
7. Vizzardi E, Zanini G, Antonioli E, D'Aloia A, Raddino R, et al. (2008) QT prolongation: a case of arsenical pericardial and pleural effusion. Cardiovasc Toxicol 8: 41–44.
8. Ducas RA, Seftel MD, Ducas J, Seifer C (2011) Monomorphic ventricular tachycardia caused by arsenic trioxide therapy for acute promyelocytic leukaemia. J R Coll Physicians Edinb 41: 117–118.
9. Li Y, Sun X, Wang L, Zhou Z, Kang YJ (2002) Myocardial toxicity of arsenic trioxide in a mouse model. Cardiovasc Toxicol 2: 63–73.
10. Hirano S, Cui X, Li S, Kanno S, Kobayashi Y, et al. (2003) Difference in uptake and toxicity of trivalent and pentavalent inorganic arsenic in rat heart microvessel endothelial cells. Arch Toxicol 77: 305–312.
11. Hwang JT, Kwon DY, Park OJ, Kim MS (2008) Resveratrol protects ROS-induced cell death by activating AMPK in H9c2 cardiac muscle cells. Genes Nutr 2: 323–326.
12. Manna P, Sinha M, Sil PC (2008) Arsenic-induced oxidative myocardial injury: protective role of arjunolic acid. Arch Toxicol 82: 137–149.
13. Cesselli D, Jakoniuk I, Barlucchi L, Beltrami AP, Hintze TH, et al. (2001) Oxidative stress-mediated cardiac cell death is a major determinant of ventricular dysfunction and failure in dog dilated cardiomyopathy. Circ Res 89: 279–286.
14. Pereira GC, Silva AM, Diogo CV, Carvalho FS, Monteiro P, et al. (2011) Drug-induced cardiac mitochondrial toxicity and protection: from doxorubicin to carvedilol. Curr Pharm Des 17: 2113–2129.

Supporting Information

Figure S1   Co-treatment of As_2O_3 and Rev on total GSH level in NB4 cells and NRLVMs (n = 6). Co-treatment of 5 μM Rev further decreased the GSH level in NB4 cells (A) but reversed that of NRLVMs (B). ***$p<0.001$ or $p = 0.001$, versus As_2O_3+Rev.

Figure S2   Result of CI calculation of the combinations of As_2O_3 and Rev on the cell viability of NB4 cells (n = 6). A. Effect of As_2O_3+Rev combinations of different concentrations on the cell viability of NB4 cells. B. CI values of As_2O_3+Rev combinations at different concentrations. A CI value of less than 1 means synergistic action by As_2O_3 and Rev.

Figure S3   Result of flow cytometric analysis of cell apoptosis in NB4 cells and NRLVMs. Co-treatment of 5 μM Rev and 2 μM As_2O_3 synergistically promoted early and late apoptosis instead of necrosis in NB4 cells (**A**). Addition of 5 μM Rev markedly relieved cardiomyocyte apoptosis that was induced by 5 μM As_2O_3 (**B**).

Author Contributions

Conceived and designed the experiments: YF WZ. Performed the experiments: YF MC JM LY YT LW KF. Analyzed the data: YF WZ. Contributed reagents/materials/analysis tools: YF WZ. Wrote the paper: YF WZ.

15. Zhang W, Guo C, Gao R, Ge M, Zhu Y, et al. (2013) The Protective Role of Resveratrol against Arsenic Trioxide-Induced Cardiotoxicity. Evid Based Complement Alternat Med 2013: 407839.
16. Fan Y, Wang C, Zhang Y, Hang P, Liu Y, et al. (2013) Genistein ameliorates adverse cardiac effects induced by arsenic trioxide through preventing cardiomyocytes apoptosis. Cell Physiol Biochem 31: 80–91.
17. Hollman PC, Katan MB (1999) Dietary flavonoids: intake, health effects and bioavailability. Food Chem Toxicol 37: 937–942.
18. Ravindranath MH, Muthugounder S, Presser N, Viswanathan S (2004) Anticancer therapeutic potential of soy isoflavone, genistein. Adv Exp Med Biol 546: 121–165.
19. Sun W, Wang W, Kim J, Keng P, Yang S, et al. (2008) Anti-cancer effect of resveratrol is associated with induction of apoptosis via a mitochondrial pathway alignment. Adv Exp Med Biol 614: 179–186.
20. Lee J, Giordano S, Zhang J (2012) Autophagy, mitochondria and oxidative stress: cross-talk and redox signalling. Biochem J 441: 523–540.
21. Lanotte M, Martin-Thouvenin V, Najman S, Balerini P, Valensi F, et al. (1991) NB4, a maturation inducible cell line with t(15;17) marker isolated from a human acute promyelocytic leukemia (M3). Blood 77: 1080–1086.
22. Chu W, Li C, Qu X, Zhao D, Wang X, et al. (2012) Arsenic-induced interstitial myocardial fibrosis reveals a new insight into drug-induced long QT syndrome. Cardiovasc Res 96: 90–98.
23. Ghaffari SH, Bashash D, Dizaji MZ, Ghavamzadeh A, Alimoghaddam K (2012) Alteration in miRNA gene expression pattern in acute promyelocytic leukemia cell induced by arsenic trioxide: a possible mechanism to explain arsenic multi-target action. Tumour Biol 33: 157–172.
24. Park SY, Sohn UD (2011) Inhibitory effect of rosiglitazone on the acid-induced intracellular generation of hydrogen peroxide in cultured feline esophageal epithelial cells. Naunyn Schmiedebergs Arch Pharmacol 383: 191–201.
25. Chou TC (2006) Theoretical basis, experimental design, and computerized simulation of synergism and antagonism in drug combination studies. Pharmacol Rev 58: 621–81.
26. Jiang S, Zu Y, Fu Y, Zhang Y, Efferth T (2008) Activation of the mitochondria driven pathway of apoptosis in human PC-3 prostate cancer cells by a novel hydrophilic paclitaxel derivative, 7-xylosyl-10-deacetylpaclitaxel. Int J Oncol 33: 103–111.
27. Gao F, Yi J, Yuan JQ, Shi GY, Tang XM (2004) The cell cycle related apoptotic susceptibility to arsenic trioxide is associated with the level of reactive oxygen species. Cell Res 14: 81–85.
28. Heiss EH, Schilder YD, Dirsch VM (2007) Chronic treatment with resveratrol induces redox stress- and ataxia telangiectasia-mutated (ATM)-dependent senescence in p53-positive cancer cells. J Biol Chem 282: 26759–26766.

29. Ullah MF, Ahmad A, Zubair H, Khan HY, Wang Z, et al. (2011) Soy isoflavone genistein induces cell death in breast cancer cells through mobilization of endogenous copper ions and generation of reactive oxygen species. Mol Nutr Food Res 55: 553–559.

30. Liou GY, Storz P (2010) Reactive oxygen species in cancer. Free Radic Res 44: 479–496.

31. Scherz-Shouval R, Shvets E, Fass E, Shorer H, Gil L, et al. (2007) Reactive oxygen species are essential for autophagy and specifically regulate the activity of Atg4. EMBO J 26: 1749–60.

32. Qian W, Liu J, Jin J, Ni W, Xu W (2007) Arsenic trioxide induces not only apoptosis but also autophagic cell death in leukemia cell lines via up-regulation of Beclin-1. Leuk Res 31: 329–339.

33. Kanamori H, Takemura G, Goto K, Tsujimoto A, Ogino A, et al. (2013) Resveratrol reverses remodeling in hearts with large, old myocardial infarctions through enhanced autophagy-activating AMP kinase pathway. Am J Pathol 182: 701–713.

34. Zhang XW, Yan XJ, Zhou ZR, Yang FF, Wu ZY, et al. (2010) Arsenic trioxide controls the fate of the PML-RARalpha oncoprotein by directly binding PML. Science 328: 240–243.

35. Jeanne M, Lallemand-Breitenbach V, Ferhi O, Koken M, Le Bras M, et al. (2010) PML/RARA oxidation and arsenic binding initiate the antileukemia response of As2O3. Cancer Cell 18: 88–98.

36. Leonard SS, Xia C, Jiang BH, Stinefelt B, Klandorf H, et al. (2003) Resveratrol scavenges reactive oxygen species and effects radical-induced cellular responses. Biochem Biophys Res Commun 309: 1017–1026.

37. Sun W, Wang W, Kim J, Keng P, Yang S, et al. (2008) Anti-cancer effect of resveratrol is associated with induction of apoptosis via a mitochondrial pathway alignment. Adv Exp Med Biol 614: 179–186.

38. Nadal-Serrano M, Pons DG, Sastre-Serra J, Blanquer-Rosselló Mdel M, Roca P, et al. (2013) Genistein modulates oxidative stress in breast cancer cell lines according to ERα/ERβ ratio: effects on mitochondrial functionality, sirtuins, uncoupling protein 2 and antioxidant enzymes. Int J Biochem Cell Biol 45: 2045–2051.

39. Xuan W, Wu B, Chen C, Chen B, Zhang W, et al. (2012) Resveratrol improves myocardial ischemia and ischemic heart failure in mice by antagonizing the detrimental effects of fractalkine*. Crit Care Med 40: 3026–3033.

40. Kanamori H, Takemura G, Goto K, Tsujimoto A, Ogino A, et al. (2013) Resveratrol reverses remodeling in hearts with large, old myocardial infarctions through enhanced autophagy-activating AMP kinase pathway. Am J Pathol. 182: 701–713.

41. Nencioni A, Cea M, Montecucco F, Longo VD, Patrone F, et al. (2013) Autophagy in blood cancers: biological role and therapeutic implications. Haematologica 98: 1335–1343.

16

Redox State and Mitochondrial Respiratory Chain Function in Skeletal Muscle of LGMD2A Patients

Mats I. Nilsson, Lauren G. Macneil, Yu Kitaoka, Fatimah Alqarni, Rahul Suri, Mahmood Akhtar, Maria E. Haikalis, Pavneet Dhaliwal, Munim Saeed, Mark A. Tarnopolsky*

Department of Pediatrics and Medicine, Neuromuscular Clinic, McMaster University Hospital, Hamilton, Ontario, Canada

Abstract

Background: Calpain-3 deficiency causes oxidative and nitrosative stress-induced damage in skeletal muscle of LGMD2A patients, but mitochondrial respiratory chain function and anti-oxidant levels have not been systematically assessed in this clinical population previously.

Methods: We identified 14 patients with phenotypes consistent with LGMD2A and performed *CAPN3* gene sequencing, CAPN3 expression/autolysis measurements, and *in silico* predictions of pathogenicity. Oxidative damage, anti-oxidant capacity, and mitochondrial enzyme activities were determined in a subset of muscle biopsies.

Results: Twenty-one disease-causing variants were detected along the entire *CAPN3* gene, five of which were novel (c.338 T>C, c.500 T>C, c.1525-1 G>T, c.2115+4 T>G, c.2366 T>A). Protein- and mRNA-based tests confirmed *in silico* predictions and the clinical diagnosis in 75% of patients. Reductions in antioxidant defense mechanisms (SOD-1 and NRF-2, but not SOD-2), coupled with increased lipid peroxidation and protein ubiquitination, were observed in calpain-3 deficient muscle, indicating a redox imbalance primarily affecting non-mitochondrial compartments. Although ATP synthase levels were significantly lower in LGMD2A patients, citrate synthase, cytochrome *c* oxidase, and complex I+III activities were not different from controls.

Conclusions: Despite significant oxidative damage and redox imbalance in cytosolic/myofibrillar compartments, mitochondrial respiratory chain function is largely maintained in skeletal muscle of LGMD2A patients.

Editor: Jianhua Zhang, University of alabama at birmingham, United States of America

Funding: Work was supported with private donations from Jessica Heikoop and family and Jay's Drive Fore MD Golf Tournament. The funders had no role in study design, data collection and analysis, decision to publish, or preparation of the manuscript.

Competing Interests: The authors have declared that no competing interests exist.

* Email: tarnopol@mcmaster.ca

Introduction

Limb-girdle muscular dystrophy (LGMD) are a heterogeneous group of genetic disorders and characterized by progressive weakness and wasting of the proximal limb girdle muscles and dystrophic muscle pathology. To date, 24 forms of LGMD have been identified with either autosomal dominant (1A-1H) or recessive (2A-2Q) inheritance patterns. Primary calpainopathy (LGMD2A, OMIM 253600), caused by mutations in the 40-kb *CAPN3* gene (OMIM 114240, mapped to 15q15.1-q21.1), is the most frequent form of recessive LGMD, with a prevalence of 1:15,000–1:150,000 depending on the population [1]. Disease onset generally occurs in early childhood to the second decade of life and is distinguished by an increase in serum creatine kinase (CK), symmetrical involvement of shoulder/pelvic girdles, and a dystrophic muscle pathology [2], ultimately causing loss of ambulation and wheel-chair dependence in adulthood [3].

The *CAPN3* gene contains 24 exons encoding for the 94-kDa Na^+/Ca^{2+}-dependent cysteine protease calpain-3 (CAPN3) [4,5], which serves both structural and proteolytic roles within sarco-meres of skeletal muscle [6,7,8], interacting mainly with α-actinin and titin to regulate myofibrillar disassembly, protein turnover, and mechanotransduction [9,10,11]. Muscle-specific CAPN3 consists of four domains (I–IV [Fig. S1]) and has three unique insertions sequences NS, IS1 (autolytic sites) and IS2 (titin-binding and nuclear translocation signal). Deficiency of CAPN3 is associated with build-up of toxic debris, oxidative damage, degeneration, and necrosis in LGMD2 patients, proving that it is indispensable for the maintenance and function of skeletal muscle. While the majority of the reported ~480 pathological *CAPN3* mutations impair autolysis and enzyme activity of calpain-3 (www.dmd.nl), titin-anchorage and substrate binding may also be affected [3], which is exemplified by the fact that 20–30% of LGMD2A patients exhibit normal calpain-3 protein levels and no loss in autolytic activity [12,13,14,15]. As such, the assessment of protein expression and Ca^{2+}-dependent autolysis of calpain-3 may be a cost-effective diagnostic approach (particularly in the absence of substrate-specific enzyme activity assays); however, *CAPN3* gene sequencing is essential for assigning a specific diagnosis in a significant portion of LGMD2A patients and remains the gold standard. Gene sequencing allows the practitioner to differentiate between primary and secondary calpainopathies and to perform genotype-phenotype correlations. Furthermore, the discovery of novel mutations improves our current understanding of molecular pathology, protein function, and may uncover previously unknown cellular roles of calpain-3.

Among the recently elucidated roles of CAPN3 is stabilization of the ryanodine receptor (RyR) and regulation of Ca^{2+} release during excitation-contraction coupling in the skeletal muscle triads. RyR expression, Ca^{2+} release, and CAMKII signaling are significantly reduced in CAPN3 knock-out (KO) mice, causing a decreased sensitivity to exercise stimuli, abnormal morphology and organization of mitochondria, decreased ATP production, and preferential involvement of slow-twitch muscle fibers [6,7,8,16]. Although proteomic studies support the notion that CAPN3 is an important regulator of mitochondrial function [16,17], and slow-twitch muscle fibers ($\uparrow$ mitochondrial abundance in slow vs. fast) are predominately affected in LGMD2A patients [7,18,19], expression and activities of rate-limiting enzymes in the Kreb's cycle and mitochondrial respiratory chain (MRC) have not been assessed in calpain-3 deficient humans to date. Furthermore, the effect of calpainopathy on mitochondrial anti-oxidants are unknown despite the fact that oxidative damage is a hallmark of LGMD2A and mitochondria are postulated to generate the majority of cellular free radicals [20]. To this end, we measured oxidative damage, anti-oxidant capacity, protein ubiquitination, and expression/activities of rate-limiting mitochondrial enzymes in skeletal muscle of genetically confirmed LGMD2A patients. From our cohort of 14 subjects, we identified 21 mutations of the CAPN3 gene, including five previously unreported sequence variants, and present biochemical data and in silico predictions of pathogenicity to strengthen genotype-phenotype correlations.

Methods

Clinical diagnosis, muscle biopsy and blood collection

All experiments were conducted according to the principles expressed in the Declaration of Helsinki. Written informed consent for muscle biopsies and approval for the use of archived patient samples were given by all subjects and the research ethics board at Hamilton Health Sciences (HIREB project # 10-327-T).

Fourteen out of 272 patients with confirmed or suspected muscular dystrophy in the Neuromuscular Disease Clinic at McMaster University Hospital exhibited clinical features consistent with LGMD2A. Major diagnostic criteria included absence of an autosomal dominant or X-linked inheritance pattern, atrophy and progressive weakness of shoulder/hip girdles, preferential posterior involvement of thighs/calves, sparing of facial, oculomotor, and cardiac muscles, and CK levels 5–80 times above normal [2,21,22]. Additional clinical features seen in some patients were waddling gate, winging scapulae, loss of ambulation, and wheelchair dependence. Upon review of clinical records, patients were further classified into Erb phenotype (scapulohumeral), early pelvifemoral phenotype (≤ 12 y), classical pelvifemoral phenotype (Leyden-Möbius; 13–29 y), late onset pelvifemoral phenotype (≥ 30 y), or asymptomatic phenotype (hyperCKemia) if possible [13,21]. To confirm clinical diagnosis, whole blood from antecubital vein (N = 14) and/or a skeletal muscle biopsy from vastus lateralis (N = 12) were obtained and sent for CAPN3 mutational testing and electron/light microscopy. Upon receiving genetic and pathology results, a sub-set of biopsies, previously snap-frozen in liquid nitrogen and stored at $-80°C$, were used for mitochondrial and CAPN3 mRNA/protein expression studies (WB and RT-PCR), oxidative damage/autolytic activity tests, and immunohistochemistry. For diagnostic purposes, those patients with one identified CAPN3 sequence variant were prioritized for biochemical analyses and compared to subjects with proven pathology and age/gender-matched controls. Control muscles were obtained from our biopsy bank, which contains specimens from healthy subjects that have previously consented to the use of their tissues in our research. Bioinformatic software tools were used to predict pathogenicity of all mutations and strengthen genotype-phenotype correlations. Molecular tests and/or gene sequencing were done to rule out Duchenne/Becker muscular dystrophy (DMD/BMD), facioscapulohumeral muscular dystrophy (FSHD), Emery Dreifuss muscular dystrophy, LGMD2B (DYSF), LGMD2C-F (sarcoglycanopathies), and LGMD2I (FKRP) in select patients.

CAPN3 mutation and in silico analyses

Whole blood samples from patients were sent to PreventionGenetics (Marshfield, WI) and Athena Diagnostics (Worcester, MA) for CAPN3 DNA sequence testing as previously described [23,24]. PreventionGenetics extracted genomic DNA using a Gentra PUREGENE kit and used PCR to amplify the full coding region (24 exons, 2466 basepairs) as well as ~50 bases of flanking intronic or other non-coding sequences. After cleaning of PCR products, cycle sequencing was carried out using the ABI Big Dye Terminator v.3.0 kit. Products were resolved by electrophoresis on an ABI 3130×l capillary sequencer and compared with reference sequences. Sequencing was performed separately in both forward and reverse directions. Similarly, Athena Diagnostics isolated highly purified genomic DNA, followed by automated unidirectional DNA sequencing of the coding region and 20 bases surrounding each exon. All abnormal variants were confirmed bidirectionally and detectable at an overall sensitivity approaching 99%. All test results were reviewed, interpreted, and reported by ABMG certified clinical molecular geneticists.

Pathogenicity of identified mutations was predicted using bioinformatics software as previously described by our laboratory [23,25]. Missense mutations were assessed by SIFT (sift.jcvi.org, SIFT sequence, UniProt-TrEMBL 2009 Mar) and PolyPhen2 (http://genetics.bwh.harvard.edu/pph2/) whereas intronic sequence variants were evaluated by the Human Splicing Finder program, version 2.4.1 (http://www.umd.be/HSF/). NetGene2 and BDGP Splite Site Prediction were used to verify the results obtained from HSF. Evolutionary conservation analysis of non-mutated nucleotides/amino acids was carried out using the UCSC Genome Browser (http://genome.ucsc.edu/cgi-bin/hgGateway). Mutations that alter highly conserved nucleotides/amino acids are likely to be deleterious, as these nucleotides/amino acids may be vital to mRNA/protein structure or function. As such, evolutionary conservation analysis was carried out with the UCSC Genome Browser using the "Feb.2009 (GRCH37/hg19)" assembly. Conservation of non-mutated nucleotides/amino acids across 46 species from the subphylum Vertebrata was assessed, including 36 mammalian species (Mammalia; 33 eutharians with chorioallontoic placenta, two metatherians with choriovitelline/yolk placenta, and one egg-laying prototherian), five species of bony fish (Osteichthyes), one jawless fish (Agnatha), two birds (Aves), one frog (Amphibia), and one lizard (Reptilia). Among these vertebrates were chimp, orangutan, rhesus, mouse, rat, guinea pig, rabbit, dolphin, cow, dog, elephant, opossum, lizard, Xenopus tropicalis, tetraodon, fugu, zebrafish, and lampreys. Mutation nomenclature adheres to the guidelines from the Human Genome Variation Society and nucleotide accession # NM000070.2 and protein accession # NP000061.1.

RNA isolation and quantitative real-time PCR (RT-PCR)

Total RNA isolation, first strand cDNA synthesis, and PCR amplification were performed as previously described with minor modifications [23]. Total RNA was extracted from approximately 25 mg of quadriceps muscle that was homogenized in 1 mL TRIzol® reagent (Invitrogen, Burlington, ON, Canada). Following homogenization, 0.2 mL of chloroform was added to each sample and the clear aqueous phase was transferred to RNeasy spin columns, followed by RNA isolation as per manufacturer's instructions (Qiagen, Germantown, Maryland, USA). The samples were DNase treated on the spin columns to prevent contamination with genomic DNA (Qiagen) and the absorbances at 230 nm (OD_{230}), 260 nm (OD_{260}), and 280 nm (OD_{280}) were determined using an ultraviolet spectrophotometer (NanoDrop 1000; Thermo Scientific). Measurements were repeated twice with a coefficient of variation of <7.5% and $OD_{260/280}$ and $OD_{260/230}$ ratios >1.5. Reverse transcription was performed on 150 ng of total RNA primed with random hexamers on a gradient thermocycler (MyCycler, Biorad, Hercules, CA, USA) as per manufacturer's instructions (Applied Biosystems, Foster City, CA, USA). Real-time polymerase chain reaction (RT-PCR) was performed with the 7300 Real-time PCR system (Applied Biosystems, Foster City, CA, USA) using SYBR® Green chemistry (PerfeCTa SYBR® Green Supermix with ROX, Quanta Biosciences, Gaithersburg, MD, USA) with standard thermocycling conditions. Primers, based on human gene sequences from GenBank (http://www.ncbi.nlm.nih.gov/genbank/), were designed for CAPN3 (NM_000070; F: 5'-atgactcggaggtgatttgc-3', R: 3'-tttgggaacctcgtagatgg-5') and β2-microglobulin (NM_004048.2; F: 5'-ggctatccagccgtactccaa-3'; R: 3'-gatgaaacccagacacatagca-5') using Primer3 software (http://biotools.umassmed.edu/bioapps/primer3_www.cgi). Melt curve analysis was performed on all primers to ensure the validity of amplification. Tm for forward and reverse CAPN3 primers was 60.08°C and 59.93°C, respectively. CAPN3 mRNA expression was thereafter quantified using the $2^{-\Delta Ct}$ method and normalized to β2-microglobulin.

Western blotting

In order to minimize CAPN3 Ca^{2+} autolysis, whole quadriceps muscle was homogenized in 1:10 wt/vol in 0.4 M Tris hydrochloride, 25 mM EGTA ($[Ca^{2+}] <10$ nM), 4% SDS, and protease inhibitor mixture (Complete Tablets, Roche) (pH 6.8) as previously described with minor modifications [11,26]. Immediately following homogenization, samples were heated to 95°C in SDS loading buffer for 10 min (0.125 M Tris hydrochloride, 10% glycerol, 4% SDS, 4 M urea, 10% mercaptoethanol, and 0.0001% bromophenol blue, pH 6.8) and stored at −80°C. A small aliquot of muscle homogenate, obtained prior to denaturation, was analyzed for protein concentration by a standard colorimetric assay [27].

The samples were loaded in equal amounts on 4–15% SDS polyacrylamide gels (10–20 μg), electrophoresed for one hour at 25 mA, and wet-transferred in Otter buffer (49.6 mM Tris, 384 mM glycine, 20% methanol, and 0.01% SDS) for 50 min at 400 mA onto 0.45 μM nitrocellulose membranes (Amersham Hybond-ECL, GE Healthcare). Following a 1-hr block step, membranes were incubated at 1:1000 (unless otherwise noted) with primary antibodies from Novacastra (CAPN 3*, NL-CALP-12A2, 1:100), Abcam (4-HNE#, ab48506, 1:3000; SOD1*, ab16831; SOD2*, ab13534), MitoSciences (total OXPHOS*, MS601), and Santa Cruz (Ub*, sc-8017; NRF-2*, C-20/sc-722; Keap-1*, sc15246) at 1:1000 overnight at 4°C. Standard HRP-linked secondary antibodies from GE Healthcare (NA931V [anti-mouse]; NA934V [anti-rabbit]) and Bio-Rad (anti-goat) diluted 1:5000 were used to detect primary IgGs, and reacted with Immobilon Western Chemiluminescent HRP Substrate from Millipore. Lastly, the membranes were developed in a dark room with Amersham Hyperfilm (GE Healthcare), and relative intensities of specific antigen bands or entire lanes (ubiquitin and 4-HNE) were quantified digitally with ImageJ 1.37v software. Blocking was performed in 1% milk* (m) or 5% m# (1×TBS), primary incubations in 1% m* or 5% BSA# (1×TBS), and secondary incubations in 1% m* or 5% m# (1×TBS). All incubation steps were followed by 3×5 min washes in TBS. CAPN3 blots were repeated twice with homogenates prepared from two separate pieces of muscle. Equal loading was verified by Ponceau S stain following wet transfer, which in our hands is a more consistent way of normalizing WB data compared to the use of single house-keeping proteins. Select membranes were probed for actin to confirm accuracy of Ponceau S.

Mitochondrial enzyme assays

Cytochrome c oxidase (COX; EC 1.9.3.1), complex I+III, and citrate synthase (CS; EC 2.3.3.1) activities were measured in quadriceps homogenates as previously described by our group [28,29,30]. All samples were analyzed in duplicate on a Cary 300 Bio UV–visible spectrophotometer (Varion, Inc., Palo Alto, CA) and the intra-assay coefficient of variation for all samples was less than 5%.

For COX activity, oxidized cytochrome c (Sigma C7752) was reduced by sodium ascorbate in 0.05 M potassium phosphate buffer (KH_2PO_4, pH 7.4). Fifteen microliters of muscle homogenate were added to 955 μL of 0.05 M potassium phosphate buffer and 15 μL of reduced cytochrome c in a 1.5 mL cuvette. The rate of oxidation of reduced cytochrome c was measured at 550 nm for 3 min at 37°C. COX activity was expressed in nmol/min/mg protein.

Complex I+III activity (NADH-cytochrome c oxidoreductase) was assessed by adding 15 μL of oxidized cytochrome c (40 mg/ml) to 1 mL of reaction buffer (0.1 M potassium phosphate and 1 mM sodium azide, pH~7.0, 37.5°C) in two 1.5 mL cuvettes. Following mixing, five μL of 1 mM rotenone (Sigma R8875) was added to a "rotenone-sensitive" cuvette (back) and 20 μl of muscle homogenate (~50–150 μg total protein) were added to both (front and back). A blank reading was done after 1 min equilibration and 5 μL of NADH was added to the front cuvette only at the start of the measurement. The reduction of oxidized cytochrome c was measured over two minutes at 550 nm. Activity was expressed in μmol cytochrome c reduced $\cdot$ min^{-1} $\cdot$ mg protein^{-1}.

CS activity was determined by measuring the formation of thionitrobenzoate anion. Fifteen microliters of muscle homogenate were added to 810 μL buffer (0.1 M Tris–HCl buffer, pH 8.0) along with 10 μL of acetyl CoA (7.5 mM in 0.1 M Tris-HCL buffer, pH 8.0) and 100 μL of 0.1 mM dithionitrobenzoic acid. The reaction was started by adding 50 μL of 9.0 mM oxaloacetate. Absorbance was measured at 412 nm for 2 min at 37°C. CS activity was expressed in nmol·min^{-1}·mg of protein^{-1}.

Calpain 3 autolytic activity immunoblots

The autolytic activity assay is based on the observation that full-length CAPN3 (94-kDa) undergoes gradual degradation into lower molecular weight products (56-, 58-, and 60-kDA [NL-CALP-12A2]) when incubated in a calcium-enriched saline solution for ≥ 5 min [14,15,31]. Cellular Ca^{2+} concentrations are ~100 nM at rest and increase to ~250 nM for 24 hrs following eccentric exercise, which is enough to activate CAPN3 autolysis [11]. As such, muscle was homogenized in 1:10 wt/vol saline solution (0.9% NaCl) with 5 mM $CaCl_2$ and incubated at room

Table 1. LGMD2A phenotypes, CAPN3 sequence variants, and *in silico* predictions.

ID	Sex	Age[A]	Pheno[B]	Mutation	Ex/In[C]	Nucleotide	Amino Acid	Dom[D]	Zyg[E]	Nov[F]	Bioinformatics[G] (missense/deletion)		
											SIFT	Poly2	Cons
*P1	M	37/31/14	Classical	Transition	10	c.1250 C>T	p.Thr417Met	III	Het	N	Y	Y	42
				Transition	4	c.500 T>C	p.Phe167Ser	II	Het	Y	Y	Y	44
*P2	M	39/38/34	Late	Transversion	22	c.2338 G>C	p.Asp780His	IV	Het	N	Y	Y	42
				Transversion	22	c.2366 T>A	p.Leu789Gln	IV	Het	Y	Y	Y	43
*P3	F	39/36/36	Asympt.	Deletion	13	c.1573_1575 del	p.Phe525del	III	Het	N	-	-	37
				Transition	20	c.2120 A>G	p.Asp707Gly	IV	Het	N	Y	Y	41
*P4	M	†56/53/18	Classical	Transversion	19i	IVS19+4 T>G	Cryptic splice site§	IV	Hom	Y	-	-	-
				(intronic)		(c.2115+4 T>G)							
P5	M	w28/23/14	Classical	Transversion	4i	IVS4+1 G>C	Donor splice site#	II	Hom	N	-	-	-
				(intronic)		(c.632+1 G>C)							
P6	F	w39/32/4	Early	Deletion (Frameshift)	4	c.550 del A	p.Thr184ArgfsX36	II	Hom	N	-	-	-
P7	F	54/50/39	Late	Transition	11	c.1477 C>T	p.Arg493Trp	III	Het	N	Y	Y	40
				Deletion (Frameshift)	4	c.550 del A	p.Thr184ArgfsX36	II	Het	N	-	-	-
P8	M	w37/33/15	Classical	Deletion (Frameshift)	3	c.483 del G	p.Ile162SerfsX17	II	Hom	N	-	-	-
P9	M	15/14/13	Classical	Transition	9	c.1162 C>T	p.Gln388stop	II	Het	N	-	-	-
				Transition	11	c.1465 C>T	p.Arg489Trp	III	Het	N	Y	Y	38
*P10	M	54/50/c	Early	Transition	13	c.1621 C>T	p.Arg541Trp	III	Het	N	Y	Y	38
				Transition	2	c.338 T >C	p.Ile113Thr	II	Het	Y	Y	N	33
*P11	M	40/33/30	Late	Transversion	10	c.1257 T>G	p.Asp419Glu	III	Het	N	Y	Y	43
*P12	F	39/32/27	Unspecified	Transversion	11i	IVS11-1 G>T	Acceptor splice site‡	III	Het	Y	-	-	-
				(intronic)		(c.1525-1 G>T)							
*P13	M	45/45/38	Late	Transition	1	c.224 A>G	p.Tyr75Cys	I	Het	N	Y	Y	35
				Transition	8	c.1099 G>A	p.Gly367Ser	II	Het	N	Y	Y	43
P14	M	30/28/15	Classical	Transition	4	c.527 T>C	p.Val176Ala	II	Het	N	Y	Y	43
				Deletion	5	c.759_761 del	p.Lys254 del	II	Het	N	-	-	41

[A] Current age/age at biopsy (or genetic confirmation)/first symptoms noted, † = deceased, w = wheelchair, c = childhood;
[B] Phenotypic classification into Erb (scapulohumeral), early pelvifemoral (Leyden-Möbius;13–29 y), classical pelvifemoral (≤12 y), late onset pelvifemoral (≥30 y), or asymptomatic phenotype (hyperCKemia);
[C] CAPN3 exon/intron;
[D] CAPN3 domains;
[E] Zygosity;
[F] Novelty;

temperature for 5 min to ensure partial autolysis. The reaction was blocked by adding 1:1 vol/vol loading buffer containing Ca^{2+}-chelating EDTA (0.05 DTT, 0.1 M EDTA, 0.125 M Tris hydrochloride, 4% SDS, 10% glycerol, and 0.005% bromophenol blue, pH 8.0), followed by immediate heating at 95°C for 10 min and storage at −80°C. Protein concentration and CAPN3 expression were measured as previously described for the conventional Western blot. CAPN3 autolytic tests were repeated twice with homogenates prepared from two separate pieces of muscle. Equal loading was verified with Ponceau S stain as previously described.

Calpain 3 immunohistochemistry

Quadriceps muscle (1.5 mm^3) was embedded in Optimal Cutting Temperature compound (OCT) and immersed in liquid nitrogen-cooled isopentane, followed by cryosectioning of 8 μm slices that were mounted on polylysine-coated slides and stored at −80°C. The slides were brought to room temperature, fixed in acetone for 10 min, rinsed 2×2 min, and stained according to manufacturer's protocol using the Vector Elite ABC detection system (Vector Laboratories, Burlingame, CA) [32]. Briefly, slides were incubated with 1:50 CAPN3 (NL-CALP-12A2) for 60 min, followed by quenching of endogenous peroxidase activity with 0.3% H_2O_2 and washing 3×2 min. A secondary biotinylated anti-mouse antibody was applied at a 1:500 dilution for 60 min and samples washed for 3×5 min. Slides were then incubated with Vectastain ABC reagent for 30 min, washed 1×5 min, and exposed to peroxidase substrate (3,3'-diaminobenzidine; DAB) for 5 min. Following a rinse in tap-water, the sections were counterstained with hematoxylin for nuclear detail, dehydrated in ascending concentrations of ethanol, and cleared in xylene to increase tissue transparency and improve focus of internal structures. Sections were cover-slipped with Permount and visualized using bright-field microscopy at 400× total magnification as previously described [29]. Antibody incubations and wash steps were done in 0.25% BSA/0.025% Triton X100/TBS solution and TBS, respectively.

Statistical analysis

Data analysis was performed using independent t-tests (Sigma Stat®, ver. 3.5). Statistical significance was set at $P \leq 0.05$. To increase reproducibility, assays were repeated twice for each patient and presented as means ± standard error.

Results

Clinical findings

We studied 14 patients (10 males and 4 females [Table 1]) that fulfilled the diagnostic criteria for LGMD2A proposed by the European Neuromuscular Centre Workshop [22], including atrophy and progressive weakness of shoulder/hip girdles, elevated CK levels, and muscle biopsies consistent with a dystrophic/myopathic process. The age at onset ranged from 4 to 39 y and the majority of patients presented with pelvic girdle weakness or asymptomatic hyperCKemia (92.9%). In this cohort we identified two subjects with early onset (14.3%), six with the classical Leyden Möbius phenotype (42.9%), four with late onset (28.6%), one asymptomatic (7.1%), and one unspecified (7.1%). Surprisingly, no patients exhibited primary shoulder-girdle involvement/onset (Erb phenotype). At the time of the investigation three subjects were wheelchair-bound (P5, P6, and P8) and one (P4) had passed away.

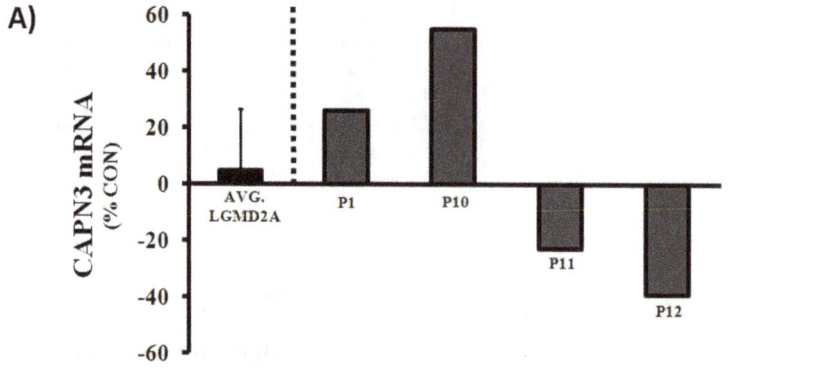

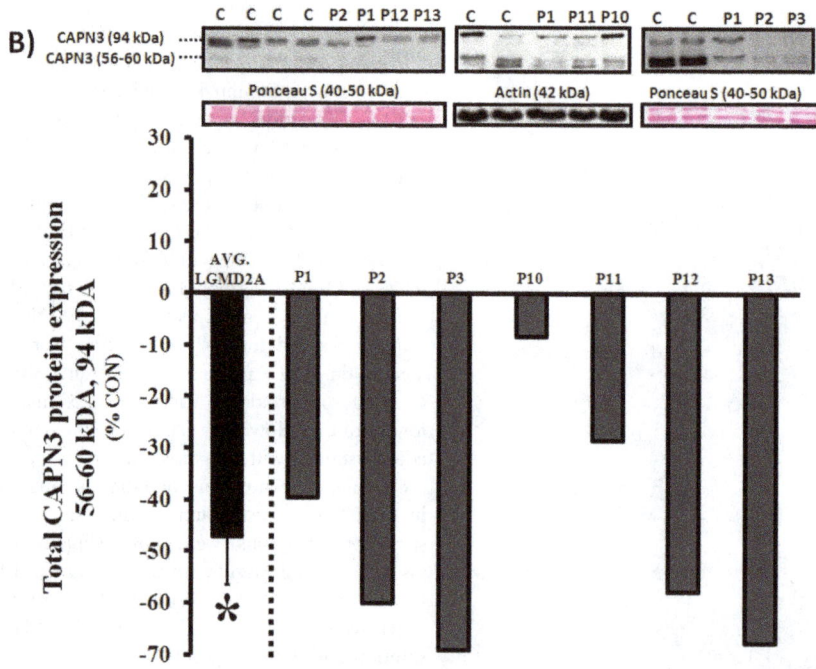

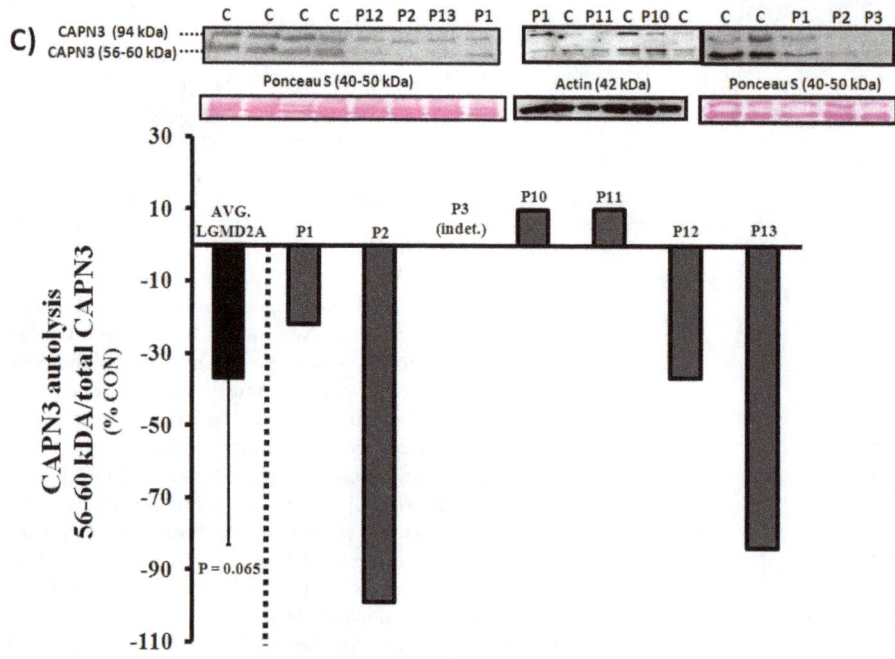

Figure 1. Expression and autolysis of CAPN3 in quadriceps muscle of LGMD2A patients. A) CAPN3 mRNA expression (RT-PCR); B) CAPN3 protein (Western blot); C) Ca^{2+}-induced autolytic activity of CAPN3 (Western blot). Calpain-3 autolytic activity is presented as a ratio between autolyzed fragments and total CAPN3 (representing *relative autolytic capacity* of protein present), but the results should also be interpreted in the context of total protein expression from regular Western blots. Logically, a reduction in total CAPN3, obtained from Ca^{2+}-free homogenates, equates to a decrease in *total autolytic capacity*. All CAPN3 data were normalized to a suitable housekeeping gene (β2-microglobulin), protein (actin), or total proteins levels (Ponceau S stain) and graphed as % age/gender-matched healthy controls. Representative images of CAPN3 blots (56–60 kDa, 94 kDa), Ponceau S stain (40–50 kDa), or actin (42 kDa) are shown in B–C. For total protein expression and autolytic activity, N = 7 (LGMD2A) and N = 8 (control), while N = 4 (LGMD2A) and N = 6 (control) for mRNA. Bars to the far left represent the average of all LGMD2A patients (AVG. LGMD2A). INDT: Indeterminate. *Significantly lower compared to controls (P≤0.05).

Pathological findings

Biopsies and/or blood were collected and used for *CAPN3* mutational analysis and muscle histopathology as described in the methods section (mean age 35.6±2.9 y, range 14–53 y) [Table 1, Figs. S1–S2]. For further diagnostic and biochemical testing, a sub-set of patients were selected (N = 8; mean age 39.8±3.0 y, range 31–50 y) and compared to age- and gender-matched controls (N = 7; mean age 36.6±3.7 y, range 25–50 y) or as noted in the figure legends. Muscle histopathology (electron microscopy and IHC) ranged from mild to moderate to acute dystrophic processes and consisted of internalized nuclei, variation in fiber size, necrosis, degeneration/regeneration, and fiber splitting. Three patients (P1, P10, and P11) were randomly chosen for fiber-type quantification and revealed selective type 1 atrophy (−16% avg. diameter vs. CON) and type II dominance in P11 (83% fast/17% slow vs. 61%/39% in CON) [Fig. S2]. PAS, Oil-Red-O, succinate dehydrogense, cytochrome *c* oxidase, and NADH dehydrogenaze stains generally showed normal triglyceride abundance, glycogen content, and activity/distribution of mitochondria in all patients. Intra-mitochondrial crystalloid inclusions were present in electron micrographs of P4, but no other mitochondrial abnormalities were observed. Unless otherwise noted, immunohistochemistry showed normal reactivity towards dystrophin, spectrin, merosin, sarcoglycans (α,β,γ,δ), beta dystroglycan, caveolin III, desmin, and dysferlin in all subjects.

Genotype-phenotype correlations

Gene sequencing of the *CAPN3* gene revealed 21 sequence variants in our cohort of 14 patients, including 13 missense mutations, 1 nonsense mutation, 4 deletions (frameshifts/premature stop), and 3 intronic mutations (Table 1). Consistent with idea of mutation clustering in specific exons of the *CAPN3* gene (i.e. 1, 4, 5, 8, 10, 11, 21), ~60% of identified variants in this study occurred in aforementioned exons (Fig. S1). The majority of patients were compound heterozygotes with the exception of four homozygous individuals (P4, P5, P6, and P8) and two subjects with one mutation identified but with a clinical and/or biochemical phenotype consistent with LGMD2A (P11 and P12). All mutations were predicted to be pathogenic with bioinformatic software programs, exchanging highly conserved amino acids in the enzyme or nucleotides indispensable for splicing of the premRNA. Five of these pathological sequence variants were novel and had not been reported in the Leiden database previously. Biochemical analyses were a priority in those patients exhibiting novel mutations (P1, P2, P4, P10, and P12) and/or one pathological sequence variant (P10 and P11), which were compared to subjects with proven pathology (P3 and P13) and age/gender-matched controls. Collectively, we confirmed the *in silico* predictions in75% of patients using WB or IHC for CAPN3 levels/autolytic activity and RT-PCR for mRNA expression, including subject P12, but not in P4 or P10 (Fig. 1A–C; Table S1; Fig. S2). Immunoblotting was the most robust test in this study, while RT-PCR and IHC were less useful

for diagnostic purposes. Gene sequencing was necessary for specific diagnosis in P4 and P10. Mutations predicted to be pathogenic are presented in Table 1 and novel variants are also described in the text.

Proband 1 is of European Canadian decent and diagnosed with classical pelvifemoral LGMD2A (Leyden-Möbius). *CAPN3* sequencing revealed a unique combination of missense mutations [c.1250 C>T (p.Thr417Met) and c.500 T>C (p.Phe167Ser)]. Upon biochemical analyses, moderate reductions in protein expression and autolytic activity of calpain-3 were noted, but no defects in mRNA abundance. The former sequence variant exchanges a highly conserved threonine for a methione in domain III and results in an absence of CAPN3 protein when combined with c.2362_2363delinsTCATCT [33]. The second mutation in proband 1 is novel and exchanges a highly conserved phenylalanine (nonpolar, neutral, and hydrophobic) for a serine (polar, neutral, and hydrophilic) in domain II, which contains the catalytic module of CAPN3. Because there is no biochemical data on either mutation in the homozygous state, individual contributions of each sequence variant to the phenotype are difficult to determine.

Proband 2 is of South-East Asian heritage and exhibited two compound heterozygous missense mutations [c.2338 G>C (p. Asp780His) and c.2366 T>A (p.Leu789Gln)] causing late-onset pelvifemoral LGMD2A. Protein expression and autolytic activity, but not mRNA levels, were significantly reduced and the biochemical phenotype was more severe than P1 despite the late-onset form. Both sequence variants exchange evolutionary conserved amino acids in domain IV of CAPN3 (exon 22), which may affect Ca^{2+}-binding with downstream effects on autolytic activity. Interestingly, c.2338 G>C was inherited from his mother and is a recently recognized founder mutation originating from northern India in the Agarwal community, whose clan members practice intra-communal exogamy and are postulated to be descendants of King Agrasen [34]. This mutation was previously shown to cause pelvifemoral LGMD2A in the homozygous state and in combination with c.2099-1 G>T or c.1106 G>A, but effects on CAPN3 expression were inconclusive (protein non-significantly reduced vs. absent) [34,35]. We speculate that the novel sequence variant c.2366 T>A has deleterious effects on protein expression and autolysis of CAPN3, although verification in a homozygous patient or through site-directed mutagenesis is preferred.

Proband 4 was born in Pakistan and died at 56 years of age due to respiratory insufficiency. The patient exhibited a classical pelvifemoral LGMD2A phenotype with an onset in his late teens and he was wheelchair-bound at the time of his death. We identified a novel homozygous transversion (c.2115+4 T>G) in intron 19, which is predicted to create a cryptic splice site that is used instead of the regular site. Activation of a previously dormant cryptic splice may result in exon skipping or intron retention, and considering that CAPN3 reactivity appeared largely normal on IHC in this patient, we surmise that the gene product is stable but that the protein is truncated or otherwise dysfunctional.

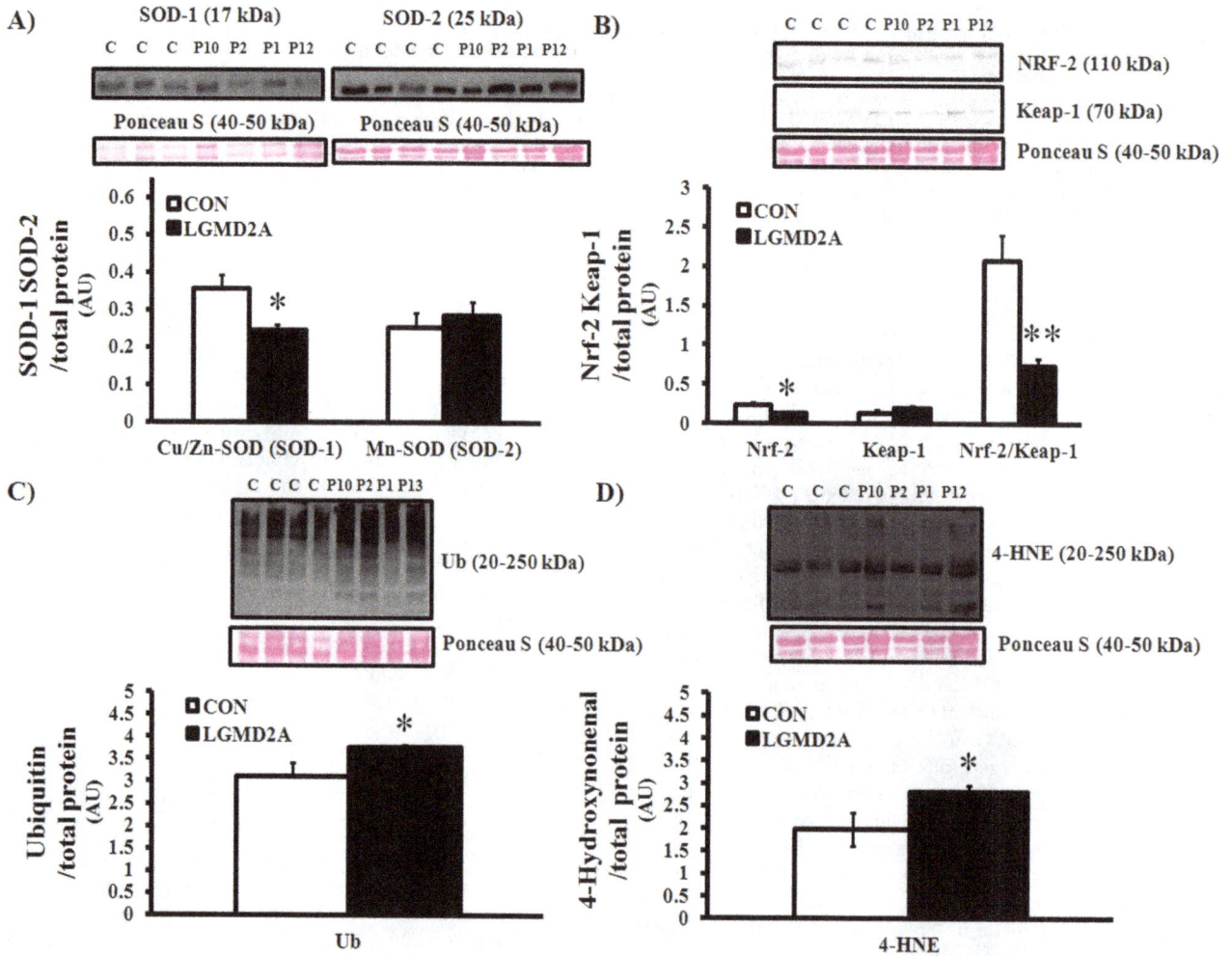

Figure 2. Western blot analyses of anti-oxidant capacity (SOD-1, SOD-2, NRF-2/Keap-1), oxidative damage (lipid peroxidation; 4-HNE), and ubiquitination (Ub) in LGMD2A patients. *P≤0.05 vs. control. **P≤0.01 vs. control. All data were normalized to total protein levels (Ponceau S stain) and represent averages of age/gender-matched controls (N=3–4; white bars) and LGMD2A patients (N=4; black bars). Representative images of blots and Ponceau S stain (40–50 kDa) are shown.

Proband 10 is of Irish decent and was clinically diagnosed with early onset pelvifemoral LGMD2A. The patient was found to be compound heterozygous for two missense mutations [c.1621 C>T (p.Arg541Trp) and c.338 T>C (p.Ile113Thr)], affecting conserved amino acids and predicted to be pathological by SIFT analysis. While the muscle biopsy showed a definite dystrophic pattern, we did not detect CAPN3 deficiency using the standard RT-PCR, WB, or IHC tests, possibly indicating that other functions, such as substrate recognition/binding or proteolytic activity, are impaired. c.1621 C>T has previously been reported in LGMD2A patients in the compound heterozygous and homozygous states and is associated with a reduction in CAPN3 expression in both Erb and Leyden-Möbius phenotypes [13,36]. c.338 T>C is a novel mutation exchanging isoleucine (nonpolar, neutral, and hydrophobic) for threonine (polar, neutral and hydrophilic), and is predicted by SIFT to be pathogenic and may impair proteolytic activity in domain II of CAPN3.

Proband 12 is of Iranian heritage and exhibited the major diagnostic criteria for primary calpainopathy, but clinical records were insufficient to pinpoint a specific LGMD2A phenotype. The mutational screen revealed a novel transversion in intron 11 (c.1525-1 G>T) that was predicted to destroy an acceptor splice site, but a second sequence variant was not identified. Canonical mutations of conserved nucleotides in positions −2, −1, +1, and +2 will significantly affect splicing (minus/plus signs indicate upstream/downstream from 5′ and 3′ ends of the exon, respectively) and may cause exon skipping or intron retention [37], ultimately affecting the mRNA stability and/or protein structure. CAPN3 protein levels, mRNA abundance, and autolytic activity were significantly reduced in P12, which strongly suggests that the mutation is pathogenic and confirms the clinical diagnosis.

Redox balance and mitochondrial function

Although structural and distributional abnormalities of mitochondria, oxidative damage, and markers of degradation may be hallmarks of the dystrophic process in calpain-3 deficient skeletal muscle [18,20,38], mitochondrial enzyme function and antioxidant defense have not been assessed in LGMD2A patients to date. As such, we measured the expression of CuZn-SOD (SOD-1), Mn-SOD (SOD-2), Nrf-2/Keap-1 and assessed the degree of oxidative damage, protein ubiquitinylation, and mitochondrial function in a sub-set of patient biopsies. Interestingly, SOD-1 and the Nrf-2/Keap-1 ratio were significantly lower in LGMD2A tissue, while SOD-2 levels were normal (Fig. 2A–B). As expected,

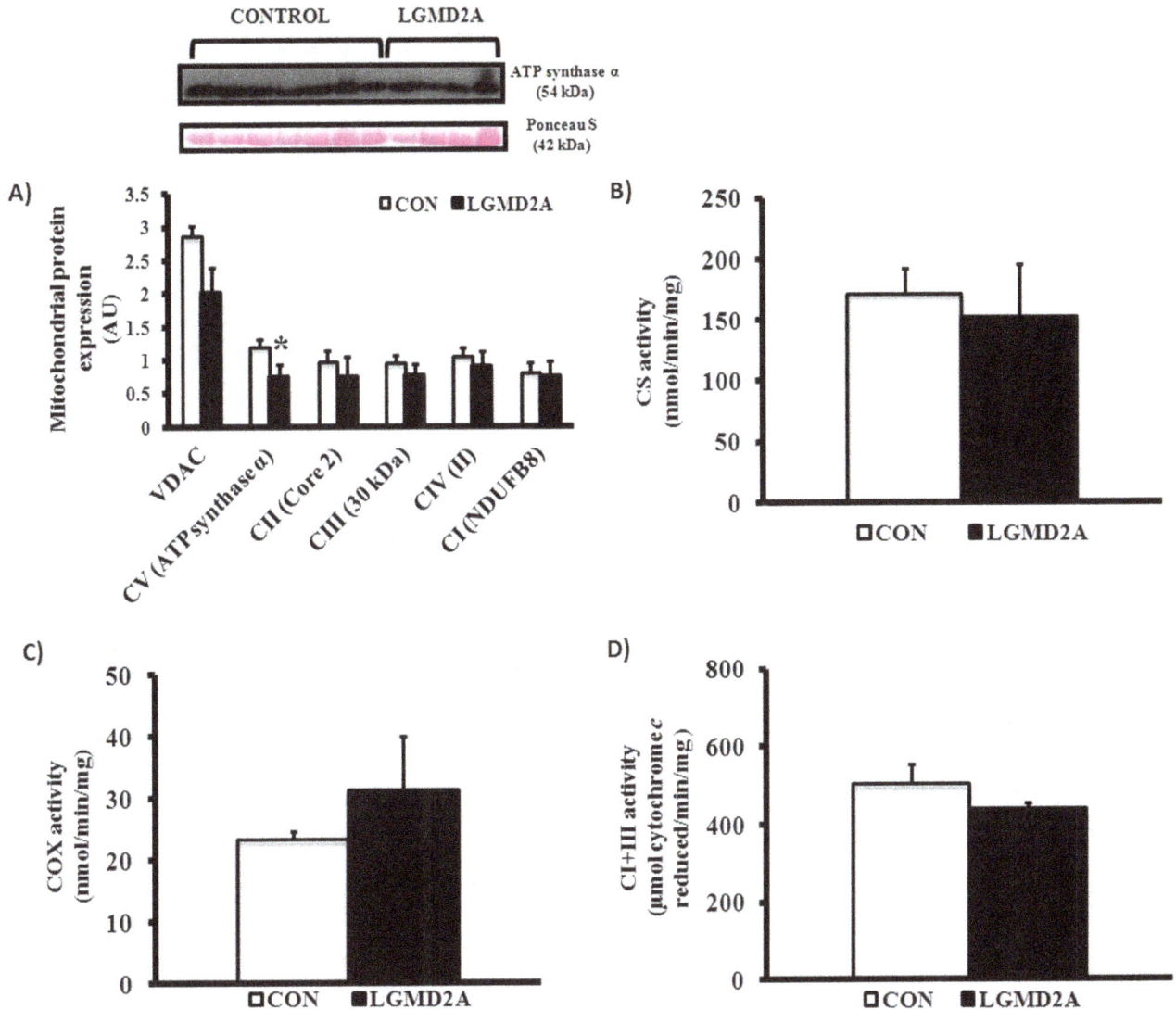

Figure 3. Western blot analyses of OXPHOS expression (complex I–V) and ETC enzyme activities (CS, COX, and complex I+III) in LGMD2A patients. *Significantly lower ATP synthase expression in calpain-3 deficient muscle (P≤0.05). All Western blot data were normalized to total protein levels (Ponceau S stain) and represent averages of age/gender-matched controls (N = 7 for OXPHOS and enzyme assays; N = 5 for VDAC) and LGMD2A patients (N = 5 for OXPHOS and VDAC; N = 2–3 for enzyme assays). Representative images of OXPHOS blots and Ponceau S stain (42 kDa) are shown.

lipid peroxidation (4-HNE) and total ubiquitin expression were elevated in calpain-3 deficient muscle (Fig. 2C–D). Activities of citrate synthase, COX, and complex I+III were not different from age/gender-matched controls, although a moderate reduction of complex V (ATP synthase) was detected on immunoblots (Fig. 3A–D).

Discussion

Herein we present five novel sequence variants that add to the mutational spectrum of LGMD2A and provide further insights into the cellular mechanisms underlying pathology in this patient population. Our results support the contention that gel-based tests (protein expression and autolytic activity) are the most important diagnostic tools next to *CAPN3* gene sequencing, while microscopy-based methods may be less useful for genotype-phenotype correlations and confirmation of clinical diagnosis.

In addition to our mutational data, we assessed oxidative damage, key anti-oxidant markers, and mitochondrial enzyme function in a subset of patient biopsies. Although the limited sample size prohibits us from making generalized statements, our findings leave open the possibility of mitochondrial enzyme dysfunction not being a universal feature of calpainopathy in humans, which appears to be the case in CAPN3 KO mice [16]. We found that the activities of rate-limiting enzymes in the Kreb's cycle (citrate synthase), mitochondrial respiratory chain (cytochrome *c* oxidase and NADH-cytochrome *c* oxidoreductase), and expression of OXPHOS proteins were largely normal in LGMD2A patients. In support of these observations, SOD-2 levels were comparable to age- and gender-matched controls, suggesting a preserved ability of mitochondria to catalyze highly reactive superoxide anions from complex I and III into hydrogen peroxide. Conversely, Nrf-2, Nrf-2/Keap1 ratio, and CuZn-SOD (SOD-1) were significantly suppressed in calpain-3 deficient skeletal muscle, collectively indicating a primary cytosolic/myofibrillar redox imbalance. Considering that Nrf-2 dissociates from its cytosolic inhibitor Keap1 and moves to the nucleus to regulate the transcription of anti-oxidant genes under stress conditions, aberrant regulation of Nrf-2 is generally synonymous with a reduction in cytoprotection, as previously shown by our group [39]. Given the results of the current study, and others [20,40,41], cellular redox imbalance appears to be compartment-specific and induces the ubiquitin-proteasome pathway, which in turn orchestrates protein degradation and muscle wasting in LGMD2A.

Calpain-3 associates with the ryanodine receptor and regulates Ca^{2+} release at the muscle triads, and calpain-3 deficiency impairs Ca^{2+} transport, RyR expression, and CAMKII signaling in CAPN3 KO mice [6,7,8]. Calcium kinetics play an important role in loading-induced muscle adaptations and maintenance of slow fiber phenotype in humans, and LGMD2A patients may exhibit lower RyR levels and a preferential involvement of slow muscle fibers [7]. Although the connection between calpain-3 and mitochondrial function remains unclear, two reports have demonstrated mitochondrial abnormalities in Japanese LGMD2A patients [18,38]. In partial agreement with aforementioned studies, ATP synthase levels were suppressed and type 1 fibers preferentially affected in our patient cohort, but we did not find general deficits in mitochondrial enzyme function, protein expression, or ultra-structure. Interestingly, ATP production is impaired in CAPN3 KO mice [16], but neither ATP synthase activity or energy status were assessed in our study. Because Ca^{2+} modulates the phosphorylation of subunit c of F_0F_1 ATPase and increased Ca^{2+} levels activates a number of nuclear genes encoding mitochondrial proteins (including ATP synthase) [42,43], calpainopathy may impair transcription of ATP synthase and/or its function. Selective type 1 fiber atrophy conceivably lowers the total amount of mitochondria in CAPN3-deficient skeletal muscle, and in light of our finding that VDAC was symmetrically reduced (albeit not significantly) compared to F_0F_1 ATPase, further research is necessary to delineate potential complex-specific deficiencies in isolated mitochondrial fractions.

In summary, we confirmed pathogenicity of *CAPN3* mutations in 75% of LGMD2A patients selected for biochemical analyses, which stresses the importance of gene sequencing in the diagnostic process. Assessment of total CAPN3 expression and autolysis by immunoblotting were the most reliable diagnostic tools (compared to RT-PCR and IHC) in the absence of substrate-specific enzymatic activity assays. We confirmed that oxidative damage is a hallmark of LGMD2A and expanded on previous studies by showing that calpain-3 deficiency is associated with cytosolic redox imbalance and a mild reduction in ATP synthase levels. Given the fact that CAPN3 regulates calcium release and Ca^{2+} is necessary for transcription and function of ATP synthase, future studies

elucidating potential deficits in ATP production and F_0F_1 ATPase activity in LGMD2A patients may be warranted.

Supporting Information

Figure S1   Localization and distribution of 21 *CAPN3* sequence variants from our cohort of 14 LGMD2A patients along pre-mRNA (top), mRNA (middle), and protein (bottom). Mutational data adhere to the guidelines proposed by the Human Genome Variation Society (www.hgvs.org/mutnomen) and nucleotide numbering reflects the cDNA sequence with +1 corresponding to the A of the ATG translation initiation codon in the reference sequence. Exons 4, 11, 13, and 22 show the highest number of mutations, affecting protein domains II (3 mutations), III (4 mutations), and IV (2 mutations). Intronic mutations mainly affect domains III and IV. Domain I has regulatory role, domain II is the proteolytic module, domain III has a C2-like domain, and domain IV binds Ca^{2+} ions. NS, IS1, and IS2 are calpain-3 specific insertions.

Figure S2   Hematoxylin and eosin stain, immunohisto-chemical determination of fiber-type, and CAPN3 reactivity on flat sections in a sub-set of LGMD2A patients (total magnification 200×−400×). Top panel: Red circles show markedly increased abundance of internalized nuclei in calpain-deficient muscle. Middle panel: Primarily slow-twitch fiber atrophy and increased variation in fiber size/shape in LGMD2A patients. Note fast-twitch fiber dominance in P11. Lower panel: Normal CAPN3 reactivity in all subjects despite pathological mutations.

Table S1 [a]Clinical diagnosis: Phenotype consistent with major criteria of LGMD2A (see methods); [b]CAPN3 mRNA expression by RT-PCR (Fig. 1A); [c]Total CAPN3 protein expression on Western blot (Fig. 1B); [d]Ca^{2+}-induced CAPN3 autolytic activity assessed on immunoblot (Fig. 1C); [e]CAPN3 reactivity on 8 μm frozen sections (Fig. S2); ND: Not done; INDT: Indeterminate.

Acknowledgments

We gratefully acknowledge the patients and the volunteers in the Neuromuscular and Neurometabolic Clinic at McMaster University Hospital.

Author Contributions

Conceived and designed the experiments: MN MT. Performed the experiments: MN FA LM MH YK MA RS PD MS. Analyzed the data: MN FA LM MH YK MA RS PD MS. Contributed reagents/materials/analysis tools: MT. Contributed to the writing of the manuscript: MN MT.

References

1. Duguez S, Bartoli M, Richard I (2006) Calpain 3: a key regulator of the sarcomere? FEBS Journal 273: 3427–3436.
2. Saeenz A, Leturcq F, Cobo AM, Poza JJ, Ferrer X, et al. (2005) LGMD2A: genotype-phenotype correlations based on a large mutational survey on the calpain 3 gene. Brain 128: 732–742.
3. Kramerova I, Beckmann JS, Spencer MJ (2007) Molecular and cellular basis of calpainopathy (limb girdle muscular dystrophy type 2A). Biochimica et Biophysica Acta (BBA) - Molecular Basis of Disease 1772: 128–144.
4. Ono Y, Ojima K, Torii F, Takaya E, Doi N, et al. (2010) Skeletal muscle-specific calpain is an intracellular Na+-dependent protease. Journal of Biological Chemistry 285: 22986–22998.
5. Richard I, Broux O, Allamand Ve, Fougerousse Fo, Chiannilkulchai N, et al. (1995) Mutations in the proteolytic enzyme calpain 3 cause limb-girdle muscular dystrophy type 2A. Cell 81: 27–40.

6. Ojima K, Ono Y, Ottenheijm C, Hata S, Suzuki H, et al. (2011) Non-proteolytic functions of calpain-3 in sarcoplasmic reticulum in skeletal muscles. Journal of Molecular Biology 407: 439–449.
7. Kramerova I, Kudryashova E, Ermolova N, Saenz A, Jaka O, et al. (2012) Impaired calcium calmodulin kinase signaling and muscle adaptation response in the absence of calpain 3. Human Molecular Genetics 21: 3193–3204.
8. Kramerova I, Kudryashova E, Wu B, Ottenheijm C, Granzier H, et al. (2008) Novel role of calpain-3 in the triad-associated protein complex regulating calcium release in skeletal muscle. Human Molecular Genetics 17: 3271–3280.
9. Ojima K, Kawabata Y, Nakao H, Nakao K, Doi N, et al. (2012) Dynamic distribution of muscle-specific calpain in mice has a key role in physical-stress adaptation and is impaired in muscular dystrophy. The Journal of Clinical Investigation 120: 2672–2683.

10. Ojima K, Ono Y, Doi N, Yoshioka K, Kawabata Y, et al. (2007) Myogenic stage, sarcomere length, and protease activity modulate localization of muscle-specific calpain. Journal of Biological Chemistry 282: 14493–14504.
11. Murphy RM, Goodman CA, McKenna MJ, Bennie J, Leikis M, et al. (2007) Calpain-3 is autolyzed and hence activated in human skeletal muscle 24 h following a single bout of eccentric exercise. Journal of Applied Physiology 103: 926–931.
12. Milic A, Daniele N, Lochmuller H, Mora M, Comi GP, et al. (2007) A third of LGMD2A biopsies have normal calpain 3 proteolytic activity as determined by an in vitro assay. Neuromuscular Disorders 17: 148–156.
13. Fanin M, Fulizio L, Nascimbeni AC, Spinazzi M, Piluso G, et al. (2004) Molecular diagnosis in LGMD2A: Mutation analysis or protein testing? Human Mutation 24: 52–62.
14. Fanin M, Nascimbeni AC, Angelini C (2007) Screening of calpain-3 autolytic activity in LGMD muscle: a functional map of CAPN3 gene mutations. Journal of Medical Genetics 44: 38–43.
15. Fanin M, Nascimbeni AC, Fulizio L, Trevisan CP, Meznaric-Petrusa M, et al. (2003) Loss of calpain-3 autocatalytic activity in LGMD2A patients with normal protein expression. The American Journal of Pathology 163: 1929–1936.
16. Kramerova I, Kudryashova E, Wu B, Germain S, Vandenborne K, et al. (2009) Mitochondrial abnormalities, energy deficit and oxidative stress are features of calpain 3 deficiency in skeletal muscle. Human Molecular Genetics 18: 3194–3205.
17. Cohen N, Kudryashova E, Kramerova I, Anderson LVB, Beckmann JS, et al. (2006) Identification of putative in vivo substrates of calpain 3 by comparative proteomics of overexpressing transgenic and nontransgenic mice. Proteomics 6: 6075–6084.
18. Chae J, Minami N, Jin Y, Nakagawa M, Murayama K, et al. (2001) Calpain 3 gene mutations: genetic and clinico-pathologic findings in limb-girdle muscular dystrophy. Neuromuscular Disorders 11: 547–555.
19. Fardeau M, Eymard B, Mignard C, Tome FMS, Richard I, et al. (1996) Chromosome 15-linked limb-girdle muscular dystrophy: Clinical phenotypes in Reunion Island and French metropolitan communities. Neuromuscular Disorders 6: 447–453.
20. Rajakumar D, Alexander M, Oommen A (2013) Oxidative stress, NF-KB and the ubiquitin proteasomal pathway in the pathology of calpainopathy. Neurochemical Research: 1–10.
21. Angelini C, Fanin M (2005) Calpainopathy. In: Pagon R, Adam M, Bird T, editors. GeneReviews™. Seattle (WA): University of Washington.
22. Beckmann J, Bushby K (1996) Advances in the molecular genetics of the limb-girdle type of autosomal recessive progressive muscular dystrophy. Curr Opin Neurol (5): 389–393.
23. Nilsson MI, Laureano ML, Saeed M, Tarnopolsky MA (2013) Dysferlin aggregation in limb-girdle muscular dystrophy type 2B/Miyoshi myopathy necessitates mutational screen for diagnosis. Muscle & Nerve 47: 740–747.
24. Wu Y, Weber JL, Vladutiu GD, Tarnopolsky MA (2011) Six novel mutations in the myophosphorylase gene in patients with McArdle disease and a family with pseudo-dominant inheritance pattern. Molecular Genetics and Metabolism 104: 587–591.
25. Nilsson MI, Kroos MA, Reuser AJ, Hatcher E, Akhtar M, et al. (2014) Novel GAA sequence variant c.1211 A>G reduces enzyme activity but not protein expression in infantile and adult onset Pompe disease. Gene 537: 41–45.
26. Murphy RM, Snow RJ, Lamb GD (2006) u-Calpain and calpain-3 are not autolyzed with exhaustive exercise in humans. American Journal of Physiology - Cell Physiology 290: C116–C122.
27. Smith PK, Krohn RI, Hermanson GT, Mallia AK, Gartner FH, et al. (1985) Measurement of protein using bicinchoninic acid. Anal Biochem 150: 76–85.
28. McKenzie S, Phillips SM, Carter SL, Lowther S, Gibala MJ, et al. (2000) Endurance exercise training attenuates leucine oxidation and BCOAD activation during exercise in humans. American Journal of Physiology - Endocrinology and Metabolism 278: E580–E587.
29. Nilsson MI, Samjoo IA, Hettinga BP, Koeberl DD, Zhang H, et al. (2012) Aerobic training as an adjunctive therapy to enzyme replacement in Pompe disease. Molecular Genetics and Metabolism 107: 469–479.
30. Safdar A, Hamadeh MJ, Kaczor JJ, Raha S, deBeer J, et al. (2010) Aberrant mitochondrial homeostasis in the skeletal muscle of sedentary older adults. PLoS ONE 5: e10778.
31. Fanin M, Nascimbeni AC, Tasca E, Angelini C (2008) How to tackle the diagnosis of limb-girdle muscular dystrophy 2A. Eur J Hum Genet 17: 598–603.
32. Kolski HK, Hawkins C, Zatz M, De Paula F, Biggar D, et al. (2008) Diagnosis of limb-girdle muscular dystrophy 2A by immunohistochemical techniques. Neuropathology 28: 264–268.
33. Krahn M, Bernard R, Pécheux C, Hammouda EH, Eymard B, et al. (2006) Screening of the CAPN3 gene in patients with possible LGMD2A. Clinical Genetics 69: 444–449.
34. Ankala A, Kohn JN, Dastur R, Gaitonde P, Khadilkar SV, et al. (2013) Ancestral founder mutations in calpain-3 in the Indian Agarwal community: Historical, clinical, and molecular perspective. Muscle & Nerve 47: 931–937.
35. Todorova A, Kress W, Mueller C (2005) Novel mutations in the calpain 3 gene in Germany. Clinical Genetics 67: 356–358.
36. Piluso G, Politano L, Aurino S, Fanin M, Ricci E, et al. (2005) Extensive scanning of the calpain-3 gene broadens the spectrum of LGMD2A phenotypes. Journal of Medical Genetics 42: 686–693.
37. Desmet F-O, Hamroun D, Lalande M, Collod-Beroud G, Claustres M, et al. (2009) Human Splicing Finder: an online bioinformatics tool to predict splicing signals. Nucleic Acids Research 37: e67.
38. Kawai H, Akaike M, Kunishige M, Inui T, Adachi K, et al. (1998) Clinical, pathological, and genetic features of limb-girdle muscular dystrophy type 2A with new calpain 3 gene mutations in seven patients from three Japanese families. Muscle & Nerve 21: 1493–1501.
39. Kitaoka Y, Ogborn DI, Nilsson MI, Mocellin NJ, MacNeil LG, et al. (2013) Oxidative stress and Nrf2 signaling in McArdle disease. Mol Genet Metab 110: 297–302.
40. Fanin M, Nascimbeni AC, Angelini C (2013) Muscle atrophy in Limb Girdle Muscular Dystrophy 2A: a morphometric and molecular study. Neuropathology and Applied Neurobiology 39: 762–771.
41. Whitehead NP, Yeung EW, Froehner SC, Allen DG (2010) Skeletal muscle NADPH oxidase is increased and triggers stretch-induced damage in the mdx mouse. PLoS ONE 5: e15354.
42. Hood DA (2001) Invited Review: Contractile activity-induced mitochondrial biogenesis in skeletal muscle. Journal of Applied Physiology 90: 1137–1157.
43. Grover GJ, Marone PA, Koetzner L, Seto-Young D (2008) Energetic signalling in the control of mitochondrial F1F0 ATP synthase activity in health and disease. The International Journal of Biochemistry & Cell Biology 40: 2698–2701.

17

Bazhen Decoction Protects against Acetaminophen Induced Acute Liver Injury by Inhibiting Oxidative Stress, Inflammation and Apoptosis in Mice

Erqun Song, Juanli Fu, Xiaomin Xia, Chuanyang Su, Yang Song*

Key Laboratory of Luminescence and Real-Time Analytical Chemistry (Ministry of Education), College of Pharmaceutical Sciences, Southwest University, Chongqing, People's Republic of China

Abstract

Bazhen decoction is a widely used traditional Chinese medicinal decoction, but the scientific validation of its therapeutic potential is lacking. The objective of this study was to investigate corresponding anti-oxidative, anti-inflammatory and anti-apoptosis activities of Bazhen decoction, using acetaminophen-treated mice as a model system. A total of 48 mice were divided into four groups. Group I, negative control, treated with vehicle only. Group II, fed with 500 mg/kg/day Bazhen decoction for 10 continuous days. Group III, received a single dose of 900 mg/kg acetaminophen. Group IV, fed with 500 mg/kg/day Bazhen decoction for 10 continuous days and a single dose of 900 mg/kg acetaminophen 30 min before last Bazhen decoction administration. Bazhen decoction administration significantly decrease acetaminophen-induced serum ALT, AST, ALP, LDH, TNF-α, IL-1β, ROS, TBARS and protein carbonyl group levels, as well as GSH depletion and loss of MMP. Bazhen decoction restore SOD, CAT, GR and GPx activities and depress the expression of pro-inflammatory factors, such as iNOS, COX-2, TNF-α, NF-κB, IL-1β and IL-6, respectively. Moreover, Bazhen decoction down-regulate acetaminophen-induced Bax/Bcl-2 ratio, caspase 3, caspase 8 and caspase 9. These results suggest the anti-oxidative, anti-inflammatory and anti-apoptosis properties of Bazhen decoction towards acetaminophen-induced liver injury in mice.

Editor: Gautam Sethi, Yong Loo Lin School of Medicine, National University of Singapore, Singapore

Funding: This work was supported by the Fundamental Research Funds for the Central Universities (XDJK2014A020, XDJK2013B009). The funders had no role in study design, data collection and analysis, decision to publish, or preparation of the manuscript.

Competing Interests: The authors have declared that no competing interests exist.

* Email: songyangwenrong@hotmail.com

Introduction

Bazhen decoction, also recognized as eight-treasure decoction or eight precious decoction, was recorded in "A Repertory of Traumatology". Bazhen decoction is a traditional Chinese medicine formula which related to a lot of symptoms, such as anemia, asthenia, breathlessness, chronic abscess, dizziness, fatigue, glare, irregular menstruation, lethargy, metrorrhagia, palpitations, poor appetite, anxiety, dull complexion, fatigue of the muscles, pale complexion, pale tongue, thin-white coating, fine-faint pulse and large-forceless-empty pulse. In traditional use, Bazhen decoction is a frequently-used prescription for the treatment of "qi and blood" deficiency. Bazhen decoction is a combination of Sijunzi decoction and Siwu decoction. The traditional use of Sijunzi decoction was to replenish or invigorate the intestine and stomach function, and promote the circulation of "qi and blood" [1]. Siwu decoction removes heat to cool blood, promotes blood flow and regulates menstruation, which has the best treatment effect for conditions of Yin blood deficiency [2]. In traditional Chinese medicine theory, "qi and blood" supplement each other, therefore, the combination of Sijunzi and Siwu decoction brings out the best in each other and appropriate for more severe conditions.

Acetaminophen (4-hydroxyacetanilide) is a clinical analgesic/antipyretic drug [3]. Although acetaminophen is safe at therapeutic doses, it causes hepatic injury in both human and experimental animals. In fact, acetaminophen overdose is a leading cause of drug-related acute liver failure [4]. The hepatotoxicity of acetaminophen has been related to many emergency hospital admissions, such as hepatitis, cirrhosis, and hepatic transplant and continues to be associated with high mortality [5].

The mechanism of acetaminophen-induced hepatotoxic effect is well known and has been extensively reviewed [6–9]. Cytochromes P450, mainly CYP2E1, catalyze acetaminophen to form corresponding reactive metabolite of acetaminophen, N-acetyl-p-benzoquinone imine, which is responsible for cytotoxicity, mutagenicity, and potential carcinogenicity. N-acetyl-p-benzoquinone imine easily reacts with cellular glutathione (GSH) and proteins. Besides protein modification, acetaminophen also contributes to the generation of reactive oxygen species (ROS) during its metabolism process. Antioxidant enzymes, such as superoxide dismutase (SOD), catalase (CAT), glutathione reductase (GR) and glutathione peroxidase (GPx), play critical roles in modulating the severity of acetaminophen-induced hepatotoxicity [10]. Lipid peroxidation (LPO) is also thought to linked with the initiation or progression of liver injury induced by acetaminophen [11]. Acetaminophen overdose trigger the transcriptional activation of pro-inflammatory factors, such as TNF-α, IL-1β and others in macrophages [12]. Previous studies have extensively demonstrated that antioxidants play important roles in scavenge ROS, inhibit oxidative stress and down-regulation of pro-inflammatory factors to against acetaminophen-induced toxicity [13–17].

The active components of Bazhen decoction were previously identified, which implied Bazhen decoction may possess antioxidative, anti-inflammatory and anti-apoptosis activities [18]. However, there is no direct evidence to support this hypothesis at this stage, which encourage us conduct the present work in order to investigate the protective effect of Bazhen decoction against acetaminophen-induced liver injury in mice. In addition, the possible mechanisms underlying these effects were also investigated.

Materials and Methods

Ethics statements

All animal experiments were performed according to the protocol approved by the Experimental Animal Ethical Committee of Southwest University. Animals were maintained in specific pathogen free laboratory under standard conditions of humidity ($50 \pm 5\%$), temperature ($25 \pm 2°C$) in a 12 h light/12 h dark cycle. They were fed standard rodent chow and had free access to water, acclimatized for at least one week prior to use. All surgery was performed under ether anesthesia, and all efforts were made to minimize suffering.

Materials and reagents

Acetaminophen (>98.0% HPLC) were purchased from Sigma-Aldrich Inc. Silymarin, 2,4-dinitrophenylhydrazine (DNPH) and 5,5',6,6'-tetrachloro-1,1',3,3'-tetraethylbenzimidazol-carbocyanine iodide (JC-1) dye were obtained from Aladdin Reagent Database Inc. Diagnostic kits used for the determination of ROS, TBARS, GSH, tumor necrosis factor-alpha (TNF-α), interleukin-1beta (IL-1β), SOD, CAT, GR and GPx, AST, ALT, ALP and LDH activities were obtained from the Nanjing Jiancheng Institute of Biotechnology (Nanjing, China). Rabbit polyclonal COX-2, iNOS, TNF-α, NF-κB, IL-1β, IL-6, Bcl-2, Bax, cytochrome c, caspase 3, caspase 8 and caspase 9 antibodies were purchased from Dingguo Biotechnology Co. Ltd (Beijing, China). All other chemicals used were of highest commercial grade.

Preparation of Bazhen decoction

Herbs were purchased from an authentic herb supplier in the local market of Chongqing. Their Chinese names, English names, Latin names, family, part used, voucher numbers and daily adult dose (g) were presented in **Table 1**. The quality of these crude drugs was controlled and processed according to the Chinese Pharmacopoeia (2005). Radix Angelicae Sinensis (10 g), Rhizoma Chuanxiong (5 g), Radix Paeoniae Alba (8 g), Radix Rehmannia Libosch (15 g), Radix Ginseng (3 g), Rhizoma Atractylodis Macrocephalae (10 g), Poria cocos (8 g) and Radix Glycyrrhiza (5 g) were immersed in 500 mL distilled water and boiled for 30 min. The aqueous part was filtered. This procedure was repeated twice and the aqueous solutions were combined and lyophilized to yield brown pellet (5.7%, w/w). The dry residue was dispersed in distilled water before use.

Animals and treatment

Male Kunming mice (20–24 g, 4 weeks old) were purchased from Chongqing Tengxin Biotechnology Co. Mice were randomly divided into five groups, each group consisting of 12 animals. (1) Negative control group, treated with vehicle only, (2) Bazhen group, 500 mg/kg/day Bazhen decoction was administered by intragastric gavage for 10 continuous days, (3) acetaminophen group, a single dose of 900 mg/kg acetaminophen (ip), (4) acetaminophen + Bazhen group, 500 mg/kg/day Bazhen decoction was administered by intragastric gavage for 10 continuous days and (5) acetaminophen + Silymarin group, 100 mg/kg/day Silymarin was administered by intragastric gavage for 10 continuous days. On the 10th day, a single dose of 900 mg/kg acetaminophen was injected (ip) 30 min before Bazhen decoction administration. After 12 h of acetaminophen injection, the animals were sacrificed under deep anesthesia. Blood was collected by cardiac puncture and allowed to clot for 45 min at room temperature. The livers were excised carefully, washed twice with saline, blotted dry on a filter paper, weighed and cut into two pieces. One halves were used for immunohistochemical analysis. Other halves were used for hepatic homogenate preparation.

Cytosolic fraction isolation

Cell lysates were added to cytosolic extraction buffer, vortexed vigorously for 15 s. After incubation for 10 min on ice, cell lysates were centrifuged at 12,000 rpm for 10 min and the cytosolic fraction supernatants were transferred to new tubes and stored at $-20°C$ until used.

Biochemical analysis

The blood samples were centrifuged (600 g for 15 min) for serum collection. Serum analysis of various liver marker enzymes, such as ALT, AST, ALP and LDH activities were measured using assay kits according to the supplier specifications (Nanjing Jiancheng). Serum TNF-α and IL-1β were determined using commercially available enzyme linked-immunosorbent assay (ELISA) kits (Nanjing Jiancheng) according to the manufacturer's instructions.

Liver were rinsed in ice-cold physiological saline and homogenized in Tris-HCl buffer (0.01 M, pH = 7.4) to give a 10% homogenate. Homogenates were centrifuged at 3,000 rpm, 4°C for 10 min and supernatants were collected for further analysis. In the tissue samples, hepatic ROS, TBARS, GSH, SOD, CAT, GR and GPx levels were determined with commercial assay kits (Nanjing Jiancheng). Protein oxidative damage was evaluated by measuring protein carbonyl formation using 2,4-dinitrophenylhydrazine (DNPH) as a probe. Carbonyl content was determined by measuring the spectra of the supernatant at 365 nm (UV-2450, SHIMADZU, Japan). The results were expressed as nmol of DNPH incorporated/mg protein based on the molar extinction coefficient of 22,000 M^{-1} cm^{-1} for aliphatic hydrazones.

Measurement of mitochondrial membrane potential (MMP)

Changes in mitochondrial membrane potential were assessed by staining with JC-1 dye. The homogenates were incubated with JC-1 staining buffer (5 μg/mL) for 20 min in the dark at 37°C. MMP were monitored by recording green (excitation/emission wavelength = 485/510–525 nm) and red (excitation/emission wavelength = 485/590 nm) fluorescence using a fluorescence microscope. Mitochondrial depolarization is indicated by an increase ratio in green fluorescence and decrease in red fluorescence.

Immunohistochemical analysis of iNOS and COX-2

The paraffin-embedded sections were deparaffinized and rehydrated and were treated with a 1 mM EDTA buffer (pH = 9.0) in a microwave for 3 min for antigen retrieval. The following steps were followed the instruction of Histostain TM-

Table 1. The compositions of Bazhen decoction.

Chinese names	English names	Latin names	Family	Part used	Voucher numbers	daily adult dose (g)
Danggui	Radix *Angelicae Sinensis*	Angelica sinensis (Oliv.) Diels	Umbelliferae	Root	20130205	10
Chuanxiong	Rhizoma *Chuanxiong*	Ligusticum striatum DC.	Apiaceae	Rhizome	20130306	5
Baishao	Radix *Paeoniae Alba*	Paeonia sterniana H.R.Fletcher	Paeoniaceae	Root	20130205	8
Shudi	Radix *Rehmannia Libosch*	Rehmannia glutinosa (Gaertn.) DC.	Plantaginaceae	Processed root tuber	20130306	15
Renshen	Radix *Ginseng*	Panax ginseng C.A.Mey	Araliaceae	Root	20130205	3
Baizhu	Rhizoma *Atractylodis Macrocephalae*	Atractylodes macrocephala Koidz	Compositae	Rhizome	20130205	10
Fuling	*Poria cocos*	Poria cocos wolf	Fungus	Sclerotium	20130401	8
Zhigancao	Radix *Glycyrrhiza*	Glycyrrhiza uralensis Fisch.	Leguminosae	Honeyed root and rhizome	20130205	5

Plus and diaminobenzidine substrate kits. Briefly, 3% H_2O_2 was used to block endogenous peroxidase activity. Nonspecific protein binding was blocked by normal goat serum. The rabbit polyclonal anti-COX-2 diluted 1:50, and rabbit polyclonal anti-iNOS diluted 1:50 were used as primary antibodies. Then, slide was incubated with biotin labeled goat-rabbit IgG and horseradish peroxidase-conjugated streptavidin for 1 h, respectively. Immunoreaction was visualized employing diaminobenzidine and counterstained by hematoxylin. Image was taken by a light microscopy (magnification, 200×, Nikon Eclipse Ti-SR).

Western blotting

Proteins were separated by 10% SDS-PAGE electrophoresis and transferred onto nitrocellulose membrane. After blocking with 10% skimmed milk, membranes were incubated with primary polyclone rabbit antibodies TNF-α, NF-κB, IL-1β, IL-6, Bcl-2, Bax, cytochrome c, caspase 3, caspase 8 and caspase 9 at room temperature for 3 h. After washing three times with PBS, membranes were further incubated with secondary antibody conjugated with horseradish peroxidase (HRP) for 1.5 h. Finally, immune-reactive protein bands were detected by diaminobenzidine method. The relative density of protein expressions were quantitated by ImageJ software. Protein levels were standardized by comparison with β-actin.

RNA isolation and real-time RT-PCR

Total cellular RNA was extracted from liver homogenate using innuPREP Micro RNA Kit according to the manufacturer's instructions (AJ Innuscreen GmbH). mRNA was reversely transcribed into cDNA (MMLV Reverse Transcriptase, Gibco/BRL) using oligo(dT) as primers and two-step real-time PCR was carried out using a LightCycler (Roche, Basel, Switzerland). Primers sequences were used as previous reported [19]. Bcl-2, 5'-GGGATGCCTTTGTGGAACTATA TG-3' (forward), 5'-TGAGCAGCGTCTTCAGAGACA-3' (reverse); Bax, 5'-GA-CACCTG AGCTGACCTTGGA-3' (forward), 5'-GA-CACTCGCTCAGCTTCTTGGT-3' (reverse); GAPDH, 5'-GCA CCG TCA AGG CTG AGA AC-3' (forward), 5'-TGG TGA AGA CGC CAG TGGA-3' (reverse). Thermocycler conditions included an initial holding period at 50°C for 2 min, then 94°C for 2 min, followed by 40 cycles of denaturation at 94°C for 30 s, annealing at 55°C for 15 s and extension at 72°C for 15 s. SYBR Green I fluorescence emission was monitored after each cycle, and mRNA levels were quantified using the second-derivative maximum method of the LightCycler software. The amount of each gene was expressed relative to the housekeeping gene, GAPDH. The products were separated by electrophoresis in 2% agarose gels and visualized by nucleic acid stain (Dingguo Biotechnology Co., Beijing, China) under ultraviolet light.

Histopathological examination

Parts of the liver tissue were fixed by immersion in 4% paraformaldehyde and dehydrated. Sections of 5 μm thickness were taken and stained with hematoxylin and eosin (H&E). Slides were observed for histopathological changes using fluorescence microscope system (TE2000, Nikon, Japan) and representative images were presented.

Statistical analysis

All experiments were repeated at least three times independently. All values were expressed as means ± SEM. The results were evaluated by one-way ANOVA and Tukey's multiple comparison tests. Differences were considered to be significant only for $p < 0.05$.

Results

Effect of Bazhen decoction on serum biochemical parameters

Serum ALT/AST/ALP activities were assessed as biochemical markers of hepatic damage (**Table 2**). Bazhen decoction (500 mg/kg/day) treatment resulted in no change in serum ALT/AST/ALP activities compare to control group. A single dose of acetaminophen (900 mg/kg) showed hepatotoxic effect with the evidence of increased in ALT/AST/ALP serum activities. In contrast, Bazhen decoction treatment prevented acetaminophen-induced elevation of ALT/AST/ALP serum activities significantly. There has no significant difference between Bazhen and control group. Serum LDH activity is a marker of generalized tissue damage as well. Our result showed a significant increase in acetaminophen group (4356.1±134.5 U/L) when compared to control group (877.4±45.6 U/L), however, acetaminophen + Bazhen group showed reduced LDH activity (1032.5±99.5 U/L, $p < 0.001$ *vs* acetaminophen group). Silymarin also showed protective effect may imply similar protective mechanism.

Table 2. Effects of Bazhen decoction on serum biochemical parameters in mice intoxicated with acetaminophen.

group	ALT (U/L)	AST (U/L)	ALP (U/L)	LDH (U/L)
control	43.2±7.0	50.3±5.9	120.1±11.9	877.4±45.6
Bazhen	35.8±6.9	41.1±8.2	123.4±22.1	822.4±62.0
acetaminophen	767.1±152.0***	1003.6±181.4***	480.3±35.9***	4356.1±134.5***
acetaminophen + Bazhen	122.2±38.4###	279.0±60.2###	184.8±24.7###	1032.5±99.5###
acetaminophen + Silymarin	81.8±15.6###	110.5±22.6###	167.8±22.9###	908.5±113.7###

Values are expressed as means ± SD of 12 animals in each group. Significance difference were ***$p<0.001$ as compared with the control; ###$p<0.001$ as compared with acetaminophen group.

Effect of Bazhen decoction on serum cytokine expressions

To investigate the effect of Bazhen decoction on the modulation of inflammatory cytokines, serum TNF-α and IL-1β were determined. As shown in **Figure 1**, Acetaminophen-administration significantly increased levels of TNF-α (56.1±11.2 pg/mL) and IL-1β (65.7±4.2 pmol/mL) compared with their levels in normal mice (17.9±2.4 pg/mL and 24.1±4.9 pmol/mL, respectively), suggesting that severe inflammatory reaction had been conducted. However, Bazhen decoction significantly inhibited serum TNF-α and IL-1β levels (36.6±4.7 pg/mL and 52.0±4.9 pmol/mL, respectively, $p<0.001$, compared with acetaminophen group.

Effect of Bazhen decoction on hepatic non-protein oxidative stress markers

Acetaminophen administration showed increased levels of ROS (121.3±8.5% vs. 100%, $p<0.001$), TBARS (4.4±0.1 vs. 3.3±0.3 μmol/g protein, $p<0.001$) and protein carbonyl group (16.6±2.1 vs. 6.5±1.2 μmol/g protein, $p<0.001$) in the mice liver, as compared to control group, **Figure 2A, 2B and 2C**. However, acetaminophen + Bazhen group had significantly inhibition of ROS (106.6±3.4%), TBARS (3.7±0.2 μmol/g protein) and

protein carbonyl group (10.7±3.0 μmol/g protein), $p<0.001$ respectively.

The endogenous antioxidant, GSH level in hepatic tissue was decreased significantly ($p<0.01$) in acetaminophen group (10.0±0.70 mg/g) as compared to control group (12.1±0.31 mg/g), while Bazhen decoction treatment significantly ($p<0.05$) reversed this acetaminophen-induced GSH reduction (11.8±0.55 mg/g), **Figure 2D**.

Effect of Bazhen decoction on hepatic antioxidant enzyme activities

Hepatic SOD (39.8±4.1 vs. 53.8±4.0 U/mg protein), CAT (51.6±4.5 vs. 74.5±6.1 U/mg protein), GR (9.4±0.8 vs. 15.3±1.0 U/g protein) and GPx (101.6±10.7 vs. 213.8±15.5 U/mg protein) activities were significantly reduced in acetaminophen-intoxicated mice, compared to normal group ($p<0.001$), as shown in **Figure 3**. However, pretreatment with Bazhen decoction significantly enhanced SOD (47.6±3.0 U/mg protein), CAT (73.3±4.4 U/mg protein), GR (12.2±1.0 U/g protein) and GPx (175.9±11.0 U/mg protein) activities compared with those of acetaminophen-intoxicated mice. Administration of Bazhen decoction alone has no significant effect on enzymatic antioxidants.

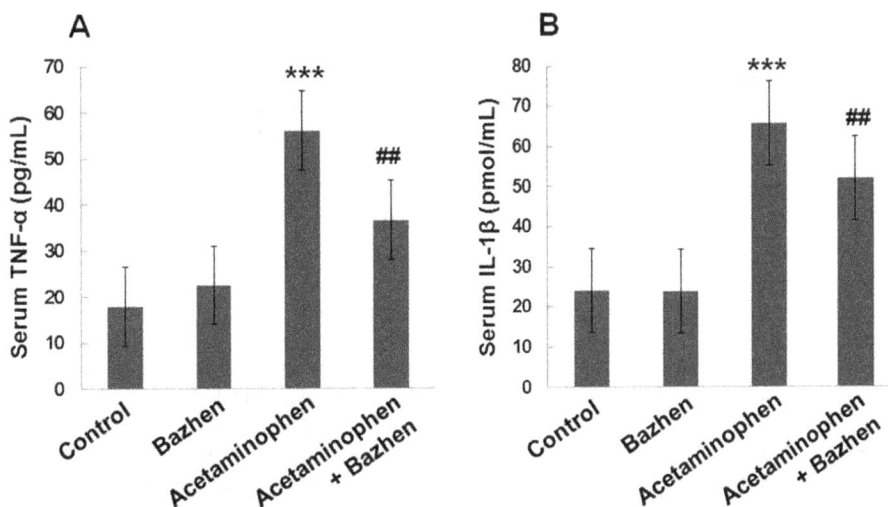

Figure 1. Effect of Bazhen decoction on serum TNF-α and IL-1β levels in acetaminophen intoxicated mice. (**A**) TNF-α and (**B**) IL-1β. Values are expressed as means ± SD of 12 animals in each group. Significance difference were ***$p<0.001$ as compared with the control; ##$p<0.01$ as compared with acetaminophen group.

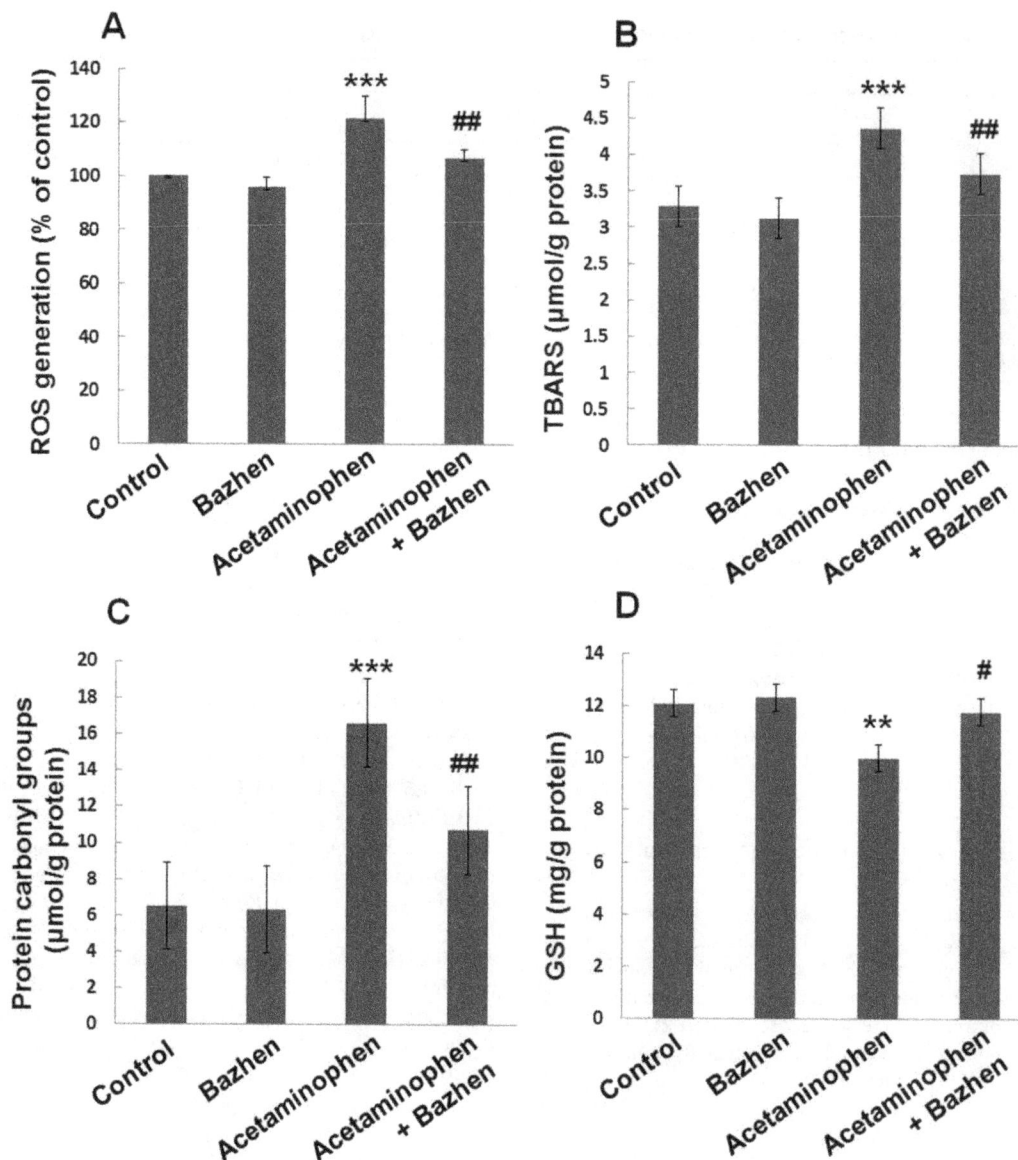

Figure 2. Effect of Bazhen decoction on hepatic ROS, TBARS, protein carbonyl group and GSH levels in acetaminophen intoxicated mice. (A) ROS, (B) TBARS, (C) protein carbonyl group and (D) GSH. Values are expressed as means ± SD of 12 animals in each group. Significance difference were ***$p<0.001$ or **$p<0.01$ as compared with the control; ##$p<0.01$ or #$p<0.05$ as compared with acetaminophen group.

Effect of Bazhen decoction on inflammatory response in mouse livers

We observed the effect of Bazhen decoction on hepatic iNOS and COX-2 levels using immunohistochemical assay. The livers of control mice did not show substantial iNOS and COX-2 immunopositivity (**Figure 4A and 4E**), and the animals receiving Bazhen decoction alone were similar to control (**Figure 4B and 4F**). However, acetaminophen-treatment dramatically increased iNOS and COX-2 immunopositivity in the livers compared with control (**Figure 4C and 4G**), which was attenuated by Bazhen decoction administration (**Figure 4D and 4H**).

Western blotting results indicated the protective effect of Bazhen decoction on the expression of TNF-α, NF-κB, IL-1β and IL-6 in hepatic tissues. All these proteins associated with inflammation showed significantly up-regulated in acetaminophen

group, but down-regulated with Bazhen decoction administration (**Figure 5**).

Effect of Bazhen decoction on apoptosis features in mouse livers

The decreased anti-apoptotic gene Bcl-2 and increased pro-apoptotic gene Bax were showed in acetaminophen-intoxicated mice liver, however, Bazhen decoction reverted these changes significantly (**Figure 6A**). It is interesting to notice that acetaminophen showed significant effect on mRNA levels of Bcl-2 and Bax, which is coordinate with their protein expressions (**Figure 6B**). To gain a better understanding of the underlying mechanism, we determined the effect of Bazhen decoction on acetaminophen-induced loss of MMP. As shown in **Figure 6C**, the loss of MMP was observed after treatment with acetaminophen. However, Bazhen decoction reversed this effect, although no statistical

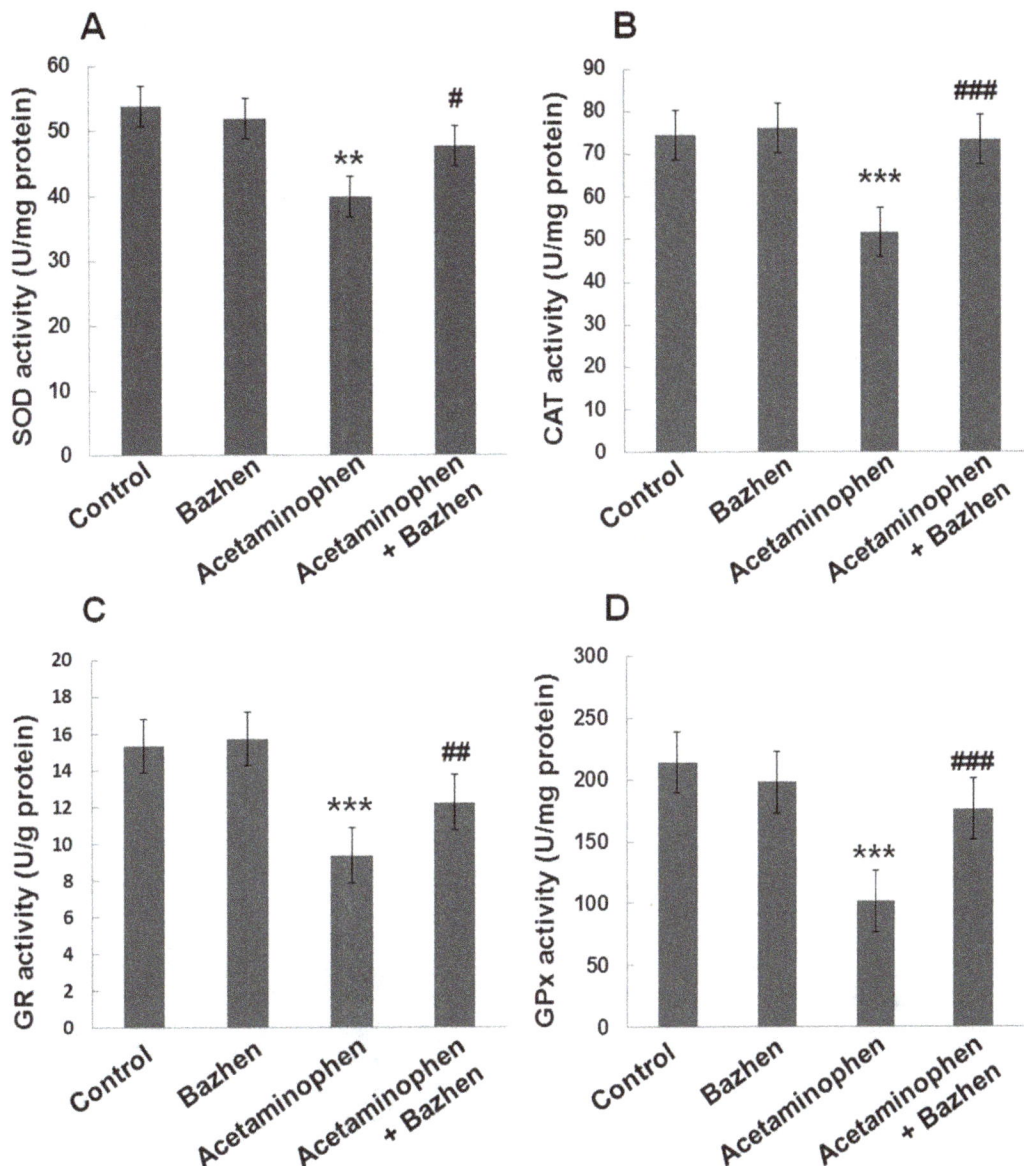

Figure 3. Effects of Bazhen decoction on the hepatic antioxidant enzymes activities in mice intoxicated with acetaminophen. (A) SOD, **(B)** CAT, **(C)** GR and **(D)** GPx. Values are expressed as means ± SD of 12 animals in each group. Significance difference were ***$p<0.001$ or **$p<0.01$ as compared with the control; ###$p<0.001$, ##$p<0.01$ or #$p<0.05$ as compared with acetaminophen group.

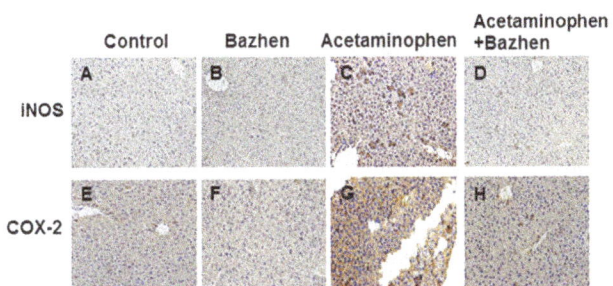

Figure 4. Effects of Bazhen decoction on acetaminophen-induced immunohistochemical stain of iNOS and COX-2 expression in liver tissue. Typical images were shown for iNOS expression in **(A)** control, **(B)** Bazhen, **(C)** acetaminophen and **(D)** acetaminophen + Bazhen group, and COX-2 expression in **(E)** control, **(F)** Bazhen, **(G)** acetaminophen and **(H)** acetaminophen + Bazhen group. Original magnification 200×.

significance was found between (Bazhen and acetaminophen + Bazhen group). In addition, the expressions of cleaved (activated) caspase family protein following the administration of acetaminophen were higher than in the control group. On the contrary, Bazhen administration attenuated the enhanced expression of activated caspase family proteins.

Histopathological changes were presented in **Figure 7** to support the effect of Bazhen decoction on acetaminophen-induced liver injury. Liver section in acetaminophen group showed cytoplasmic vacuolation and degeneration of hepatocytes, along with necrosis and inflammatory cells, compare with control group. Bazhen effectively limits the acetaminophen-induced acute liver injury.

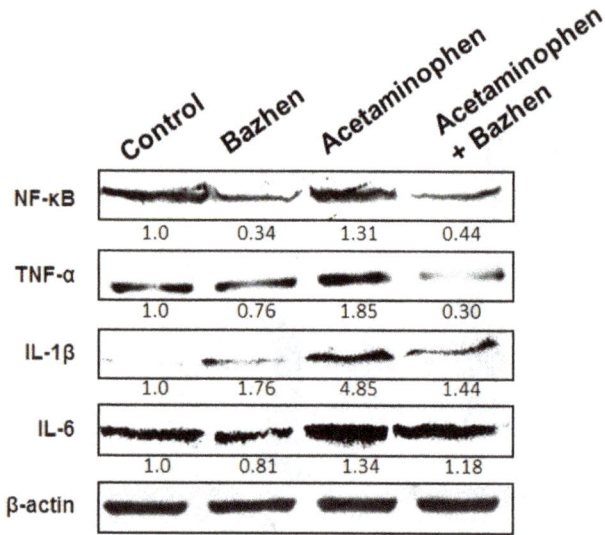

Figure 5. Effects of Bazhen decoction on the hepatic NF-κB, TNF-α, IL-6 and IL-1β expressions in mice intoxicated with acetaminophen. Data were normalized to β-actin used as control.

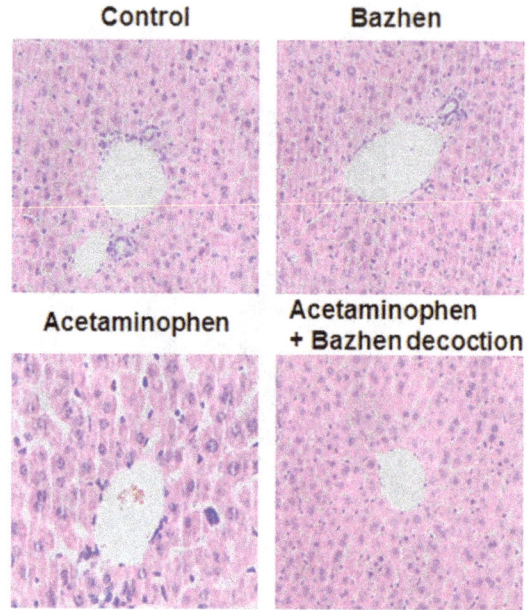

Figure 7. Effect of Bazhen decoction on acetaminophen-induced histopathological change in the liver tissue. Original magnifications were 200x.

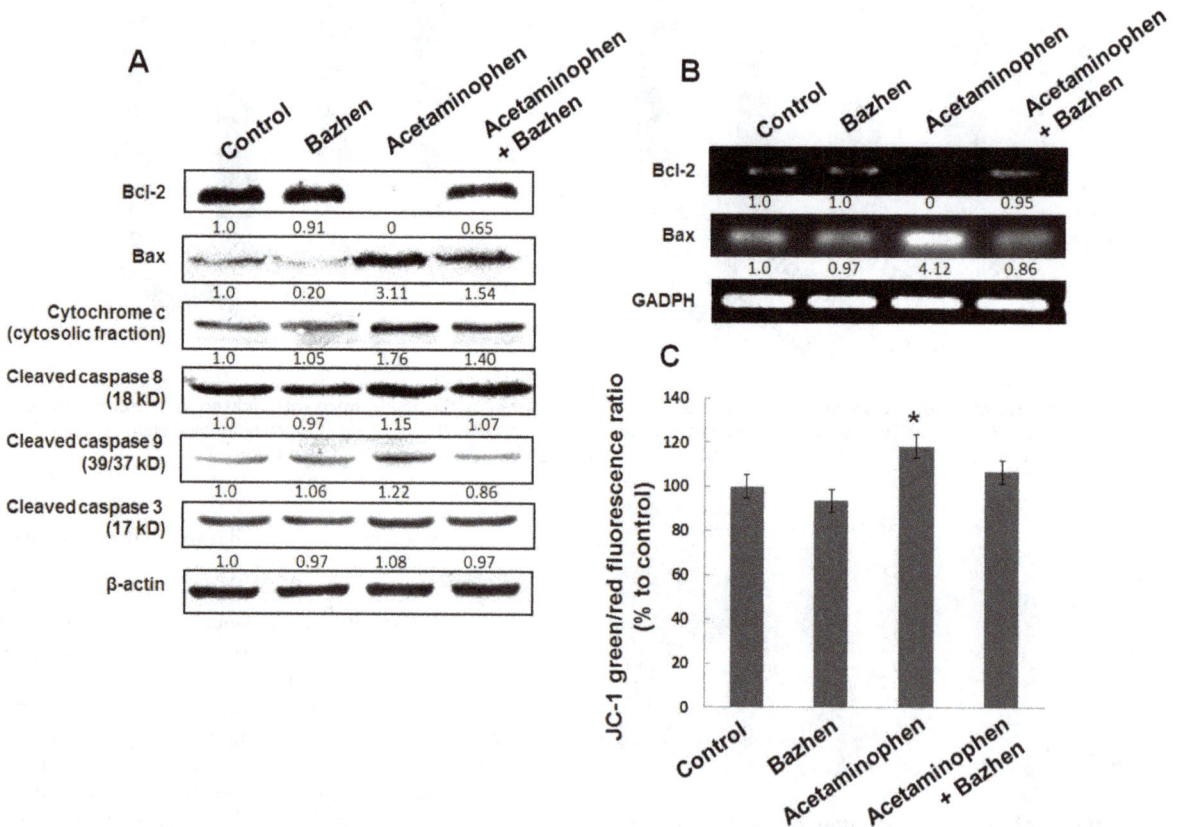

Figure 6. Effects of Bazhen decoction on apoptotic features in mice intoxicated with acetaminophen. (**A**) Western blotting of Bcl-2, Bax, cytochrome c (cytosolic fraction), cleaved caspase 8, 9 and 3 expressions. Data were normalized to β-actin used as control, (**B**) mRNA expression of Bcl-2 and Bax. GAPDH was used as internal control and (**C**) Fluorimetric quantified the green to red fluorescence ratio of JC-1. The value of control group was set as 100%.

Discussion

Early study identified the metabolites of Bazhen decoction from rat feces using a high performance liquid chromatography/mass spectrometry (HPLC/MS) technique [18]. A total of 29 major fragments were found and 19 chemical constituents were identified in Bazhen decoction, including Paeoniflorin, Atractylenolide II, Benzoyl-paeoniflorin, Liquiritin, Pachymic acid, Ginsenoside Re, Ginsenoside Rg_1, Ginsenoside Rb_1, Ginsenoside Rd, Glycyrrhizic acid, Paeonimetabolin I, Aucubinine A, 20-O-β-D-glucopyrano-syl-20 (S)-protopanaxadiol, 20 (S)-Protopanaxatriol, 16 α-hydroxy acids perforation, 20 (S)-Protopanaxadiol, Licorice saponine, 18 β-Glycyrrhetinic acid and Ginsenoside Rh_1. Liu *et al* identified three types of active components, ginsenoside, flavonoid and triterpe-noid in Sijunzi decoction, using HPLC-coupled tandem mass spectrometry (HPLC/MS^n) [1]. Su *et al* identified eighty-four components in Siwu decoction, including ten organic acids, thirty glycosides, fourteen lactones, eighteen flavonoids and eleven alkaloids using ultra-high performance liquid chromatography coupled time-of-flight mass spectrometry (UPLC-QTOF-MS^n) and HPLC-DAD [20]. Many investigators illustrated these constituents have promising anti-oxidative and anti-inflammatory activities. For example, Paeoniflorin protects human EA.hy926 endothelial cells against gamma-radiation induced oxidative injury by activating the NF-E2-related factor 2/heme oxygenase-1 pathway and it also protect against LPS-induced liver inflamma-tion [21,22], liquiritin exerts neuroprotective effect against focal cerebral ischemia/reperfusion in mice *via* its anti-oxidative properties [23], pachymic acid improves bone disturbance against AH plus-induced inflammation in MC-3T3 E1 cells for its anti-oxidative property [24], ginsenoside analogs have great potential on anti-oxidative and anti-inflammatory applications for Alzhei-mer's disease and other neurodegenerative disorders [25–27]. Paeoniflorin showed effective effect on the protection of hypoxia-induced apoptosis in endothelial cells [28]. These results strongly suggested the protective effect of Bazhen decoction.

Liver is a major organ for metabolism, which has a number of functions including glycogen storage, decomposition of red blood cells, plasma protein synthesis and detoxification. However, it is also an important target for the toxicity of drugs in terms of oxidative stress. The accumulation of ROS, including superoxide, hydroxyl, and hydrogen peroxide cause oxidative stress and DNA, proteins and lipids damages. Acetaminophen-induced hepatotox-icity is characterized as increased oxidative stress and the massive impairment of antioxidant defense systems [7]. Lipid peroxidation is also associated with acetaminophen-induced toxicity [29]. The level of TBARS and protein carbonyl group, which indicate the degree of lipid and protein peroxidation, respectively. On the other hand, cellular antioxidant enzymes, including SOD, CAT, GR and GPx were impaired with acetaminophen treatment [30]. The present study showed TBARS/protein carbonyl group level was significantly increased and the activities of SOD/CAT/GR/GPx in mice liver were dramatically decreased by the treatment of acetaminophen. Interestingly, Bazhen decoction could markedly inhibit TBARS and protein carbonyl group formations and restore the activities of those antioxidant enzymes in the livers of acetaminophen-treated mice. In addition, Bazhen decoction remarkably reduced serum ALT/AST/ALP/LDH levels, which coincided with the reduction of acetaminophen-induced oxidative injury. These results, for the first time, indicate that Bazhen decoction protected the liver against oxidative stress through the inhibitions of ROS production and lipid/protein peroxidation.

Inflammation has been considered as a protective reaction to against invading pathogens or chemicals in order to maintain body health [31]. However, the inflammatory process, also mediate the progression of tissue damage and resulting in a number of neurodegenerative diseases, *e.g.*, Alzheimer's disease and Parkin-son's disease [32]. Inhibition of inflammatory cytokine production play a central role in therapeutic potential for treatment of inflammatory diseases. During inflammation, many cytokines were up-regulated and accumulated in the liver, among them, TNF-α [33] and IL-1β [34] have been recently implicated as critical mediators of acetaminophen-induced hepatotoxicity. In the current study, we demonstrated that Bazhen decoction exhibits anti-inflammatory properties by inhibiting the activities of TNF-α and IL-1β in serum and the expression of iNOS, COX-2, TNF-α, NF-κB, IL-1β and IL-6 in liver. Inflammation mediated damage also attributed to over-production iNOS and COX-2 [35]. iNOS is essential in immune and inflammatory response to a variety of xenobiotics, which reflect the degree of inflammation. COX-2, an inducible isoform of cyclooxygenases, has been associated with inflammatory response in many different diseases [36]. Both iNOS and COX-2 were up-regulated in response to inflammation challenge, have been shown to be the major factors in mediating inflammatory processes. These results implied that the protective effect of Bazhen decoction may also due to its anti-inflammatory ability.

Massive evidences demonstrated acetaminophen induced trans-location of Bcl-2 family proteins [37], release of cytochrome c [38] and positive cells staining for TUNEL assay [39]. Therefore, we also investigated the effect of Bazhen decoction on acetamino-phen-induced apoptotic signals. Our results revealed that acetaminophen down-regulated Bcl-2 and up-regulated Bax in hepatocytes, which is in line with previous studies [40,41]. Accordingly, acetaminophen-induced release of cytochrome c from the mitochondria to the cytoplasm with the breakdown of MMP, and the activation of caspase 8, caspase 9 and caspase 3 were showed in previous works [41–43]. However, we first showed that Bazhen decoction administration dramatically reversed acetaminophen-induced elevation of Bax/Bcl-2 ratio on protein and mRNA level respectively. It also alleviated the release of cytochrome c, as well as the activation of caspase 8, caspase 9 and caspase 3. It is worth to mention that only slight up-regulation of cleaved caspase family proteins were detected in acetaminophen-treated animals. Some arguments claimed that acetaminophen-induced Bax translocation or cytochrome c release are not specific for apoptosis features, and there has no evidence for caspase activation [37,38], therefore, acetaminophen-induced liver injury may *via* necrosis rather than apoptosis mechanism. Indeed, histopathological examination showed necrosis and inflammatory cells in the current study. However, controversial results also presented, acetaminophen was found not only down-regulated Bcl-2 and up-regulated Bax, release of cytochrome c, but also the activation of caspase 9/3 [40,41]. Interestingly, Ray et al first reported that 40% of hepatocytes actually die by apoptosis after acetaminophen overdose [44], however, a detailed morphological study clearly demonstrated that >95% of injured hepatocytes die through oncotic necrosis in vivo [39]. Therefore, the mechanism of acetaminophen induced cell death may base on their corresponding experimental model, and need further investiga-tion.

In conclusion, our results confirmed the anti-oxidative, anti-inflammatory and anti-apoptosis effects of Bazhen decoction in acetaminophen-treated mice. The protective mechanism of Bazhen decoction is, at least in part, associated with the up-regulation of anti-oxidative enzyme activities and down-regulation of pro-inflammatory factors resulting from acetaminophen admin-istration. In addition, Bazhen decoction disrupted the mitochondrial apoptotic pathway by up-regulating Bcl-2 and down-regulating Bax expression, preventing caspase 8, caspase 9 and caspase 3 activation. Taking together, Bazhen decoction might be used as a potential therapeutic strategy to prevent acute liver injury encountered with acetaminophen overdose. Furthermore, our results indicated the possible usage of Bazhen decoction in the treatment of toxic acute liver failure.

References

1. Liu Y, Yang J, Cai Z (2006) Chemical investigation on Sijunzi decoction and its two major herbs Panax ginseng and Glycyrrhiza uralensis by LC/MS/MS. J Pharm Biomed Anal 41: 1642–1647.
2. Shang X, He X, He X, Li M, Zhang R, et al. (2010) The genus Scutellaria an ethnopharmacological and phytochemical review. J Ethnopharmacol 128: 279–313.
3. Lores Arnaiz S, Llesuy S, Cutrin JC, Boveris A (1995) Oxidative stress by acute acetaminophen administration in mouse liver. Free Radic Biol Med 19: 303–310.
4. Botta D, Shi S, White CC, Dabrowski MJ, Keener CL, et al. (2006) Acetaminophen-induced liver injury is attenuated in male glutamate-cysteine ligase transgenic mice. J Biol Chem 281: 28865–28875.
5. Colle D, Arantes LP, Gubert P, da Luz SC, Athayde ML, et al. (2012) Antioxidant properties of Taraxacum officinale leaf extract are involved in the protective effect against hepatoxicity induced by acetaminophen in mice. J Med Food 15: 549–556.
6. Jaeschke H, McGill MR, Ramachandran A (2012) Oxidant stress, mitochondria, and cell death mechanisms in drug-induced liver injury: lessons learned from acetaminophen hepatotoxicity. Drug Metab Rev 44: 88–106.
7. Jaeschke H, McGill MR, Williams CD, Ramachandran A (2011) Current issues with acetaminophen hepatotoxicity–a clinically relevant model to test the efficacy of natural products. Life Sci 88: 737–745.
8. Hinson JA, Roberts DW, James LP (2010) Mechanisms of acetaminophen-induced liver necrosis. Handb Exp Pharmacol: 369–405.
9. Jaeschke H (2005) Role of inflammation in the mechanism of acetaminophen-induced hepatotoxicity. Expert Opin Drug Metab Toxicol 1: 389–397.
10. Michael Brown J, Ball JG, Wright MS, Van Meter S, Valentovic MA (2012) Novel protective mechanisms for S-adenosyl-L-methionine against acetaminophen hepatotoxicity: improvement of key antioxidant enzymatic function. Toxicol Lett 212: 320–328.
11. Li G, Chen JB, Wang C, Xu Z, Nie H, et al. (2013) Curcumin protects against acetaminophen-induced apoptosis in hepatic injury. World J Gastroenterol 19: 7440–7446.
12. Jaeschke H, Williams CD, Ramachandran A, Bajt ML (2012) Acetaminophen hepatotoxicity and repair: the role of sterile inflammation and innate immunity. Liver Int 32: 8–20.
13. Liu WX, Jia FL, He YY, Zhang BX (2012) Protective effects of 5-methoxypsoralen against acetaminophen-induced hepatotoxicity in mice. World J Gastroenterol 18: 2197–2202.
14. Wu YL, Jiang YZ, Jin XJ, Lian LH, Piao JY, et al. (2010) Acanthoic acid, a diterpene in Acanthopanax koreanum, protects acetaminophen-induced hepatic toxicity in mice. Phytomedicine 17: 475–479.
15. Choi JH, Choi CY, Lee KJ, Hwang YP, Chung YC, et al. (2009) Hepatoprotective effects of an anthocyanin fraction from purple-fleshed sweet potato against acetaminophen-induced liver damage in mice. J Med Food 12: 320–326.
16. Olaleye MT, Rocha BT (2008) Acetaminophen-induced liver damage in mice: effects of some medicinal plants on the oxidative defense system. Exp Toxicol Pathol 59: 319–327.
17. Lee KJ, You HJ, Park SJ, Kim YS, Chung YC, et al. (2001) Hepatoprotective effects of Platycodon grandiflorum on acetaminophen-induced liver damage in mice. Cancer Lett 174: 73–81.
18. Li w, Bai J, Wang M, Ji Y (2012) Identification of the chemical constituents of bazhen decoction in rat feces by high performance liquid chromatography electro spray ionization mass spectrometry (HPLC-ESI/MS) [n]. Journal of Medicinal Plants Research 6: 2601–2605.
19. Xu Y, Wang H, Bao S, Tabassam F, Cai W, et al. (2013) Amelioration of liver injury by continuously targeted intervention against TNFRp55 in rats with acute-on-chronic liver failure. PLoS One 8: e68757.
20. Su S, Cui W, Zhou W, Duan JA, Shang E, et al. (2013) Chemical fingerprinting and quantitative constituent analysis of Siwu decoction categorized formulae by UPLC-QTOF/MS/MS and HPLC-DAD. Chin Med 8: 5.
21. Yu J, Zhu X, Qi X, Che J, Cao B (2013) Paeoniflorin protects human EA.hy926 endothelial cells against gamma-radiation induced oxidative injury by activating the NF-E2-related factor 2/heme oxygenase-1 pathway. Toxicol Lett 218: 224–234.
22. Kim ID, Ha BJ (2010) The effects of paeoniflorin on LPS-induced liver inflammatory reactions. Arch Pharm Res 33: 959–966.
23. Sun YX, Tang Y, Wu AL, Liu T, Dai XL, et al. (2010) Neuroprotective effect of liquiritin against focal cerebral ischemia/reperfusion in mice via its antioxidant and antiapoptosis properties. J Asian Nat Prod Res 12: 1051–1060.
24. Kim TG, Lee YH, Lee NH, Bhattarai G, Lee IK, et al. (2013) The antioxidant property of pachymic acid improves bone disturbance against AH plus-induced inflammation in MC-3T3 E1 cells. J Endod 39: 461–466.
25. Cheng Y, Shen LH, Zhang JT (2005) Anti-amnestic and anti-aging effects of ginsenoside Rg1 and Rb1 and its mechanism of action. Acta Pharmacol Sin 26: 143–149.
26. Wang L, Zhang Y, Wang Z, Li S, Min G, et al. (2012) Inhibitory effect of ginsenoside-Rd on carrageenan-induced inflammation in rats. Can J Physiol Pharmacol 90: 229–236.
27. Kim TW, Joh EH, Kim B, Kim DH (2012) Ginsenoside Rg5 ameliorates lung inflammation in mice by inhibiting the binding of LPS to toll-like receptor-4 on macrophages. Int Immunopharmacol 12: 110–116.
28. Ji Q, Yang L, Zhou J, Lin R, Zhang J, et al. (2012) Protective effects of paeoniflorin against cobalt chloride-induced apoptosis of endothelial cells via HIF-1alpha pathway. Toxicol In Vitro 26: 455–461.
29. Sener G, Toklu HZ, Sehirli AO, Velioglu-Ogunc A, Cetinel S, et al. (2006) Protective effects of resveratrol against acetaminophen-induced toxicity in mice. Hepatol Res 35: 62–68.
30. O'Brien PJ, Slaughter MR, Swain A, Birmingham JM, Greenhill RW, et al. (2000) Repeated acetaminophen dosing in rats: adaptation of hepatic antioxidant system. Hum Exp Toxicol 19: 277–283.
31. Wang YH, Shen YC, Liao JF, Lee CH, Chou CY, et al. (2008) Anti-inflammatory effects of dimemorfan on inflammatory cells and LPS-induced endotoxin shock in mice. Br J Pharmacol 154: 1327–1338.
32. Amor S, Puentes F, Baker D, van der Valk P (2010) Inflammation in neurodegenerative diseases. Immunology 129: 154–169.
33. Ghosh J, Das J, Manna P, Sil PC (2010) Acetaminophen induced renal injury via oxidative stress and TNF-alpha production: therapeutic potential of arjunolic acid. Toxicology 268: 8–18.
34. Williams CD, Farhood A, Jaeschke H (2010) Role of caspase-1 and interleukin-1beta in acetaminophen-induced hepatic inflammation and liver injury. Toxicol Appl Pharmacol 247: 169–178.
35. Muir KW, Tyrrell P, Sattar N, Warburton E (2007) Inflammation and ischaemic stroke. Curr Opin Neurol 20: 334–342.
36. Huang ZF, Massey JB, Via DP (2000) Differential regulation of cyclooxygenase-2 (COX-2) mRNA stability by interleukin-1 beta (IL-1 beta) and tumor necrosis factor-alpha (TNF-alpha) in human in vitro differentiated macrophages. Biochem Pharmacol 59: 187–194.
37. Adams ML, Pierce RH, Vail ME, White CC, Tonge RP, et al. (2001) Enhanced acetaminophen hepatotoxicity in transgenic mice overexpressing BCL-2. Mol Pharmacol 60: 907–915.
38. El-Hassan H, Anwar K, Macanas-Pirard P, Crabtree M, Chow SC, et al. (2003) Involvement of mitochondria in acetaminophen-induced apoptosis and hepatic injury: roles of cytochrome c, Bax, Bid, and caspases. Toxicol Appl Pharmacol 191: 118–129.
39. Gujral JS, Knight TR, Farhood A, Bajt ML, Jaeschke H (2002) Mode of cell death after acetaminophen overdose in mice: apoptosis or oncotic necrosis? Toxicol Sci 67: 322–328.
40. Kumari A, Kakkar P (2012) Lupeol protects against acetaminophen-induced oxidative stress and cell death in rat primary hepatocytes. Food Chem Toxicol 50: 1781–1789.
41. Kumari A, Kakkar P (2012) Lupeol prevents acetaminophen-induced in vivo hepatotoxicity by altering the Bax/Bcl-2 and oxidative stress-mediated mitochondrial signaling cascade. Life Sci 90: 561–570.
42. Boulares AH, Zoltoski AJ, Stoica BA, Cuvillier O, Smulson ME (2002) Acetaminophen induces a caspase-dependent and Bcl-XL sensitive apoptosis in human hepatoma cells and lymphocytes. Pharmacol Toxicol 90: 38–50.
43. Yuan HD, Jin GZ, Piao GC (2010) Hepatoprotective effects of an active part from Artemisia sacrorum Ledeb. against acetaminophen-induced toxicity in mice. J Ethnopharmacol 127: 528–533.
44. Ray SD, Mumaw VR, Raje RR, Fariss MW (1996) Protection of acetaminophen-induced hepatocellular apoptosis and necrosis by cholesteryl hemisuccinate pretreatment. J Pharmacol Exp Ther 279: 1470–1483.

Author Contributions

Conceived and designed the experiments: ES YS. Performed the experiments: ES JF XX CS. Analyzed the data: ES JF XX CS. Contributed reagents/materials/analysis tools: ES JF XX YS. Contributed to the writing of the manuscript: ES YS.

18

Matrix Metalloproteinase 2 Contributes to Pancreatic Beta Cell Injury Induced by Oxidative Stress

Chongxiao Liu[1,9], Xiaoyu Wan[1,9], Tingting Ye[1], Fang Fang[1], Xueru Chen[1], Yuanwen Chen[2], Yan Dong[1*]

1 Department of Endocrinology, Xinhua Hospital, Shanghai Jiao Tong University School of Medicine, Shanghai, China, **2** Department of Gastroenterology, Xinhua Hospital, Shanghai Jiao Tong University School of Medicine, Shanghai, China

Abstract

Objective: To investigate the role of matrix metalloproteinase 2 (MMP2) in pancreatic beta cell injury induced by oxidative stress.

Methods: Rat pancreatic beta cell line INS-1 cells were treated with advanced glycation end-products (AGE) to induce intracellular oxidative stress. Intracellular MMP2 expression and activity were determined by quantitative reverse transcription polymerase chain reaction (RT-PCR), Western blotting, and zymography, respectively. MMP2 expression and activity were manipulated by over-expression with recombinant MMP2 plasmids or knockdown with either MMP2 specific siRNA or inhibitors, and effects on apoptosis and insulin-secretion were measured by flow cytometry and ELISA.

Results: AGE treatment induced intracellular oxidative stress in INS-1 cells, as indicated by elevated ROS levels, apoptotic cell death, and suppressed insulin secretion. This was accompanied by increased MMP2 expression and activity. However, Antioxidant N-acetylcysteine (NAC) treatment inhibited MMP2 expression and activity, and partially reversed cell apoptosis and insulin secretion dysfunction induced by AGE. Forced expression of MMP2 mimicked the effects of AGE treatment while inhibition of MMP2 either by a specific MMP2 inhibitor or MMP2 siRNA protected oxidative stress induced by AGE.

Conclusion: MMP2 expression and intracellular activity are increased by oxidative stress, contributing to cellular dysfunction and apoptosis in INS-1 cells after AGE challenge.

Editor: Bridget Wagner, Broad Institute of Harvard and MIT, United States of America

Funding: This work was supported by the grants from the National Natural Science Foundation of China (No. 81170757) and the Fund of Shanghai Jiao Tong University School of Medicine (No 09xj21011). The author YD received the funding. The funders had no role in study design, data collection and analysis, decision to publish, or preparation of the manuscript.

Competing Interests: The authors have declared that no competing interests exist.

* Email: yandong00@hotmail.com

9 These authors contributed equally to this work.

Introduction

Type 2 diabetes mellitus (T2DM) is generally considered to be caused by the dysfunction of pancreatic beta cells and insulin resistance. Failure of pancreatic beta cells by their progressive loss is regarded as a critical step in the pathogenesis of T2DM [1,2]. However, the mechanisms underlying pancreatic beta cell dysfunction and loss are still unclear.

Accumulating evidence has indicated that pancreatic beta cell loss in T2DM partially results from oxidative stress [3,4,5]. Pancreatic beta cells are more vulnerable to oxidative stress because of low antioxidase activity [6,7]. The factors responsible for pancreatic beta cell damage that lead to cell dysfunction via oxidative stress remain unknown. It is generally believed that direct chemical modification contributes to that process. Reactive oxygen species (ROS) can oxidize or nitrify proteins, lipids and DNA by direct chemical modification, leading to dysfunction of crucial proteins including signal transduction factors, ribosomal subunits, DNA repair enzymes, and proteases associated with energy metabolism in pancreatic beta cells [8]. Nevertheless, whether factors other than direct chemical modification might contribute to pancreatic beta cell dysfunction in oxidative stress is largely unknown.

Intracellular matrix metalloproteinases (MMPs) including MMP2 are involved in myocardial cell damage via oxidative stress [9]. MMPs belong to a family of zinc-dependent endopeptidases which degrade extracellular matrix and contribute to tissue remodeling in angiogenesis, embryogenesis, atherosclerosis, aortic aneurysm and myocardial infarction [10,11,12,13]. Given that MMP2, a member of the gelatinase family of proteases, also plays vital roles in myocardial ischemia-reperfusion injury [14], it is hypothesized that MMP2 may also have biological functions besides degrading extracellular matrix. Increased MMP2 activity has been reported to result in proteolysis of cytoskeletal proteins including myocardial troponin, myosin, and actin which causes oxidative stress and mitochondrial injury, and ultimately leads to cardiomyocyte dysfunction. Additionally, inhibition of MMP2 activity has been found to attenuate myocardial damage [15,16]. Similarly, elevated MMP2 has been implicated in the development

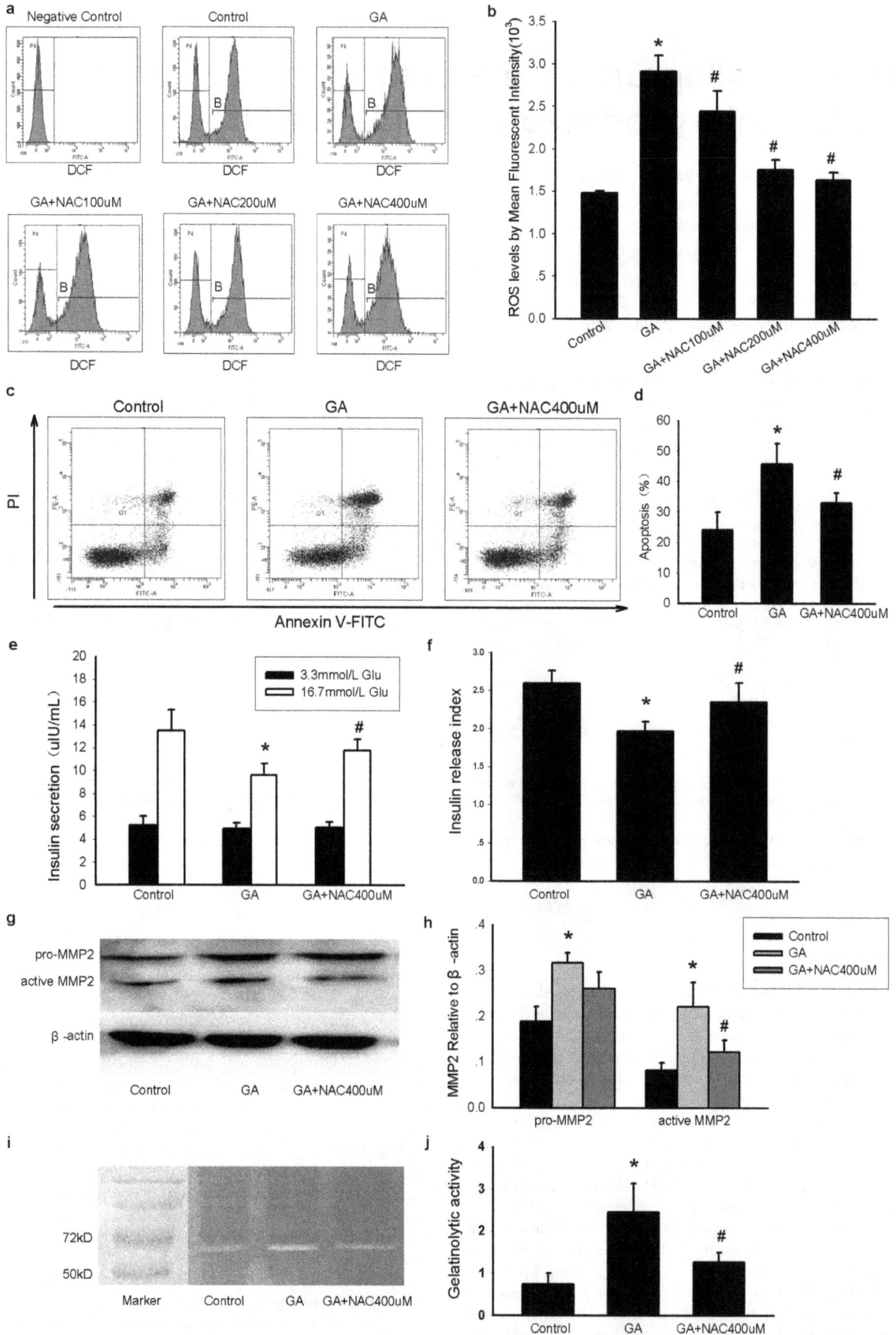

Figure 1. Oxidative stress increases MMP2 expression and activity in INS-1 cells. INS-1 cells were treated with GA (200 mg/L) or BSA (200 mg/L) for 24 h. Antioxidant NAC was dissolved in sterile double-distilled water and used in different final concentrations with GA (200 mg/L). The antioxidant effect of NAC was measured by DCFH-DA through flow cytometer. The concentration with better antioxidant effect was used for following experiments. (a, b) The level of cytosolic ROS in different groups. The mean fluorescence intensity (MFI) of DCF is used to measure cellular ROS levels. BSA–treated cells without DCFH-DA incubation serve as negative control. (c) Apoptotic cells in different groups. Annexin V positive cells (including Annexin V single positive population and the Annexin V and PI double positive population) representing apoptotic cells were mainly located in the right upper quadrant and right lower quadrant. (d) Average apoptotic rate in the three groups. (e) Insulin secretion of INS-1 cells stimulated with 3.3 mmol/L glucose or 16.7 mmol/L glucose in the different groups. *$P<0.05$ vs the corresponding control group; #$P<0.05$ vs the corresponding GA group. (f) Insulin release index (IRI) of each group. The IRI was adopted as an index to estimate the insulin secretion function of INS-1 cells. IRI = insulin concentration of high glucose stimulation (16.7 mmol/L)/insulin concentration of low glucose stimulation (3.3 mmol/L). (g, h) Protein expression of MMP2 in different groups, including both pro-MMP2($\sim$72 kD) and active MMP2($\sim$62 kD). (i, j) The gelatinolytic activity of MMP2 in different groups. The white band in gray background was the location of MMP2, band intensity was used to represent the activity of MMP2 in each group. Data are shown as means $\pm$ SD, $P<0.05$ indicates a statistically significant difference. *$P<0.05$ vs the control group; #$P<0.05$ vs the GA group.

of diabetes mellitus, and a MMP inhibitor, PD166793, reduces blood glucose in Zucker diabetic rats [17]. However, it remains unclear whether suppression of MMPs activity is associated with remission of pancreatic beta cell damage.

In the present study, we aim to investigate the role of MMP2 in pancreatic beta cell injury induced by oxidative stress.

Materials and Methods

1. INS-1 Cells Culture

Rat pancreatic beta cell line INS-1 cells were donated by Shanghai Institute of Endocrine and Metabolic Diseases and cultured in Roswell Park Memorial Institute (RPMI) medium1640 as previous described [18].

2. Cytosolic ROS generation in INS-1 cells

To determine the effects of oxidative stress in intracellular MMP2 expression and activity, INS-1 cells were challenged by an intracellular oxidative stress with Glycated bovine serum albumin (GA), which acts as an Advanced glycation end-products (AGE). The control group was treated with BSA. A third group was co-treated with GA and an antioxidant NAC (Sigma-Aldrich, St. Louis, Missouri, USA) in different concentrations to block intracellular ROS generation.

Cytosolic ROS levels were analyzed by 2′,7′-dichlorodihydro-flurescein diacetate (DCFH-DA, Sigma-Aldrich, St. Louis, Missouri, USA) through flow cytometry. The INS-1 cells were washed and incubated with 10 μM of DCFH-DA for 40 min. INS-1 cells were then harvested, washed twice with cold PBS, and directly collected before detection of the mean fluorescence intensity (MFI) of 2′,7′-dichlorofluorescein (DCF) for 10^5 cells per sample to measure cellular ROS levels (excitation 490 nm, emission 530 nm).

3. Inhibition of MMP-2 activity

To determine the protective role of MMP2 inhibition in beta cell dysfunction induced by oxidative stress, INS-1 cells were co-treated with GA and a MMP2 specific inhibitor (cis-9-Octadece-noyl-N- hydroxylamide, OA-Hy, Santa Cruz Biotechnology, Dallas, Texas, USA) for 24 h, the other two groups were treated with GA or BSA.

4. Forced expression of MMP-2

A 2.1-kb fragment containing the open reading frame of the rat pro-MMP2 gene was obtained by RT-PCR using the following primers, which contained restriction endonuclease sites XhoI and KpnI. The sense primer was 5′- TCCGCTCGAGATGGAGG-CACGATTGGTCTG-3′, and the anti-sense primer was 5′-ATGGGGTACCTCAGCAGCCCAGCCAGTCC-3′. After se-quence confirmation, MMP2 was subcloned into the XhoI and

KpnI sites of the eukaryotic expression plasmid pcDNA3.1(+) vector. INS-1 cells were transfected with the pcDNA3.1-MMP2 and pcDNA3.1 plasmid. Prior to transfection, INS-1 cells were seeded in 12-well plates at a density of 10^5/mL and were maintained in medium RPMI 1640 without antibiotics. When the density reached 50%–70%, the cells were grown in Opti-MEM I reduced serum medium (Invitrogen, Life Technologies, Carlsbad, California, USA) during transfection for 6 h. Then, the medium was replaced with normal medium. Transient transfection of INS-1 cells was performed using lipofectimine 2000 reagent (Invitro-gen) as per the manufacturer's instructions.

5. Transfection of INS-1 cells with MMP2-siRNA

INS-1 cells were transfected with MMP2 siRNA using a transfection reagent kit (Santa Cruz Biotechnology) according to the manufacturer's instructions. The transfection complexes, prepared by adding MMP2 siRNA and siRNA transfection reagent, were incubated for 30 min at room temperature, and the cells were incubated with this transfection complex for 8 h at 37°C. Parallel incubations were performed using non-targeting scrambled siRNA. After transfection for 48 h, INS-1 cells were rinsed with PBS and incubated with GA or BSA for 24 h to test the protective effect of MMP2 knockdown in oxidative stress injury. Annealed double-stranded small-interfering RNA (siRNA) for rat MMP2 were designed and synthesized by Genepharma (Shanghai, China) following the sequence 5′-CUGCCUUUAA-CUGGAGUAATT-3′.

6. Determination of MMP2 expression

The mRNA expression level of MMP2 was determined by quantitative reverse transcription polymerase chain reaction (RT-PCR). In brief, total RNA of INS-1 cells was extracted, and cDNA was synthesized from 1 μg RNA with PrimeScript RT Master Mix (TaKaRa, Osaka, Japan). RT-PCR analyses were performed using SYBR Premix Ex Taq (TaKaRa). The standard PCR conditions consisted of 95°C for 30 sec, followed by 40 cycles of 95°C for 5 sec and 60°C for 34 sec, with a final dissociation stage, and the samples were run on an ABI 7500 detector (Applied Biosystems, Foster City, CA, USA). The primer sequences for the rat cells were as follows: Fwd 5′-GAGTAAGAACAAGAAGACATACATC-3′ and Rev 5′-GTAATAAGCACCCTTGAAGAAATAG-3′ for MMP2; and Fwd 5′-GC AAGTTCAACGGCACAG-3′ and Rev 5′-GCCAGTAGA CTCCACGAGAT-3′ for GAPDH.

Protein expression levels of MMP2 were determined by Western blot analysis. Total proteins were extracted using a radioimmu-noprecipitation assay (RIPA) lysis buffer and were subsequently separated by 10% SDS-PAGE gels. Proteins were then electro-phoretically transferred onto PVDF membranes and probed with the corresponding antibodies (Abcam, Cambridge, MA, USA) overnight at 4°C after blocking in 5% non-fat milk in Tris-buffered

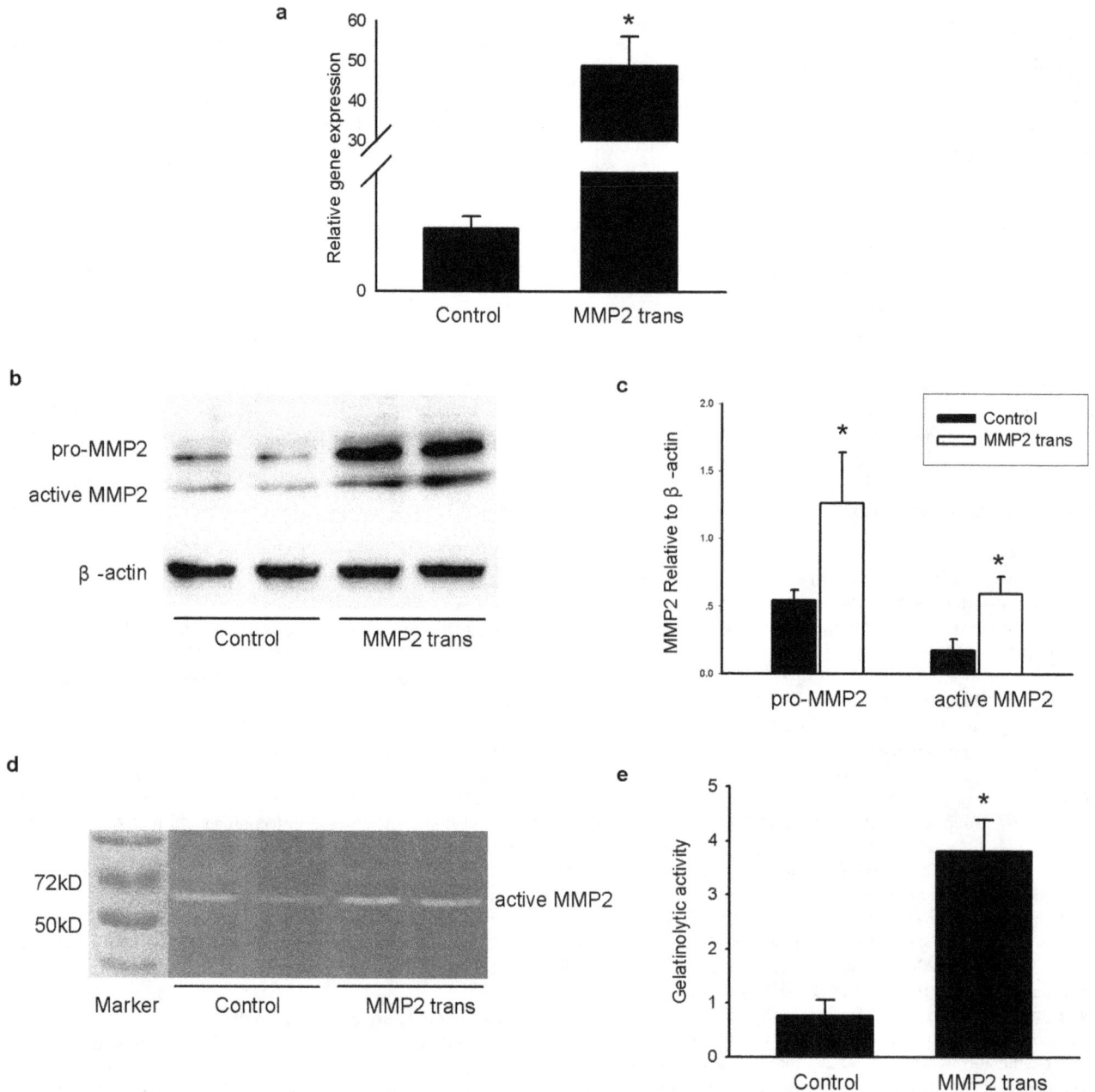

Figure 2. Forced expression of MMP2 in transient transfection of INS-1 cells groups. INS-1 cells were transfected with 1.6 µg MMP2 recombination plasmids and 4 µL Lipofectmine 2000 in each well. An empty vector served as control. After 48 h incubation, the mRNA, protein and gelatinolytic activity of MMP2 were evaluated. (a) Relative mRNA level of MMP2 after 48 h transfection in each group. (b, c) Protein expression (including pro-MMP2 and active MMP2) after 48 h of transfection in each group. (d, e) Gelatinolytic activity of MMP2 after 48 h of transfection in each group. Data are shown as means ± SD, $P<0.05$ indicates a statistically significant difference. *$P<0.05$ vs the control group.

saline with Tween-20 (TBST) for 2 h. Secondary peroxidase-coupled antibodies were applied, and a chemiluminescent substrate system was used to detect the signals. Band intensity was analyzed using ChemiDoc XRS+ software (Bio-Rad Laboratories, Hercules, CA, USA).

7. Gelatinolytic activity of MMP2

Gelatinolytic activity of MMP2 was measured in INS-1 cells by zymography. Proteins were extracted using the same protocol described above but without denaturation. An equal amount of protein was loaded on the 10% SDS-PAGE gels containing 1 mg/

mL gelatin. The gels were equilibrated in the Novex zymogram renaturing buffer (Invitrogen) for 30 min at room temperature with gentle agitation, before being incubated in Novex zymogram developing buffer (Invitrogen) at 37°C overnight. The gels were then stained with Coomassie Blue dye (Invitrogen) and photographed after destaining in double-distilled water for at least 7 h. Band intensity was analyzed by Bio-Rad ChemiDoc XRS+ software.

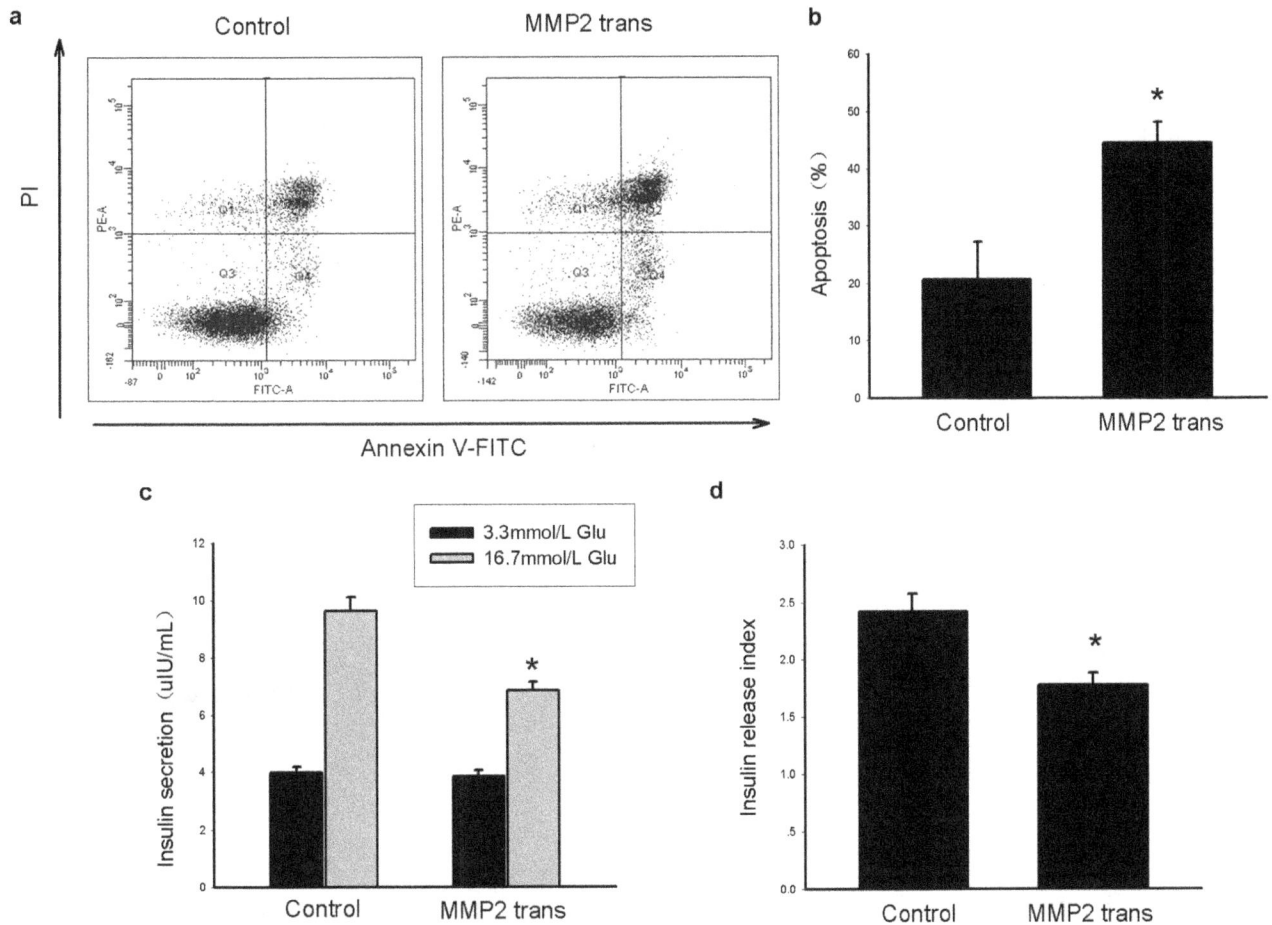

Figure 3. Forced expression of MMP2 increases apoptosis and leads to reduced insulin secretion in INS-1 cells. INS-1 cells were transfected with 1.6 μg MMP2 recombination plasmid and 4 μL Lipofectmine 2000 in each well. An empty vector served as control. The apoptosis and insulin-secretion function of INS-1 cells were evaluated in each group after 48 h of incubation. (a) Apoptotic cells in the control group. Annexin V positive cells (including Annexin V single positive population and the Annexin V and PI double positive population) representing apoptotic cells were mainly located in the right upper quadrant and right lower quadrant. (b) Average apoptotic rate of each group. (c) Insulin secretion stimulated under 3.3 mmol/L or 16.7 mmol/L glucose in each group. *$P<0.05$ compared to the corresponding control group. (d) Insulin release index (IRI) of each group. Data are shown as means ± SD, $P<0.05$ indicates a statistically significant difference. *$P<0.05$ vs the control group.

8. Apoptosis of INS-1 cells

Apoptosis of INS-1 cells was detected by flow cytometry using an Annexin V- FITC/PI apoptosis assay kit (Becton, Dickinson and Company, Franklin Lakes, NJ, USA) following the manufacturer's instructions. Briefly, the cells were harvested, washed twice with cold PBS, and stained with Annexin V-FITC/PI for 15 min in the dark. The cells were then measured by flow cytometry.

9. Insulin secretion of INS-1 cells

For each experimental group, INS-1 cells were pre-incubated in Kreb's buffer containing: NaCl 140 mM, KCl 4.6 mM, MGAO₄ 1 mM, NaHPO₄ 0.15 mM, NaHCO₃ 5 mM, CaCl₂ 2 mM, and HEPES 30 mM, pH 7.4, and mixed with 0.2% BSA and 3.3 mmol/L of glucose at 37°C for 30 min. After that, the INS-1 cells were stimulated with either 3.3 or 16.7 mmol/L of glucose for 1 h. The medium was collected, and insulin was measured using the rat insulin ELISA kit (Roche Applied Science, Indianapolis, IN, USA) following the manufacturer's instructions.

10. Statistical analysis

Each experiment was conducted in either duplicate or triplicate, and a total of three independent experiments were performed. Data were expressed as mean ± standard deviation (SD). Student's t test was applied for comparisons between two groups, while one-way ANOVA with Tukey's or Dunnett's test was applied to compare all groups or specific groups with the control. Statistical analyses were conducted using SPSS 19.0 statistical software (SPSS Inc. USA). P values less than 0.05 were considered to be statistically significant.

Results

1. Oxidative stress increases MMP-2 expression and activity in INS-1 cells

AGE (GA) treatment significantly increased cytosolic ROS levels, indicating that oxidative stress occurred by this treatment (Fig. 1a and 1b). In addition, apoptosis and insulin secretion dysfunction were also observed after GA treatment (Fig. 1c–f). Interestingly, the protein levels of MMP2 were also elevated in

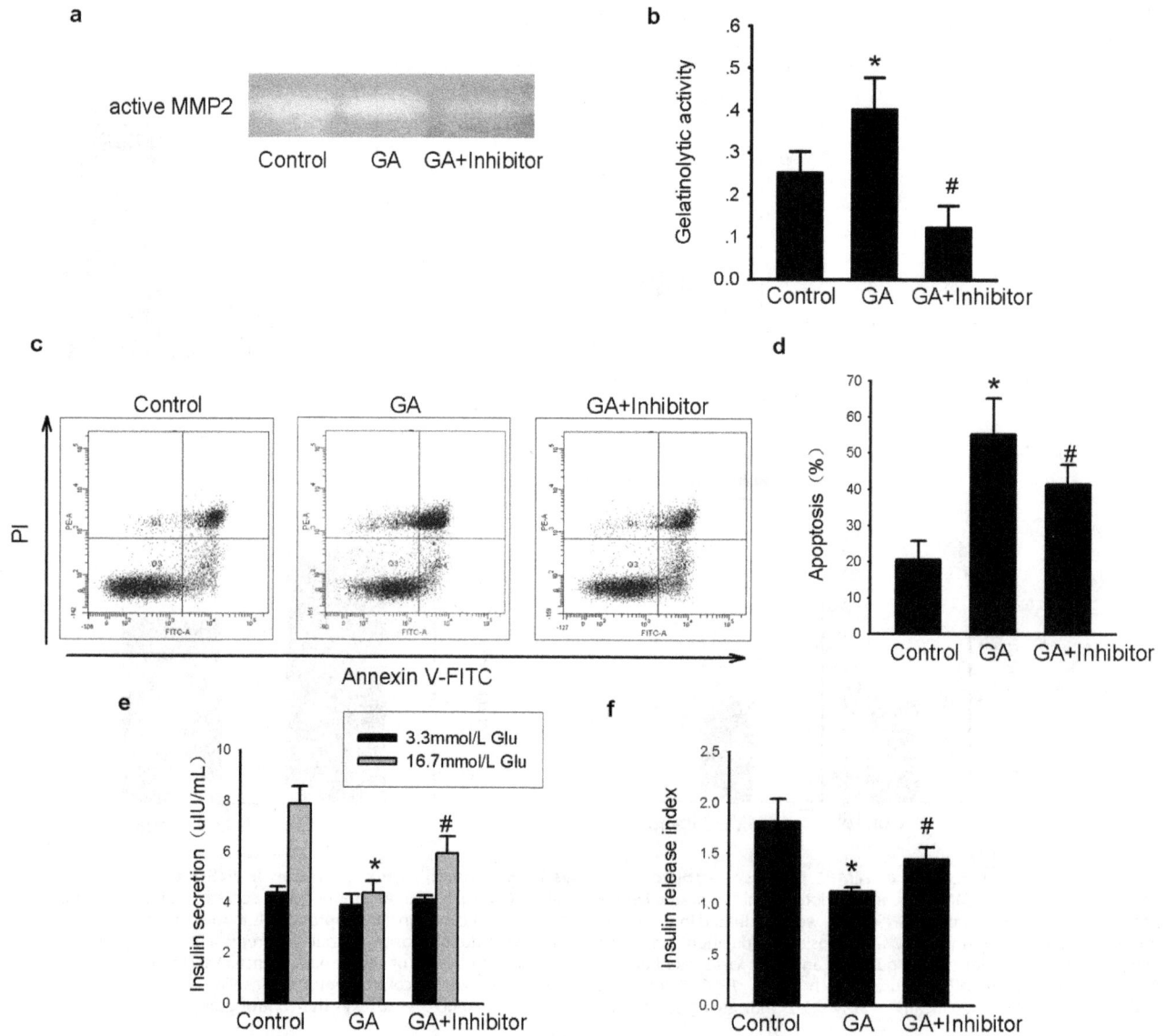

Figure 4. Inhibition of MMP2 decreases apoptosis and attenuates insulin secretion dysfunction caused by oxidative stress in INS-1 cells. INS-1 cells were treated with GA (200 mg/L) or BSA (200 mg/L) for 24 h. MMP2 inhibitor (OA-Hy) was dissolved in DMSO and used at a final concentration of 20 µmol/L with GA for 24 h. (a, b) The gelatinolytic activity of MMP2 in different groups. (c) Apoptotic cells in different groups. Annexin V positive cells (including Annexin V single positive population and the Annexin V and PI double positive population) representing apoptotic cells were mainly located in the right upper quadrant and right lower quadrant. (d) Average apoptotic rate in the three groups. (e) Insulin secretion of INS-1 cells stimulated with 3.3 mmol/L glucose or 16.7 mmol/L glucose in the different groups. *$P<0.05$ vs the corresponding control group; #$P<0.05$ vs corresponding GA-treated group (f) Insulin release index (IRI) of each group. Data are shown as means ± SD, $P<0.05$ indicates a statistically significant difference. *$P<0.05$ vs the control group; #$P<0.05$ vs GA-treated group.

GA-treated cells (Fig. 1 g–h). Moreover, gelatinolytic activity was also increased in INS-1 cells exposed to GA (Fig. 1i and 1j).

However, the antioxidant NAC treatment sharply decreased intracellular ROS level with dose-dependent effect. The cytosolic ROS level even declined near to basal level (control group) when co-treated with GA and 400 uM NAC. Correspondingly, the active MMP2 expression and activity were significantly decreased under NAC treatment (400 uM) compared to GA-treatment group, which further confirmed the effects of oxidative stress on intracellular MMP2 expression and activity. Besides, there was also a decline in INS-1 cell apoptosis and a recovery of insulin secretion function with antioxidant NAC treatment. These results

indicated that MMP2 might contribute to the oxidative stress damage in INS-1 cells.

2. Forced expression of MMP2 increases apoptosis and leads to dysfunctional insulin secretion in INS-1 cells

To determine if forced expression of MMP2 is sufficient to mimic the effects of GA treatment, full-length pro-MMP2 cDNA was overexpressed in INS-1 cells. Increased expression levels of MMP2 at the mRNA and protein levels were confirmed (Fig. 2a–c) and MMP2 gelatinolytic activity was also elevated (Fig. 2d, 2e).

MMP2 overexpression increased the apoptosis rate of INS-1 cells by at least two fold (Fig. 3a, 3b). Although the basal insulin

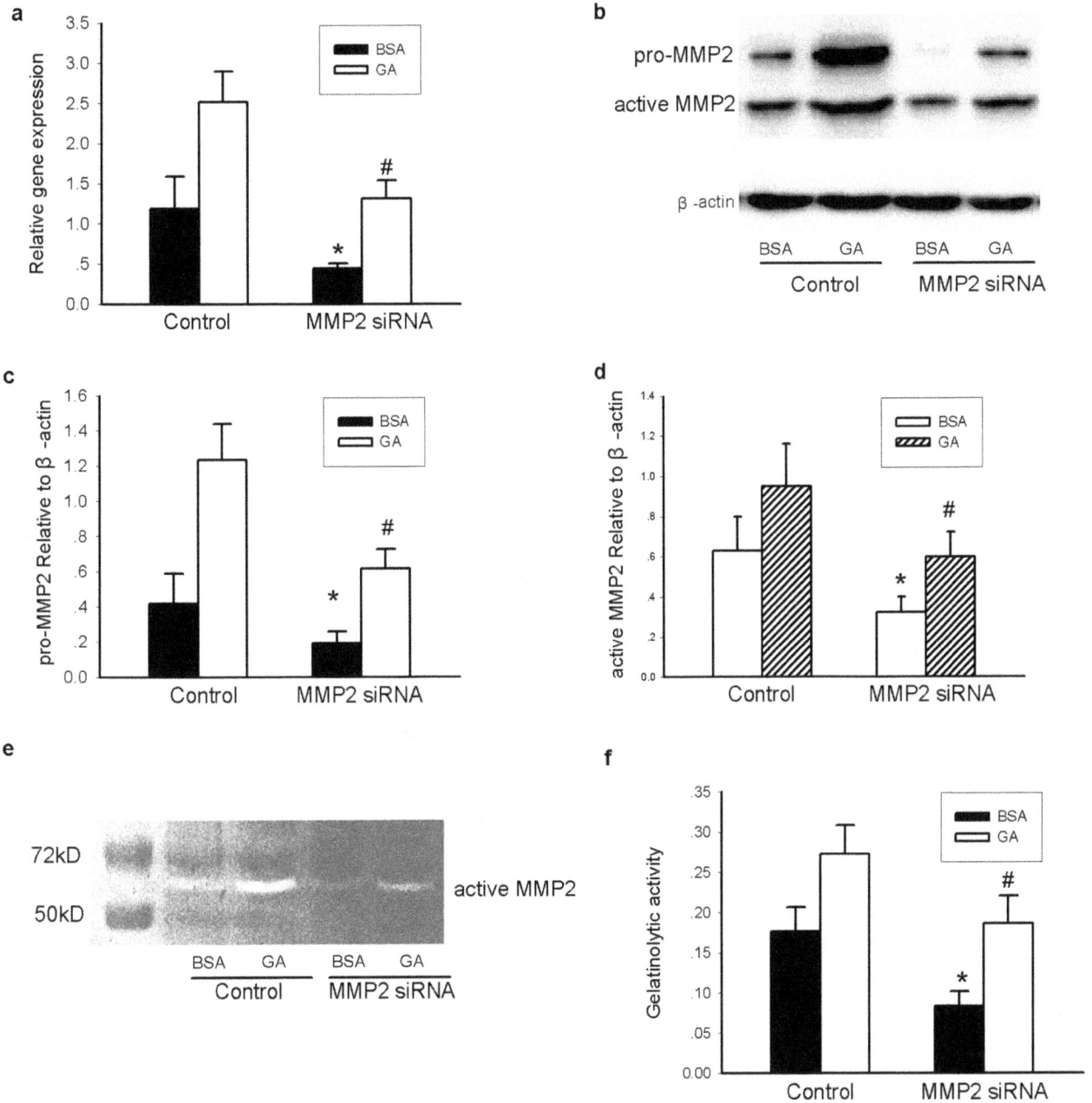

Figure 5. Transient transfection of MMP2 siRNA decreased intracellular MMP2 expression and gelatinolytic activity in INS-1 cells.
INS-1 cells of each well were transfected with 40 pmol MMP-2 siRNA by 2 μL Lipofectmine 2000 in each well. A scrambled siRNA was used as control. 48 h after siRNA transfection, INS-1 cells were then treated with GA (200 mg/L) or BSA (200 mg/L) for another 24 h. (a) mRNA expression of MMP2 in different groups; (b–d) Protein expression (including pro-MMP2 and active MMP2) in each group; (e, f) Gelatinolytic activity of MMP2 in each group. Data are shown as means ± SD, $P<0.05$ indicates a statistically significant difference. * $P<0.05$, #$P<0.05$ vs corresponding control.

secretion (3.3 mmol/L glucose stimulation) in INS-1 cells was not affected by MMP2 overexpression (Fig. 3c), insulin secretion declined when exposure to high amounts of glucose (16.7 mmol/L) (Fig. 3c). This result was consistent with a decreased insulin release index (IRI) (Fig. 3d).

3. Inhibition of MMP2 decreases apoptosis and attenuates dysfunctional insulin secretion caused by oxidative stress in INS-1 cells

To determine if the up-regulation of MMP2 is necessary for the effects of GA treatment, a MMP2 inhibitor, OA-Hy, was used. The effect of OA-Hy as a MMP2 inhibitor was confirmed by gelatin zymography (Fig. 4a, 4b). OA-Hy significantly decreased apoptosis in GA-treated cells (Fig. 4c, 4d). In addition, insulin

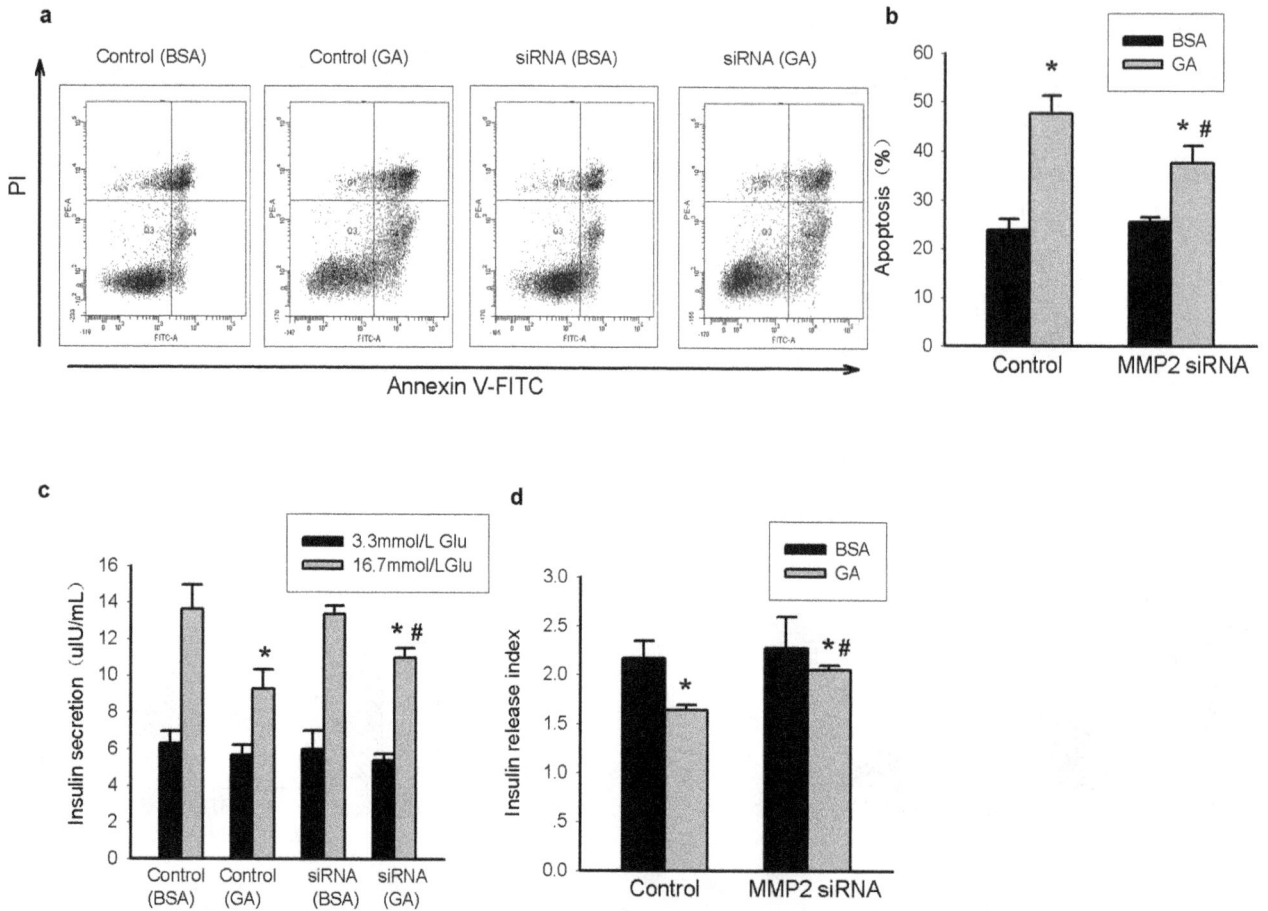

Figure 6. Decreased expression of MMP2 attenuates beta cell dysfunction caused by oxidative stress in INS-1 cells. INS-1 cells were transfected with 40 pmol MMP-2 siRNA. A scramble siRNA was used as control. 48 h after siRNA transfection, INS-1 cells were then treated with GA (200 mg/L) or BSA (200 mg/L) for another 24 h. (a) Apoptotic cells in different groups. Annexin V positive cells (including Annexin V single positive population and the Annexin V and PI double positive population) representing apoptotic cells were mainly located in the right upper quadrant and right lower quadrant. (b) Average apoptotic rate of each group. (c) The insulin secretion stimulated under 3.3 mmol/L glucose or 16.7 mmol/L glucose in each group. *$P<0.05$ vs BSA-treated subgroup under 16.7 mmol/L glucose stimulation. #$P<0.05$ vs corresponding control (treated with GA) under 16.7 mmol/L glucose stimulation. (d) Insulin release index (IRI) of each group. Data are shown as means ± SD, $P<0.05$ indicates a statistically significant difference. *$P<0.05$ vs BSA-treated subgroup, #$P<0.05$ vs corresponding control (treated with GA).

secretion of INS-1 cells increased with the administration of the MMP2 inhibitor after treatment with GA (Fig. 4e, 4f).

To exclude non-specific effects of the MMP2 inhibitor OA-Hy, MMP2 siRNA was used. Decreased MMP2 mRNA and protein expression levels and decreased MMP2 activity confirmed that this siRNA was effective in INS-1 cells (Fig. 5). Consistent with our results with the MMP2 inhibitor, MMP2 siRNA ameliorated insulin secretion dysfunction and apoptosis of INS-1 cells induced by oxidative stress (Fig. 6), further confirming that MMP2 is required for the effects of GA treatment in INS-1 cells.

Discussion

The major findings of the present study are as follows. First, oxidative stress increases MMP-2 expression and activity in INS-1 cells. Second, forced expression of MMP2 increases apoptosis and leads to dysfunctional insulin secretion in INS-1 cells. Finally, inhibition of MMP2 either by pharmacologic means or siRNA decreases apoptosis and attenuates insulin secretion dysfunction caused by oxidative stress in INS-1 cells. To the best of our

knowledge, this study shows for the first time that MMP2 controls pancreatic beta cell injury induced by oxidative stress.

MMP2, a gelatinase family MMP, is expressed in almost all cells and can degrade collagen IV and other ECM components. Recent findings have indicated that intracellular MMP2 might play an important role in cell injury, especially caused by oxidative stress. ROS has been reported to increase pro-MMP2 release in vascular smooth cells through NAD(P)H oxidase in response to mechanical stretch [19]. In addition, MMP2 in retinal capillary cells was activated by superoxide in the development of diabetic retinopathy [20]. Moreover, MMP2 has been shown to be expressed in pancreatic islets of Zucker diabetic fatty (ZDF) rats, and the expression and activity of MMP2 were increased along with the onset of islet dysfunction and diabetes [17]. All this evidence strongly suggests that MMP2 may also be involved in pancreatic beta cell injury induced by increased oxidative stress. Here, we show that oxidative stress increases MMP-2 expression and activity in INS-1 cells while antioxidant NAC attenuates this increase in MMP2 expression/activity by blocking ROS level, indicating that increased expression of MMP2 is consistent with increased oxidative stress in INS-1 cells. Actually, our results from western blot show that there is only a slight attenuation in the expression of pro-MMP2 without statistical significant, whereas the expression of active MMP2 in NAC-treatment group drastically decreases compared to GA-treatment group. Although unproven, we assume that enhanced oxidative stress might also aggravate cleavage of proenzyme into active form of MMP2 in addition to regulating expression of intracellular MMP2. Giving further support to this assumption, similar findings have also been reported that the increase in active MMP2 other than pro-MMP2 has been partially reversed in aortic tissue of diabetic rats treated with antioxidant [21]. Meanwhile, forced expression of MMP2 mimics the effects of oxidative stress induced in INS-1 cells in our study, suggesting that MMP2 overexpression is sufficient to mimic the effects of oxidative stress-induced damage in INS-1 cells. PD-166793, a broad-spectrum MMP inhibitor, has been shown to prevent female ZDF rats on a high-fat diet from beta-cell dysfunction and diabetes, though the subfamily of MMP responsible for this effect is unclear [17]. In the present study, we show that a MMP2-selective inhibitor OA-Hy can improve INS-1 cell insulin secretion function and reduce apoptosis induced by oxidative stress. Moreover, specific down-regulation of MMP2 by MMP2 siRNA shows the same beneficial effects as the MMP2 chemical inhibitor. These results indicate that up-regulation of MMP2 is necessary for the effects of GA treatment in pancreatic beta cells.

Still we have no conclusions on the mechanism of beta cell dysfunction induced by AGE. Recent evidence suggests that there exist several pathways which may mediate AGE-induced beta cell dysfunction. It was reported that AGE could impair insulin synthesis and secretion of INS-1 cells through enhancing glycogen synthase kinase-3 (GAK-3) activation to further decrease PDX-1 expression other than increasing ROS production [22]. Another proapoptotic mechanism of AGE was also discovered that autophagy deficiency as well as increased endoplasmic reticulum stress and oxidative stress, resulting in nuclear factor-κB (p65)-

iNOS-caspase-3 cascade activation, contributed to AGE-mediated pancreatic beta cell apoptosis and dysfunction [23]. The results in our study showed that inhibiting intracellular MMP2 activity could significantly reduce GA-induced beta cell apoptosis and improve insulin secretion, although not totally reversed, which suggested that MMP2 played an important role in one of oxidative stress-activated pathways induced by AGE. However, the downstream target of MMP2 responsible for the pancreatic beta cell dysfunction induced by oxidative stress remains unclear. In cardiomyocytes, oxidative stress-induced MMP2 expression is due to the activation of activator protein-1 (AP-1) and/or nuclear factor-kappa B (NF-κB) [24,25]. In addition, whether intracellular MMP2 serves as a protease or only as a signaling protein to induce apoptosis, or both, in pancreatic beta cell oxidative injury, is worthy of further study. It has been reported that intracellular MMP2 was responsible for the loss of mitochondrial potential and increased mitochondrial membrane permeability in retinal endothelial cells, which induced the translocation of Bax and cytochrome C from the mitochondria to the cytoplasm to activate intracellular apoptotic mechanisms [26,27]. Nevertheless, this study gives direct evidence that MMP2 is necessary and sufficient for pancreatic beta cells injury induced by oxidative stress.

In conclusion, this study shows that MMP2 expression and intracellular activity are increased by oxidative stress, contributing to cellular dysfunction and apoptosis in INS-1 cells after AGE challenge. Inhibition of intracellular MMP2 may represent a new therapeutic approach for the protection of pancreatic beta cells from oxidative injury and the prevention of diabetes.

Author Contributions

Conceived and designed the experiments: YD YWC. Performed the experiments: CXL XYW. Analyzed the data: TTY FF. Contributed reagents/materials/analysis tools: XRC. Contributed to the writing of the manuscript: CXL.

References

1. Jonas JC, Bensellam M, Duprez J, Elouil H, Guiot Y, et al. (2009) Glucose regulation of islet stress responses and beta-cell failure in type 2 diabetes. Diabetes Obes Metab 11 Suppl 4: 65–81.
2. Rhodes CJ (2005) Type 2 diabetes-a matter of beta-cell life and death? Science 307: 380–384.
3. Pitocco D, Zaccardi F, Di Stasio E, Romitelli F, Santini SA, et al. (2010) Oxidative stress, nitric oxide, and diabetes. Rev Diabet Stud 7: 15–25.
4. Drews G, Krippeit-Drews P, Dufer M (2010) Oxidative stress and beta-cell dysfunction. Pflugers Arch 460: 703–718.
5. Robertson R, Zhou H, Zhang T, Harmon J (2007) Chronic oxidative stress as a mechanism for glucose toxicity of the beta cell in type 2 diabetes. Cell Biochem Biophys 48: 139.
6. Abdul-Ghani MA, DeFronzo RA (2008) Mitochondrial dysfunction, insulin resistance, and type 2 diabetes mellitus. Curr Diab Rep 8: 173–178.
7. Mulder H, Ling C (2009) Mitochondrial dysfunction in pancreatic beta-cells in Type 2 diabetes. Mol Cell Endocrinol 297: 34–40.
8. Baines CP, Kaiser RA, Purcell NH, Blair NS, Osinska H, et al. (2005) Loss of cyclophilin D reveals a critical role for mitochondrial permeability transition in cell death. Nature 434: 658–662.
9. Kandasamy AD, Chow AK, Ali MA, Schulz R (2010) Matrix metalloproteinase-2 and myocardial oxidative stress injury: beyond the matrix. Cardiovasc Res 85: 413–423.
10. Roy R, Zhang B, Moses MA (2006) Making the cut: protease-mediated regulation of angiogenesis. Exp Cell Res 312: 608–622.
11. Vu TH, Werb Z (2000) Matrix metalloproteinases: effectors of development and normal physiology. Genes Dev 14: 2123–2133.
12. Deryugina EI, Quigley JP (2006) Matrix metalloproteinases and tumor metastasis. Cancer Metastasis Rev 25: 9–34.
13. Mohammed FF, Smookler DS, Khokha R (2003) Metalloproteinases, inflammation, and rheumatoid arthritis. Ann Rheum Dis 62 Suppl 2: ii43–47.
14. Wang W, Sawicki G, Schulz R (2002) Peroxynitrite-induced myocardial injury is mediated through matrix metalloproteinase-2. Cardiovascular research 53: 165–174.
15. Wang W, Schulze CJ, Suarez-Pinzon WL, Dyck JR, Sawicki G, et al. (2002) Intracellular action of matrix metalloproteinase-2 accounts for acute myocardial ischemia and reperfusion injury. Circulation 106: 1543–1549.
16. Sawicki G, Leon H, Sawicka J, Sariahmetoglu M, Schulze CJ, et al. (2005) Degradation of myosin light chain in isolated rat hearts subjected to ischemia-reperfusion injury: a new intracellular target for matrix metalloproteinase-2. Circulation 112: 544–552.
17. Zhou YP, Madjidi A, Wilson ME, Nothhelfer DA, Johnson JH, et al. (2005) Matrix metalloproteinases contribute to insulin insufficiency in Zucker diabetic fatty rats. Diabetes 54: 2612–2619.
18. Lin N, Zhang H, Su Q (2012) Advanced glycation end-products induce injury to pancreatic beta cells through oxidative stress. Diabetes & metabolism 38: 250–257.
19. Grote K, Flach I, Luchtefeld M, Akin E, Holland SM, et al. (2003) Mechanical stretch enhances mRNA expression and proenzyme release of matrix metalloproteinase-2 (MMP-2) via NAD(P)H oxidase-derived reactive oxygen species. Circ Res 92: e80–86.
20. Kowluru RA, Kanwar M (2009) Oxidative stress and the development of diabetic retinopathy: contributory role of matrix metalloproteinase-2. Free Radical Biology and Medicine 46: 1677–1685.
21. Martinez ML, Rizzi E, Castro MM, Fernandes K, Bendhack LM, et al. (2008) Lercanidipine decreases vascular matrix metalloproteinase-2 activity and protects against vascular dysfunction in diabetic rats. Eur J Pharmacol 599: 110–116.
22. Fiory F, Lombardi A, Miele C, Giudicelli J, Beguinot F, et al. (2011) Methylglyoxal impairs insulin signalling and insulin action on glucose-induced insulin secretion in the pancreatic beta cell line INS-1E. Diabetologia 54: 2941–2952.
23. Song YM, Song SO, You YH, Yoon KH, Kang ES, et al. (2013) Glycated albumin causes pancreatic beta-cells dysfunction through autophagy dysfunction. Endocrinology 154: 2626–2639.
24. Alfonso-Jaume MA, Bergman MR, Mahimkar R, Cheng S, Jin ZQ, et al. (2006) Cardiac ischemia-reperfusion injury induces matrix metalloproteinase-2 expression through the AP-1 components FosB and JunB. Am J Physiol Heart Circ Physiol 291: H1838–1846.

25. Yoshida M, Korfhagen TR, Whitsett JA (2001) Surfactant protein D regulates NF-κB and matrix metalloproteinase production in alveolar macrophages via oxidant-sensitive pathways. The Journal of Immunology 166: 7514–7519.

26. Mohammad G, Kowluru RA (2010) Matrix metalloproteinase-2 in the development of diabetic retinopathy and mitochondrial dysfunction. Laboratory Investigation 90: 1365–1372.

27. Mohammad G, Kowluru RA (2011) Novel role of mitochondrial matrix metalloproteinase-2 in the development of diabetic retinopathy. Investigative ophthalmology & visual science 52: 3832–3841.

19

SERPINA3K Plays Antioxidant Roles in Cultured Pterygial Epithelial Cells through Regulating ROS System

Chengpeng Zhu[1,9], **Fangyu Pan**[1,9], **Lianping Ge**[1], **Jing Zhou**[1], **Longlong Chen**[1], **Tong Zhou**[1], **Rongrong Zong**[1], **Xinye Xiao**[1], **Nuo Dong**[2], **Maomin Yang**[3], **Jian-xing Ma**[4], **Zuguo Liu**[1,2], **Yueping Zhou**[1]*

1 Eye Institute of Xiamen University, Fujian Provincial Key Laboratory of Ophthalmology and Visual Science, Xiamen, Fujian, China, 2 Affiliated Xiamen Eye Center of Xiamen University, Xiamen, Fujian, China, 3 Xiamen Kehong Eye Hospital, Xiamen, Fujian, PR China, 4 Department of Physiology, The University of Oklahoma Health Sciences Center, Oklahoma City, Oklahoma, United States of America

Abstract

We recently demonstrated that SERPINA3K, a serine proteinase inhibitor, has antioxidant activity in the cornea. Here we investigated the antioxidant effects of SERPINA3K on the pterygial, which is partially caused by oxidative stress in pathogenesis. The head part of primary pterygial tissue was dissected and then cultured in keratinocyte serum-free defined medium (KSFM). The cultured pterygial epithelial cells (PECs) were treated with SERPINA3K. The cell proliferation and migration of PECs were measured and analyzed. Western blot and quantitative real-time polymerase chain reaction (PCR) assay were performed. It showed that SERPINA3K significantly suppressed the cell proliferation of PECs in a concentration-dependent manner, compared with cultured human conjunctival epithelial cells. SERPINA3K also inhibited the cell migration of PECs. Towards its underlying mechanism, SERPINA3K had antioxidant activities on the PECs by significantly inhibiting NADPH oxidase 4 (NOX4), which is an important enzyme of ROS generation, and by elevating the levels of key antioxidant factors of ROS: such as NAD(P)H dehydrogenase (quinone 1) (NQO1), NF-E2–related factor-2 (NRF2) and superoxide dismutases (SOD2). Meanwhile, SERPINA3K down-regulated the key effectors of Wnt signaling pathway: β-catenin, nonphospho-β-catenin, and low-density lipoprotein receptor-related protein 6 (LRP6). We provided novel evidence that SERPINA3K had inhibitory effects on pterygium and SERPINA3K played antioxidant role via regulating the ROS system and antioxidants.

Editor: Masaru Katoh, National Cancer Center, Japan

Funding: This project was supported by a grant from Natural Science Foundation of China (grant No. 81170818) and by a grant from National High Technology Research and Development Program of China (grant No. 2012AA020507). The funders had no role in study design, data collection and analysis, decision to publish, or preparation of the manuscript.

Competing Interests: The authors have declared that no competing interests exist.

* Email: ypzhou@yahoo.com

9 These authors contributed equally to this work.

Introduction

Pterygium is a common ocular surface disease with the characteristics of triangle shape pathologic tissue of fibrovascular neoformation, which originates from conjunctiva, eventually invades cornea and will block the vision in severe cases. Pterygium often happens in the specific geographic regions with strong ultraviolet light, such as, South-East Asia, South-East China, Australia, and so on. Extensive research has been done on the pathogenesis of pterygium. Oxidative stress is considered a major pathogenesis of pterygium, there are other causes, for example, ultraviolet radiation-induced DNA injury, limbal stem cells deficiency (LSCD) [1–5] while the mechanism of pterygium is not fully understood. Meanwhile, there is no effective medication to treat pterygium or prevent the development of pterygium, the current main treatment is to remove the pterygium by surgery and the relapse rate after surgery is high [6,7].

Multiple recent investigations suggest that the epithelial cells of pterygium are highly proliferative, with tumor cell like cell property [8–10]. This high cell proliferation leads to the rapid development and high rate of relapse of pterygium in the clinic. It needs better elucidation on the mechanism of pterygium and exploration of new inhibitory agents to hamper the development of pterygium.

SERPINA3K is a member of the family of serine proteinase inhibitors. SERPINA3K is expressed in the liver, kidney, and ocular tissues. SERPINA3K was first identified as a specific inhibitor of tissue kallikrein, also known as kallikrein-binding protein, since it specifically binds with tissue kallikrein to form a covalent complex and inhibits its proteolytic activities [11]. We recently reported that SERPINA3K has antiinflammatory, anti-angiogenic and antioxidant activity in the corneal epithelium [12,13]. SERPINA3K is also believed to be an inhibitor of Wnt signaling pathway [14]. In this present study, we, for the first time, investigated the inhibitory effects of SERPINA3K on the epithelial cells of pterygium and the underlying mechanism by focusing on reactive oxygen species (ROS) system and Wnt signaling pathway.

Methods

Patients

Seventy-six primary pterygium patients were recruited, irrespective of sex (18 cases of men and 58 cases of women) and age (25–76 years old, mean of age: 50±3.4). The conjunctiva samples were collected from 10 strabismus patients, irrespective of sex and age (2–18 years old). All cases were carefully diagnosed clinically with routine examinations and slit-lamp observation. The patients were not found any severe ocular complications, for example, corneal ulcer, and so on, when recruited. The patients underwent surgery at Xiamen Eye Center. All investigations were conducted in accordance with the tenets of the Declaration of Helsinki and were approved by the Ethics Committee of Xiamen Eye Center (an affiliated hospital of Xiamen University). A written informed consent was acquired from all participating patients. The head part of the pterygium tissue, that is, the part invading cornea, was excised for the cell culture experiment.

Materials

The CCK-8 assay kits were purchased from Dojindo (Tokyo, Japan). The antibodies of anti-NOX4, anti-NQO1, anti-NRF2, anti-β-catenin, anti-nonphospho-β-catenin, and anti-LRP-6 were purchased from Abcam (Cambridge, MA). AlexaFluor488-conjugated IgG was purchased from Invitrogen (Carlsbad, CA).

Purification of SERPINA3K

The SA3K/pET28 construct was introduced into Escherichia coli strain BL21. The purification procedure of SERPINA3K has been previously reported [12]. The purity of recombinant SERPINA3K was examined by SDS PAGE. Endotoxin concentration was monitored by using a limulus amebocyte kit. Activity was checked by MTT assay with HUVEC cells.

Cell Culture

The culture experiments were performed within two hours after surgical removal of pterygium or collection of conjunctiva samples. Fresh head part of pterygial specimens was dissected and conjunctiva tissue was collected. The dissected specimens were then cut into small pieces (1–2 mm in diameter), washed in keratinocyte serum-free defined medium (KSF-M) (GIBCO, Carlsbad, CA) and placed in a culture dish. The culture dish was placed in a CO_2-regulated incubator with 5% CO_2. The KSF-M medium was replaced every 2 days for about 15 days until the appearance of an outgrowth of pterygial or conjunctival epithelial cells. The procedures of pterygium epithelial cell culture and identification were previously described and followed [15].

Experimental Procedures

First passage of pterygial epithelial cells (PECs) or conjunctival epithelial cells collected from explant culture were cultured and used in the formal experiments until the cells were cultured to 75% confluency for cell viability measurement and 90% confluency for the cell migration test, respectively. SERPINA3K at concentrations given was added in the media for 12 or 24 hours in the treatment groups before experimental measurements and assays.

Cell Viability

The cultured pterygial epithelial cells (PECs) and conjunctival epithelial cells were used. Cell viability or cell proliferation of PECs and conjunctival epithelial cells was measured by the CCK-8 assay. CCK-8 assay was conducted with the protocol of the manufacturer. Briefly, after incubation in conditional media for 24 hours, the media were replaced by CCK-8 constituted in culture media, followed by incubation for 4 hours at 37°C in the dark. The CCK-8 containing medium was detected directly after incubation. The absorbance was measured spectrophotometrically at 570 nm with a Bio Tek ELX800 microplate reader (Bio-Tek Instruments, Winooski, VT).

Cell Migration

A scratch wound test was conducted to detect the cell migration of PECs. Briefly when PECs cells were cultured to 90% confluency, a scratch was applied in the center of the culture dish. The cell images were recorded at 0 and 12 hours. The length of the unmigrated or uninvading area was measured and analyzed to represent the cell migration of PECs.

Western Blot

Total cellular proteins of the harvested PECs cells were extracted. The standard Western blot protocol was applied. The specific primary antibodies of anti-NOX4, anti-NQO1, anti-NRF2, anti-β-catenin, anti-nonphospho-β-catenin, anti-LRP-6, and a horseradish peroxidase–conjugated secondary antibody were used. Finally, the specific bands were visualized by enhanced chemiluminescence reagents and recorded on film.

Quantitative Real-time Polymerase Chain Reaction (PCR) Assay

Total RNA was extracted from the cultured PECs cells by using TRIzol reagent (Invitrogen, Carlsbad, CA.). Reverse transcription was performed with Oligo 18T primers and reverse transcription reagents according to the manufacturer's protocol (TaKaRa, Shiga, Japan). Quantitative real-time polymerase chain reaction (PCR) was performed with mRNA special primers. The following primers were used for the PCR assay: for NOX4, 5′-TATC-CAGTCCTTCCGTTGGTT-3′ (forward) and 5′-CTGAGGTA-CAGCTGGATGTTGA-3′ (reverse); for SOD2, 5′-GAGAAG-TACCAGGAGGCGTTG-3′ (forward) and 5′-GAGCCTTGG-ACACCAACAGAT-3′ (reverse) and for NRF-2, 5′-AAACCA-GTGGATCTGCCAAC-3′(forward) and 5′-GACCGGGAATA-TCAGGAACA-3′(reverse). PCR reactions were performed on a BIO-RAD CFX-96 Real Time system with SYBR Premix Ex Taq (TaKaRa, Shiga, Japan) at 95°C for 10 minutes, followed by 45 cycles of 95°C for 10 seconds, 57°C for 30 seconds, and 75°C for 10 seconds, after which melt curve analysis was performed at once from 65°C to 95°C. All reactions were performed in triplicate and the average cycle threshold (Ct) values greater than 38 were treated as negative. The level of GAPDH mRNA was used as an internal control.

Statistical Analysis

One-way analysis of variance test (ANONA) was conducted to analyze the data of CCK-8 assay, scratch wound test, Western blot, and quantitative real-time PCR assay followed by a post hoc analysis Tukey test to compare the differences between the groups or a Student's t-test. A value of $p < 0.05$ was considered statistically significant.

Results

SERPINA3K Suppressed Cell Viability and Migration of Pterygium Epithelial Cells

Since the epithelial cells of pterygium are highly proliferative [8–10], we first evaluated the inhibitory effects of SERPINA3K (SA3K) on the cell viability or cell proliferation of cultured

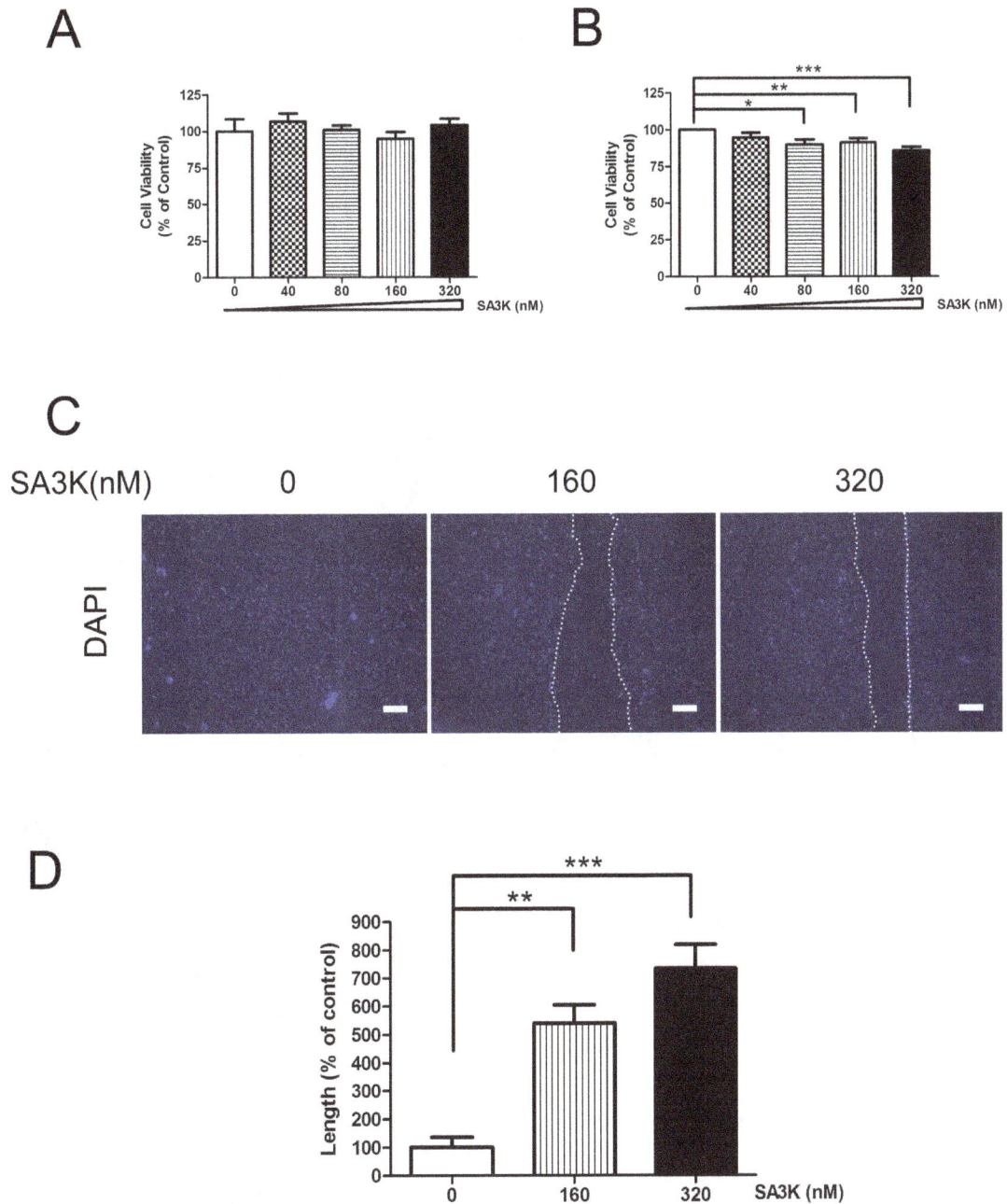

Figure 1. SERPINA3K (SA3K) suppressed the cell proliferation and cell migration of pterygial epithelial cells (PECs). Comparison of the effects of SERPINA3K on the cell proliferation of conjunctival epithelial cells (**A**) and PECs (**B**). Conjunctival epithelial cells and PECs were cultured in keratinocyte serum-free defined medium (KSF-M) and treated with SA3K at concentrations of 0, 40, 80, 160, and 320 nM for 24 hours. Data were presented as mean±SEM; n = 9–10; *: $p<0.05$, **: $p<0.01$, ***: $p<0.001$. (**C**) Representative images of cell migration of PECs after treatment of SA3K (0, 160 and 320 nM) for 12 hours. The central dotted area demonstrated the unmigrated or uninvading area of PECs. Scale bar,100 μm (**D**) Statistic analysis of the length of the unmigrated or uninvading area between control, 160 nM and 320 nM SA3K groups. Data were presented as mean ±SEM; n = 4; **: $p<0.01$, ***: $p<0.001$.

pterygial epithelial cells (PECs) and compared PECs with cultured human conjunctival epithelial cells. It demonstrated that SA3K statistically significantly suppressed the cell proliferation of PECs at concentration of 80, 160 and 320 nM after treatment of 24 hours (Figure 1B). Meanwhile, SA3K at same concentrations did not influence the cell proliferation of cultured human conjunctival epithelial cells significantly (Figure 1A), indicating that SERPI-NA3K may selectively and specifically suppress the cell prolifer-

ation of pterygial epithelial cells. We next investigated the effects of SA3K on the cell migration of cultured PECs using scratch wound test. SA3K at concentration of 160 nM and 320 nM significantly inhibited the cell migration of PECs after treatment of 12 hours. (Figure 1C, 1D) These data indicated that SERPINA3K has inhibitory effects on pterygium.

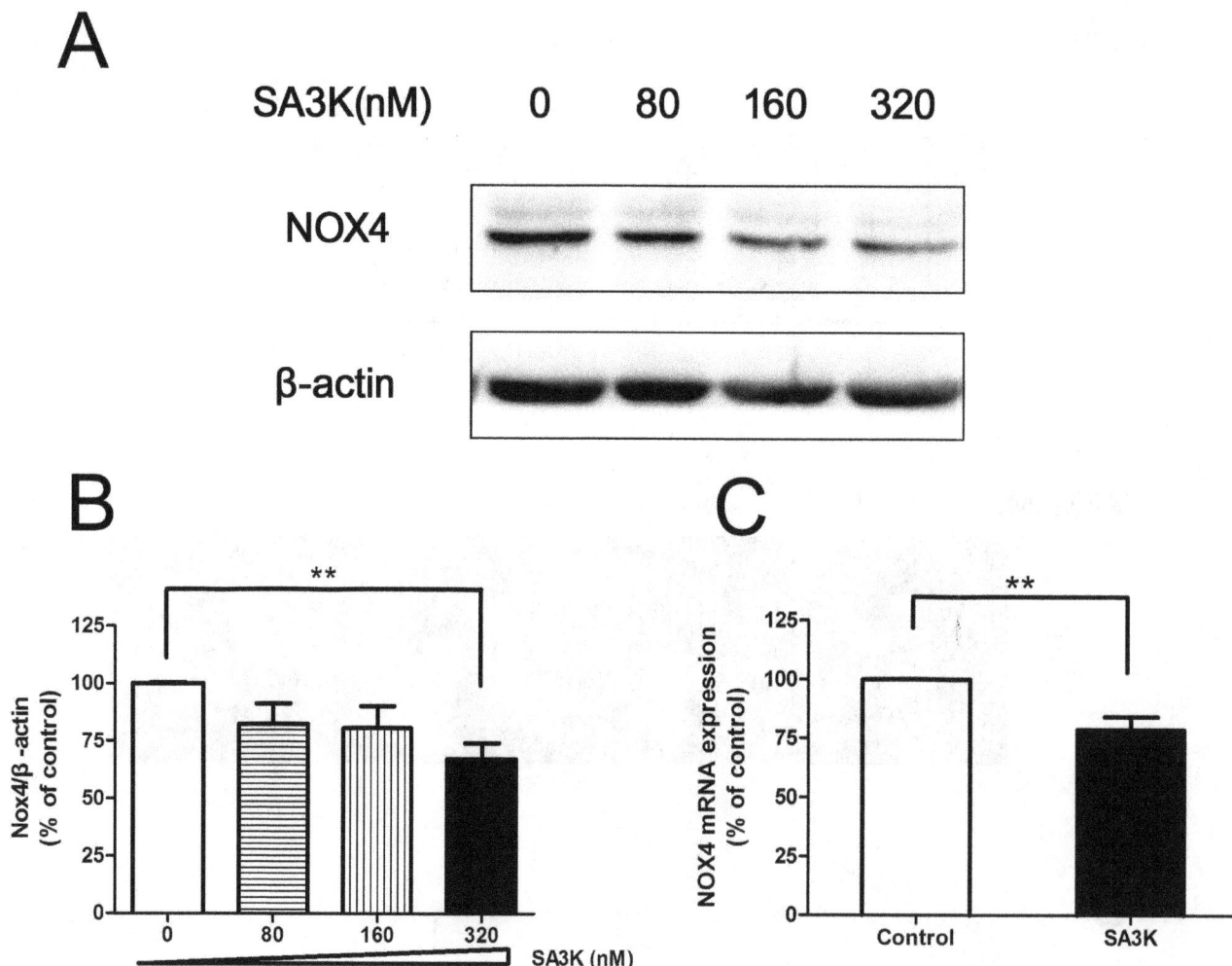

Figure 2. SERPINA3K (SA3K) inhibited the key ROS generation enzyme: NOX4. (**A**) Representative images of Western blot with anti-NOX4 antibody in the PECs after treatment of SA3K at concentration of 0, 80, 160, and 320 nM for 24 hours. (**B**) Statistic analysis of the Western blot data. Data were presented as mean±SEM; n = 5; **: p<0.01. (**C**) Quantitative real-time PCR assay data of NOX4 in the PECs after treatment of 320 nM SA3K for 24 hours. Data were presented as mean±SEM; n = 5; **: p<0.01.

SERPINA3K Regulated the ROS Generation Enzyme and Antioxidants

Oxidative stress is the major pathogenesis of pterygium [1–5], we recently reported that SERPINA3K plays an antioxidant role in the corneal epithelium [13], we then identified if SERPINA3K inhibited PECs through targeting the reactive oxygen species (ROS) system, for example, regulations of the key enzyme of the ROS generation system: NADPH oxidase 4 (NOX4) [16–18] and the antioxidants of the ROS system: such as, NAD(P)H dehydrogenase (quinone 1) (NQO1), NF-E2–related factor-2 (NRF2) and superoxide dismutases (SOD2) [19–23].

We first examined the effect of SERPINA3K on the ROS generation enzyme NOX4 by Western blot with specific anti-NOX4 antibody. It showed that SA3K significantly downregulated the protein level of NOX4 after treatment of 24 hours (Figure 2A, 2B). In addition, we also detected the gene expression of NOX4 by quantitative real-time PCR assay. SA3K significantly inhibited the gene expression of NOX4 in the PECs after treatment of 24 hours. (Figure 2C).

On the other hand, we evaluated the effects of SA3K on the antioxidants of ROS system: NQO1, NRF2 and SOD2. It was demonstrated by Western blot that SA3K significantly increased the protein level of NQO1 after treatment of 24 hours (Figure 3A, 3B). We also detected the changes of gene expression and protein level of antioxidant NRF2 in the PECs after treatment of SA3K for 24 hours. The Western blot results revealed that SA3K significantly increased the protein level of NRF2 in the PECs (Figure, 3C, 3D). Furthermore, it was also shown by quantitative real-time PCR assay that the gene expression of NRF2 was significantly increased in the PECs (Figure 3E). Moreover, SA3K also statistically significantly elevated the gene expression of another antioxidant SOD2 in the PECs after treatment of 24 hours (Figure 3F).

These data suggested that SERPINA3K protects against oxidative stress of PECs via blocking the ROS generation enzyme and increasing the antioxidants.

SERPINA3K Downregulated Wnt Signaling Pathway

We previously demonstrated that SERPINA3K is a Wnt signaling pathway inhibitor via binding and blocking the Wnt pathway upstream effector: low-density lipoprotein receptor-related protein 6 (LRP6) [14], we then determined if the inhibitory

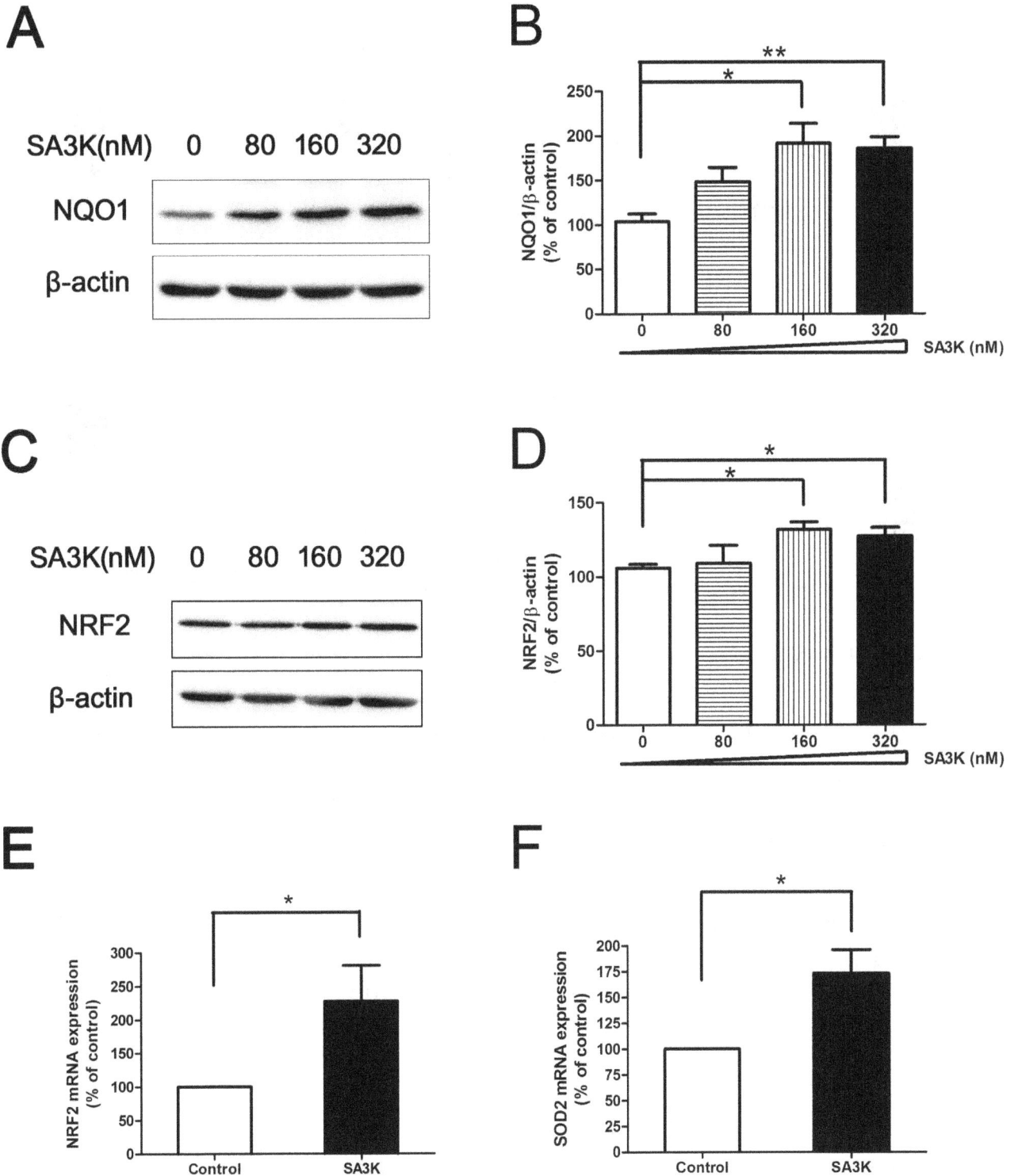

Figure 3. SERPINA3K (SA3K) increased the levels of antioxidants: NQO1, NRF2 and SOD2. (A) Representative images of Western blot with anti-NQO1 antibody in the PECs after treatment of SA3K at concentration of 0, 80, 160, and 320 nM for 24 hours. (B) Statistic analysis of Western blot data of NQO1. Data were presented as mean±SEM; n = 3; *: p<0.05, **: p<0.01. (C) Representative images of Western blot with anti-NRF2 antibody in the PECs after treatment of SA3K at concentration of 0, 80, 160 and 320 nM for 24 hours. (D) Statistic analysis of the western blot data of NRF2. Data were presented as mean±SEM; n = 3; *: p<0.05. (E) Quantitative real-time PCR assay data of NRF2 in the PECs after treatment of 320 nM SA3K for 24 hours. Data were presented as mean±SEM; n = 6; *: p<0.05. (F) Quantitative real-time PCR assay data of SOD2 in the PECs after treatment of 320 nM SA3K for 24 hours. Data were presented as mean±SEM; n = 3; *: p<0.05.

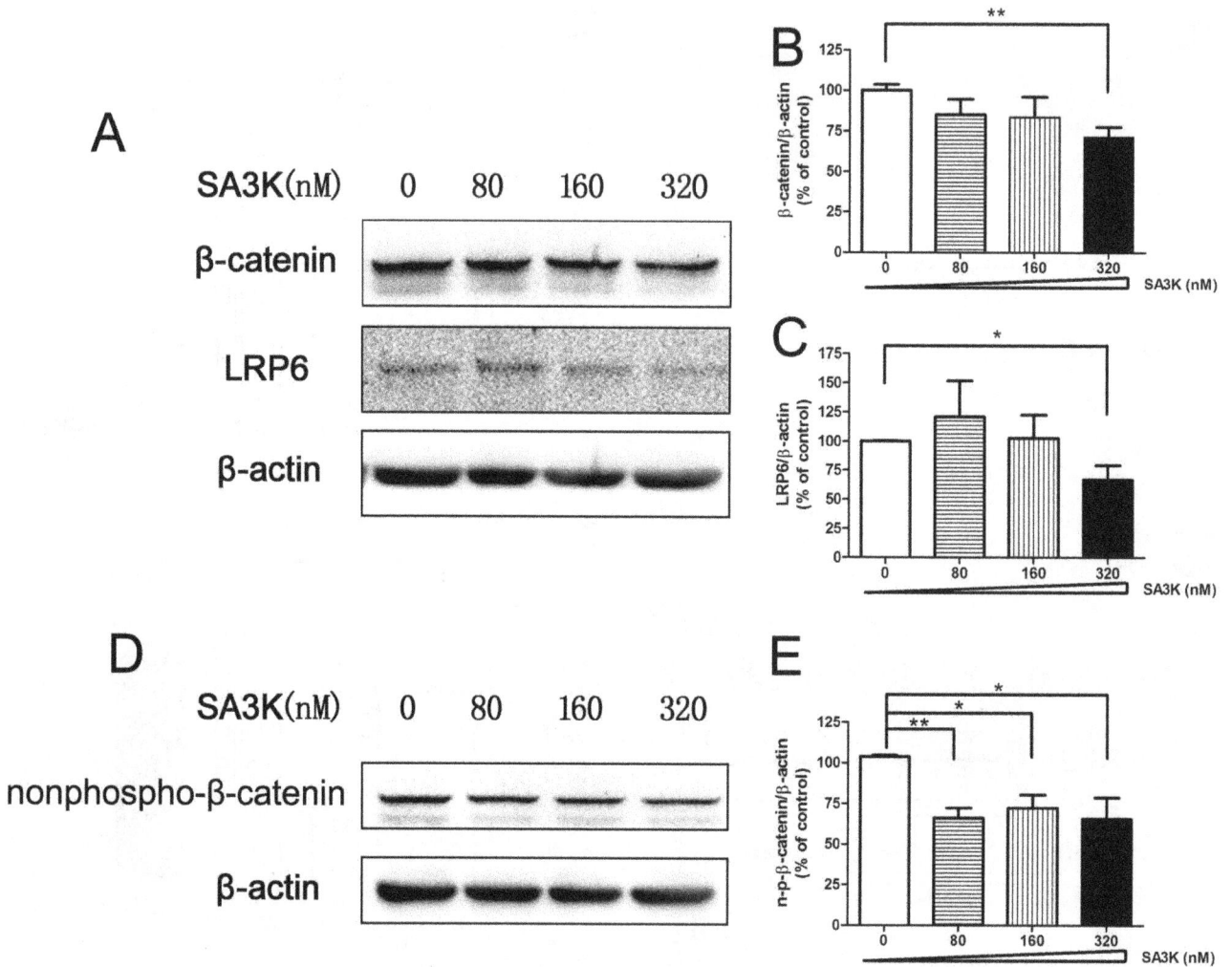

Figure 4. SERPINA3K (SA3K) downregulated Wnt signaling pathway. (**A**) Representative images of Western blot with anti-β-catenin and anti-LRP6 antibodies in the PECs after treatment of SA3K at concentration of 0, 80, 160, and 320 nM for 24 hours. (**B**) Statistic analysis of the western blot data of β-catenin. Data were presented as mean±SEM; n = 4; **: p<0.01. (**C**) Statistic analysis of the Western blot data of LRP6. Data were presented as mean±SEM; n = 5; *: p<0.05. (**D**) Representative images of Western blot with anti-nonphospho-β-catenin antibody in the PECs after treatment of SA3K at concentration of 0, 80, 160 and 320 nM for 24 hours. (**E**) Statistic analysis of the Western blot data of nonphospho-β-catenin. Data were presented as mean±SEM; n = 3; *: p<0.05, **: p<0.01.

effects of SERPINA3K on the PECs are associated with the downregulation of Wnt signaling pathway in the present study. To evaluate the downregulation of Wnt pathway in the PECs, we conducted Western blot of the key effectors of Wnt pathway: β-catenin and LRP6. The Western blot data showed that the protein levels of β-catenin and LRP6 were decreased in the PECs after treatment of SA3K for 24 hours (Figure 4A, 4B, 4C). To further confirm the association of SA3K with the Wnt pathway in the PECs, we also measured another key Wnt pathway effector: nonphospho-β-catenin by Western blot. SA3K at concentration of 80, 160 and 320 nM statistically significantly decreased the protein level of nonphospho-β-catenin after treatment of 24 hours (Figure 4D, 4E). These results suggested that SA3K downregulates the Wnt signaling pathway.

Discussion

Pterygium is a pathologic ocular surface tissue with highly proliferative cells [8–10] and it still lacks of effective medication

except the surgical removal. In this study, we, for the first time, demonstrated that SERPINA3K, a serine proteinase inhibitor, suppresses the cell proliferation and migration of pterygial epithelial cells. Moreover, we also revealed that the underlying mechanism of SERPINA3K is through regulations of ROS system and the blockade of Wnt signaling pathway. Our experimental data may contribute to the exploration of new therapeutic agents to antagonize the formation and development of pterygium.

SERPINA3K has been demonstrated to have antiinflammation and antioxidatant activities in the eyes including corneas and retina [12,13,24,25]. It has not been reported about the effect of SERPINA3K on the pterygium, which is associated with oxidative stress and inflammation in pathogenesis. The experimental evidence from this study supported our previous findings of antiinflammatory and antioxidant effects of SERPINA3K in another ocular pathologic tissue and status. It suggested that SERAPINA3K, as an endogenous protein with multiple functions including antiinflammatory, antiangiogenic and antioxidant effects, may have an advantage to treat pterygium and prevent the development of pterygium compared with the current application of antiinflammatory medication after surgical removal of pterygium.

A pterygium originates from conjunctiva and it invades cornea in many cases, it is necessary to determine if SERPINA3K selectively and specifically targets the pterygial epithelial cells, by comparison of the effects of SERPINA3K on conjunctival epithelial cells and corneal epithelial cells. It was revealed by the present investigation that SERPINA3K did not suppress the cell proliferation of cultured human conjunctival epithelial cells. In addition, we previously demonstrated that SERPINA3K at various concentrations did not inhibit the cell proliferation of human corneal epithelial cells (HCEs) [12]. These data suggest that SERPINA3K can specifically suppress the cell proliferation of pterygial epithelial cells. On the other hand, as a pterygium is composed of epithelial layer and the basal layer, which contains lots of fibroblasts or stroma cells, we just demonstrated that SERPINA3K has inhibitory effects on the cell proliferation and migration of epithelial cells of pterygium in this study, it needs further investigation to elucidate the effect of SERPINA3K on pterygial fibroblasts or stroma cells.

Due to the limitation of application of SERPINA3K on human pterygium patients in clinic and the lack of good in vivo animal models of pterygium at present time, we only performed the investigation of SERPINA3K in the cultured pterygial cells, a further investigation on the efficacy of local application of SERPINA3K on animal model of pterygium in vivo and human pterygium should be conducted when available. Furthermore, we mainly focused on the effect of SERPINA3K in primary pterygium in this study, it is of worth to elucidate the effect of SERPINA3K on recurrent pterygium in the future.

Oxidative stress is believed to play a vital role in the pathogenesis and development of pterygium [1–5]. Oxidative stress is also a major pathogenesis of other eye diseases, for example, other ocular surface diseases, age-related eye diseases, and so on. [28–30] Oxidative stress is a pathologic state of excessive ROS production or abnormal balance of the ROS system or ROS pathway [31,32]. In this study, we demonstrated that SERPINA3K suppresses the generation enzyme of ROS: NOX4, which is a key enzyme of ROS generation [16–18], meanwhile, SERPINA3K also elevated the levels of various antioxidant factors, such as NQO1, NRF2 and SOD2 [19–23].

This present study is consistent with our previous report about the antioxidant activity of SERPINA3K in the corneal epithelium [13]. Since we mainly focused on the antioxidant role of SERPINA3K in pterygium, it is necessary to make a further comparison of the antioxidant activities of SERPINA3K between the pterygium, conjunctiva and corneas with same range and stages of age to better understand and evaluate the antioxidant role of SERPINA3K in the formation and development of pterygium.

It is reported that SERPINA3K is an inhibitor of Wnt signaling pathway, the target and binding site of SERPINA3K is the upstream effector of Wnt pathway: LRP6 [14]. Thus we evaluated the alteration of Wnt pathway after treatment of SERPINA3K in the cultured pterygial epithelial cells, we demonstrated that SERPINA3K down-regulated the Wnt pathway, including the effectors: LRP6, β-catenin and nonphospho-β-catenin. This result also supports the hypothesis that SERPINA3K is an inhibitor of Wnt signaling pathway in different ocular tissue and cells, while the more detailed molecular mechanistic needs further elucidated, for example, how SERPINA3K affects the activities of downstream factors of Wnt pathway in the pterygial epithelial cells, such as transcription factor 4 (TCF4), and so on. It also requires a better understanding of the role of Wnt pathway in the formation and development of pterygium and to compare the effects of SERPINA3K on Wnt pathway between pterygium, conjunctiva as well as cornea, while there are multiply reports indicating that Wnt signaling pathway is highly expressed or activated in the pterygium [26,27].

Taken together, we provided novel experimental evidence that SERPINA3K may inhibit the formation and development of pterygium and SERPINA3K has antioxidant activity in pterygium, indicating that SERPINA3K is of the potential to be used as a therapeutic agent in the treatment of pterygium or to prevent the relapse of pterygium after surgical removal in clinic.

Author Contributions

Conceived and designed the experiments: CZ FP YZ. Performed the experiments: CZ LG JZ LC TZ RZ FP. Analyzed the data: CZ FP ZT XX JxM ZL YZ. Contributed reagents/materials/analysis tools: ND MY. Wrote the paper: CP YZ.

References

1. Cimpean AM, Sava MP, Raica M (2013) DNA damage in human pterygium: one-shot multiple targets. Mol Vis 19: 348–356.
2. Balci M, Şahin S, Mutlu FM, Yağci R, Karanci P, et al. (2011) Investigation of oxidative stress in pterygium tissue. Mol Vis 2011; 17: 443–447.
3. Tsai YY, Cheng YW, Lee H, Tsai FJ, Tseng SH, et al. (2005) Oxidative DNA damage in pterygium. Mol Vis11: 71–75.
4. Perra MT, Maxia C, Corbu A, Minerba L, Demurtas P, et al. (2006) Oxidative stress in pterygium: relationship between p53 and 8-hydroxydeoxyguanosine. Mol Vis 12: 1136–1142.
5. Chui J, Coroneo MT, Tat LT, Crouch R, Wakefield D, et al. (2011) Ophthalmic pterygium: a stem cell disorder with premalignant features. Am J Pathol 178: 817–827.
6. Ozgurhan EB, Agca A, Kara N, Yuksel K, Demircan A, et al. (2013) Topical application of bevacizumab as an adjunct to recurrent pterygium surgery. Cornea 32: 835–838.
7. Nakasato H, Uemoto R, Mizuki N (2012) Treatment of pterygium by ligation and bevacizumab injection. Cornea 31: 1339–1341.
8. Chowers I, Pe'er J, Zamir E, Livni N, Ilsar M, et al. (2001) Proliferative activity and p53 expression in primary and recurrent pterygia. Ophthalmology 108: 985–988.
9. Kase S, Takahashi S, Sato I, Nakanishi K, Yoshida K, et al. (2007) Expression of p27 (KIP1) and cyclin D1, and cell proliferation in human pterygium. Br J Ophthalmol 91: 958–961.
10. Liang K, Jiang Z, Ding B, Cheng P, Huang DK, et al. (2011) Expression of cell proliferation and apoptosis biomarkers in pterygia and normal conjunctiva. Mol Vis 17: 1687–1693.
11. Chai KX, Ma JX, Murray SR, Chao J, Chao L (1991) Molecular cloning and analysis of the rat kallikrein-binding protein gene. J Biol Chem 266: 16029–16036.
12. Liu X, Lin Z, Zhou T, Zong R, He H, et al. (2011) Anti-angiogenic and antiinflammatory effects of SERPINA3K on corneal injury. PLoS ONE 6: e16712.
13. Zhou T, Zong R, Zhang Z, Zhu C, Pan F, et al. (2012) SERPINA3K protects against oxidative stress via modulating ROS generation/degradation and KEAP1-NRF2 pathway in the corneal epithelium. Invest Ophthalmol Vis Sci 53: 5033–5043.
14. Zhang B, Abreu JG, Zhou K, Chen Y, Hu Y, et al. (2010) Blocking the Wnt pathway, a unifying mechanism for an angiogenic inhibitor in the serine proteinase inhibitor family. Proc Natl Acad Sci U S A 107: 6900–6905.
15. Xu K, Tao T, Jie J, Lu X, Li X, et al. (2013) Increased importin 13 activity is associated with the pathogenesis of pterygium. Mol Vis 19: 604–613.
16. Bedard K, Krause KH (2007) The NOX family of ROS-generating NADPH oxidases: physiology and pathophysiology. Physiol Rev 87: 245–313.
17. Petry A, Djordjevic T, Weitnauer M, Kietzmann T, Hess J, et al. (2006) NOX2 and NOX4 mediate proliferative response in endothelial cells. Antioxid Redox Signal 8: 1473–1484.
18. Block K, Gorin Y, Abboud HE (2009) Subcellular localization of Nox4 and regulation in diabetes. Proc Natl Acad Sci U S A 106: 14385–14390.

19. Siegel D, Ross D (2000) Immunodetection of NAD(P)H: quinone oxidoreductase 1 (NQO1) in human tissues. Free Radic Biol Med 29: 246–253.

20. Schelonka LP, Siegel D, Wilson MW, Meininger A, Ross D (2000) Immunohistochemical localization of NQO1 in epithelial dysplasia and neoplasia and in donor eyes. Invest Ophthalmol Vis Sci 41: 1617–1622.

21. Nguyen T, Nioi P, Pickett CB (2009) The Nrf2-antioxidant response element signaling pathway and its activation by oxidative stress. J Biol Chem 284: 13291–13295.

22. Li W, Kong AN (2009) Molecular mechanisms of Nrf2-mediated antioxidant response. Mol Carcinog 48: 91–104.

23. Kaspar JW, Niture SK, Jaiswal AK (2009) Nrf2: INrf2 (Keap1) signaling in oxidative stress. Free Radic Biol Med 47: 1304–1309.

24. Zhang B, Hu Y, Ma JX (2009) Anti-inflammatory and antioxidant effects of SERPINA3K in the retina. Invest Ophthalmol Vis Sci 50: 3943–3952.

25. Zhang B, Ma JX (2008) SERPINA3K prevents oxidative stress induced necrotic cell death by inhibiting calcium overload. PLoS ONE 3: e4077.

26. Zhou T, Zhou KK, Lee K, Gao G, Lyons TJ, et al. (2011) The role of lipid peroxidation products and oxidative stress in activation of the canonical wingless-type MMTV integration site (WNT) pathway in a rat model of diabetic retinopathy. Diabetologia 54: 459–468.

27. Kato N, Shimmura S, Kawakita T, Miyashita H, Ogawa Y, et al. (2007) Beta-catenin activation and epithelial-mesenchymal transition in the pathogenesis of pterygium. Invest Ophthalmol Vis Sci 48: 1511–1517.

28. Giacco F, Brownlee M (2010) Oxidative stress and diabetic complications. Circ Res 107: 1058–1070.

29. Khandhadia S, Lotery A (2010) Oxidation and age-related macular degeneration: insights from molecular biology. Expert Rev Mol Med 12: e34.

30. Buddi R, Lin B, Atilano SR, Zorapapel NC, Kenney MC, et al. (2002) Evidence of oxidative stress in human corneal diseases. J Histochem Cytochem 50: 341–351.

31. Wasserman WW, Fahl WE (1997) Functional antioxidant responsive elements. Proc Natl Acad Sci U S A 94: 5361–5366.

32. Kietzmann T (2010) Intracellular redox compartments: mechanisms and significances. Antioxid Redox Signal 13: 395–398.

20

Melatonin Enhances Photo-Oxidation of 2′, 7′-Dichlorodihydrofluorescein by an Antioxidant Reaction That Renders N1-Acetyl-N2-Formyl-5-Methoxykynuramine (AFMK)

David Hevia[1,2], Juan C. Mayo[1,2], Dun-Xian Tan[3], Aida Rodriguez-Garcia[1,2], Rosa M. Sainz[1,2]*

1 Departamento de Morfologia y Biologia Celular, School of Medicine, University of Oviedo, Oviedo, Spain, 2 Instituto Universitario Oncologico del Principado de Asturias (IUOPA), Oviedo, Spain, 3 Department of Cellular and Structural Biology, University of Texas Health Science Center at San Antonio, San Antonio, Texas, United States of America

Abstract

The indolamine melatonin (MEL) is described as an antioxidant and a free radical scavenger. However occasionally, the indoleamine has been reported to increase free radicals with insufficient mechanistic explanation. In an attempt to find a reason for those controversial results, a potential mechanism that explains MEL prooxidant activity is investigated. The current controversy about redox detection methods has prompted us to search a possible interaction between MEL and dichlorodihydrofluorescein ($DCFH_2$), perhaps the most widely fluorescence probe employed for free radicals detection in cellular models. Here, it is demonstrated that melatonin potentiates the photooxidation of $DCFH_2$ in a cell-free system, increasing the production of its fluorescent metabolite. Indeed, MEL works as an antioxidant scavenging hydroxyl radicals in this system. Thus, this reaction between MEL and $DCFH_2$ produces N1-acetyl-N2-formyl-5-methoxykynuramine (AFMK), a biogenic amine with antioxidant properties too. This reaction is O_2 and light dependent and it is prevented by antioxidants such as N-acetylcysteine or ascorbic acid. Furthermore, when $DCFH_2$ has been employed to evaluate antioxidant or prooxidant activities of MEL in cellular models it is confirmed that it works as an antioxidant but these results can be modulated by light misleading to a prooxidant conclusion. In conclusion, here is demonstrated that $DCFH_2$, light and melatonin interact and results obtained using these fluorescence probes in studies with melatonin have to be carefully interpreted.

Editor: Sayuri Miyamoto, Instituto de Química, Universidade de São Paulo, Brazil

Funding: This work has been supported by an ISCIII (FISS-09-PS09/02204) grant. ARG acknowledges support from the "Severo Ochoa" fellowship program (FICYT). DH and JCM acknowledge sponsorship from Instituto Universitario Oncologico del Principado de Asturias (IUOPA). The funders had no role in study design, data collection and analysis, decision to publish, or preparation of the manuscript.

Competing Interests: The authors have declared that no competing interests exist.

* Email: sainzrosa@uniovi.es

Introduction

Oxidative stress has an important impact in human health. Its implication in several disorders including atherosclerosis, diabetes, neurodegeneration or cancer has been widely investigated. The principal components of oxidative stress are a variety of chemical species such as nitric oxide (NO), superoxide anions ($O_2^{\bullet-}$), hydroxyl radicals ($^{\bullet}OH$) and hydrogen peroxide (H_2O_2) among others. Some of these molecules are generated exogenously or produced endogenously from several sources including oxidative phosphorylation in mitochondria. Given its important role in physiology and pathology, there is an increasing interest in developing accurate methods to measure free radical production in cells.

One of the principal drawbacks of oxidative stress research has been the accuracy when measuring ROS production in *in vivo* systems. There are currently several methods developed for measuring free radicals inside cells including chemiluminescence of luminol or lucigenin [1], cytochrome c reduction [2] or ferrous oxidation of xylenol orange [3] as well as some other commercially available fluorescence probes. However, among all of them, 2′,7′-dichlorofluorescein (DCF) staining is by far the most widely employed for the analysis of ROS and cellular oxidative stress [4,5]. To measure ROS in cells [6], $DCFH_2$-DA is used because it can be easily taken up and it is more resistant to oxidation than $DCFH_2$. Upon internalization it is rapidly de-acetylated and after that it reacts with ROS to produce a fluorescence product [7]. Given its simplicity and sensitivity, $DCFH_2$-DA [4] has been employed to study the production of H_2O_2 [8] in several reports by using microplate reader [9] or flow cytometry methods [10].

N-acetyl-5-methoxy-tryptamine or melatonin is an indolamine produced endogenously and secreted into circulation mainly by pineal gland though it is also synthesized in many other locations. In all species studied thus far, its synthesis from tryptophan occurs during darkness [11,12]. Considering its nocturnal synthesis, melatonin has been linked to sleep promotion [13], a chemical signal of light:dark cycle [14], and a regulator of reproductive physiology in seasonal breeding mammals among others [15]. Besides regulating circadian and circannual rhythms, melatonin is a major endogenous antioxidant and a free radical scavenger [16]. Melatonin functions as a direct-scavenging molecule and it also stimulates indirectly gene expression and activities of antioxidant enzymes [17]. As a direct scavenger, melatonin reacts with different free radicals including ${}^{\bullet}OH$, $O_2^{\bullet-}$, $NO^{\bullet}$ and alkyl-peroxyl radicals [18–20] and indirectly, it stimulates glutathione production and the activities of both, glutathione peroxidase and superoxide dismutase [21,22]. There is an inverse relationship between melatonin levels and tumour growth, in terms of initiation but also, of progression and metastasis [23]. Although numerous mechanisms have been identified to explain melatonin inhibition of cancer [24], its role as an intracellular redox regulator has been well documented as one of the mechanism by which it could modulate cancer growth [25]. Melatonin has been mostly reported to inhibit cell growth by reducing free radicals production or activity [26] but also, it has been suggested that melatonin by itself promotes cell toxicity and death of some tumour cells through a prooxidant pathway [27–30].

Antioxidant and prooxidant activities of melatonin have been previously evaluated by using $DCFH_2$ or $DCFH_2$-DA staining by other researchers. Furthermore, there are several cases of interactions between $DCFH_2$ or $DCFH_2$-DA with other molecules. So, a set of experiments to assess any potential interaction between melatonin with $DCFH_2$ or $DCFH_2$-DA are performed to clarify discrepancies observed about antioxidant or prooxidant properties of the pineal neuroindoleamine when this probe are used.

Material and Methods

Chemicals and solutions

2′-7′-dichlorodihydrofluorescein diacetate ($DCFH_2$-DA) was purchased from Invitrogen (Life Technologies, Alcobendas, Madrid, Spain). All other chemicals were purchased from Sigma-Aldrich (Tres Cantos, Madrid, Spain). Melatonin (Merck, Darmstadt, Germany) stock (1 M) was prepared in DMSO and then diluted until desired concentration directly in phosphate buffer saline (PBS). Other reagents including catalase (CAT), superoxide dismutase (SOD), ascorbic acid (AA), N-acetyl cysteine (NAC) or H_2O_2 were freshly prepared in PBS and used immediately for all assays.

Light-dark experiments

Light-dark experiments were performed in a hermetic box protected from external light and equipped with a light bulb located at 15 cm from samples. Light used was a 6W linear fluorescent (F6T5/D, GE lighting # 10028) with the following features: Initial Lumen (NOM) 230, Median Lumen (NOM) 185, Colour temperature 6500 K, Nominal initial lumen per Watt (NOM) 38. Other specific parameters such as spectral, power distribution or electric characteristic can be checked at the company web site (www.gelighting.com). Light power reaching samples was 25000 lux. All the experiments were performed at RT. All solutions were placed in open tubes and at the same time for each experiment. Dark experiments were carried out in the same conditions than light experiments but in this case light of box was turned off.

DCFH₂ preparation

For cell-free experiments $DCFH_2$-DA was deacetilated to $DCFH_2$ prior to each experiment following the method described

before [31]. Briefly, 0.5 ml $DCFH_2$-DA (1.0 mM in methanol) was mixed with 2 ml of NaOH (0.01 M) for 30 minutes at RT. Then, mixture was neutralized by adding 10 ml of NaH_2PO_4 (25 mM, pH 7.4). Final solution 1 mM $DCFH_2$ was employed within 15 minutes after dilution.

Fluorescence and absorbance spectroscopy

Absorption spectra of samples containing $DCFH_2$-DA or $DCFH_2$ in PBS at pH 7.4 with or without MEL, H_2O_2, AA, SOD or CAT were measured by using a Cary 50 Bio UV-Vis spectrophotometer (Agilent Technologies, Santa Clara, CA, USA) at room temperature. Changes in absorption were quantified at 501 nm (λ_{max} of DCF).

Fluorescence were measured in quartz cuvettes using a Cary Eclipse fluorimeter (Agilent Technologies, Santa Clara, CA USA) at RT ($\lambda_{exc} = 480$ nm, $\lambda_{em} = 500–700$ nm). Voltage was set between 400 and 800 V. Since voltage was changed to get enough acquisition, all groups from the same set of experiments were measured at the same time, using the same voltage intensity. For studies under a N_2 atmosphere, an atmosbag glove bag (Sigma-Aldrich) was used.

HPLC measurements

HPLC analysis was performed on 1260 Infinity HPLC system (Agilent Technologies, USA) equipped with a binary pump with solvent selection valves, online degasser and a programmable autosampler. A tracer Extrasil ODS1 column (250 mm×0.46 mm, 5 μm) (Teknokroma, Barcelona, Spain), operating at 35°C was used. An ODS guard column was placed previously to protect the analytical column. Mobile phase solution was always filtered through a 0.45 μm membrane filter. Identification of the compounds was determined by their retention time (RT) and UV spectrum. All measurements were performed using Chemstation software.

HPLC analysis of MEL, N1-acetyl-N2-formyl-5-methoxykynuramine (AFMK), N1-acetyl-5-methoxykynuramine (AMK) or cyclic 3-hydroxymelatonin (3-COHM) was performed as previously described [32]. Briefly, sodium acetate (20 mM, pH 5.1) in 35% methanol was used as mobile phase. A flow of 0.9 ml/min and different wavelengths (190 at 800 nm) were employed to obtain the spectrum of absorbance for each compound. The elution order was 3-COHM, AMK, MEL and AFMK and absorbance was set at 230/279 nm (absolute/relative maximum) for MEL, 233/380 nm for AMK, 233/337 nm for AFMK and 231/306 for 3COHM. Quantification was performed at 231 nm. Standards of AFMK, AMK and 3COHM were synthesized by using the method reported by Tan et al [33]. Thus, H_2O_2 was diluted to 50 mM with PBS (50 mM, pH 7.0) and deferoxamine was dissolved in this solution at a final concentration of 1 mM to chelate any possible trace of free iron. MEL was then added to this solution to make a final concentration of 1 mM. The mixture was incubated for 2 h at RT. The majority components of this solution were then mixed with an equal volume of dichloromethane and shaken horizontally for 10 min. The water phase was discarded and the organic phase was dried under vacuum. The residue was dissolved in a small volume of methanol and fractionated by analytical thin layer chromatography with silica gel on polyester, fluorescent indicator, layer of 250 mm and 20 3 20 cm (TLC) using ethyl acetate as the solvent. The major spot (about 90% in all metabolites), which migrated with an RF of 0.2 (detected with UV lamp at 254 nm) was scraped from the TLC plate and extracted with methanol. The TLC purification was repeated two additional times. The purified product was identified to be AFMK by simple 1H-NMR. For AMK synthesis, the above purified AFMK was

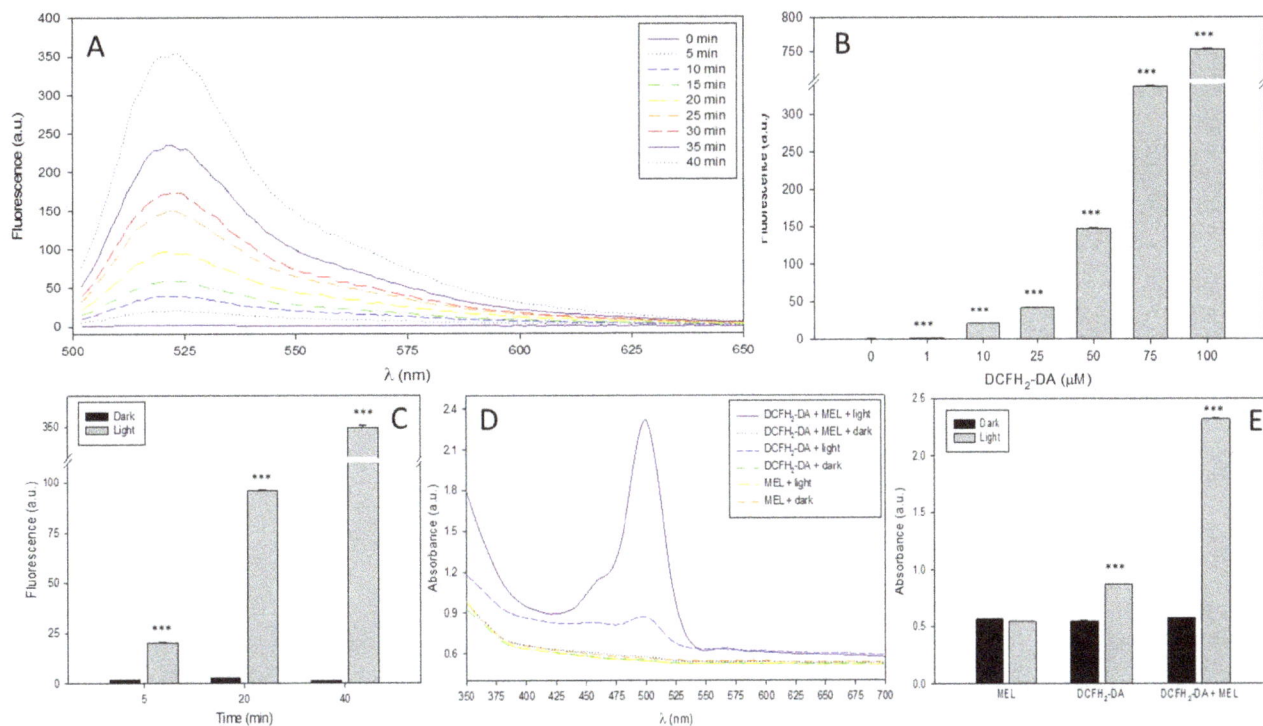

Figure 1. Effect of melatonin on light-induced DCFH$_2$-DA oxidation. A) Fluorescence spectrum ($\lambda_{exc} = 485$ nm, $\lambda_{em} = 500$–700 nm) of DCFH$_2$-DA (100 µM) plus MEL (1 mM) under light (0–40 min). B) Fluorescence of several concentrations of DCFH$_2$-DA plus MEL (1 mM) and light 60 minutes. ***p<0.001 vs no treat. C) Fluorescence of DCFH$_2$-DA plus MEL (1 mM) during 5, 20 or 40 minutes under light or dark conditions. ***p<0.001 vs Darkness. D) Absorbance Spectrum (350–700 nm) of DCFH$_2$-DA (100 µM) or MEL (1 mM) alone or mixed under 30 minutes of dark or light conditions. E) Absorbance measurement at 505 nm of MEL (1 mM), DCFH$_2$-DA (100 µM), alone or mixed under 30 minutes of light or dark conditions. ***p< 0.001 vs Darkness.

dissolved in PBS buffer (50 mM, pH 7.0) at a final concentration of 7 mM and incubated with catalase (2500 U/ml) at room temperature for 24 h. The solution was mixed with two portions of dichloromethane (per volume) and shaken horizontally for 10 min. The water phase was discarded and the organic phase was dried under vacuum. The residue was then dissolved in a small volume of methanol and the enzyme metabolite was fractionated by analytical TLC using ethyl acetate as the solvent. The single metabolite produced by catalase was isolated from TLC plate as described above and identified to be the AMK by 1H-NMR.

DCFH$_2$ and DCF were separated by HPLC in an isocratic mode following the method previously reported [34]. A mixture of NaH$_2$PO$_4$ (20 mM, pH 6.8) and methanol (43:57) was used as mobile phase. Flow was set at 1 ml/min, at RT and 20 µl of sample were injected. Wavelengths between 190 and 800 nm were used.

HPLC-MS was used to confirm presence of AFMK in samples. Agilent 1290 Infinity (HPLC) and Agilent 6460 triple quad (MS) equipped with a Zorbax Eclipse Plus C18 column (Agilent, 2.1×50 mm, 1.8 µm particle) were used. Mobile phase consisting in two components (A 0.1% formic acid; B ACN with 0.1% formic acid) in gradient mode (5% B to 90% B, 1 to 6 min) with a flow of 250 µl/min at 30°C and 2 µl of injection volume were the optimal parameters chosen. Flow of 5 L/min and temperature of 300°C of nebulization gas was chosen. ESI positive at 3500 V, product ion mode (m/z ion 265 $(M+H)^+$) and 10 eV as Collision Energy to fragment precursor ion was used.

Cell culture experiments

Hippocampal neuronal (HT22) and prostate cancer (PC3) cell lines were cultured in DMEM and DMEM/F12 respectively, supplemented with 10% FBS and 1% antibiotic-antimycotic cocktail. Cells were grown at 37°C in a humidified 5% CO$_2$ environment, seeded at a density of 25,000 cell/mL of complete media in 6 or 96 well plates and allowed to attach overnight before experiments. Cells were incubated 24 hours with or without 1 mM MEL. Thereafter, medium was replaced and KRH buffer (50 mM HEPES, 137 mM NaCl, 4.7 mM KCl, 1.85 mM CaCl$_2$, 1.3 mM MgSO$_4$, 0.1% BSA, pH: 7.4) with 10 µM of 2,7-dichlorofluorescein diacetate (DCFH-DA) was added for 30 min at 37°C in darkness. Fluorescence was measured after 30 min in a microplate reader (λex 485 nm, λem 530 nm - µQuant, Biotek) or from flow cytometer (Beckman-Coulter EPICS-XL Cytometer) as previously described [9,35].

Results

Evaluation of DCFH$_2$-DA photooxidation in the presence of melatonin

DCFH$_2$-DA is one of the most widely employed fluorescence probe to measure redox state inside cells. It is a cell permeable precursor of DCFH$_2$ that can readily cross membrane. After internalization, it is cleaved by intracellular esterases giving DCFH-DA obtaining DCFH$_2$. Therefore, to evaluate a possible interference in the fluorescence of DCF caused by MEL and light reaction, both molecules (DCFH$_2$ and DCFH$_2$-DA) were employed. Thus, DCFH$_2$-DA photooxidation was evaluated by

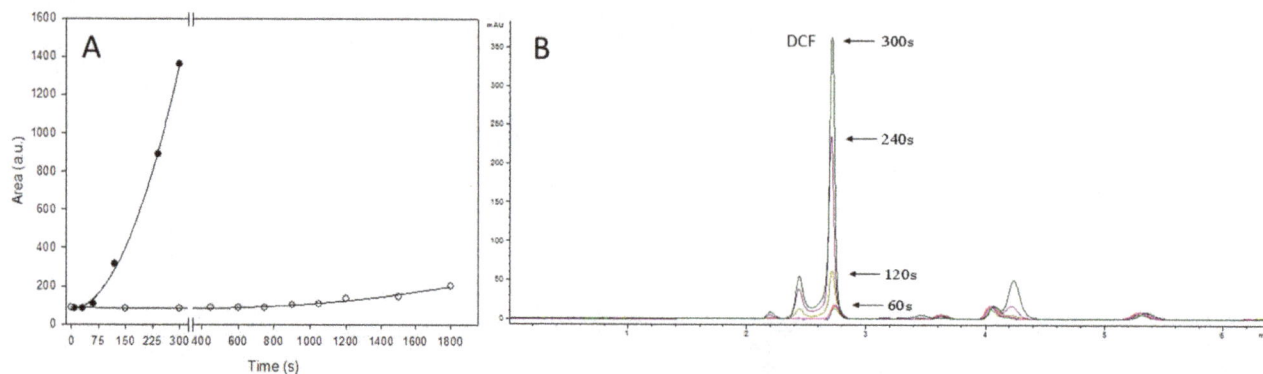

Figure 2. Time-dependence in melatonin effect on DCFH$_2$ photooxidation. A) Time course of DCF production by DCFH$_2$ (10 μM) alone (-○-) or plus MEL 1 mM (-●-) under light. B) Chromatogram of DCF after DCFH$_2$ (10 μM) plus MEL (1 mM) were exposed to light for 60, 120, 240 or 300 seconds.

measuring fluorescence emission of its oxidant product in the presence or absence of MEL in both, under light or in darkness. When DCFH$_2$-DA was mixed with MEL and exposed to light at different times, a significant increase in fluorescence emission was observed (Fig. 1A). This increase of fluorescence was clearly dependent on time, DCFH$_2$-DA concentration (Fig. 1B) and light (Fig. 1C). Similarly, when DCFH$_2$-DA alone or plus MEL were exposed to light/dark and absorbance was measured, MEL increased significantly the absorbance of DCFH$_2$-DA (Fig. 1D, E).

Evaluation of DCFH$_2$ photooxidation in the presence of melatonin

Once it was observed the enhancement of DCFH$_2$-DA photooxidation by MEL, the interaction of DCFH$_2$ and MEL was also studied. DCFH$_2$-DA was deacetylated to DCFH$_2$ which was then mixed with MEL under light. As reported above, a significant increase of time-dependent fluorescence when 100 μM DCFH$_2$ was exposed to light was observed. By using 10 μM DCFH$_2$ plus 1 mM MEL under light, fluorescence was rapidly increased after few seconds (Fig. 2A). Chromatogram presented in figure 2B showed a production of DCF compound after 60, 120, 240 and 300 seconds plus light and MEL. As shown, after only

60 seconds of exposition to MEL and light, DCF peak is 10 times higher than control.

Evaluation of DCFH$_2$ and DCFH$_2$-DA photooxidation in the presence of melatonin under UV light or in a N$_2$ atmosphere

In addition to visible light, UV light was employed to evaluate the photooxidation of DCFH$_2$ and DCFH$_2$-DA. After DCFH$_2$ exposure to UV light, there was an increase in fluorescence, and again, that increase was dependent on time. Similarly to what happens under visible light, when DCFH$_2$ was incubated with MEL under UV light, fluorescence emission was significantly higher (Fig. 3A). The increment of fluorescence under UV light is much higher than under visible light since even lower compound concentration gives a much faster time of reaction. The spectrum of fluorescence after light exposure at different times is shown in supplementary material. The increment of fluorescence is 10 times higher when DCFH$_2$ was combined with MEL under UV light than when DCFH$_2$-DA was employed (Figure S1A). Likewise, MEL was able to increase by 100 fold the fluorescence of DCFH$_2$ when they were exposed to UV light for several minutes (Figure S1B).

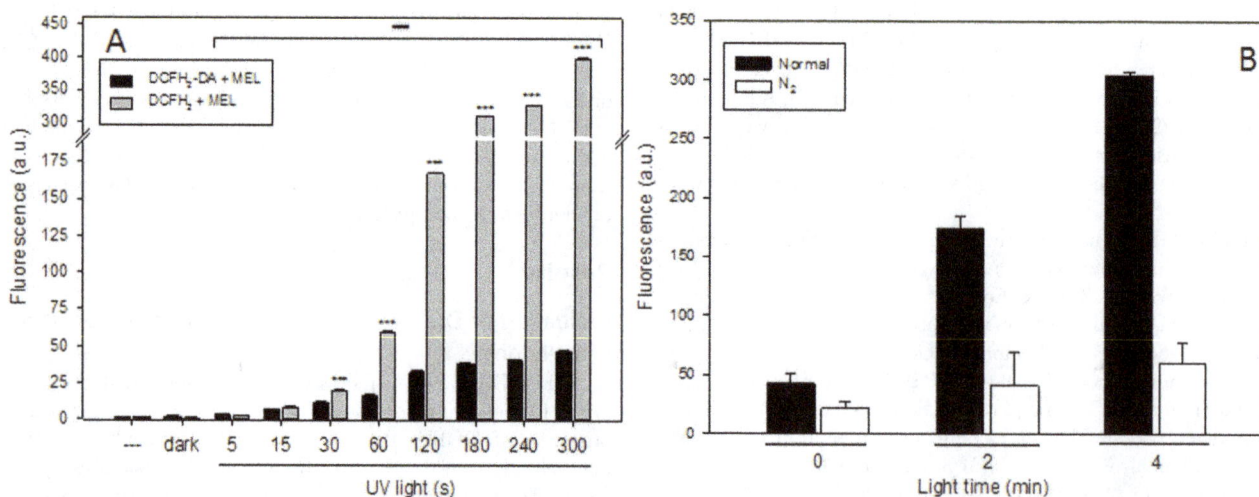

Figure 3. Role of UV light and O$_2$ in DCFH$_2$-DA and DCFH$_2$ photooxidation. A) Fluorescence of DCFH$_2$ (10 μM) or DCFH$_2$-DA (100 μM) plus MEL (1 mM) under UV light. B) Fluorescence of DCFH$_2$ (10 μM) plus MEL (1 mM) under N$_2$ or normal atmosphere.

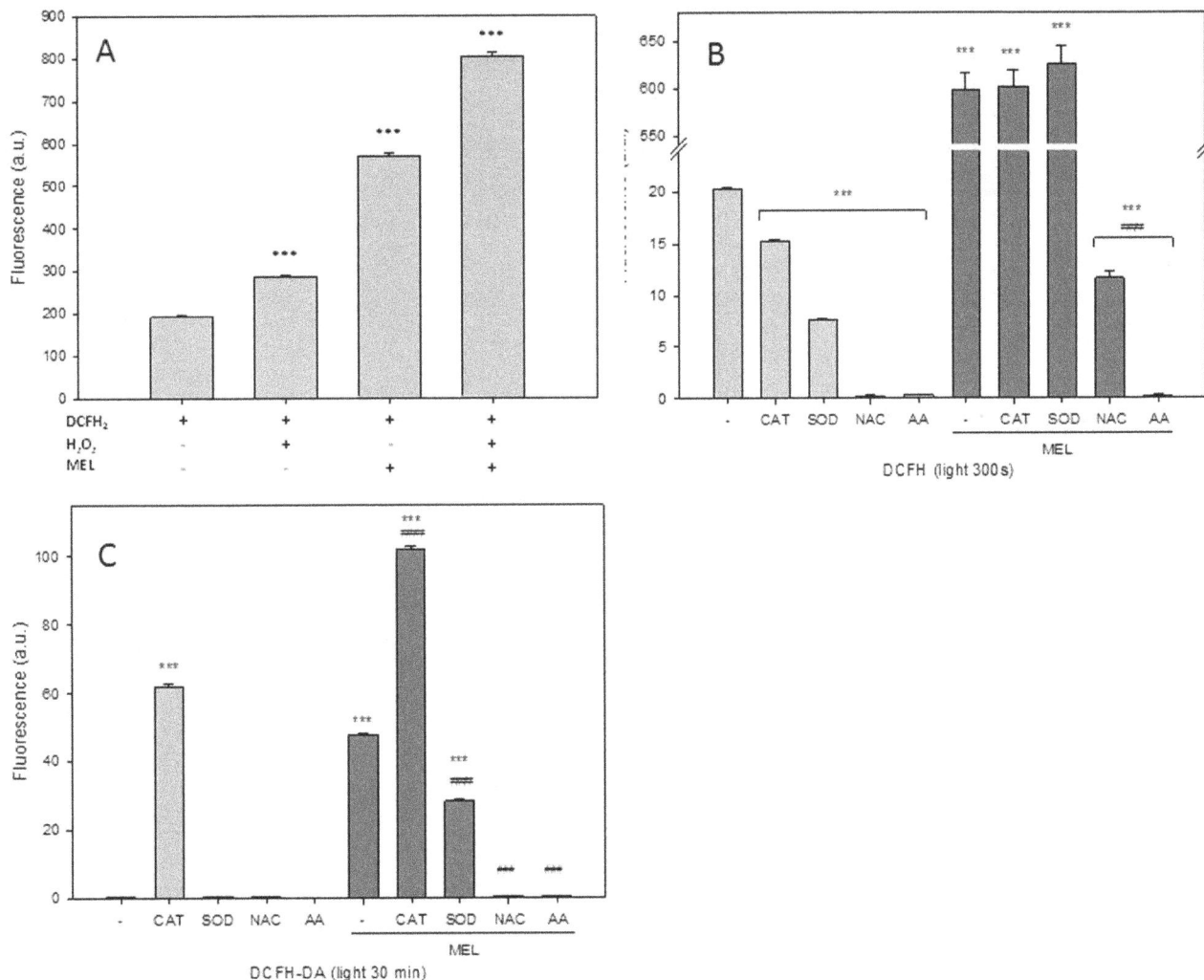

Figure 4. Impact of antioxidants on melatonin enhancement of DCFH$_2$ and DCFH$_2$-DA photooxidation. A) Fluorescence of DCFH$_2$ (10 µM), MEL (1 mM), H$_2$O$_2$ (10 µM) alone or in combination under light for 300 second. B) Evaluation of fluorescence of DCFH$_2$ (10 µM) with CAT (200 U), SOD (200 U), NAC (10 mM) and AA (10 mM) with or without supplementation of MEL (1 mM) under light for 300 seconds. C) Evaluation of fluorescence of DCFH$_2$-DA (100 µM) with CAT (200 U), SOD (200 U), NAC (10 mM) and AA (10 mM) with or without supplementation of MEL (1 mM) under 30 min seconds of light exposure.

To check if atmospheric O$_2$ has an important role in photooxidation of DCFH$_2$ by MEL, an experiment under N$_2$ was performed. When O$_2$ was eliminated from solution fluorescence did not increase. After 2 minutes under light, fluorescence intensity under N$_2$ atmosphere is clearly lower than under normal atmosphere (Fig. 3B). For these experiment it is possible to conclude that O$_2$ plays an instrumental role in the photooxidation process.

Participation of H$_2$O$_2$ generation by melatonin in DCFH$_2$ or DCFH$_2$-DA photooxidation

In order to understand the mechanism of DCFH$_2$ photooxidation by MEL, H$_2$O$_2$ was included in the DCFH$_2$ plus MEL mixture solution. After 300 seconds under visible light, the increment of fluorescence was measured. As previously described by others [7], an increment of DCF was observed after either H$_2$O$_2$ or MEL addition (Fig. 4A). In previous reports [7,36,37], the activity of antioxidant enzymes in preventing DCF formation was studied to demonstrate its dependence on ROS production.

Consequently, catalase (CAT), superoxide dismutase (SOD), N-acetyl-cysteine (NAC) or ascorbic acid (AA) were employed to inhibit DCF formation after DCFH$_2$ or DCFH$_2$-DA plus MEL under light. CAT or SOD did not inhibit DCF formation after DCFH$_2$ plus MEL exposure under light but they clearly reduced its formation after DCFH$_2$ exposure alone (Fig. 4B). On the contrary, antioxidants such as AA or NAC inhibited DCF fluorescence when both DCFH$_2$ (Fig. 4B) or DCFH$_2$-DA (Fig. 4C) were incubated alone or plus MEL under light [38,39].

Production of kynureamines after DCFH$_2$ and melatonin reaction

Previous studies focused on photooxidation of MEL by protoporphyrin IX [40] or by 2-hydroxyquinoxaline [41] showed the presence of several kynureamines as metabolites. For this reason, N1-acetyl-N2-formyl-5-methoxykynuramine (AFMK), N1-acetyl-5-methoxykynuramine (AMK) or cyclic 3-hydroxymelatonin (3-COHM) were studied after DCFH$_2$ exposure to light in the presence of MEL. When DCFH$_2$ plus MEL was exposed for

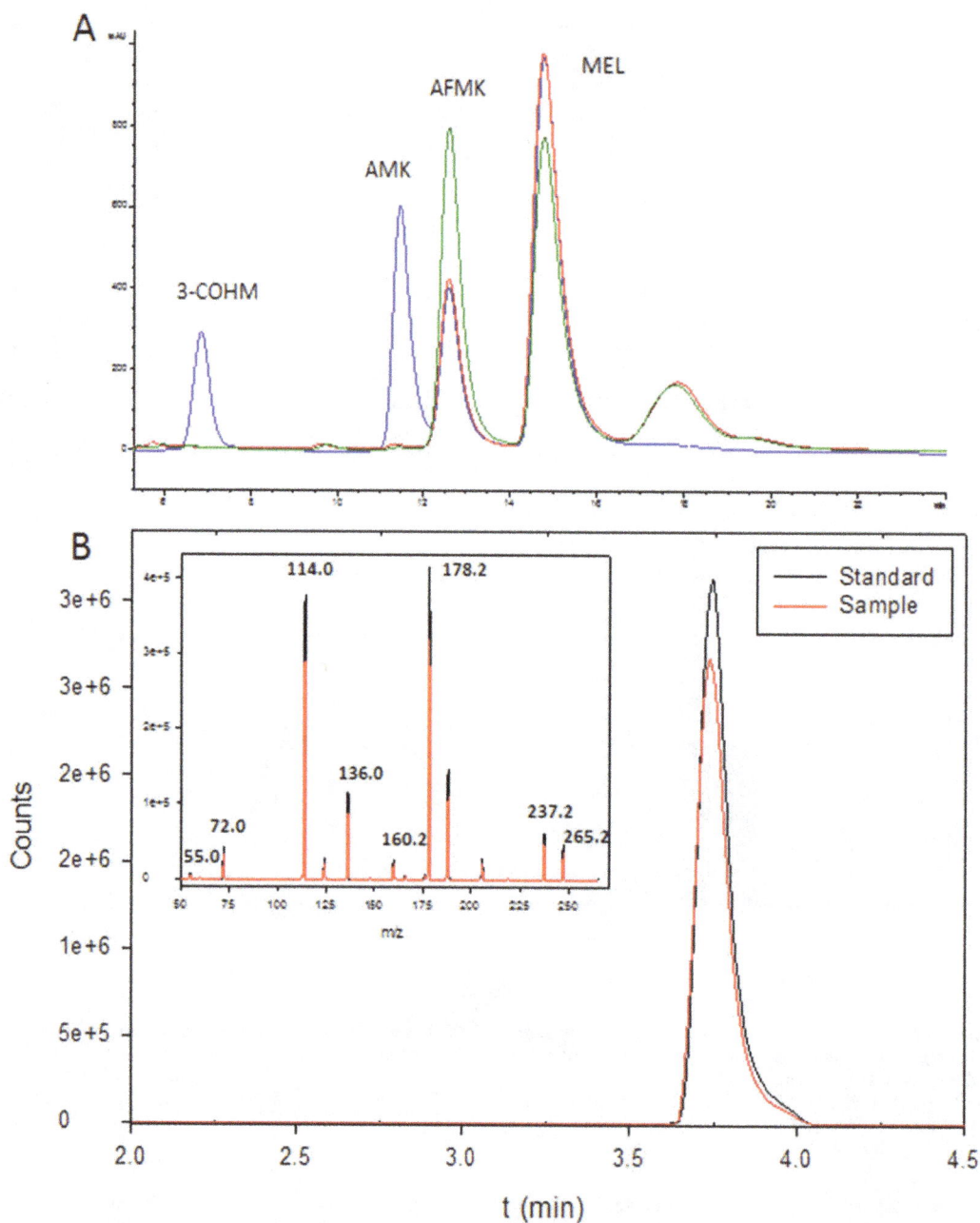

Figure 5. Presence of melatonin metabolites in DCFH$_2$ photooxidation enhanced by melatonin. A) Chromatogram of standards of 3-COHM, AMK, AFMK and MEL (blue line), chromatogram of MEL (1 mM) with DCFH (10 μM) under light 5 min (red) or 10 min (green). B) Chromatogram and mass-spectrum obtained by HPLC-MS of AFMK standard (black) and AFMK present in sample (red) after MEL (1 mM) incubation with DCFH (10 μM) after 5 min of exposure to light.

30 seconds under light, we found a significant reduction of MEL concomitant with the presence of some new products. By comparing retention time as well as uv-spectrum with AFMK, AMK or 3-COHM standards, it was confirmed that AFMK was found after DCFH$_2$ plus MEL were exposed to light (Fig. 5A). To ensure that AFMK is the compound generated in this reaction, a molecules produced and AFMK standard were compared by HPLC-MS obtained a positive confirmation of AFMK generation (Fig. 5B). The formation of AFMK requires the presence of two oxygen atom. Thus, when these experiments were performed in pure DMSO, DCF fluorescence was not found (data not shown).

Dose response study of DCFH$_2$ photooxidation by melatonin

A dose response study was made by using 0.1 μM of DCFH$_2$ and 3 μM MEL, the concentration of the indole found inside prostate LNCaP cells when they are incubated with 1 mM MEL for 6 hours [42]. Under these conditions, an increase of fluorescence was observed even after only 30 seconds (Fig. 6A). In addition, by using AA as antioxidant, there was a clear reduction in DCF formation also in a dose dependent manner (Fig. 6B). Furthermore a higher dose response study was done. So,

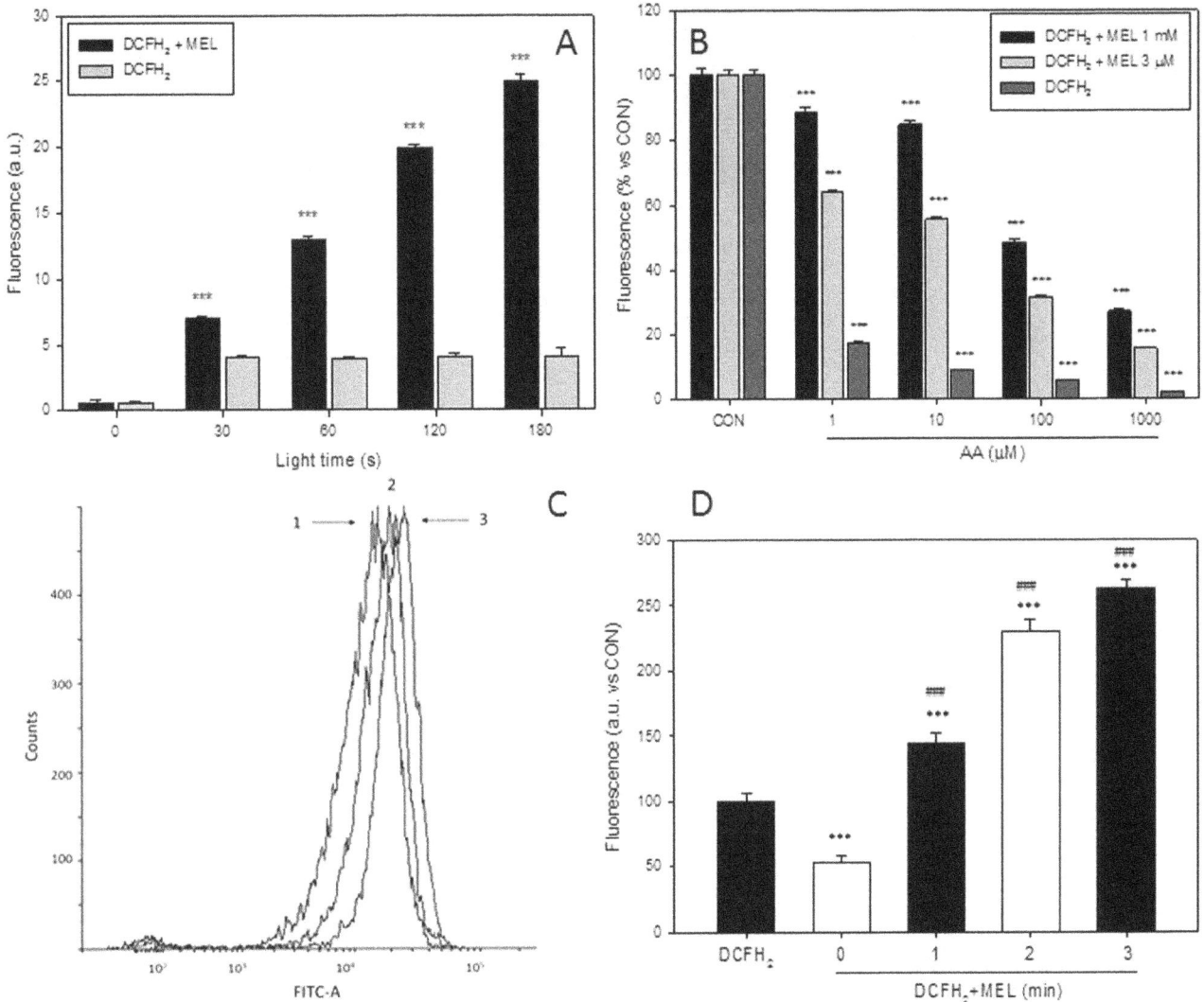

Figure 6. Dose dependence of DCFH₂ in melatonin enhancement of photooxidation *in vitro* and in cellular models. A) Fluorescence of DCFH₂ (0.1 μM) alone or plus MEL (3 μM) under light. B) Fluorescence of DCFH₂ (0.1 μM) alone plus MEL (3 μM) or MEL (1 mM) in combination with AA (1–1000 μM) under light exposure for 60 seconds. C) Fluorescence, detected by flow cytometer, of HT22 cells incubated with 10 μM DCFH₂ alone (1) or with 1 mM MEL plus 10 μM DCFH₂ in darkness (2) or after 2 minutes of light exposure (3). D) Fluorescence, detected by microplate fluorimeter, of PC3 cells incubated with DCFH₂ (10 μM) alone or with 1 mM MEL plus DCFH₂ (10 μM) in darkness or after 1, 2 and 3 minutes of light exposure.

in all MEL concentrations studied −1 nM to 1 mM- an increase in fluorescence was observed (Figure S2).

DCFH₂ photooxidation by MEL in culture cells

Prostate cancer (PC3) and hippocampal neuronal (HT22) cells were incubated with or without 1 mM MEL for 24 hours. Then, 10 μM of DCFH₂-DA was added for 30 min prior to cytometer or fluorometric measurement. Those experimental conditions were chosen because there were normally employed by investigations describing pro-oxidant activity of the indoleamine [27,43–45]. Changes in fluorescence among experimental groups were detected in both cell lines. Thus, when cells are incubated with MEL, a decrease in fluorescence is observed only when all experiment is performed in complete darkness (Fig. 6 C,D). When HT22 cells were exposed to light only for 1 minute, an increase of fluorescence and therefore DCF formation was observed. Same results were found in PC3 cells but light effect was lower. Thus,

after 2 min under light an increase in fluorescence was also observed.

According to our results, a hypothetical pathway describing the potential reactions between DCFH₂ and MEL are shown in Figure 7.

Discussion

This study tried to understand an apparent dual role of MEL as pro-oxidant or anti-oxidant molecule. Mostly, the indolamine has been considered to scavenges free radicals or stimulates cell antioxidant defense [11,17] while some reports described a pro-oxidant activity that in some context might induce cell death [27,28]. The number of references that describe MEL as a pro-oxidant factor are considerably fewer that those describing antioxidant properties of the indole and also, few mechanistic explanations are proposed to explain its activity in promoting free radicals.

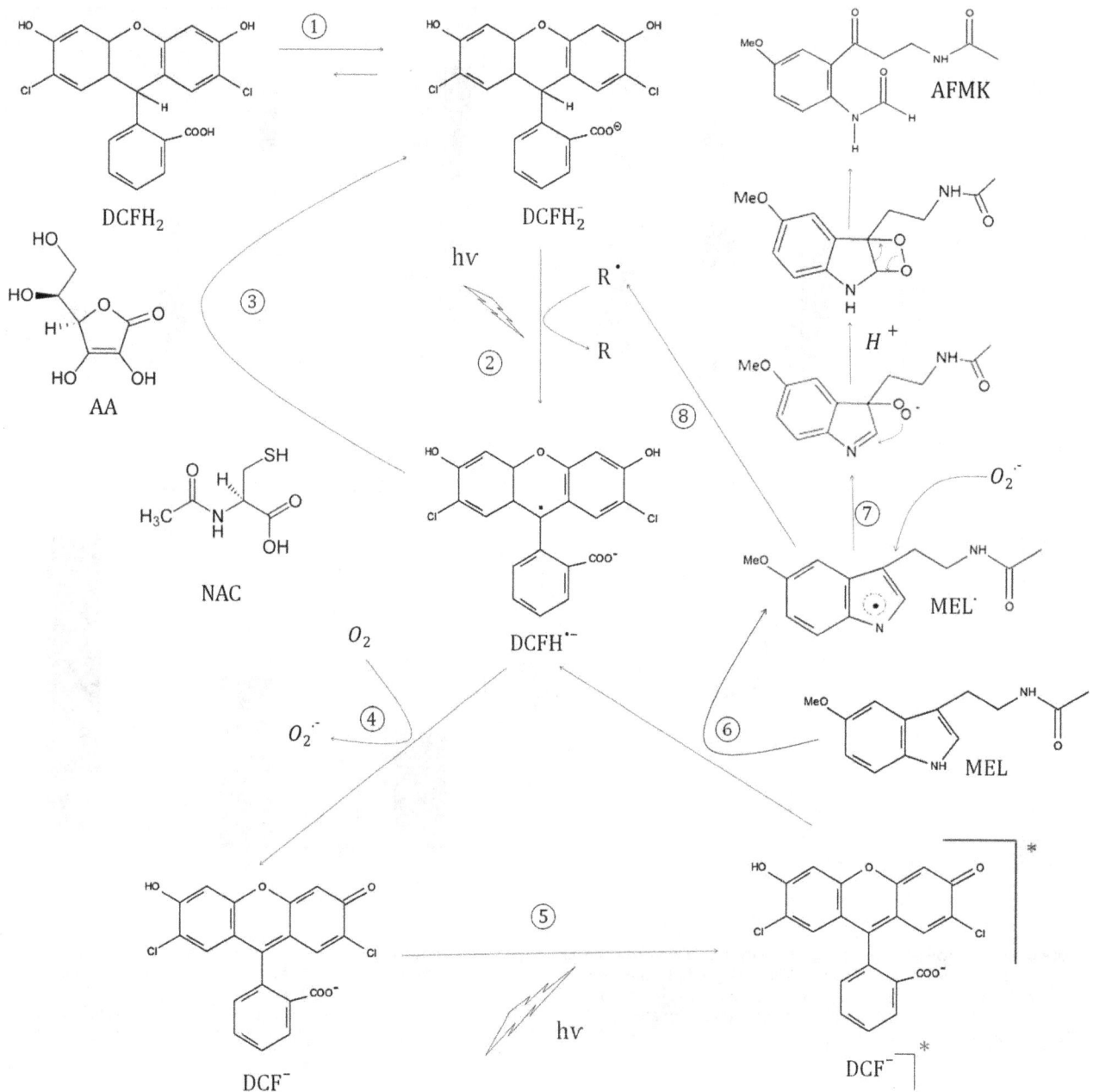

Figure 7. Diagram of proposal hypothesis about the mechanism of DCFH₂, MEL and light reactions.

There is a clear controversy about the challenges and limitations of assay methods for measuring ROS [46]. In fact, some investigators considered essential to keep this limitations in mind for proper interpretation of data obtained [47]. Several reports have showed that DCFH₂ is even oxidized in processes that do not actually involve ROS. Also, photo-irradiation incidental to spectrofluorometric or fluorescence microscopy observation has also been reported, therefore causing serious problems for the correct interpretation of DCFH₂ as an indicator of ROS production [39]. For this reason and in order to evaluate the convenience of using DCFH₂ in the evaluation of ROS production by melatonin, here it was performed an *in vitro* study about possible interactions between both, DFCH₂-DA or DCFH₂ and

MEL, since those are probably the most widely employed probes for ROS analysis inside living cells.

Photo-oxidation of MEL has been previously reported in several occasions [40,41,48]. But while there was no increase in fluorescence when MEL was exposed to light alone in a free cell system, a clear increment was found when DCFH₂-DA alone was exposed to light for a long time as previously described by others [38,39,49,50].

The mechanism of DCFH₂ oxidation is not clear yet [47,51,52]. In a previous report, Wrona et al. [53] have shown that a radical product DCFH·⁻ occur as an intermediate. DCFH·⁻ is necessary since its elimination by reaction with AA or NAC results in no DCF formation. Accordingly, when DCFH₂ and MEL were incubated together in the absence of light, DCF was not detected, thus indicating that light is necessary for fluorescence enhancement.

On the other hand, high concentrations of $DCFH_2$-DA (100 μM) and MEL (1 mM) are necessary to increase fluorescence in a cell-free system. Interestingly those experimental conditions are normally employed by investigations describing pro-oxidant activity of the indoleamine [27,43–45]. This might explain the increment observed in DCF after MEL incubation under some situations without any net increase in ROS production. Our results prove this fact since antioxidants such as CAT or SOD are unable to inhibit DCF formation after MEL incubation. Furthermore, our results by using two different cell lines showed that under light, DCF assay might induce wrong in conclusions. Thus, MEL is inhibiting DCF formation when the experiment was performed in complete darkness but after a short exposition to light DCF fluorescence increase.

An accumulation of $DCFH_2$ in V79 hamster cells after incubation with 10 μM of $DCFH_2$ has been documented [46,54]. Considering that we have used high concentrations of both, $DCFH_2$ (10 μM) and MEL (1 mM) and the uptake of high concentrations of MEL might be compromised, being intracellular concentrations of the indole much lower than those applied in the culture media [55]. Here we studied the ability of MEL to increase DCF formation when employed at micromolar range concentration to assure that these observations were feasible to occur in the intracellular environment. In vitro experiments when MEL increases DCF fluorescence, high concentration of MEL (1 mM) in culture medium was used. For this reason, photooxidation of $DCFH_2$ by MEL is possible as shown here.

Results obtained suggest that the mechanism by which DCF is produced from $DCFH_2$ and $DCFH_2$-DA is mechanistically different. As expected, these results confirmed that $DCFH_2$ and $DCFH_2$-DA are not the most adequate probes to test the ability of MEL to depurate free radicals in biological systems since fluorescence is a consequence of a side reaction that do not involve ROS participation. Also, considering mechanistic differences between $DCFH_2$ and $DCFH_2$-DA, it seems that $DCFH_2$-DA could be a better choice since it is necessary a longer light exposure and a higher concentration to obtain less than 10 times of fluorescence when employed.

In conclusion, by using $DCFH_2$ staining to measure redox control by MEL, it could be concluded than MEL might be a pro-oxidant molecule, while the real situation is very different since it is still working as an antioxidant compound and scavenging free radicals as shown in the diagram (Fig. 7). Most of the reactions shown in the depicted diagram (1–5) have already been demonstrated in previous reports. Thus, step 1 is due to physiological pH and step 2 was also previously described [53,56]. By the effect of radical species or light, $DCFH_2^-$ is rapidly converted into $DCFH^{\bullet-}$ (2). AA and NAC acting as direct scavengers react with $DCFH^{\bullet-}$ (3) and inhibit DCF^- formation. DCF^- is generated from $DCFH^{\bullet-}$ when it reacts with oxygen to form superoxide (4). Under light, DCF^- absorbs energy and changes to the excited state $DCF^-]^*$ (5) and MEL would be able to react with it to give $DCFH^{\bullet-}$ and $MEL^{\bullet}$ (6). This last reaction has been described when other molecules [57], such as GSH, are employed and it might be the reason why MEL is able to augment DCF fluorescence without increasing ROS production. Furthermore $MEL^{\bullet}$ can react with H_2O, O_2 or $O_2^{\bullet-}$ to render AFMK (7). Other possibility is the role of this $MEL^{\bullet}$ as catalyst of the reaction 2 obtained MEL as product ($R^{\bullet}$ to R) (8). Thus, the increment in DCF production by MEL might not be a result of a pro-oxidant activity, but rather it seems that MEL is still working as an antioxidant in this context (6).

Altogether results presented here led us to propose that unless performed under dim red light all time of the performance of the assay, $DCFH_2$ should not be employed for ROS measuring when working with melatonin since depending on time, $DCFH_2$ or MEL concentration, it is possible to detect an increment in DCF^- fluorescence without any increment of ROS more on the contrary, while melatonin is still working as an antioxidant and a radical scavenger. Results published in the literature concerning pro-oxidant activity of melatonin in certain cell types should be re-evaluated, as this pro-oxidant action does not seem to be the underlying mechanism by which the indole induces cell death.

Supporting Information

Figure S1 Fluorescence spectrum (λ_{exc} = 480 nm, λ_{em} = 500–700 nm) of $DCFH_2$-DA (100 μM) plus MEL (1 mM) under UV light (A), $DCFH_2$ (10 μM) alone (C) or plus MEL (1 mM) under UV light at short times (B) or long times (D).

Figure S2 Fluorescence of $DCFH_2$ (10 μM) plus several concentrations of MEL under light exposure (120 s).

Acknowledgments

The authors would like to thank Dr. Sergio Cueto for performing HPLC-MS analysis. We are grateful to Javier Iglesias and Javier Fernandez for their helpful technical assistance with the light chamber.

Author Contributions

Conceived and designed the experiments: DH RMS DXT. Performed the experiments: DH ARG. Analyzed the data: JCM DH. Contributed reagents/materials/analysis tools: JCM DH. Wrote the paper: DH JCM RMS.

References

1. Gyllenhammar H (1987) Lucigenin chemiluminescence in the assessment of neutrophil superoxide production. J Immunol Methods 97: 209–213.

2. Dahlgren C, Karlsson A (1999) Respiratory burst in human neutrophils. J Immunol Methods 232: 3–14.

3. Nourooz-Zadeh J (1999) Effect of dialysis on oxidative stress in uraemia. Redox Rep 4: 17–22.

4. Brandt R, Keston AS (1965) Synthesis of Diacetyldichlorofluorescin: A Stable Reagent for Fluorometric Analysis. Anal Biochem 11: 6–9.

5. LeBel CP, Ischiropoulos H, Bondy SC (1992) Evaluation of the probe 2′,7′-dichlorofluorescin as an indicator of reactive oxygen species formation and oxidative stress. Chem Res Toxicol 5: 227–231.

6. Bass DA, Parce JW, Dechatelet LR, Szejda P, Seeds MC, et al. (1983) Flow cytometric studies of oxidative product formation by neutrophils: a graded response to membrane stimulation. J Immunol 130: 1910–1917.

7. Hempel SL, Buettner GR, O'Malley YQ, Wessels DA, Flaherty DM (1999) Dihydrofluorescein diacetate is superior for detecting intracellular oxidants: comparison with 2′,7′-dichlorodihydrofluorescein diacetate, 5(and 6)-carboxy-2′,7′-dichlorodihydrofluorescein diacetate, and dihydrorhodamine 123. Free Radic Biol Med 27: 146–159.

8. Keston AS, Brandt R (1965) The Fluorometric Analysis of Ultramicro Quantities of Hydrogen Peroxide. Anal Biochem 11: 1–5.

9. Wang H, Joseph JA (1999) Quantifying cellular oxidative stress by dichlorofluorescein assay using microplate reader. Free Radic Biol Med 27: 612–616.

10. Hafer K, Iwamoto KS, Schiestl RH (2008) Refinement of the dichlorofluorescein assay for flow cytometric measurement of reactive oxygen species in irradiated and bystander cell populations. Radiat Res 169: 460–468.

11. Tan DX, Hardeland R, Manchester LC, Paredes SD, Korkmaz A, et al. (2010) The changing biological roles of melatonin during evolution: from an

antioxidant to signals of darkness, sexual selection and fitness. Biol Rev Camb Philos Soc 85: 607–623.

12. Stehle JH, Saade A, Rawashdeh O, Ackermann K, Jilg A, et al. (2011) A survey of molecular details in the human pineal gland in the light of phylogeny, structure, function and chronobiological diseases. J Pineal Res 51: 17–43.

13. Lemoine P, Zisapel N (2012) Prolonged-release formulation of melatonin (Circadin) for the treatment of insomnia. Expert Opin Pharmacother 13: 895–905.

14. Reiter RJ (1991) Melatonin: the chemical expression of darkness. Mol Cell Endocrinol 79: C153–158.

15. Reiter RJ, Tan DX, Manchester LC, Paredes SD, Mayo JC, et al. (2009) Melatonin and reproduction revisited. Biol Reprod 81: 445–456.

16. Galano A, Tan DX, Reiter RJ (2011) Melatonin as a natural ally against oxidative stress: a physicochemical examination. J Pineal Res 51: 1–16.

17. Mayo JC, Sainz RM, Antoli I, Herrera F, Martin V, et al. (2002) Melatonin regulation of antioxidant enzyme gene expression. Cell Mol Life Sci 59: 1706–1713.

18. Tan DX, Reiter RJ, Manchester LC, Yan MT, El-Sawi M, et al. (2002) Chemical and physical properties and potential mechanisms: melatonin as a broad spectrum antioxidant and free radical scavenger. Curr Top Med Chem 2: 181–197.

19. Hardeland R, Reiter RJ, Poeggeler B, Tan DX (1993) The significance of the metabolism of the neurohormone melatonin: antioxidative protection and formation of bioactive substances. Neurosci Biobehav Rev 17: 347–357.

20. Allegra M, Reiter RJ, Tan DX, Gentile C, Tesoriere L, et al. (2003) The chemistry of melatonin's interaction with reactive species. J Pineal Res 34: 1–10.

21. Quiros I, Sainz RM, Hevia D, Garcia-Suarez O, Astudillo A, et al. (2009) Upregulation of manganese superoxide dismutase (SOD2) is a common pathway for neuroendocrine differentiation in prostate cancer cells. Int J Cancer 125: 1497–1504.

22. Fischer TW, Kleszczynski K, Hardkop LH, Kruse N, Zillikens D (2012) Melatonin enhances antioxidative enzyme gene expression (CAT, GPx, SOD), prevents their UVR-induced depletion, and protects against the formation of DNA damage (8-hydroxy-2'-deoxyguanosine) in ex vivo human skin. J Pineal Res.

23. Blask DE, Sauer LA, Dauchy RT (2002) Melatonin as a chronobiotic/anticancer agent: cellular, biochemical, and molecular mechanisms of action and their implications for circadian-based cancer therapy. Curr Top Med Chem 2: 113–132.

24. Blask DE, Hill SM, Dauchy RT, Xiang S, Yuan L, et al. (2011) Circadian regulation of molecular, dietary, and metabolic signaling mechanisms of human breast cancer growth by the nocturnal melatonin signal and the consequences of its disruption by light at night. J Pineal Res 51: 259–269.

25. Sainz RM, Mayo JC, Tan DX, Lopez-Burillo S, Natarajan M, et al. (2003) Antioxidant activity of melatonin in Chinese hamster ovarian cells: changes in cellular proliferation and differentiation. Biochem Biophys Res Commun 302: 625–634.

26. Mediavilla MD, Sanchez-Barcelo EJ, Tan DX, Manchester L, Reiter RJ (2010) Basic mechanisms involved in the anti-cancer effects of melatonin. Curr Med Chem 17: 4462–4481.

27. Osseni RA, Rat P, Bogdan A, Warnet JM, Touitou Y (2000) Evidence of prooxidant and antioxidant action of melatonin on human liver cell line HepG2. Life Sci 68: 387–399.

28. Wolfler A, Caluba HC, Abuja PM, Dohr G, Schauenstein K, et al. (2001) Prooxidant activity of melatonin promotes fas-induced cell death in human leukemic Jurkat cells. FEBS Lett 502: 127–131.

29. Zhang HM, Zhang Y, Zhang BX (2011) The role of mitochondrial complex III in melatonin-induced ROS production in cultured mesangial cells. J Pineal Res 50: 78–82.

30. Bejarano I, Espino J, Barriga C, Reiter RJ, Pariente JA, et al. (2011) Pro-oxidant effect of melatonin in tumour leucocytes: relation with its cytotoxic and pro-apoptotic effects. Basic Clin Pharmacol Toxicol 108: 14–20.

31. Cathcart R, Schwiers E, Ames BN (1983) Detection of picomole levels of hydroperoxides using a fluorescent dichlorofluorescein assay. Anal Biochem 134: 111–116.

32. Hevia D, Botas C, Sainz RM, Quiros I, Blanco D, et al. (2010) Development and validation of new methods for the determination of melatonin and its oxidative metabolites by high performance liquid chromatography and capillary electrophoresis, using multivariate optimization. J Chromatogr A 1217: 1368–1374.

33. Tan DX, Manchester LC, Reiter RJ, Plummer BF, Limson J, et al. (2000) Melatonin directly scavenges hydrogen peroxide: a potentially new metabolic pathway of melatonin biotransformation. Free Radic Biol Med 29: 1177–1185.

34. Possel H, Noack H, Augustin W, Keilhoff G, Wolf G (1997) 2,7-Dihydrodi-chlorofluorescein diacetate as a fluorescent marker for peroxynitrite formation. FEBS Lett 416: 175–178.

35. Eruslanov E, Kusmartsev S (2010) Identification of ROS using oxidized DCFDA and flow-cytometry. Methods Mol Biol 594: 57–72.

36. Liochev SI, Fridovich I (2001) Copper,zinc superoxide dismutase as a univalent NO(-) oxidoreductase and as a dichlorofluorescin peroxidase. J Biol Chem 276: 35253–35257.

37. Kim YM, Lim JM, Kim BC, Han S (2006) Cu,Zn-superoxide dismutase is an intracellular catalyst for the H(2)O(2)-dependent oxidation of dichlorodihydro-fluorescein. Mol Cells 21: 161–165.

38. Bilski P, Belanger AG, Chignell CF (2002) Photosensitized oxidation of 2',7'-dichlorofluorescin: singlet oxygen does not contribute to the formation of fluorescent oxidation product 2',7'-dichlorofluorescein. Free Radic Biol Med 33: 938–946.

39. Afzal M, Matsugo S, Sasai M, Xu B, Aoyama K, et al. (2003) Method to overcome photoreaction, a serious drawback to the use of dichlorofluorescin in evaluation of reactive oxygen species. Biochem Biophys Res Commun 304: 619–624.

40. Hardeland R, Balzer I, Poeggeler B, Fuhrberg B, Uria H, et al. (1995) On the primary functions of melatonin in evolution: mediation of photoperiodic signals in a unicell, photooxidation, and scavenging of free radicals. J Pineal Res 18: 104–111.

41. Behrends A, Riediger S, Grube S, Poeggeler B, Haldar C, et al. (2007) Photocatalytic mechanisms of indoleamine destruction by the quinalphos metabolite 2-hydroxyquinoxaline: a study on melatonin and its precursors serotonin and N-acetylserotonin. J Environ Sci Health B 42: 599–606.

42. Hevia D, Mayo JC, Quiros I, Gomez-Cordoves C, Sainz RM (2010) Monitoring intracellular melatonin levels in human prostate normal and cancer cells by HPLC. Anal Bioanal Chem 397: 1235–1244.

43. Sanchez-Sanchez AM, Martin V, Garcia-Santos G, Rodriguez-Blanco J, Casado-Zapico S, et al. (2011) Intracellular redox state as determinant for melatonin antiproliferative vs cytotoxic effects in cancer cells. Free Radic Res 45: 1333–1341.

44. Albertini MC, Radogna F, Accorsi A, Uguccioni F, Paternoster L, et al. (2006) Intracellular pro-oxidant activity of melatonin deprives U937 cells of reduced glutathione without affecting glutathione peroxidase activity. Ann N Y Acad Sci 1091: 10–16.

45. Buyukavci M, Ozdemir O, Buck S, Stout M, Ravindranath Y, et al. (2006) Melatonin cytotoxicity in human leukemia cells: relation with its pro-oxidant effect. Fundam Clin Pharmacol 20: 73–79.

46. Wardman P (2007) Fluorescent and luminescent probes for measurement of oxidative and nitrosative species in cells and tissues: progress, pitfalls, and prospects. Free Radic Biol Med 43: 995–1022.

47. Kalyanaraman B, Darley-Usmar V, Davies KJ, Dennery PA, Forman HJ, et al. (2012) Measuring reactive oxygen and nitrogen species with fluorescent probes: challenges and limitations. Free Radic Biol Med 52: 1–6.

48. Poeggeler B, Hardeland R (1994) Detection and quantification of melatonin in a dinoflagellate, Gonyaulax polyedra: solutions to the problem of methoxyindole destruction in non-vertebrate material. J Pineal Res 17: 1–10.

49. Chignell CF, Sik RH (2003) A photochemical study of cells loaded with 2',7'-dichlorofluorescin: implications for the detection of reactive oxygen species generated during UVA irradiation. Free Radic Biol Med 34: 1029–1034.

50. Marchesi E, Rota C, Fann YC, Chignell CF, Mason RP (1999) Photoreduction of the fluorescent dye 2'-7'-dichlorofluorescein: a spin trapping and direct electron spin resonance study with implications for oxidative stress measurements. Free Radic Biol Med 26: 148–161.

51. Myhre O, Andersen JM, Aarnes H, Fonnum F (2003) Evaluation of the probes 2',7'-dichlorofluorescin diacetate, luminol, and lucigenin as indicators of reactive species formation. Biochem Pharmacol 65: 1575–1582.

52. Halliwell B, Whiteman M (2004) Measuring reactive species and oxidative damage in vivo and in cell culture: how should you do it and what do the results mean? Br J Pharmacol 142: 231–255.

53. Wrona M, Wardman P (2006) Properties of the radical intermediate obtained on oxidation of 2',7'-dichlorodihydrofluorescein, a probe for oxidative stress. Free Radic Biol Med 41: 657–667.

54. Wrona M, Patel K, Wardman P (2005) Reactivity of 2',7'-dichlorodihydro-fluorescein and dihydrorhodamine 123 and their oxidized forms toward carbonate, nitrogen dioxide, and hydroxyl radicals. Free Radic Biol Med 38: 262–270.

55. Hevia D, Sainz RM, Blanco D, Quiros I, Tan DX, et al. (2008) Melatonin uptake in prostate cancer cells: intracellular transport versus simple passive diffusion. J Pineal Res 45: 247–257.

56. Rota C, Chignell CF, Mason RP (1999) Evidence for free radical formation during the oxidation of 2'-7'-dichlorofluorescin to the fluorescent dye 2'-7'-dichlorofluorescein by horseradish peroxidase: possible implications for oxidative stress measurements. Free Radic Biol Med 27: 873–881.

57. Wrona M, Patel KB, Wardman P (2008) The roles of thiol-derived radicals in the use of 2',7'-dichlorodihydrofluorescein as a probe for oxidative stress. Free Radic Biol Med 44: 56–62.

21

The Role of miR-34a in the Hepatoprotective Effect of Hydrogen Sulfide on Ischemia/Reperfusion Injury in Young and Old Rats

Xinli Huang, Yun Gao, Jianjie Qin, Sen Lu*

Center of Liver Transplantation, The First Affiliated Hospital of Nanjing Medical University, The Key Laboratory of Living Donor Liver Transplantation, Ministry of Health, Nanjing, China

Abstract

Hydrogen sulfide (H_2S) can protect the liver against ischemia-reperfusion (I/R) injury. However, it is unknown whether H_2S plays a role in the protection of hepatic I/R injury in both young and old patients. This study compared the protective effects of H_2S in a rat model (young and old animals) of I/R injury and the mechanism underlying its effects. Young and old rats were assessed following an injection of NaHS. NaHS alone reduced hepatic I/R injury in the young rats by activating the nuclear erythroid-related factor 2 (Nrf2) signaling pathway, but it had little effect on the old rats. NaHS pretreatment decreased miR-34a expression in the hepatocytes of the young rats with hepatic I/R. Overexpresion of miR-34a decreased Nrf-2 and its downstream target expression, impairing the hepatoprotective effect of H_2S on the young rats. More importantly, downregulation of miR-34a expression increased Nrf-2 and the expression of its downstream targets, enhancing the effect of H_2S on hepatic I/R injury in the old rats. This study reveals the different effects of H_2S on hepatic I/R injury in young and old rats and sheds light on the involvement of H_2S in miR-34a modulation of the Nrf-2 pathway.

Editor: Edward J. Lesnefsky, Virginia Commonwealth University, United States of America

Funding: This work was supported by grant from the Priority Academic Program of Jiangsu Higher Education Institutions. The funders had no role in study design, data collection and analysis, decision to publish, or preparation of the manuscript.

Competing Interests: The authors have declared that no competing interests exist.

* Email: senlusen@163.com

Introduction

Hepatic warm ischemia-reperfusion (I/R) injury is a dynamic process that frequently occurs during a variety of clinical situations, including liver transplantation and liver surgery [1]. A series of events, such as the formation of reactive oxygen species (ROS), depletion of ATP, production of inflammatory mediators, and apoptosis of hepatocytes are involved in the pathophysiology of hepatic I/R [2]. Several risk factors (aging and liver steatosis) can exacerbate liver failure during I/R [3]. Therefore, effective treatment of hepatic I/R injury is difficult.

The gasotransmitter hydrogen sulfide (H_2S), similar to nitric oxide and carbon monoxide, is implicated in a wide range of physiological activities [4]. Endogenous H_2S can be produced from L-cysteine in several organs, such as the brain, heart, kidney, and liver [5]. H_2S has been reported to protect these tissues against I/R injury by maintaining mitochondrial function, inhibiting proinflammatory factors, neutralizing ROS and reducing apoptosis [6]. Treatment with H_2S can be via inhalation of H_2S or administration of NaHS by intravenous injection. However, it is difficult to control the concentration of inhaled H_2S, resulting in potential toxicity to animals [7]. The administration of NaHS by intravenous injection has become the common treatment method in I/R injury because the concentration can be controlled [8].

MicroRNAs (miRNAs) are 20–25 nucleotides long non-coding RNAs that modulate a variety of biological processes, such as development, apoptosis, metabolism, and proliferation [9]. Aberrant miRNA expression is associated with a large number of pathophysiological conditions, including liver diseases [10]. In recent years, the role of miR-34a in the regulation of liver function and survival has received a great deal of attention [11–12]. An increase in the expression of miR-34a was reported to be involved in age-dependent loss of oxidative defense in the liver [13]. In addition, miR-34a expression was regulated in a partial hepatectomy model, which resulted in the inhibition of hepatocyte proliferation [14]. However, the role of miR-34a in hepatic I/R damage remains largely unknown.

As a target gene of miR-34a, nuclear erythroid-related factor 2 (Nrf-2) is involved in the detoxification process. Studies have shown that this transcription factor exerts an antioxidant effect by regulating the expression of antioxidant enzymes genes, such as glutathione S-transferase (GST), superoxide dismutases (SODs) and heme oxygenase-1 (HO-1), and NAD(P)H: quinine oxidoreductase-1 (NQO1) [15–17]. Nrf-2 provides cytoprotection by inducing an anti-inflammatory response [18]. It is activated by a variety of factors, including oxidative stress. The activation of Nrf-2 predominantly occurs via the release of the Nrf-2/Keap1 (Kelch-like ECH associating protein 1) complex in the cytosol of cells [19]. It has been reported that the administration of H_2S can have beneficial effects on cardiac I/R injury by activating Nrf-2 [20]. In the liver, activation of Nrf-2 was reported to prevent or ameliorate toxin-induced injury and fibrosis [21].

Due to decreased endogenous antioxidants production and an increased inflammatory response, the ability of the liver cells of aged animals to combat I/R injury is significantly weakened [22]. Increasing evidence has shown that hepatic I/R injury is enhanced in aged animals and patients [23]. Although the effect of age on I/R-induced hepatic damage is well known, it is unknown whether the effect of therapy differs in aged and young patients with I/R injury. Here, we investigated if H_2S protected the liver against I/R damage both in aged and young rats and whether miR-34a was involved in this effect.

Materials and Methods

Ethics statement

All the animals were treated humanely, using approved procedures in accordance with the guidelines of the Institutional Animal Care and Use Committee at Nanjing Medical University. The study was approved by the Experimental Animal Ethics Committee of Nanjing Medical University and the animal protocol was approved by the Ethics Review of Lab Animal Use Application of Nanjing Medical University (Permit Number: NJMU-ERLAUA-20120107).

Chemicals and reagents

RPMI 1640 and DMEM were obtained from GIBCO (Invitrogen Company). Fetal bovine serum (FBS) was obtained from Hyclone (Logan, UT, USA). Lipofectamine 2000 transfection reagent was obtained from Invitrogen Life Technologies (Grand Island, NY, USA). NaHS was purchased from Sigma Aldrich (St. Louis, MO, USA). Antibodies against Nrf-2, GST, SOD, HO-1, and β-Actin were purchased from Santa Cruz Biotechnology (Santa Cruz, CA, USA). The Detergent Compatible (DC) Protein Assay kit was purchased from Bio-Rad Laboratories (Hercules, CA, USA).

Animals and surgery

Young and old male Sprague-Dawley (SD) rats aged 3 months and 20 months, respectively, were obtained from Vital River Laboratories (VRL) in China. The young rats (3 months) were randomly and equally divided into six groups: sham, hepatic I/R, hepatic I/R +20 µmol/kg of NaHS, hepatic I/R+ a negative control oligonucleotide (NC), hepatic I/R+ an miR-34a mimic, hepatic I/R+NaHS+NC, and hepatic I/R+NaHS+an miR-34a mimic. The old rats (20 months) were also randomly and equally divided into six groups: sham, hepatic I/R, hepatic I/R + 20 µmol/kg of NaHS, hepatic I/R+ anti-NC, hepatic I/R+ an miR-34a inhibitor, hepatic I/R+NaHS+anti-NC, and hepatic I/R+NaHS+an miR-34a inhibitor. The rats in the sham group underwent laparotomy, and the abdominal cavity was closed without hepatic I/R. Hepatic warm I/R was induced according to the previous reports [24]. Briefly, the rats were subjected to overnight fasting (with free access to water) before the surgery, and they were anaesthetized with 7% chloral hydrate (1 ml per 100 g of 7% chloral hydrate, intraperitoneal injection). After the midline laparotomy and anatomy of the hepatic portal, the left and median hepatic artery and the portal vein branches were blocked by no-damage artery clips to create a model of partial ischemia (70%). The right hepatic artery was opened to prevent the mesenteric venous congestion by permitting portal decompression through the right and caudate lobes. Under such circumstances of occluding, liver lobes were subjected to warm ischemia for 90 min. Reperfusion for 120 min was initiated by the removal of the clamp. The rats in the hepatic I/R+NaHS group received an intraperitoneal injection of 1 ml of NaHS solution 30 min before

hepatic I/R. An miR-34a mimic (5'-UGGCAGUGUCUUAG-CUGGUUGU-3', 10 nmol) or miR-34a inhibitor (5'-ACAAC-CAGCUAAGACACUGCCA-3', 10 nmol) in 0.1 ml of saline buffer was injected into the tail vein of the rats for 48 h before the administration of NaHS and subsequent liver I/R. A cholesterol-conjugated miR-34a mimic or an miR-34a inhibitor (both from RiboBio, Guangzhou, China) was used for in vivo RNA delivery. At each of the indicated time points (1, 3, 6 and 24 hours after I/R), six rats (per group) were randomly sacrificed, and blood and liver samples were collected.

Measurement of serum H2S concentrations

Serum H_2S concentrations were measured according to a previously reported method [24]. Briefly, 75 µl of sera were mixed with 300 µl of 10% trichloroacetic acid, 100 µL of distilled water and 150 µl of 1% zinc acetate. Then, 133 µl of N-dimethyl-p-phenylenediamine sulfate (20 µmol/L) and 133 µl of $FeCl_3$ (30 µmol/L) were added to the mixture. After incubation at room temperature (25°C) for 15 min, the absorbance of the resulting solution was read at 670 nm. All the samples were assayed in duplicate, and serum H_2S concentrations were calculated based on the calibration curve of NaHS.

Measurement of serum ALT and AST

The serum samples were separated from rat blood by centrifugation at 1500 g for 15 min, and aspartate aminotransferase (AST) and alanine aminotransferase (ALT) were measured using an automated biochemistry analyzer (HITACHI 7600-020, Tokyo, Japan) to assess the hepatic function.

Histopathological evaluation

Liver samples were frozen first and fixed in 10% neutral buffered formalin, embedded in paraffin, sliced into 5 µm thickness, and stained with hematoxylin-eosin. The histopathological scoring analysis was performed blindly according to previously described methods [25].

Isolation of rat hepatocytes

Hepatocytes were isolated from the young and old rats according to a previous report [26]. Briefly, the liver was perfused retrogradely with 250 ml of 135 mmol/l NaCl, 7 mmol/l KCl, 12 mmol/l glucose, and 10 mmol/l HEPES, pH 7.4, followed by 250 ml of the same medium supplemented with collagenase (150 U/ml) and 1 mmol/l $CaCl_2$. The Hepatocytes were diluted into William's E medium supplemented with 10% fetal calf serum, 50 mg/ml penicillin-streptomycin, 5 mg/ml insulin and 4 ng/ml dexamethasone, 10 mmol/l HEPES and 1 mmol/l $CaCl_2$.

Western blot analysis

The rat hepatocytes and liver tissue samples were lysed with ice-cold lysis buffer containing the following: 50 mmol/l Tris-HCl, pH 7.4; 1% NP-40; 150 mmol/l NaCl; 1 mmol/l EDTA; 1 mmol/l phenylmethylsulfonyl fluoride; and complete proteinase inhibitor mixture (one tablet per 10 ml; Roche Molecular Biochemicals, Indianapolis, IN, USA). The lysates were sonicated using the Sonicator VCX130 (Sonics & Materials) on ice, followed by centrifuging at 12000 g for 10 minutes at 4°C and the supernatants were retained. The protein concentration in the cell lysate was quantified using the DC protein assay kit (Bio-Rad). After determination of the protein content with the DC Protein Assay kit. Western blot analysis was performed.

Real-time PCR Assay

Mature miRNAs were isolated and purified using Trizol reagent (Invitrogen, USA), according to the manufacturer's protocol. The levels of miRNAs (miR-34a, miR-28, miR-155, miR-27a, miR-144 and miR-153) were quantified with a TaqMan PCR kit. Real-time PCR was performed with LightCycler 480, using U6 small nuclear RNA as an internal normalized reference. The mature miRNAs were amplified using specific miR primers and an miScript universal primer (Qiagen, Hilden, Germany). The average expression levels of the miRNAs were normalized against U6 using the $2^{-\Delta\Delta Ct}$ method. Differences between the groups were presented as ΔCt, indicating the difference between the Ct value of the miRNAs and the Ct value of U6. To ensure consistent measurements throughout all the assays, for each PCR amplification reaction, three independent RNA samples were loaded as internal controls to account for any plate-to-plate variation, and the results from each plate were normalized against internal normalization controls.

The mRNA expression of Nrf-2, HO-1, NQO1, SOD2 and GST was assessed using SYBR GREEN PCR Master Mix (Applied Biosystems). The specific primers were as follows: Nrf-2 5'-GCTATTTTCCATTCCCGAGTTAC-3' (forward), 5'-ATTG CTGTCCATCTCTGTCAG-3' (reverse); HO-1 5'-CTTTCAGAAGGGTCAGGTG TC-3' (forward), 5'-TGCTTGTTTCGCTCTATCTCC-3' (reverse); NQO1 5'-CATCATTTGGGCAAGTCC-3' (forward), 5'-ACAGCCGTGGCAGAACTA-3' (reverse); SOD2 5'-GAGAAGTACCAGGAGGCGTTG-3' (forward), 5'-GAGCCTTG-GACACCAACAGAT-3' (reverse); GST,5'-GCTCTATGG-GAAG GACCAG-3' (forward), 5'-CTCAAAAGGCTTCAGTTGC-3' (reverse); GAPDH 5'-TATCGGACGCCTGGTTAC-3' (forward), 5'-CTGTGCCGTTGAACTTGC-3' (reverse). All the data were analyzed using GAPDH gene expression as an internal standard.

Statistical analysis

The statistical analysis was performed with the statistical analysis software SPSS 13.0. Statistical analyses were performed using either an analysis of variance (ANOVA) or a Student's t-test. Data were expressed as the mean $\pm$ standard deviation. $P<0.05$ was considered significant.

Results

H$_2$S reduced hepatic I/R injury in young rats but has no effect in old rats

To identify the effect of H$_2$S on hepatic injury according to the age of the rats, the animals were treated with 20 μmol/kg NaHS. The serum levels of H$_2$S, ALT and AST were measured 1, 3, and 6 hours after I/R. Treatment with NaHS 30 minutes prior to the ischemia markedly increased the serum concentration of H$_2$S both in young and in old rats (Figure 1A and B, $P<0.01$). NaHS significantly reduced the serum levels of ALT and AST in young rats after 6 h reperfusion (Figure 1C, $P<0.01$). However, NaHS only slightly decreased the serum levels of ALT and AST in old rats (Figure 1D, $P>0.05$). These results imply that the protective effect of H$_2$S on the hepatic I/R-induced damage differs in young and old rats. The level of ALT or AST in old rats was significantly higher than that of young rats without NaHS treatment, suggesting that old rats were prone to damage after hepatic I/R.

Hematoxylin and Eosin (HE) staining was performed on the liver tissues after 24 h of reperfusion. As shown in figure 1E and F, NaHS could improve liver damage in young rats ($P<0.01$) but had little effect in old rats ($P>0.05$).

H$_2$S stimulated Nrf-2-mediated signaling pathway in the hepatocytes of the young rats but has no effect in old rats

The antioxidant effects of the transcription factor Nrf-2 play a crucial role in the protection of hepatic I/R damage [27]. To measure whether Nrf-2 was involved in the effect of H$_2$S on hepatic I/R, we measured the expression of Nrf-2 in the hepatocytes of young and old rats. The results showed that the mRNA level of Nrf-2 was significantly decreased in the hepatocytes of the young rats after 6 h I/R, and this decrease was reversed by NaHS treatment ($P<0.01$). The mRNA level of Nrf-2 was slightly changed in the hepatocytes of the old rats following I/R and the NaHS treatment compared to that of the untreated animals (Figure 2A, $P>0.05$). Consistent with the observed alteration in mRNA levels, NaHS treatment increased Nrf-2 protein levels in the hepatocytes of the young rats after I/R (Figure 2B). More importantly, the protein level of Nrf-2 in the hepatocytes of the young rats was significantly higher than that from old rats at baseline (Figure 2B).

It has been well documented that the transcription factor Nrf-2 up-regulates the expression of NQO1, GST and HO-1 [17]. Thus, we measured mRNA and protein levels of NQO1, GST and HO-1. After I/R, the expression of NQO1, GST and HO-1 was significantly reduced in the livers of the young rats, and the reduction was reversed by NaHS treatment (Figure 2C and 2D, $P<0.01$). However, no differences were observed in mRNA and protein levels of NQO1, GST and HO-1 in the old rats (Figure 2E and 2F, $P>0.05$). These results indicate that H$_2$S can stimulate Nrf-2-mediated signaling pathway to protect the liver against I/R injury in young rats.

H$_2$S reduced miR-34a expression in hepatocytes of the young rats but has no effect in old rats

To further study the mechanism of H$_2$S on Nrf-2 expression in the liver after I/R, we detected the expression of many miRNAs including miR-34a, miR-28, miR-155, miR-27a, miR-144 and miR-153, which may be involved in regulating the expression of this transcription factor [28]. Real-time PCR assays showed that, among these miRNAs, miR-34a was significantly up-regulated in the hepatocytes of the young and old rats after I/R (Figure 3A and B). Interestingly, the level of miR-34a was remarkably increased in the old rats compared to that in the young rats in the sham group and the I/R group (Figure 3C and D, $P<0.01$).

We also measured the expression of miR-34a in the liver following I/R and treatment with NaHS. As shown in Figure 3E and 3F, NaHS significantly decrease miR-34a expression in hepatocytes from young rats after I/R, but it had no effect on miR-34a expression in the hepatocytes of the old rats.

Overexpression of miR-34a could inhibit hepatoprotective effect of H$_2$S on young rats

Next, the role of miR-34a in the hepatoprotective effect of H$_2$S on young rats was further explored. After a tail vein injection of the cholesterol-conjugated miR-34a mimic, a slight increase in the serum levels of ALT and AST was observed in hepatic I/R young rats. However, the miR-34a mimic significantly reversed the effect of H$_2$S on hepatic I/R injury (Figure 4A, $P<0.01$). In addition, the expression of miR-34a was significantly increased in the hepatocytes of the young rats administered NaHS and the miR-34a mimic (Figure 4B, $P<0.01$). These results indicate that miR-34a was involved in the hepatoprotective effect of H$_2$S on hepatic I/R in the young rats.

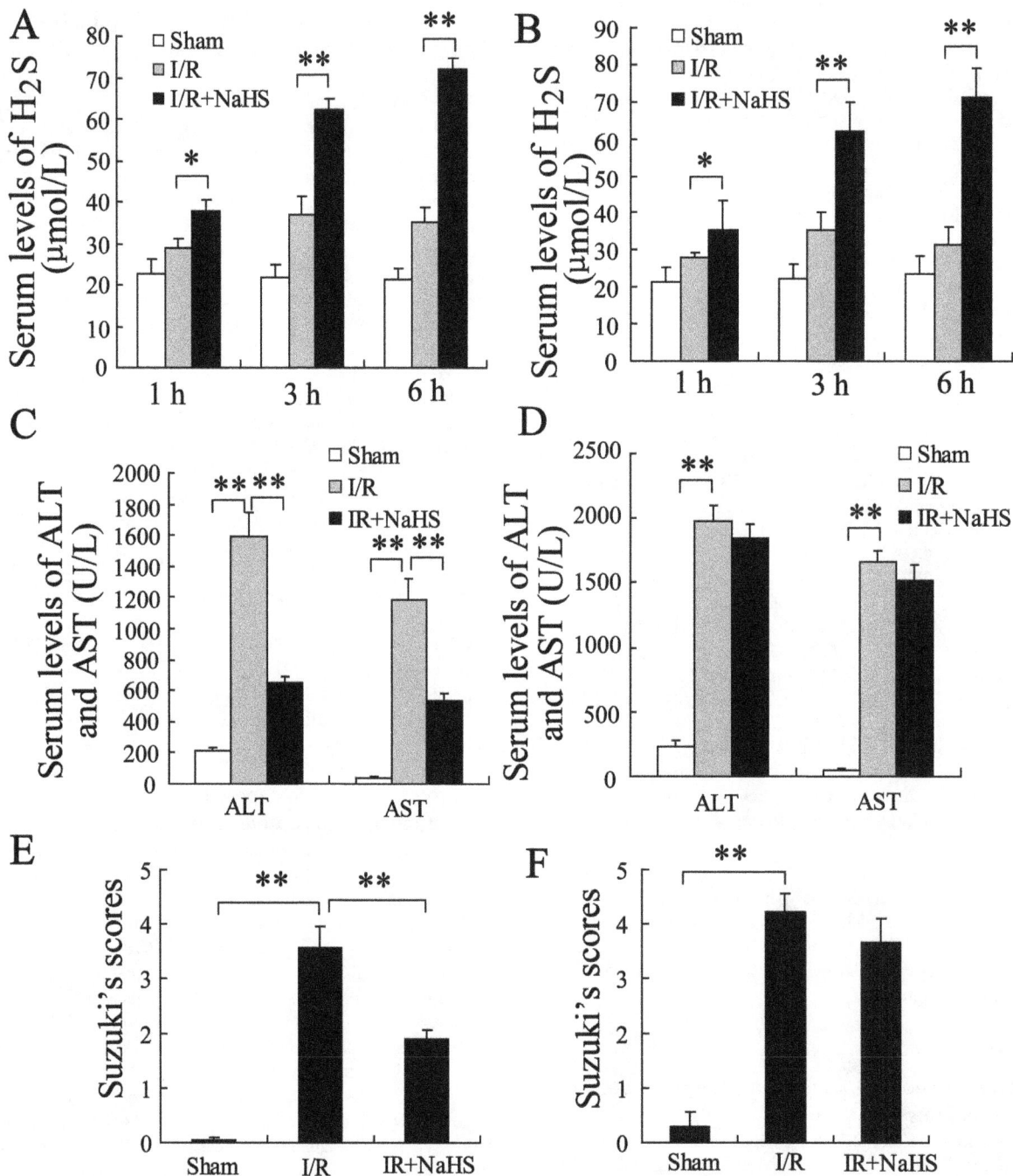

Figure 1. The effect of H₂S on hepatic I/R injury in young and old rats. (A) The serum levels of H2S were significantly increased in the young rats that received a preconditioning dose of 20 µmol/kg NaHS compared to rats in the I/R group. (B) The serum levels of H2S were significantly increased in the old rats that received a preconditioning dose of 20 µmol/kg NaHS compared to the rats in the I/R group. (C) The serum levels for alanine aminotransferase (ALT) and aspartate aminotransferase (AST) were determined in the young rats after 6 h of reperfusion. (D) The serum levels for ALT and AST were determined in the old rats after 6 h of reperfusion. (E) Suzuki's scores for the livers of the young rats after 24 h of reperfusion. (F) Suzuki's scores for the livers of the old rats after 24 h of reperfusion. **P<0.01, indicates significant differences from the respective control groups.

Knockout of miR-34a expression enhanced the hepatoprotective effect of H₂S on old rats

As the expression of miR-34a is abundant in hepatocytes of the old rats, we wondered whether the hepatoprotective effect of H₂S would be enhanced if its expression was down-regulated by an miR-34a inhibitor. As expected, the administration of the miR-34a inhibitor administration decreased serum levels of ALT and

AST in the old rats with hepatic I/R. Hepatoprotective effect were improved in the I/R group treated with NaHS and the miR-34a inhibitor compared to those in the miR-34a inhibitor-only group (Figure 5A, P<0.01), with the inhibitor further attenuating the pathological changes in the livers of the NaHS-treated old rats (Figure 5B, P<0.01).

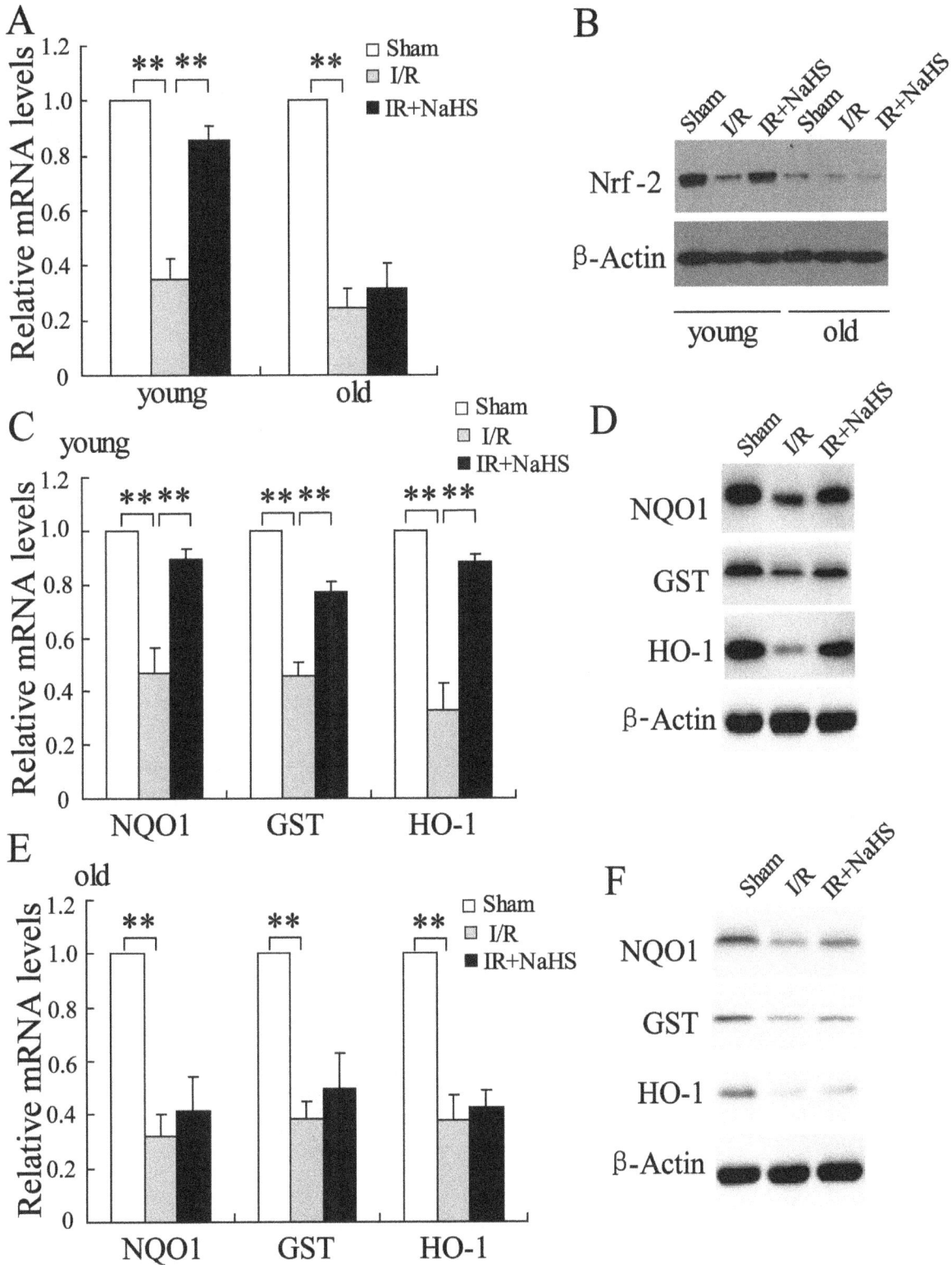

Figure 2. The effect of H₂S on Nrf-2-mediated signaling pathway. Relative mRNA levels of Nrf-2 were assayed in the young and old rats. Pretreatment with NaHS (20 μmol/kg) significantly increased Nrf-2 mRNA (A) and protein (B) levels in the young rats treated with I/R, but it had little effect on those in the old rats. Pretreatment with 20 μmol/kg NaHS significantly increased mRNA (C) and protein (D) levels of NQO1, GST, and HO-1 in the young rats treated with I/R. Pretreatment of 20 μmol/kg NaHS slightly increased mRNA (E) and protein (F) levels of NQO1, GST and HO-1 in the old rats treated with I/R. **P<0.01, indicate significant differences from the respective control groups.

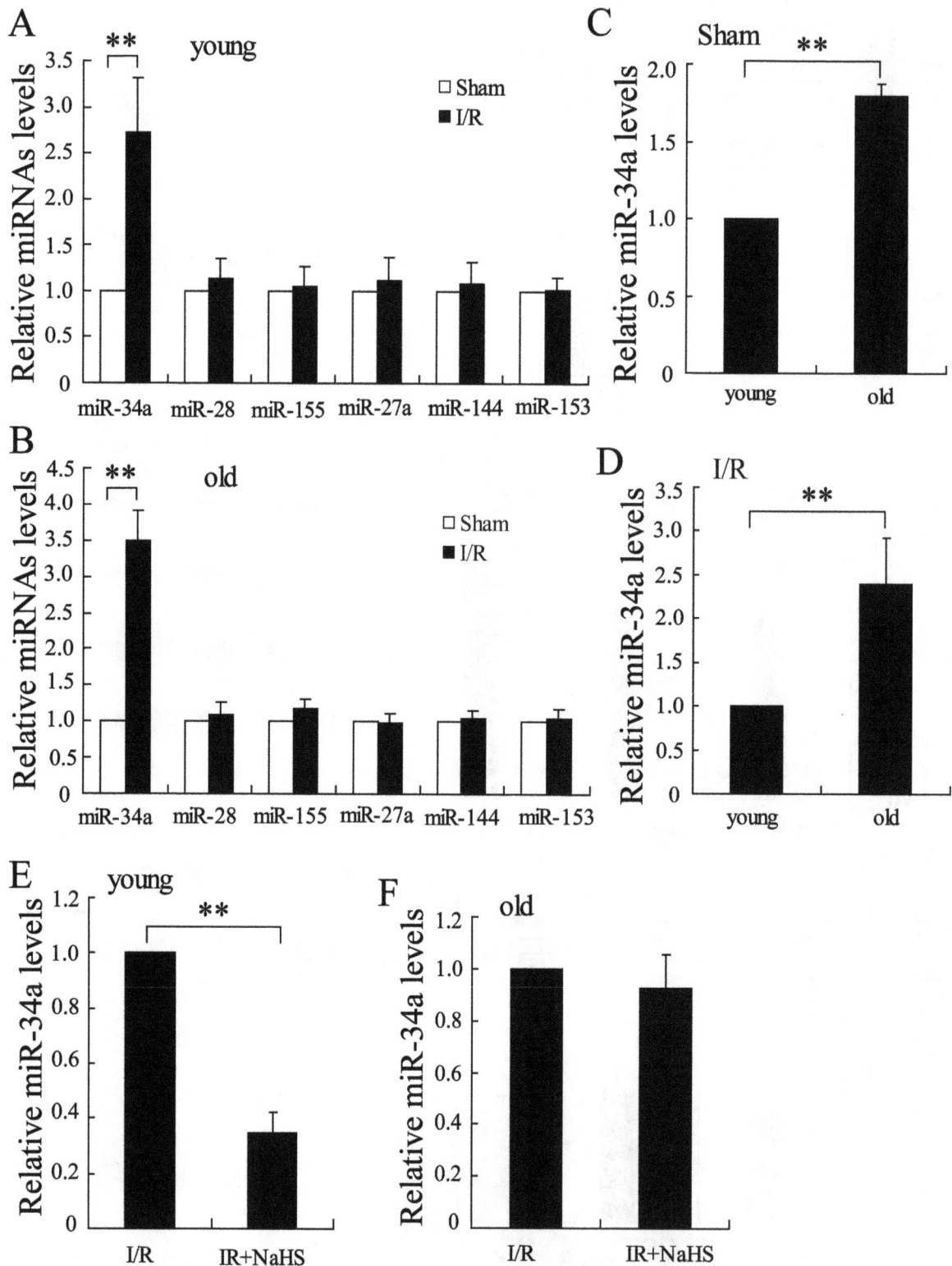

Figure 3. The effect of H₂S on miR-34a expression in the I/R liver. Relative levels of miR-34a, miR-28, miR-155, miR-27a, miR-144, and miR-153 were assayed in young rats (A) and old rats (B) after I/R. Levels of miR-34a were lower in the young rats in the sham group (C) and the in I/R group (D) than in the old rats. (E and F) Pretreatment with 20 μmol/kg NaHS significantly decreased miR-34a levels in the young rats (E), but it had little effect on those in the old rats. **P<0.01, indicates significant differences from the respective control groups.

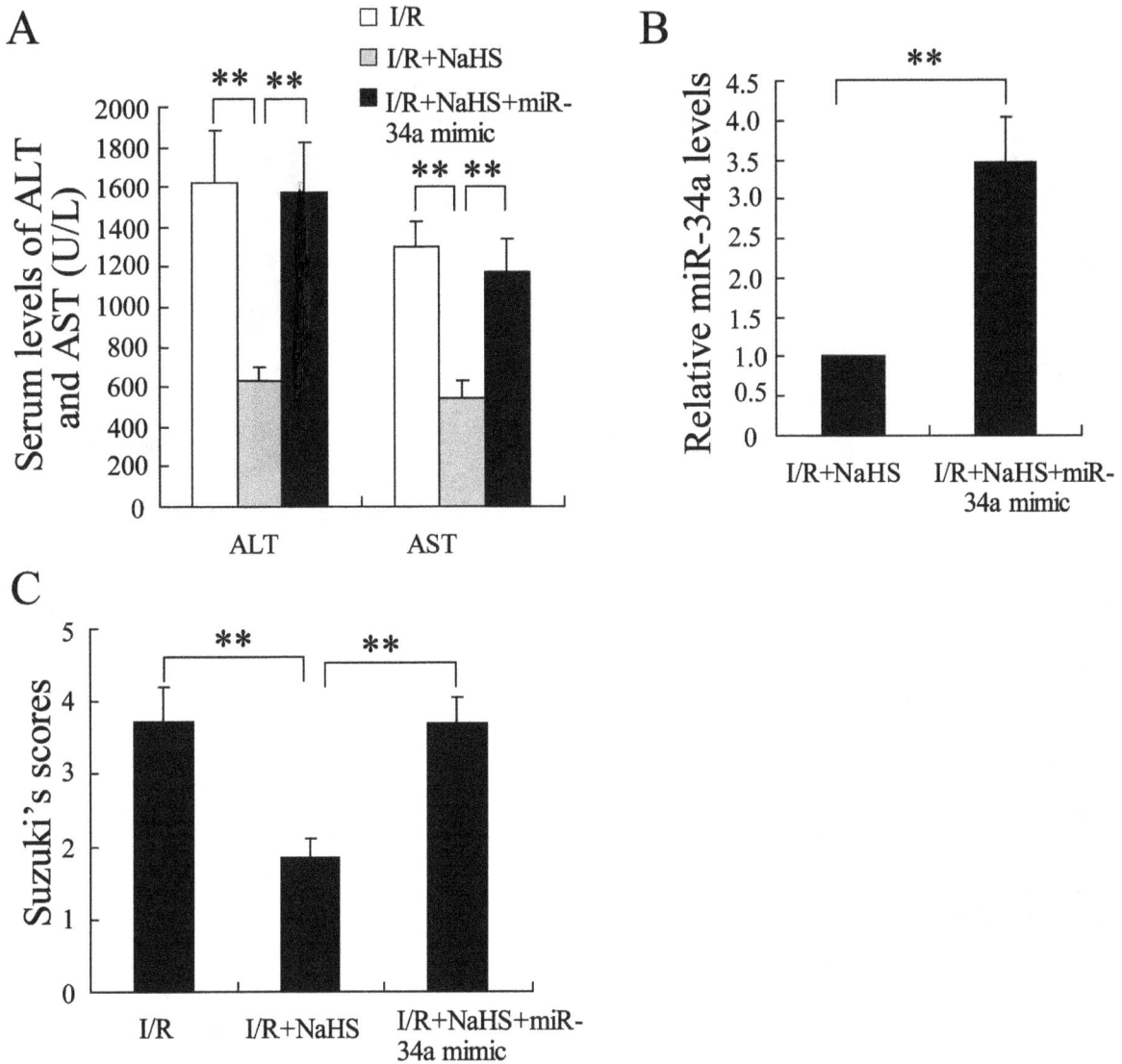

Figure 4. Overexpression of miR-34a inhibited the hepatoprotective effect of H₂S on young rats. (A) The serum levels of ALT and AST were assayed in the young rats. The serum levels of ALT and AST were significantly decreased in the young rats following the pretreatment with NaHS, and this decrease was reversed by miR-34a mimic. (B) The injection of miR-34a mimic clearly increased miR-34a levels. (C) Suzuki's scores for the livers of the young rats. **P<0.01, indicates significant differences from the respective control groups.

miR-34a mediation of Nrf-2 signaling pathway was implicated in the hepatoprotective effects of H₂S

To explore the mechanism of miR-34a in the hepatoprotective effects of H₂S, the expression of Nrf-2, NQO1, GST and HO-1 was measured in the young and old rats after injection of miR-34a mimic or inhibitor. As shown in Figure 6A and 6B, miR-34a mimic could reduce the expressions of Nrf-2, NQO1, GST and HO-1 in the young rats after hepatic I/R pretreated with NaHS, suggesting that the promotion of Nrf-2-mediated signaling pathway by NaHS might act through down-regulation of the miR-34a level. On the other hand, miR-34a inhibitor significantly increased the expressions of Nrf-2, NQO1, GST and HO-1 in the old rats after hepatic I/R injury with NaHS treatment (Figure 6C and 6D), suggesting that miR-34a-mediated Nrf-2 signaling pathway is involved in hepatoprotective effects of H₂S.

Discussion

The gasotransmitter H₂S can protect several tissues including the liver against I/R injury [29]. Previous study focused on the protective effect of H₂S on the tissues of young animals. The present study explored the hepatoprotective effect of H₂S on young (3 months) and old rats (20 months). We found that NaHS alone could reduce hepatic I/R injury in young rats, but it had little effect on hepatic I/R injury in old rats. In addition, NaHS pretreatment decreased miR-34a expression in the hepatocytes of the young rats treated with hepatic I/R. Our data also showed that miR-34a was implicated in H₂S-induced prevention of liver damage in the young rats. More importantly, the inhibition of miR-34a expression enhanced the effect of H₂S on hepatic I/R injury in the old rats. H₂S might promote Nrf-2-mediated signaling pathway through the down-regulation of the expression of miR-34a. The levels of miR-34a were higher in the hepatocytes of the old rats than in those of the young rats.

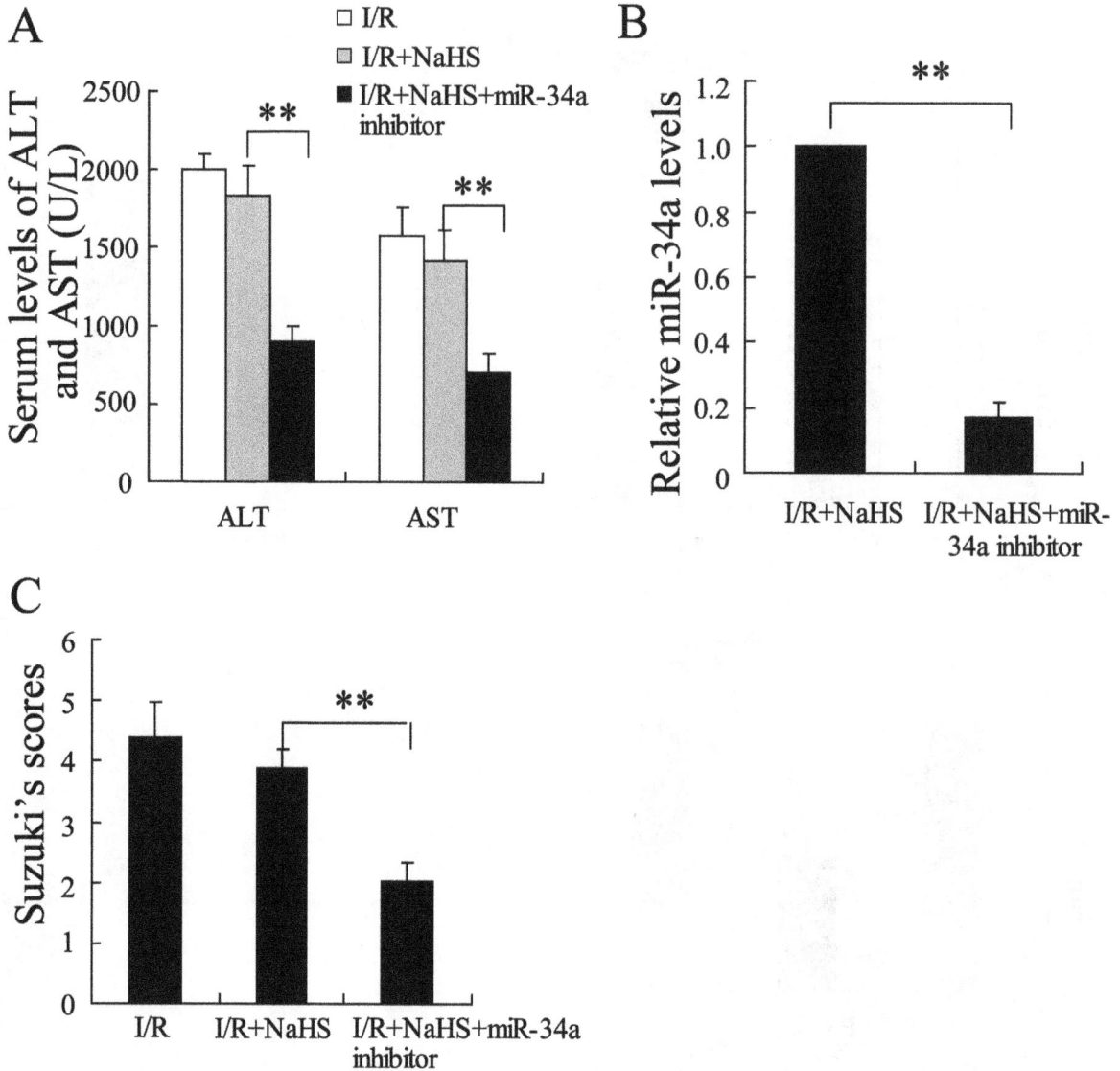

Figure 5. Knockout of miR-34a expression enhanced the hepatoprotective effect of H₂S on the old rats. (A) The serum levels of ALT and AST were assayed in the old rats. Pretreatment with NaHS had little effect on the serum levels of ALT and AST, which were significantly decreased by miR-34a inhibitor in the old rats with I/R. (B) The injection of miR-34a inhibitor clearly decreased miR-34a levels. (C) Suzuki's scores for the livers of the old rats. **P<0.01, indicates significant differences from the respective control groups.

Due to its anti-inflammatory, antioxidative, and cytoprotective activity, H₂S is capable of protecting tissues from I/R-induced injury [30]. The present study has for the first time explored the effect of H₂S on hepatic I/R injury in young and old rats. Our data showed that the administration of NaHS, a donor of H₂S, significantly decreased serum levels of AST and ALT, as well as histopathological alterations after hepatic I/R in young rats. However, NaHS had little effect on I/R-induced liver injury in the old rats. The different effect of NaHS on I/R injury was due to decreased production of endogenous antioxidants with increasing age. Our data demonstrated that NaHS stimulated the expression of Nrf-2 and its downstream target gene in young rats but that it had little effect on the expression of these molecules in old rats.

MiR-34a was previously reported to be involved in the regulation of liver function and survival [11]. In this study, we found that the level of miR-34a was remarkably higher in the hepatocytes of the old rats compared to that of the young rats,

which was consistent with previous findings [12]. NaHS significantly decreased miR-34a expression in the hepatocytes of the young rats but had little effect on miR-34a expression in the old rats due to the hepatoprotective effect of H₂S. To investigate the relationship between miR-34a and the effect of NaHS on hepatic I/R, we used miR-34a mimic and miR-34a inhibitor. Injection with miR-34a mimic diminished the protective effect of NaHS on hepatic I/R injury in the young rats. In the old rats, the combination of NaHS and the miR-34a inhibitor prevented the damage caused by hepatic I/R. MiR-34a has been implicated in liver oxidative stress during aging [12]. Based on that, we believe that the oxidative stress defense function of NaHS might rely on the regulation of miR-34a expression.

Our data also indicated that miR-34a mediation of the Nrf-2 signaling pathway was implicated in the hepatoprotective effect of H₂S. There are several lines of evidence to support this. First, in the young rats, miR-34a mimic reduced the expression of Nrf-2

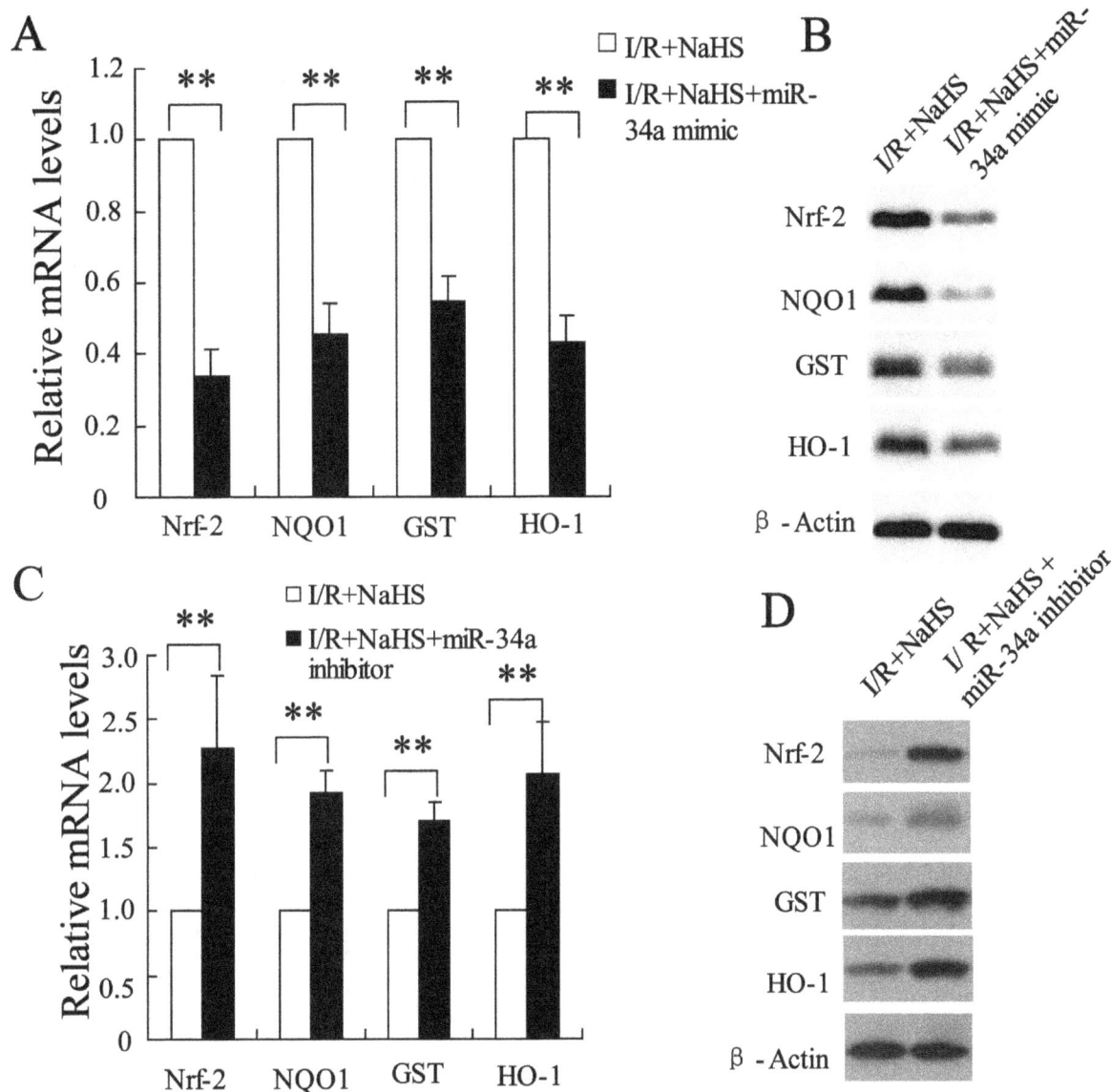

Figure 6. miR-34a mediated Nrf-2 signaling pathway was implicated in the hepatoprotective effects of H₂S. The injection of miR-34a mimic decreased the mRNA (A) and protein (B) levels of Nrf-2, NQO1, GST and HO-1 in the young rats in the I/R+pretreatment with NaHS group. The injection of miR-34a inhibitor increased the mRNA (C) and protein (D) levels of Nrf-2, NQO1, GST and HO-1 in the old rats in the with I/R+pretreatment with NaHS group. **P<0.01, indicates significant differences from the respective control groups.

and its downstream target gene in hepatic I/R pretreated with NaHS. Second, miR-34a inhibitor significantly increased the expression of Nrf-2 and its downstream target gene in the old rats with or without NaHS pretreatment. Third, miR-34a level was negatively correlated with Nrf-2 expression, which is consistent with the finding of a previous report [13].

Our data demonstrated that I/R stress decreased HO-1 mRNA and protein expressions in rat liver (Figure 2), which is inconsistent with the previous report [31]. It is possible that chloral hydrate treatment instead of pentobarbital treatment might affect the expression of some antioxidant gene in the liver. However, more clarification of the specific molecular mechanism involved is needed.

In summary, we demonstrated that NaHS had a different effect on hepatic I/R damage in young and old rats. Our results also

suggested that the hepatoprotective effect of NaHS in the young rats was due to decreased miR-34a expression, which resulted in the promotion of Nrf-2 signaling pathway. The protective effect of NaHS when it was combined with miR-34a inhibitor in the old rats provided further evidence for the role of miR-34a in hepatic I/R. These results may lead to the development of therapeutic strategies to minimize injury after I/R during liver transplantation and liver surgery both in young and aged patients.

Author Contributions

Conceived and designed the experiments: SL. Performed the experiments: XH. Analyzed the data: YG. Contributed reagents/materials/analysis tools: JQ. Contributed to the writing of the manuscript: SL.

References

1. Berrevoet F, Schäfer T, Vollmar B, Menger MD (2003) Ischemic preconditioning: enough evidence to support clinical application in liver surgeryand transplantation? Acta Chir Belg 103: 485–489.

2. Papadopoulos D, Siempis T, Theodorakou E, Tsoulfas G (2013) Hepatic ischemia and reperfusion injury and trauma: current concepts. Arch Trauma Res 2: 63–70.

3. Jaeschke H, Woolbright BL (2012) Current strategies to minimize hepatic ischemia-reperfusion injury by targeting reactive oxygen species. Transplant Rev 26: 103–114.

4. Lisjak M, Teklic T, Wilson ID, Whiteman M, Hancock JT (2013) Hydrogen sulfide: environmental factor or signalling molecule? Plant Cell Environ 36: 1607–1616.

5. Kimura H (2013) Physiological role of hydrogen sulfide and polysulfide in the central nervous system. Neurochem Int 63: 492–497.

6. Guo W, Kan JT, Cheng ZY, Chen JF, Shen YQ, et al. (2012) Hydrogen sulfide as an endogenous modulator in mitochondria and mitochondria dysfunction. Oxid Med Cell Longev 2012: 878052.

7. Wagner F, Asfar P, Calzia E, Radermacher P, Szabó C (2009) Bench-to-bedside review: Hydrogen sulfide-the third gaseous transmitter: applications for critical care. Crit Care 13: 213.

8. Henderson PW, Weinstein AL, Sohn AM, Jimenez N, Krijgh DD, et al. (2010) Hydrogen sulfide attenuates intestinal ischemia-reperfusion injury when delivered in the post-ischemic period. J Gastroenterol Hepatol 25: 1642–1647.

9. Inui M, Martello G, Piccolo S (2010) MicroRNA control of signal transduction. Nat Rev Mol Cell Biol 11: 252–263.

10. Miska EA (2005) How microRNAs control cell division, differentiation and death. Curr Opin Genet Dev 15: 563–568.

11. McDaniel K, Herrera L, Zhou T, Francis H, Han Y, et al. (2014) The functional role of microRNAs in alcoholic liver injury. J Cell Mol Med 18: 197–207.

12. Fu T, Choi SE, Kim DH, Seok S, Suino-Powell KM, et al. (2012) Aberrantly elevated microRNA-34a in obesity attenuates hepatic responses to FGF19 by targeting a membrane coreceptor β-Klotho. Proc Natl Acad Sci U S A 109: 16137–16142.

13. Li N, Muthusamy S, Liang R, Sarojini H, Wang E (2011) Increased expression of miR-34a and miR-93 in rat liver during aging, and their impact on the expression of Mgst1 and Sirt1. Mech Ageing Dev 132: 75–85.

14. Chen H, Sun Y, Dong R, Yang S, Pan C, et al. (2011) Mir-34a is upregulated during liver regeneration in rats and is associated with the suppression of hepatocyte proliferation. PLoS One 6: e20238.

15. Suzuki T, Takagi Y, Osanai H, Li L, Takeuchi M, et al. (2005) Pi class glutathione S-transferase genes are regulated by Nrf 2 through an evolutionarily conserved regulatory element in zebrafish. Biochem J 388: 65–73.

16. Sahin K, Orhan C, Tuzcu M, Sahin N, Ali S, et al. (2014) Orally Administered Lycopene Attenuates Diethylnitrosamine-Induced Hepatocarcinogenesis in Rats by Modulating Nrf-2/HO-1 and Akt/mTOR Pathways. Nutr Cancer [Epub ahead of print].

17. Zeng T, Zhang CL, Song FY, Zhao XL, Yu LH (2013) The activation of HO-1/Nrf-2 contributes to the protective effects of diallyl disulfide (DADS) against ethanol-induced oxidative stress. Biochim Biophys Acta 1830: 4848–4859.

18. Park SY, Kim JH, Lee SJ, Kim Y (2013) Involvement of PKA and HO-1 signaling in anti-inflammatory effects of surfactin in BV-2 microglial cells. Toxicol Appl Pharmacol 268: 68–78.

19. MacLeod AK, McMahon M, Plummer SM, Higgins LG, Penning TM, et al. (2009) Characterization of the cancer chemopreventive NRF2-dependent gene battery in human keratinocytes: demonstration that the KEAP1-NRF2 pathway, and not the BACH1-NRF2 pathway, controls cytoprotection against electrophiles as well as redox-cycling compounds. Carcinogenesis 30: 1571–1580.

20. Peake BF, Nicholson CK, Lambert JP, Hood RL, Amin H, et al. (2013) Hydrogen sulfide preconditions the db/db diabetic mouse heart against ischemia-reperfusion injury by activating Nrf2 signaling in an Erk-dependent manner. Am J Physiol Heart Circ Physiol 304: H1215–H1224.

21. Lu YF, Liu J, Wu KC, Qu Q, Fan F, et al. (2014) Overexpression of Nrf2 Protects against Microcystin-Induced Hepatotoxicity in Mice. PLoS One 9: e93013.

22. Schiesser M, Wittert A, Nieuwenhuijs VB, Morphett A, Padbury RT, et al. (2009) Intermittent ischemia but not ischemic preconditioning is effective in restoring bile flow after ischemia reperfusion injury in the livers of aged rats. J Surg Res 152: 61–68.

23. van der Bilt JD, Kranenburg O, Borren A, van Hillegersberg R, Borel Rinkes IH (2008) Ageing and hepatic steatosis exacerbate ischemia/reperfusion-accelerated outgrowth of colorectal micrometastases. Ann Surg Oncol 15: 1392–1398.

24. Zhang Q, Fu H, Zhang H, Xu F, Zou Z, et al. (2013) Hydrogen sulfide preconditioning protects rat liver against ischemia/reperfusion injury by activating Akt-GSK-3β signaling and inhibiting mitochondrial permeability transition. PLoS One 8: e74422.

25. Suzuki S, Toledo-Pereyra LH, Rodriguez FJ, Cejalvo D (1993) Neutrophil infiltration as an important factor in liver ischemia and reperfusion injury. Modulating effects of FK506 and cyclosporine. Transplantation 55: 1265–1272.

26. Tulsawani R, Gupta R, Misra K (2013) Efficacy of aqueous extract of Hippophae rhamnoides and its bio-active flavonoids against hypoxia-induced cell death. Indian J Pharmacol 45: 258–263.

27. Ke B, Shen XD, Zhang Y, Ji H, Gao F, et al. (2013) KEAP1-NRF2 complex in ischemia-induced hepatocellular damage of mouse liver transplants. J Hepatol. 2013; 59(6): 1200–1207.

28. Cheng X, Ku CH, Siow RC (2013) Regulation of the Nrf2 antioxidant pathway by microRNAs: New players in micromanaging redox homeostasis. Free Radic Biol Med 64: 4–11.

29. Kimura H, Shibuya N, Kimura Y (2012) Hydrogen sulfide is a signaling molecule and a cytoprotectant. Antioxid Redox Signal 17: 45–57.

30. Nicholson CK, Calvert JW (2010) Hydrogen sulfide and ischemia-reperfusion injury. Pharmacol Res 62: 289–297.

31. Tanaka Y, Maher JM, Chen C, Klaassen CD (2007) Hepatic ischemia-reperfusion induces renal heme oxygenase-1 via NF-E2-related factor 2 in rats and mice. Mol Pharmacol 71: 817–825.

22

Coenzyme Q10 Protects Hair Cells against Aminoglycoside

Kazuma Sugahara*, Yoshinobu Hirose, Takefumi Mikuriya, Makoto Hashimoto, Eiju Kanagawa, Hirotaka Hara, Hiroaki Shimogori, Hiroshi Yamashita

Department of Otolaryngology, Yamaguchi University Graduate School of Medicine, Ube, Yamaguchi, Japan

Abstract

It is well known that the production of free radicals is associated with sensory cell death induced by an aminoglycoside. Many researchers have reported that antioxidant reagents protect sensory cells in the inner ear, and coenzyme Q10 (CoQ10) is an antioxidant that is consumed as a health food in many countries. The purpose of this study was to investigate the role of CoQ10 in mammalian vestibular hair cell death induced by aminoglycoside. Cultured utricles of CBA/CaN mice were divided into three groups (control group, neomycin group, and neomycin + CoQ10 group). In the neomycin group, utricles were cultured with neomycin (1 mM) to induce hair cell death. In the neomycin + CoQ10 group, utricles were cultured with neomycin and water-soluble CoQ10 (30–0.3 μM). Twenty-four hours after exposure to neomycin, the cultured tissues were fixed, and vestibular hair cells were labeled using an anti-calmodulin antibody. Significantly more hair cells survived in the neomycin + CoQ10 group than in the neomycin group. These data indicate that CoQ10 protects sensory hair cells against neomycin-induced death in the mammalian vestibular epithelium; therefore, CoQ10 may be useful as a protective drug in the inner ear.

Editor: Berta Alsina, Universitat Pompeu Fabra, Spain

Funding: This work was supported by a grant from the Japanese Ministry of Education, Culture, Sports, Science, and Technology. The funder had no role in study design, data collection and analysis, decision to publish, or preparation of the manuscript.

Competing Interests: The authors have declared that no competing interests exist.

* Email: kazuma@yamaguchi-u.ac.jp

Introduction

Sensory hair cells are easily damaged by chemicals such as aminoglycosides, infection, and ischemia [1]. After hair cells are damaged, auditory and vestibular dysfunction is permanent; therefore, it is important to prevent the loss of hair cells of patients with inner ear diseases. Previous studies indicated that hair cell death was related to oxidative stress. Aminoglycosides are well-known ototoxic agents, and their ototoxicity is mediated by the generation of free radicals [2].

Recently, coenzyme Q10 (CoQ10) has attracted a great deal of public attention as a nutritional supplement; it is used world-wide for health promotion and anti-aging as an anti-oxidant agent. However, CoQ10 is extremely lipid-soluble and not easily absorbed by the body. Recently, water-soluble CoQ10 was developed to improve absorption of CoQ10 in the body [3]. Therefore, in the present study, we investigated the protective effect of water-soluble CoQ10 against hair cell degeneration induced by neomycin.

Materials and Methods

Animal Use and Care

CBA/N mice obtained from Kyushu Animal Company (Kumamoto, Japan) were used in this study. All mice (4–6 weeks old) were male and had normal Preyer's reflexes. The experimental protocol was reviewed and approved by the Committee for Ethics on Animal Experiments at the Yamaguchi University School of Medicine. Experiments were conducted in accordance with these guidelines, Japanese federal law (No. 105), and Notification No. 6 of the Japanese government.

Organ Culture of Utricles and Induction of Hair Cell Death

All animals were deeply anesthetized with an overdose of pentobarbital and immediately decapitated. The temporal bones were quickly removed and the individual vestibular organs were dissected in basal Eagle medium (Invitrogen, Carlsbad, CA) supplemented with Earle's balanced salt solution (Invitrogen) (2:1, v/v). Isolated utricles were moved into the culture medium, which consisted of basal Eagle medium supplemented with Earle's balanced salt solution (2:1, v/v) and 5% fetal bovine serum (Invitrogen). The free-floating utricles were incubated in 24-well tissue culture plates for 12 or 24 h at 37°C in a 5% CO_2 and 95% air environment. To induce hair cell death, neomycin solution (10 mg/mL; Sigma, St. Louis, MO) was added into the culture wells to a final concentration of 1.0 mM. After the culture protocols were completed, the utricles were fixed with 4% paraformaldehyde (PFA) for 1 h at room temperature. Otoconia were gently removed from fixed utricles by a stream of phosphate buffered saline (PBS) applied via a 28 G needle and syringe. After rinsing with PBS, the samples were used in the assays outlined below.

Preparation of coenzyme Q10 solution

Water soluble CoQ10 (Eisai Co., Tokyo, Japan) was used in this study and dissolved in the medium before initiation of culture.

| Neomycin | - | 1 mM | 1 mM | 1 mM |
| CoenzymeQ10 | - | - | 3 μM | 30 μM |

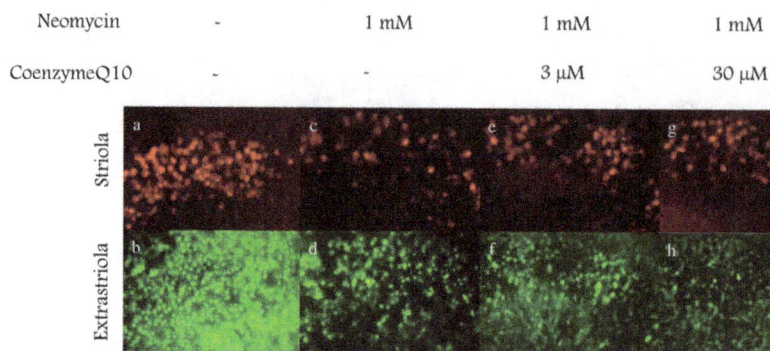

Figure 1. Protective effect of coenzyme Q10 against neomycin-induced cell death. Utricles were cultured for 24 h without neomycin (a, b), with neomycin (c, d) or with both neomycin and coenzyme Q10 (e–h). Death of striolar hair cells (red: calbindin) and extrastriolar hair cells (green: calmodulin) was inhibited by coenzyme Q10.

Immunohistochemistry for hair cell labeling

Fixed utricles were incubated in blocking solution (1% bovine serum albumin, 0.4% normal goat serum, 0.4% normal horse serum, and 0.4% Triton X-100 in PBS) overnight at 4°C. To label hair cells, a monoclonal antibody against calmodulin (Sigma) and a polyclonal antibody against calbindin (Chemicon, Temecula, CA) were used. Samples were incubated overnight at 4°C in the primary antibody solution (calmodulin 1:150 or calbindin 1:250 in the blocking solution). After washing with the blocking solution, the specimens were incubated in secondary antibodies diluted in blocking solution as follows: biotinylated horse anti-mouse IgG (1:100; Vector Laboratories, Burlingame, CA) or Alexa 488-conjugated goat anti-mouse IgG (1:500; Molecular Probes, Eugene, OR) in addition to Alexa 594-conjugated goat anti-rabbit IgG (1:500; Molecular Probes). After rinsing with blocking solution, the utricles were mounted in Vectashield (Vector Laboratories) and coverslipped.

Immunohistochemistry for production of 4-HNE

To evaluate the production of reactive oxygen species, 4-hydroxy-2-nonenal (4-HNE) production was investigated. The samples were fixed with 4% PFA after dissection. Next, utricles were incubated in a 1:100 dilution of anti-4-HNE mouse monoclonal antibody (OXIS International, Inc., Portland, OR) overnight in a refrigerator (4°C). After the rinsing in the blocking solution, the samples were incubated with Alexa 488-conjugated goat anti-mouse IgG and Texas red-conjugated phalloidin (1:100, Sigma) for 4 hours at room temperature. The fluorescence intensity of the immunohistochemistry was evaluated with the image analysis software: ImageJ. Six samples were used for the experiment. The average of the fluorescence intensity derived from utricles cultured with normal medium was defined as 1. The intensities in the other groups were shown by the relative value.

Evaluation of the number of residual sensory hair cells

Utricles were examined under a fluorescence microscope (XF-EHD2, Nikon, Tokyo, Japan) to evaluate the survival of hair cells. Calbindin-positive and calmodulin-positive cells were counted as hair cells in the striolar region and extrastriolar region, respectively. The labeled hair cells were counted in two squares, 20 μm on a side, which were determined randomly in each utricle. Eight striolar and eight extrastriolar hair cell counts were averaged to produce one striolar and one extrastriolar hair cell density for each utricle examined. At least six utricles were examined for each experimental condition. All data were expressed in mean ±

standard error. Data were analyzed with StatView version 5.0J for Macintosh (SAS institute Inc, Cary, NC). These hair cell dinsities were compared with Mann-Whitney's U test to determine significant values. A level of $P<0.05$ was accepted as statistically significant.

Results

Effect of coenzyme Q10 on hair cell survival

To evaluate the effect of CoQ10 on the survival of hair cells treated with neomycin, utricles were cultured with neomycin (1 mM) and CoQ10 (1–30 μM) for 24 hours. The utricles were incubated for 2 hours with or without CoQ10 before exposure to neomycin. Calmodulin and calbindin were immunolabeled to detect residual hair cells (Fig. 1). In the medium with neomycin, the density of hair cells was reduced after 24 hours. More hair cells survived in the medium with both neomycin and CoQ10 than in the medium with neomycin alone. The density of hair cells in the cultured utricles is shown in Fig. 2. and Table 1. CoQ10 significantly suppressed the reduction of hair cell density induced by neomycin at concentrations of 10 and 30 μM.

Coenzyme Q10 suppresses the production of 4-HNE

To detect the production of hydroxy radicals, immunohisto-chemistry was performed using an antibody against 4-HNE, which is the metabolic product of hydroxy radicals. Six cultured utricles were divided into three groups. Two utricles were cultured in the conventional medium described above for 14 hours. Two utricles were cultured in the conventional medium for 2 hours, and followed by culture for 12 hours after addition of neomycin (1 mM) into the medium. The other two utricles were cultured in medium containing neomycin (1 mM) and CoQ10 (30 μM) for 12 hours following culture in the normal medium (2 h). ß-actin was labeled with phalloidin conjugated with Texas Red to indicate the hair cell layer, and the fluorescence microscope was focused on the hair cell layer. Hair cells containing 4-HNE were not seen in utricles cultured for 12 hours without neomycin (Fig. 3b). Many hair cells containing 4-HNE appeared in utricles cultured with 1 mM neomycin (Fig. 3d). The 4-HNE signal was decreased in utricles cultured with neomycin and CoQ10 for 12 hours (Fig. 3f). These results indicate that CoQ10 suppressed the production of hydroxy radicals by utricles exposed to neomycin. The evaluation of the fluorescence intensity of the immunohistochemistry was shown in Fig. 4. The fluorescence intensity derived from 4-HNE was significantly stronger in the utricles cultured with neomycin

Table 1. The density of surviving hair cells in the utricles cultured with CoQ10 and neomycin.

	Striolar (cells/400 μm²)	Extrastriolar (cells/400 μm²)
Control	3.18±0.24	5.26±0.17
Neomycin (1 mM)	1.70±0.34	3.00±0.38
Neomycin (1 mM), CoQ10 (1.0 μM)	1.58±1.23	2.83±0.20
Neomycin (1 mM), CoQ10 (3.0 μM)	1.83±0.11	3.88±0.72
Neomycin (1 mM), CoQ10 (10.0 μM)	2.73±0.38	4.93±0.50
Neomycin (1 mM), CoQ10 (30.0 μM)	2.38±0.31	5.38±0.65

than without neomycin. The existance of coenzyme Q10 can inhibited the fluorescence intensity.

Discussion

Reactive oxygen species play an important role in hair cell death induced by aminoglycosides [4]. Many researchers have reported a relationship between the production of reactive oxygen species and hair cell damage induced by aminoglycosides [5]. Aminoglycosides are a class of compounds that are well known as specific ototoxic agents [6], and recent research suggests that hair cell death induced by these chemicals is closely related to apoptosis [7]. Therefore, many types of antioxidants are used to inhibit hair cell death induced by aminoglycosides, and antioxidant molecules are a candidate for the treatment of patients suffering from aminoglycoside-induced hearing loss and vestibular dysfunction [8].

In this study, we showed that the anti-oxidative agent CoQ10 suppresses hair cell death induced by neomycin. To elucidate the mechanism underlying the antioxidant activity of CoQ10, we assessed the production of 4-HNE, which is the metabolite of the hydroxy radical. In hair cells exposed to aminoglycoside, strong 4-HNE signals were observed, and CoQ10 inhibited this production

of 4-HNE remarkably. This scavenging of free radicals is thought to have protected the hair cells from cell death.

Several studies have reported the effect of CoQ10 on inner ear function. Sato reported that CoQ10 was effective in promoting recovery from damage to auditory hairs caused by hypoxia [9]. Sergi reported an antioxidant function of idebenone (synthetic analogue of CoQ10) in protection from noise-induced hearing loss [10]. Recently, we reported that oral administration of CoQ10 suppressed inner ear damage after intense noise exposure [2]. In the present study, the direct activity of CoQ10 was determined using utricle organ cultures. CoQ10 has already been used for clinical trials; oral administration slowed the progressive deterioration of function in Parkinson's disease [11], and CoQ10 prevented progressive hearing loss and improved blood lactate levels after exercise in patients with maternally inherited diabetes mellitus and deafness [12]. In these studies, CoQ10 was not associated with major side effects; therefore, it can safely be used for inner ear diseases.

We used a water-soluble form of CoQ10, which has traditionally been known as a lipid-soluble molecule and thus has been difficult to dissolve in medium. In addition, bioavailability of CoQ10 was low after oral administration. Recently, water-soluble

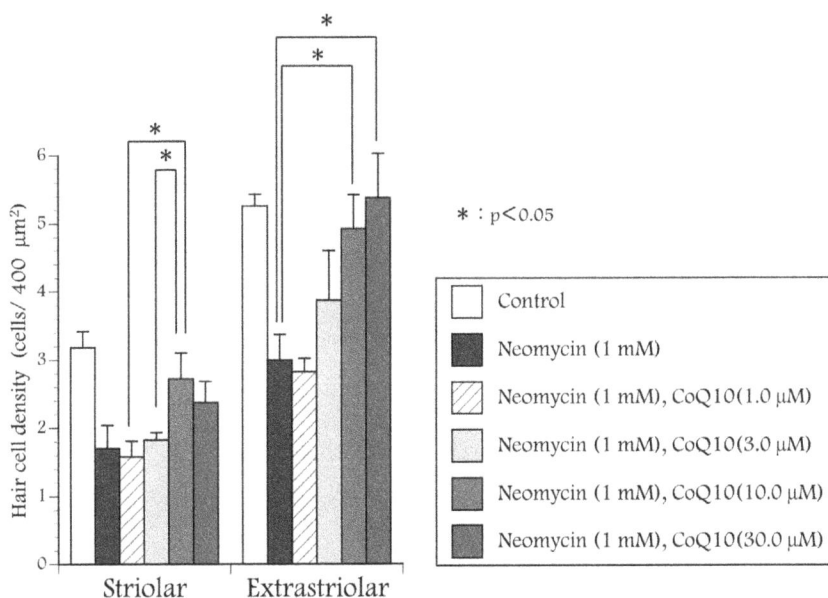

Figure 2. Relationship between the concentration of coenzyme Q10 and neomycin. The density of surviving hair cells was significantly higher in utricles treated with 10 μM and 30 μM of coenzyme Q10 and neomycin than in those treated with only 1 mM of neomycin. The protective effect of coenzyme Q10 was shown to be concentration-dependent; *: $p < 0.05$.

| Neomycin | - | 1 mM | 1 mM |
| CoenzymeQ10 | ~ | ~ | 30 μM |

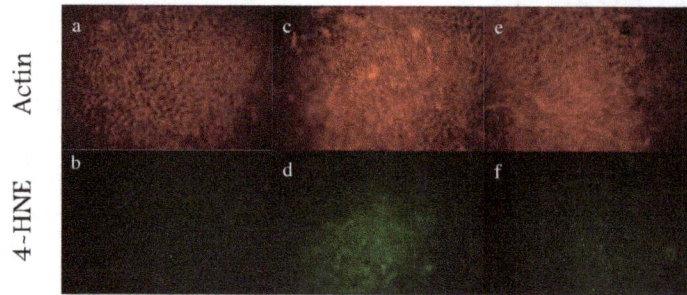

Figure 3. Inhibition of the production of 4-HNE in hair cells. Utricles were cultured for 12 h without neomycin (a, b), with neomycin (c, d), or with both neomycin and coenzyme Q10 (e, f). The hair cell layer was identified using Texas Red-conjugated phalloidin (red). 4-HNE was labeled using a specific antibody (green). Signals of 4-HNE were seen in utricle hair cells 12 h after exposure to neomycin. These 4-HNE signals were strongly inhibited by coenzyme Q10 treatment.

CoQ10 was developed to improve absorption of CoQ10. Water-soluble CoQ10 showed higher uptake when administered in a fasting state or with food compared to lipid-soluble CoQ10 in a rat and human study [3,13]. Fentoni et al. has reported the protective effect of another water-soluble CoQ10 in vivo experiments [14]. The water-soluble type of CoQ10 can be the tool for the treatment for inner ear diseases with hair cell damage.

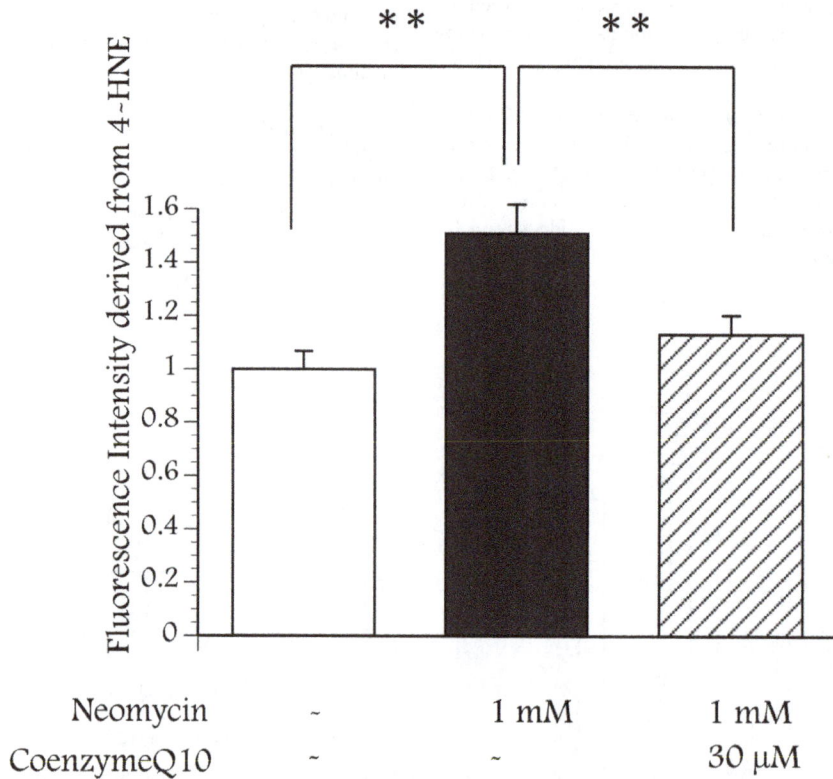

| Neomycin | ~ | 1 mM | 1 mM |
| CoenzymeQ10 | ~ | ~ | 30 μM |

$* * : p < 0.01$

Figure 4. Fluorescence Intensity derived from 4-HNE. Fluorescence intensity of the immunohistochemistry was evaluated with the image analysis software: ImageJ. The fluorescence intensity derived from 4-HNE was significantly stronger in the utricles cultured with neomycin than without neomycin. The existance of coenzyme Q10 can inhibit the fluorescence intensity.

Conclusion

In the present study performed using cultured mice utricles, water-soluble CoQ10 protected sensory hair cells against neomycin-induced death in the mammalian vestibular epithelium. These results show that CoQ10 may be useful as a protective drug in the inner ear.

References

1. Duckert LG, Rubel EW (1993) Morphological correlates of functional recovery in the chicken inner ear after gentamycin treatment. J Comp Neurol 331: 75–96.
2. Hirose Y, Sugahara K, Mikuriya T, Hashimoto M, Shimogori H, et al. (2008) Effect of water-soluble coenzyme Q10 on noise-induced hearing loss in guinea pigs. Acta Otolaryngol 128: 1071–1076.
3. Nukui K, Yamagishi T, Miyawaki H, Kettawan A, Okamoto T, et al. (2007) Comparison of uptake between PureSorb-Q40 and regular hydrophobic coenzyme Q10 in rats and humans after single oral intake. J Nutr Sci Vitaminol (Tokyo) 53: 187–190.
4. Ryals B, Westbrook E, Schacht J (1997) Morphological evidence of ototoxicity of the iron chelator deferoxamine. Hear Res 112: 44–48.
5. Kopke R, Allen KA, Henderson D, Hoffer M, Frenz D, et al. (1999) A radical demise. Toxins and trauma share common pathways in hair cell death. Ann N Y Acad Sci 884: 171–191.
6. Wu W-J, Sha S-H, Schacht J (2002) Recent advances in understanding aminoglycoside ototoxicity and its prevention. Audiol Neurootol 7: 171–174.
7. Matsui JI, Haque A, Huss D, Messana EP, Alosi JA, et al. (2003) Caspase inhibitors promote vestibular hair cell survival and function after aminoglycoside treatment in vivo. J Neurosci 23: 6111–6122.
8. Yamasoba T, Schacht J, Shoji F, Miller JM (1999) Attenuation of cochlear damage from noise trauma by an iron chelator, a free radical scavenger and glial cell line-derived neurotrophic factor in vivo. Brain Res 815: 317–325.
9. Sato K (1988) Pharmacokinetics of coenzyme Q10 in recovery of acute sensorineural hearing loss due to hypoxia. Acta Otolaryngol Suppl 458: 95–102.
10. Sergi B, Fetoni AR, Paludetti G, Ferraresi A, Navarra P, et al. (2006) Protective properties of idebenone in noise-induced hearing loss in the guinea pig. Neuroreport 17: 857–861.
11. Shults CW, Oakes D, Kieburtz K, Beal MF, Haas R, et al. (2002) Effects of coenzyme Q10 in early Parkinson disease: evidence of slowing of the functional decline. Arch Neurol 59: 1541–1550.
12. Suzuki S, Hinokio Y, Ohtomo M, Hirai M, Hirai A, et al. (1998) The effects of coenzyme Q10 treatment on maternally inherited diabetes mellitus and deafness, and mitochondrial DNA 3243 (A to G) mutation. Diabetologia 41: 584–588.
13. Nukui K, Yamagishi T, Miyawaki H, Kettawan A, Okamoto T, et al. (2008) Blood CoQ10 levels and safety profile after single-dose or chronic administration of PureSorb-Q40: animal and human studies. Biofactors 32: 209–219.
14. Fetoni AR, Eramo SLM, Rolesi R, Troiani D, Paludetti G (2012) Antioxidant treatment with coenzyme Q-ter in prevention of gentamycin ototoxicity in an animal model. Acta Otorhinolaryngol Ital 32: 103–110.

Acknowledgments

We would like to thank Dr. Akira Nakai for his valuable suggestions for the organ culture.

Author Contributions

Conceived and designed the experiments: KS YH TM MH HY. Performed the experiments: KS YH. Analyzed the data: KS EK HH HS. Contributed reagents/materials/analysis tools: KS MH HH. Wrote the paper: KS.

23

Diapocynin, a Dimer of the NADPH Oxidase Inhibitor Apocynin, Reduces ROS Production and Prevents Force Loss in Eccentrically Contracting Dystrophic Muscle

Hesham M. Ismail, Leonardo Scapozza, Urs T. Ruegg*, Olivier M. Dorchies

School of Pharmaceutical Sciences, University of Geneva and University of Lausanne, Geneva, Switzerland

Abstract

Elevation of intracellular Ca^{2+}, excessive ROS production and increased phospholipase A_2 activity contribute to the pathology in dystrophin-deficient muscle. Moreover, Ca^{2+}, ROS and phospholipase A_2, in particular $iPLA_2$, are thought to potentiate each other in positive feedback loops. NADPH oxidases (NOX) have been considered as a major source of ROS in muscle and have been reported to be overexpressed in muscles of mdx mice. We report here on our investigations regarding the effect of diapocynin, a dimer of the commonly used NOX inhibitor apocynin, on the activity of $iPLA_2$, Ca^{2+} handling and ROS generation in dystrophic myotubes. We also examined the effects of diapocynin on force production and recovery ability of isolated EDL muscles exposed to eccentric contractions *in vitro*, a damaging procedure to which dystrophic muscle is extremely sensitive. In dystrophic myotubes, diapocynin inhibited ROS production, abolished $iPLA_2$ activity and reduced Ca^{2+} influx through stretch-activated and store-operated channels, two major pathways responsible for excessive Ca^{2+} entry in dystrophic muscle. Diapocynin also prevented force loss induced by eccentric contractions of mdx muscle close to the value of wild-type muscle and reduced membrane damage as seen by Procion orange dye uptake. These findings support the central role played by NOX-ROS in the pathogenic cascade leading to muscular dystrophy and suggest diapocynin as an effective NOX inhibitor that might be helpful for future therapeutic approaches.

Editor: James M. Ervasti, University of Minnesota, United States of America

Funding: This work was supported by grants from the Swiss National Science Foundation number 3100A0 109981 (http://www.snf.ch/E/Pages/default.aspx), the Association Française contre les myopathies number 15093 and 15558 (AFM, France, http://www.afm-telethon.fr/), the Duchenne Parent Project-The Netherlands number DPPnl 2010–2012 (DPP-NL, http://www.duchenne.nl/) and the Parent Project Muscular Dystrophy number 329(PPMD, USA, http://www.parentprojectmd.org/site/PageServer?pagename=nws_inde. The funders had no role in study design, data collection and analysis, decision to publish, or preparation of the manuscript.

Competing Interests: The authors have declared that no competing interests exist.

* Email: urs.ruegg@unige.ch

Introduction

Duchenne muscular dystrophy (DMD) is a very severe muscle disease characterized by progressive skeletal muscle wasting. It is provoked by mutations in the gene encoding the protein dystrophin, leading to its absence in skeletal muscles of DMD patients [1], causing loss of the dystrophin-glycoprotein complex and improper mechano-transduction. Dystrophin-deficient myofibers are more susceptible to contraction-induced injury, leading to necrosis, muscle wasting and premature death [2].

There are numerous consequences of the absence of dystrophin on cellular signalling affecting muscle function and homeostasis of the myofiber. Of primary concern is the upregulated influx of Ca^{2+} through channels and transient breaks in the membrane [3]. Indeed, a number of studies have reported chronic elevation in intracellular Ca^{2+} concentrations in skeletal muscle fibers or in cultured myotubes from DMD patients and mdx mice, a mouse model for DMD. Stretch-activated channels (SACs) and store-operated channels (SOCs) are considered as candidates for mediating such an influx [4]. Another consequence of the lack of dystrophin is increased activity of the calcium-independent isoform of phospholipase A_2 ($iPLA_2$), observed in biopsies from DMD patients [5] and mdx mice [6]. This enzyme has been reported to activate SOCs and SACs as evidenced by $iPLA_2$ inhibition [7].

Another downstream consequence of the lack of dystrophin is increased reactive oxygen species (ROS) production. Markers of oxidative stress and lipid peroxidation are elevated in dystrophic muscles, even before the first symptoms of the disease appear (reviewed in Tidball and Wehling-Henricks [8]). Furthermore, ROS have been proposed as possible mediators of dystrophic muscle damage as they can activate several Ca^{2+} channels and promote lipid peroxidation, resulting in sarcolemmal fragility and subsequent Ca^{2+} influx through micro-ruptures, seen in dystrophic muscle [3]. In fact, reciprocal amplification of Ca^{2+} influx and ROS production results in a vicious cycle that appears to be central in the dystrophic pathology [9,10]. Several studies over the past decade were conducted in mdx mice to evaluate the effectiveness of anti-oxidants in ameliorating the pathological process, all of which showed benefit on selected parameters [10–14]. On the other hand, clinical trials conducted with anti-oxidants did not show an improvement and some even resulted in deterioration of the condition, which was attributed to lack of selectivity of the chosen anti-oxidant interventions against a defined target [15].

For a long time, mitochondria have been considered the main source of ROS in skeletal muscle during exercise. NADPH oxidases (NOXes), lipoxygenases, monoamine oxidase and xanthine oxidase have been proposed as other relevant sources of ROS in muscle cells (reviewed in [16]). It was recently shown that NOXes contribute to ROS production in skeletal muscle to a larger extent than mitochondria [9,17,18], which makes NOXes attractive targets to treat DMD.

The NOX family members are transmembrane proteins that transport electrons across biological membranes to reduce oxygen to superoxide or H_2O_2 [19]. Total mRNA from skeletal muscle contains NOX4 and NOX2. NOX4 is a constitutively active monomeric enzyme, whereas NOX2 requires the translocation of several regulatory subunits (p22^{phox}, p47^{phox} and p67^{phox}) to the membrane-spanning subunit gp91^{phox} to be active [19]. NOX2 and all of its subunits, except p22, are overexpressed in skeletal muscles from 19-day old mdx mice, just before the onset of necrosis, suggesting an early involvement of NOX in the pathology seen in DMD [20]. Another study showed that NOX4 mRNA is increased 5-fold in the left ventricles from 9–10 months old mdx mice [21].

In view of the importance of NOXes in various pathologies, a search for potent, efficacious, selective and non-toxic NOX inhibitors has been started. Several classes of compounds such as pyrazolopyridine, pyrazolopyrimidine, triazolopyrimidine, tetrahydroindole, and fulvalene analogues have been shown to inhibit NOX activity (for a review see Kim *et al.* [22]), and the synthetic peptide gp91ds-*tat* has also been shown to potently inhibit NOX2 [23]. However, the most commonly used experimental NOX inhibitor to date is apocynin. Apocynin was found to inhibit ROS production by NOXes in phagocytic cells, whereas it failed to do so and even promoted ROS production in non-phagocytic cells [24]. One explanation for this discrepancy is that phagocytic cells efficiently convert inactive apocynin monomers into active diapocynin through a peroxidase-mediated dimerization that is not operating in other cell types [24–26].

In the current study, we synthetized diapocynin and evaluated its effect on key mediators in the pathogenesis of DMD, namely ROS production, iPLA$_2$ activity and Ca^{2+} influx through SOC and SAC in dystrophic skeletal muscle cells. We also investigated its effect on force loss induced by eccentric contractions of isolated dystrophic fast twitch muscles. Not only did diapocynin inhibit ROS production in dystrophic myotubes, but also iPLA$_2$ activity and Ca^{2+} influx. In addition, it reduced force loss induced by eccentric contractions to near-control values.

Materials and Methods

Pharmacological treatments

The present investigations used a combination of pharmacological, cell biological and functional assays. In preliminary experiments, diapocynin showed significant alterations of the readouts at concentrations of 100 and 300 µM and were selected for further evaluations. For comparative purposes, apocynin was tested at a concentration 300 µM. The other compounds (BEL, BTP2, colchicine, DPI, GsMTx-4, streptomycin) were used at concentrations commonly reported in previous investigations in the field. These concentrations are around 3–10 times their IC$_{50}$ at the targets in order to ensure maximal inhibitory effects [20,27–29].

Diapocynin synthesis and characterization

Diapocynin was synthetized from apocynin (Sigma, Buchs, Switzerland) through an oxidative coupling reaction in the presence of ferrous sulfate and sodium persulfate as described [30]. The brown precipitate formed after this reaction was dissolved in 3N ammonia, re-crystallized in 6N HCl and washed 3 times with boiling water to yield pure diapocynin, as verified by NMR and mass spectrometry.

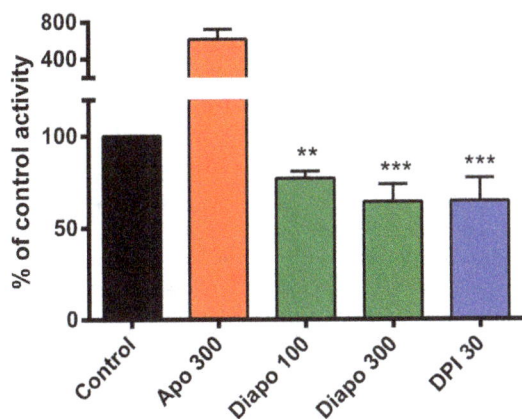

Figure 1. Diapocynin inhibits ROS production in dystrophic myotubes. ROS production in cultured dystrophic myotubes was monitored using DCFH-DA. Fluorescence increments over a period of 20 minutes were quantified in the presence of vehicle or test compounds. Diapocynin (Diapo) caused a concentration-dependent inhibition of ROS production amounting to about 40% at 300 µM, whereas apocynin (Apo) led to a 6-fold increase of fluorescence. The broad flavo-enzyme inhibitor, DPI, commonly used as NOX inhibitor, caused a similar inhibition as 300 µM diapocynin. Concentrations shown on the graph are in µM. ** $P \leq 0.01$, *** $P \leq 0.001$ compared to untreated mdx control (n = 3−7).

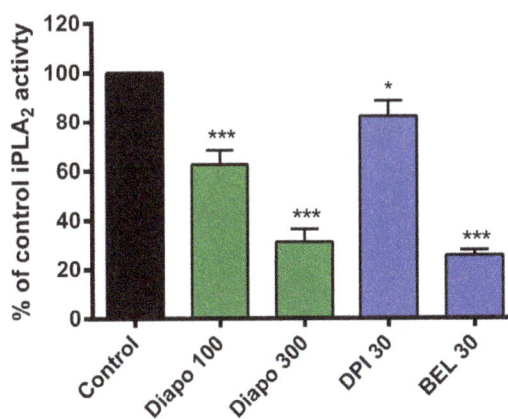

Figure 2. Diapocynin displays potent inhibition of iPLA$_2$ in dystrophic myotubes. PED-6 was used as a probe to monitor iPLA$_2$ activity in myotubes. Cellular phospholipases cleave this probe to release the fluorescent BODIPY; the rate of formation of this moiety was monitored for 20 minutes. Experiments were performed in the absence of extracellular Ca^{2+} in order to facilitate the activity of iPLA$_2$ over other phospholipase isoforms. Diapocynin (Diapo) potently inhibited the iPLA$_2$ signal to levels similar to those of the suicide inhibitor, BEL. Note the absence of significant inhibition with DPI. Concentrations shown on the graph are in µM. * $P \leq 0.05$, *** $P \leq 0.001$ compared to untreated mdx control (n = 3−8).

Cell culture

Myotubes were prepared from EDL-MDX-2 myoblasts co-cultured on a feeder layer of 10T½ fibroblasts as described previously [29,31]. Briefly, EDL-MDX-2 and 10T½ were propagated on collagen-treated and on uncoated Petri dishes (Falcon, Becton Dickinson), respectively, in high-mitogen containing proliferation media. Cells were detached with trypsin and suspensions containing 80,000 EDL-MDX-2 myoblasts and 60,000 mitomycin C-inactivated 10T½ fibroblasts per ml were seeded in 24-well plates coated with 1 μg/cm^2 Matrigel (Becton Dickinson), 0.5 ml per well. After 2 days, myotube formation was induced by changing the proliferation medium to a low-mitogen containing differentiation medium. After 3–4 days contracting myotubes were obtained.

Determination of ROS production

ROS production was measured using 2′,7′-dichlorohydrofluorescein-diacetate (DCFH-DA, Invitrogen, Zug, Switzerland), a probe that readily enters cells, which, upon de-acetylation by cellular esterases reacts with a variety of reactive oxygen/nitrogen species to yield fluorescent 2′,7′-dichlorofluorescein (DCF). To perform these experiments, myotube cultures were washed twice with Ca^{2+}-free physiological salt solution (PSS−; composition in mM: HEPES 5, KCl 5, MgCl$_2$ 1, NaCl 145, glucose 10, EGTA 0.2) and incubated with 20 μM of DCFH-DA for 1 h to allow sufficient loading of the cells. Subsequently, compounds to be tested were added and the development of the fluorescent signal was monitored with a FLUOStar Galaxy fluorimeter (BMG Laboratories, Offenburg, Germany) as described [6].

Determination of PLA$_2$ activity

PLA$_2$ activity was measured using the probe PED-6 (Invitrogen), which is cleaved by PLA$_2$ to release BODIPY, a green fluorescent compound. Briefly, EDL-MDX-2 myotube cultures were washed twice with PSS− and incubated with test compounds

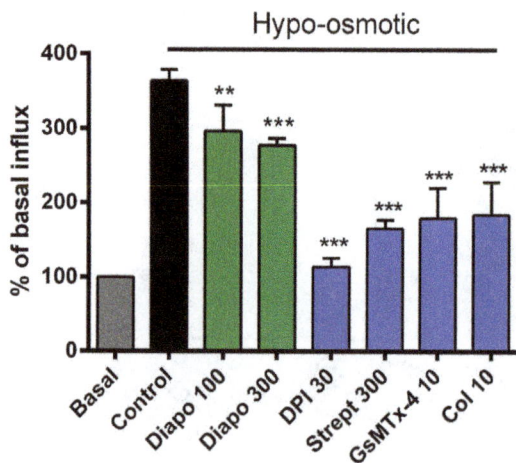

Figure 3. Modulation of hypo-osmotic shock induced Ca^{2+}-influx in dystrophic myotubes. Exposing myotubes to a hypotonic PSS containing 1 μCi ^{45}Ca^{2+} induced a 3.7-fold increase in ^{45}Ca^{2+}-influx compared to isotonic PSS. Diapocynin (Diapo) treatment resulted in a 30% inhibition of the stimulated influx, whereas DPI caused an inhibition to control levels. The SAC blockers, streptomycin (Strept) and Grammatoxin (GsMTx-4), or the microtubule disruptor, colchicine (Col), caused a similar inhibition of about 70%. Concentrations shown on the graph are in μM. ** $P \leq 0.01$, *** $P \leq 0.001$ compared to untreated mdx control (n = 4–7).

for 20 min. Subsequently, PED-6 (1 μM) was added and the fluorescence increment was measured over a period of 30 min at 37°C as described [32].

^{45}Ca^{2+} influx triggered by store depletion and hypo-osmotic shock

^{45}Ca^{2+} uptake was quantified as described by Ismail et al. [29]. To measure the activity of SACs, myotube cultures were washed twice with PSS containing 1.2 mM Ca^{2+} (PSS+), pre-incubated at 37°C for 15 min with test compounds and then exposed for 5 min to 200 μl/well of a hypo-osmotic PSS+ (100 mOsm obtained by decreasing the NaCl concentration from 145 to 25 mM) containing 1 μCi/ml of ^{45}Ca^{2+}. Plates were then placed on ice, and cultures were washed 4 times with ice-cold PSS− to remove remaining extracellular ^{45}Ca^{2+} before being lysed with 0.5 ml of 1N NaOH. The radioactivity in the lysates was determined by scintillation counting (Ultima Gold, Packard, Groningen, NL) using a beta-counter (LKB Wallac 1217 Rackbeta, Turku, Finland).

To study the activity of SOCs, the cultures were washed twice with PSS+, pre-incubated for 15 min at 37°C with test compounds in 200 μl Ca^{2+}-free PSS, and further exposed to 5 μM thapsigargin to deplete intracellular Ca^{2+} stores, in the presence of test compounds. After 10 min, PSS+ containing 1 μCi/ml ^{45}Ca^{2+} was added and uptake was measured after another 10 min. ^{45}Ca^{2+} was quantified as above.

Isolated muscle experiments

To evaluate whether diapocynin modulates force loss in eccentrically contracting muscles, a method described earlier [29] was used. Dystrophic (mdx^{5Cv}) and wild type (C57BL/6J) mice were maintained in the animal facility of the Geneva-Lausanne School of Pharmaceutical Sciences and used in compliance with the local rules on animal experimentation and welfare (Authorization #106/3626/0 delivered by the Cantonal Veterinary Office of Geneva and approved by the Swiss Veterinary Office). Mice between 8 and 12 weeks of age were anesthetized, the *extensor digitorum longus* (EDL) muscles were exposed, and their proximal and distal tendons were tied with silk sutures. Then, EDL muscles were excised and transferred to a 10 ml horizontal chamber of a muscle-testing device designed for delivering eccentric contractions (model 305C-LR, Aurora Scientific Inc., Ontario, Canada). The muscle chamber was filled with a physiological Ringer solution (composition in mM: NaCl 137, NaHCO$_3$ 24, glucose 11, KCl 5, CaCl$_2$ 2, MgSO$_4$ 1, NaH$_2$PO$_4$ 1, pH 7.4) that contained 25 μM D-tubocurarine and was continuously bubbled with 95% O$_2$-5% CO$_2$. Muscles were stimulated by 0.2 ms square wave pulses generated by a Grass S88X stimulator (Grass Technologies, West Warwick, RI, USA), delivered via platinum electrodes on both sides of the muscles. The optimum stimulating voltage and optimal muscle length (L_0) were set and muscles were exposed to 10 contractions of 400 ms each at 100 Hz, 30 s apart. One hundred and fifty ms after the initiation of each contraction, muscles were stretched by 9% of L_0 over a period of 100 ms at a speed of 0.9 L_0/s and maintained at that level for another 100 ms before returning to the original length. Force loss during the eccentric contraction procedure as well as recovery after 20 min of rest were expressed for every muscle. Test compounds or vehicle were added to the bath 20 min before initiation of the contraction protocol.

In experiments designed to assess membrane permeability, Procion orange (0.2%, w/v) was added to the bath 5 min before the eccentric contraction procedure. After performing the full protocol described above, muscles were briefly washed twice in

Ringer solution, blotted, quickly embedded in 5% Tragacanth gum and snap frozen in isopentane cooled in liquid nitrogen. Twenty µm thick sections were cut around the mid-belly of each muscle, fixed in acetone at −20°C, and incubated with wheat germ agglutinin conjugated to AlexaFluor 488 (WGA-AF$_{488}$, Invitrogen), 1 µg/ml in PBS for 1 hour as described to label the extracellular matrix [33]. The amount of Procion orange positive fibers was expressed as a percentage of the total number of fibers, determined from the WGA-AF$_{488}$ counterstain.

Data presentation and statistical analyses

Results are reported as mean ± S.E.M. Statistical differences between groups were assessed by 1-way ANOVA followed by Fisher LSD multiple comparison post-tests using the GraphPad Prism software, version 6. Differences were considered significant at values of $P \le 0.05$. For consistency, all the graphs show the untreated dystrophic and wild-type values as black and light grey columns, respectively. Values obtained with diapocynin, apocynin and blockers of specific pathways appear in green, red and blue, respectively.

Results

Diapocynin but not apocynin inhibits ROS production in dystrophic myotubes

Treating EDL-MDX-2 myotubes with 100 or 300 µM of diapocynin resulted in a reduction of the total ROS produced. Diapocynin at 300 µM reduced ROS by 36.9±9.6%, a value that was indistinguishable from that of DPI, a potent non-selective NOX inhibitor (Figure 1). By contrast, apocynin caused a 6-fold increase of ROS production.

Diapocynin but not DPI potently inhibits iPLA$_2$ in dystrophic myotubes

In order to minimize the contribution of Ca^{2+}-dependent isoforms of PLA$_2$, measurements were made on EDL-MDX-2 myotubes in a Ca^{2+}-free buffer (PSS−). Diapocynin treatment resulted in an inhibition of the PED-6 signal, amounting to 31.2±5.25% of the control values at 100 µM (Figure 2). At 300 µM, the inhibition reached a level of about 75%, similar to that obtained by 30 µM BEL, a specific iPLA$_2$ inhibitor. Interestingly, DPI failed to show a similarly extensive inhibition of PLA$_2$ (Figure 2).

Diapocynin affects ^{45}Ca^{2+} influx through SAC and SOC

Due to the central role of Ca^{2+} influx in the pathology in DMD, we evaluated the effect of diapocynin on Ca^{2+} influx through SAC and SOC. Treating the myotubes with 100 or 300 µM of diapocynin resulted in a small but significant inhibition of SAC influx with a value of 25.6±12.9% and 32.8±3.6% of control values, respectively (Figure 3). DPI, however, led to an almost complete inhibition of the influx. The classical SAC inhibitors, streptomycin and grammatoxin (GsMTx-4, a peptide isolated from the venom of the tarantula spider *Grammostola spatulata*), as well as the microtubule disruptor, colchicine, inhibited about 70% of the SAC influx (Figure 3).

When SOC influx was studied using thapsigargin, similar patterns of inhibition were observed with the test compounds. Diapocynin at 300 µM inhibited about 34% of the induced influx whereas DPI inhibited it to a level of un-stimulated cells (Figure 4). Similarly, a reference SOC blocker, BTP2, and the iPLA$_2$ inhibitor, BEL, efficaciously blocked the induced influx down to basal levels (Figure 4).

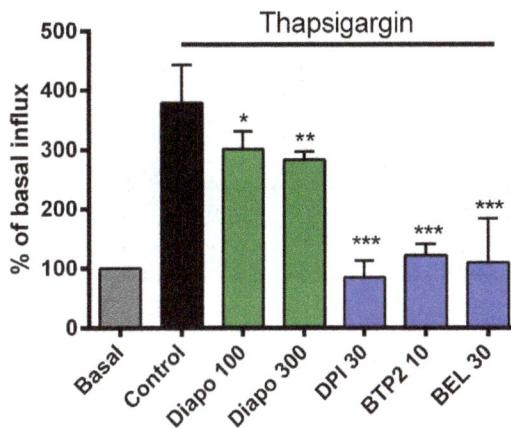

Figure 4. Modulation of Ca^{2+} influx in dystrophic myotubes induced by store-depletion. Thapsigargin (5 µM) treatment was used to deplete the sarcoplasmic Ca^{2+} stores leading to activation of SOC influx. Re-addition of ^{45}Ca^{2+}-containing buffer resulted in an almost 4-fold increase in ^{45}Ca^{2+}-influx compared to non-treated cells. Diapocynin (Diapo) treatment had a small effect, whereas DPI showed a complete inhibition, similar to the one observed with BTP2, a commonly used SOC blocker, or BEL. Concentrations shown on the graph are in µM. * $P \le 0.05$, ** $P \le 0.01$, *** $P \le 0.001$ compared to untreated mdx control (n = 3−10).

Diapocynin prevents eccentric contraction-induced damage

Exposing dystrophic EDL muscles to 10 repeated eccentric contractions resulted in a greater force loss compared to their wild-type counterparts. Incubation of the muscles with 300 µM of diapocynin prior to the contractions prevented force loss to near wild-type levels (Figure 5A). However, such a protective effect was not observed in the groups treated with streptomycin, as judged immediately after the last eccentric contraction.

Then muscles were allowed to recover from the damaging protocol for 20 minutes and the force was measured subsequently. Again, wild-type muscles recovered almost two times better than dystrophic ones: the force recovered was about 15% of pre-exercise values (Figure 5B). Streptomycin-treated muscles displayed a striking recovery compared to dystrophic and wild-type controls while it failed to prevent force loss during the active phase of the assay (Figure 5B).

To investigate sarcolemmal integrity after damaging contractions, experiments were performed in the presence of the vital dye Procion orange, which was equilibrated into the buffer 5 min before the initiation of the contraction protocol and kept till the end of the recovery phase. Exposing dystrophic EDL muscles to 10 eccentric contractions resulted in a 2-fold increased dye uptake compared to wild-type muscles (Figure 6). Diapocynin reduced this uptake to the value of non-dystrophic muscle, whereas apocynin had no significant effect. The SAC blocker, streptomycin, also had a protective effect, probably by rendering the sarcolemma more resilient to stretch-induced damage (Figure 6).

Discussion

Our study demonstrates the ability of diapocynin, but not of apocynin, to inhibit ROS production in skeletal muscle cells. We also show that diapocynin inhibits iPLA$_2$, reduces Ca^{2+} influx through SOC and SAC and protects muscle from eccentric contraction-induced force loss.

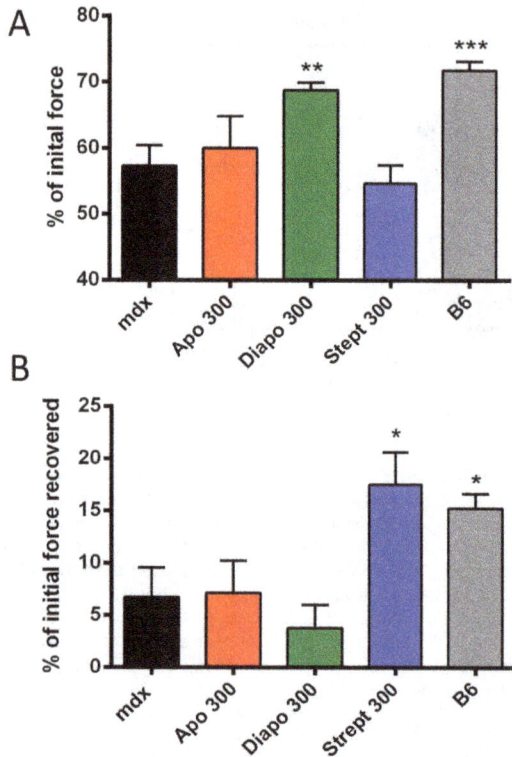

Figure 5. Diapocynin abrogates force loss in eccentrically contracted EDL muscles whereas streptomycin promotes the recovery of force loss after a period of rest. EDL muscles from wild-type (B6) and dystrophic mice were exposed to 10 eccentric contractions at 100 Hz lasting 400 ms during which they were stretched to a value of 109% of their optimal length. (A) Remaining force after 10 eccentric contractions. Note the increased force loss in dystrophic muscle (mdx) compared to wild type (B6) muscle. Of the tested compounds, only diapocynin (Diapo) abrogated the force loss seen in this assay while apocynin (Apo) failed to show such an effect. (B) Force recovered after 20 minutes of rest. Streptomycin (Strept) caused a marked recovery exceeding the one of wild-type muscles. Concentrations shown on the graph are in μM. * $P \leq 0.05$, ** $P \leq 0.01$ compared to untreated mdx control (n = 4–9).

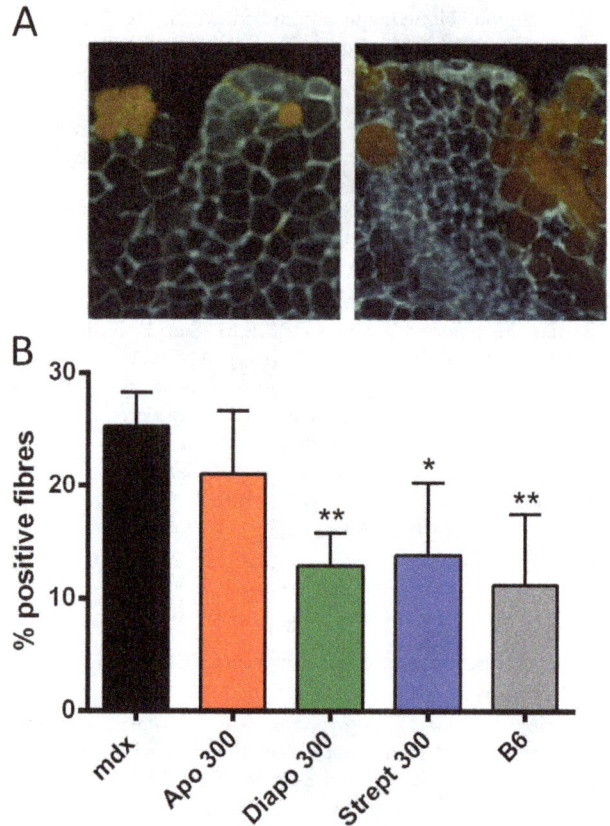

Figure 6. Protection of sarcolemmal integrity by diapocynin in eccentrically contracted EDL muscles. Procion orange is a membrane-impermeable dye that enters only cells with damaged membranes. In this assay, EDL muscles were exposed to 10 eccentric contractions in physiological buffer containing 0.2% Procion orange. Muscles were subsequently rinsed twice in physiological buffer and embedded in tragacanth gum. Twenty micrometer thick sections were made around the mid-belly region of the muscles and the percentage of Procion orange-positive fibers were quantified. Representative section of wild type (A, left) and dystrophic (A, right) EDL muscles exposed to eccentric contractions in the presence of Procion orange. (B) Quantification of Procion orange-positive fibers in the experimental groups. Dystrophic muscle (mdx) displayed a 2-fold increase in dye uptake as compared to wild-type muscle (B6). Diapocynin (Diapo) or streptomycin (Strept) treatment protected the muscle from increased membrane damage, thus lowering the values of the stained fibers down to those of the non-dystrophic controls. Apocynin (Apo) did not offer a protection in this assay. Concentrations shown on the graph are in μM. * $P \leq 0.05$, ** $P \leq 0.01$ compared to untreated mdx control (n = 4–8).

There is a lack of selective, non-toxic NOX inhibitors, the best known being apocynin. It was first isolated by Schmiedeberg in 1883 from the roots of *Apocynum cannabinum*, but it was only in the 1990's that apocynin was found to inhibit NOX-dependent ROS production (for a review see [34]). Apocynin's ability to reduce NOX-mediated ROS generation results from both altered translocation of regulatory subunits to the membranes and prevention of their proper assembly with the transmembrane core protein gp91^{phox} [35]. This inhibition was observed only in activated phagocytic cells but was completely lacking in other cell types and even had a ROS-promoting effect in non-phagocytic cells [24]. In attempts to explain these findings, apocynin was proposed to act as a pro-drug undergoing two different metabolic pathways, namely oxidative dimerization by myeloperoxidases in activated phagocytic cells to form diapocynin, which is thought to be the active moiety inhibiting the enzyme [26,36], or generation of a transient pro-oxidant apocynin radical that can subsequently oxidize sensitive sulfhydryl groups of NOXes [37]. Diapocynin was found to be superior to apocynin in inhibiting not only NOX activity acutely [36], but also gp91^{phox} expression, TNF-α and IL-

10 production in response to LPS challenge in non-phagocytic cells following a 24 hours incubation [25].

Diapocynin inhibited ROS production in skeletal muscle myotubes whereas apocynin showed a 6-fold increase in ROS output (Figure 1). This finding is in accordance with a report on non-phagocytic cells [24]. The pro-oxidant activity of apocynin depends on its prior oxidation to transient free radicals, such as apocynin radicals [37]. Such radicals have been reported to cause a 7-fold increase in glutathione oxidation and an even 100-fold increase in NADPH oxidation [38]. These results reinforce previous reports that diapocynin is the active species inhibiting NOX and that apocynin primarily serves as pro-drug of its oxidized dimer [36].

Both diapocynin and DPI inhibited ROS production in our cellular model to a similar extent (Figure 1). DPI is not a selective NOX inhibitor but a wide-spectrum flavo-enzyme inhibitor causing also inhibition of CytP450, nitric oxide synthases and xanthine oxidase [39]. The similar extent of inhibition of ROS production exhibited by DPI and diapocynin in myotube cultures (about 40%) is consistent with the fact that NOXes are major ROS contributors in skeletal muscle tissue [17,18]. A docking model for apocynin and some of its analogues into the complex p67^{phox}-p47^{phox} was recently proposed and it was shown that diapocynin had the highest affinity score of all tested compounds [40]. This supports earlier reports that diapocynin and apocynin might have the same inhibitory mechanism on NOX, namely binding to p47^{phox}, thus preventing the assembly of the subunits required for NOX2 activity [36]. Whether diapocynin inhibits NOX4, which does not require translocation of subunits, remains to be investigated.

We have shown previously the involvement of iPLA$_2$ in modulating Ca^{2+} entry into dystrophic myotubes and fibers and that pharmacological inhibition of iPLA$_2$ blocks the enhanced Ca^{2+} entry [6,31]. Diapocynin treatment fully inhibited iPLA$_2$ in our dystrophic myotubes to levels indistinguishable from those elicited by the suicide iPLA$_2$ inhibitor BEL (Figure 2). Likely targets of diapocynin could be NOXes, located in close proximity of the sarcolemma. Their inhibition would lead not only to decreased superoxide anion radical (O$_2^{\bullet-}$) formation, but also to a lower production of lipid peroxides. Such peroxides are known to be superior substrates for iPLA$_2$ compared to native phospholipids [41]. Alternatively, a direct inhibition of iPLA$_2$ by diapocynin cannot be ruled out. One important consideration in the effect of diapocynin on its targets is lipophilicity. Diapocynin is 13 times more lipophilic than apocynin [42], enabling it to cross membranes freely. Such a characteristic can lead to membrane accumulation, which could bring the compound into close vicinity of its targets. By contrast, the lack of potent iPLA$_2$ inhibition by DPI might be attributed to its reduced ability to accumulate in biological membranes and therefore the lack of potent inhibitory action in this specific cellular compartment. Also, DPI is known to be a "dirty" compound, therefore, non-specific actions of DPI on other targets may ultimately mitigate the cellular response [43,44].

Diapocynin inhibited calcium influx through SAC to a lesser extent than the classical inhibitors, streptomycin and GsMTx-4 (Figure 3). In an elegant series of papers, Lederer, Ward and colleagues showed that membrane stretch activates NOXes to produce ROS, which subsequently activate SAC [28,45]. Diapocynin, through its ability to inhibit NOX2, would lead to the disruption of this cascade and eventually block cation influx through SAC. The same authors also proposed the microtubular network to convey the mechanical stretch to NOX and that colchicine, a microtubule disruptor, leads to the inhibition of SAC influx in dystrophic FDB fibres [28]. Our present results confirm these findings in dystrophic myotubes, as colchicine inhibited SAC influx to the same extent as streptomycin or GsMTx-4 (Figure 3).

SOC influx using thapsigargin as a trigger revealed that diapocynin partially inhibited this influx but this inhibition became significant only at 300 μM (Figure 4). This can be attributed to iPLA$_2$ inhibition, as evidenced by the inhibition of the influx by BEL and is in line with our previous report [46]. Of note, BEL does not only inhibit SOC as an iPLA$_2$ inhibitor, but might also inhibits directly several TRP channels, an effect that might contribute to its full blockade seen here, as well as previously, in our hands [47]. This can explain why BEL appeared to be more efficacious than diapocynin in preventing SOC-mediated Ca^{2+} influx in our hands.

DPI caused full inhibition of both SAC and SOC, exceeding the levels reached by the most selective inhibitors of the targeted channel types, namely GsMTx-4 and BTP2, respectively (Figures 3 and 4). This cannot be explained by the sole ability of DPI to inhibit flavo-enzymes, such as NOXes. In earlier work, in which patch-clamp techniques were used on isolated pulmonary smooth muscles, it was reported that DPI inhibited both Ca^{2+} and K$^+$ channels at concentrations of 3 and 10 μM, independent of its NOX modulating activity [43]. Since the concentrations used in this study are 3–10 times higher than those reported to have channel modulating activity, such an inhibition of channels might well play a role. To the best of our knowledge, this is the first report showing that DPI has such a potent inhibitory effect on Ca^{2+}-influx stimulated by membrane stretch and by internal store emptying. However, considering the effect of DPI on SAC and SOC influx, and its broad inhibitory profile on flavo-enzymes, we suggest that DPI should not be used as an experimental tool for blocking NOXes in a similar context.

Exposing isolated EDL muscles to 10 repeated eccentric contractions resulted in an increased force loss of dystrophic muscle compared to its wild-type counterpart. This has been first reported 20 years ago by Petrof et al., who also showed enhanced membrane disruption and dye uptake as a consequence of such contractions [48]. Numerous attempts were carried out to investigate the mechanisms causing this force loss, which led to the notion that the two major determinants involved are disruption of Ca^{2+} homeostasis and myofibrillar disorganization [49]. In line with an inhibition of increased Ca^{2+} influx, SAC blockers, such as streptomycin or GsMTx-4, or removal of extracellular Ca^{2+} have been shown to be beneficial in promoting force recovery following eccentric contractions [27,50]. Recently, ROS came into play as mediators carrying an essentially cytotoxic message, as evidenced by increased resistance to eccentric damage in mdx mice by N-acetylcysteine treatment or by transgenic overexpression of catalase [10,51]. A recent study has also shown that DPI decreased force loss induced by eccentric contractions in isolated FDB fibers [20]. In the current study, we show that diapocynin was the only compound investigated that abolished force loss occurring during eccentric contractions, whereas streptomycin failed to do so (Figure 5). However, when measured after 20 minutes of recovery, streptomycin-treated muscle recovered to an extent similar to the one of diapocynin. These results support earlier findings that both SAC and ROS contribute to the force loss induced by eccentric contractions in dystrophic muscles; however, their specific roles in the different stages of force loss and recovery might be different. In support to this, it has been convincingly proposed recently that ROS production by NOXes precedes SAC activation seen in stretching conditions [28,45]. This can explain our findings that diapocynin prevented force loss whereas streptomycin promoted the recovery after the contractions. Gervasio et al. showed that increased levels of pro-oxidants, such as H$_2$O$_2$, lead to autophosphorylation of Src kinase and subsequent activation of SAC and that the anti-oxidant tiron or the Src kinase inhibitor PP2 inhibited increased Ca^{2+} influx after eccentric contractions [52]. Another study showed that addition of SAC blockers just after eccentric contractions was sufficient to obtain a protective effect [50]. Taken together, these findings point towards increased ROS production in eccentrically contracting muscle having a dual role, the first one promoting force loss by increasing ROS above the levels that are required for optimal force production [53], and the second one activating Ca^{2+} influx through SAC, promoting membrane damage and finally enhancing dye uptake. NOX inhibitors would prevent the first step of the cascade while SAC blockers would inhibit the final step. This is

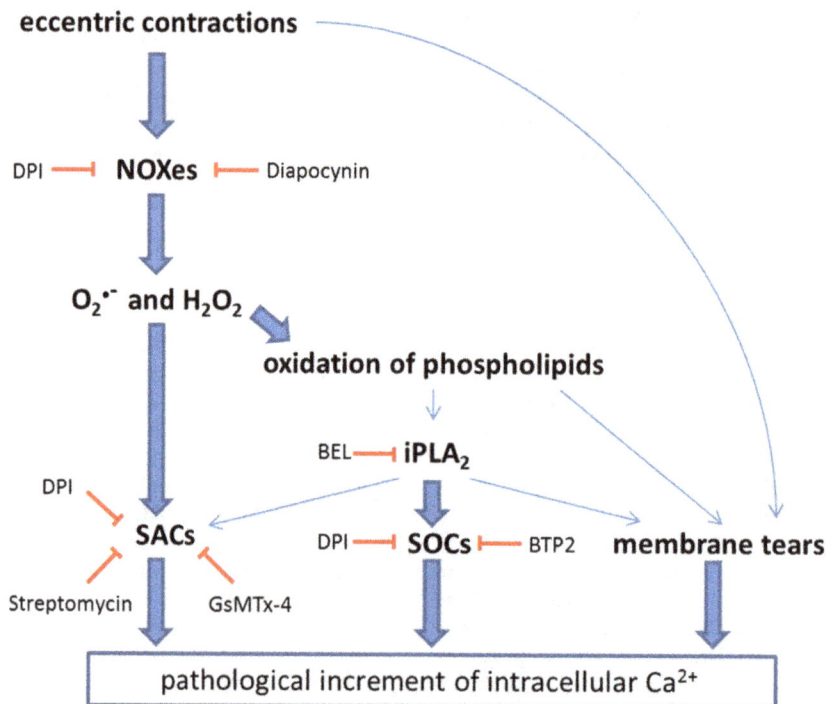

Figure 7. Proposal for the cascade implicated in the force loss in eccentrically contracting dystrophic muscles. The illustration shows a possible cascade of the events taking place in eccentrically contracting dystrophic muscle. Thick arrows highlight pathways reported to play a major role in muscle function, namely NOX-SACs, iPLA2-SOCs and membrane tears. Thin arrows point to suggested links between the main pathways involved. The blunted red arrows show the inhibitory effect of compounds used in the current study. The suggested cascade results in an elevation of intracellular Ca^{2+}, an event known to activate multiple downstream pathways playing a role in the dystrophic pathology.

illustrated in Figure 7. Our results with Procion orange dye uptake re-enforces these finding and shows that both diapocynin, and to a lesser extent streptomycin, protected the muscles form membrane damage induced by stretching contractions.

ROS contribute to normal cellular homeostasis and fine tuning of metabolic processes [54]. Many anti-oxidants tested so far in dystrophic mice are global ROS scavengers that do not discriminate between sources of ROS. Their ability to alter the cells' redox status instead of targeting a specific source of ROS might explain why such anti-oxidant therapies showed only limited improvement of the dystrophic condition. Targeting overactive NOXes with diapocynin might confer higher experimental and therapeutic potential compared to global anti-oxidants. In additions, a recent study showed that diapocynin has a good pharmacokinetic profile when administered orally and that such a treatment resulted in a neuroprotective effect in models of Parkinson's disease [55]. Another study revealed that diapocynin has a powerful anti-inflammatory activity independent of its ROS modulating capability [56]. Another consideration is the possibility that diapocynin act as a direct anti-oxidant through ROS

scavenging thanks to the presence of 2 phenolic groups [57–59]. Thus diapocynin would have a dual mechanism of action, both contributing to ROS reduction.

Altogether, our results and data by others suggest that diapocynin is a promising compound with potential for treating dystrophic muscle diseases and is worthy of further evaluation. Towards this goal we currently are performing an *in vivo* investigation of diapocynin in mdx mice.

Acknowledgments

We would like to thank Dr. Andreas Nievergelt and Prof. Muriel Cuendet for their help in diapocynin synthesis and purification.

Author Contributions

Conceived and designed the experiments: HI OMD. Performed the experiments: HI OMD. Analyzed the data: HI LS UR OMD. Contributed reagents/materials/analysis tools: LS UR. Wrote the paper: HI LS UR OMD.

References

1. Koenig M, Hoffman EP, Bertelson CJ, Monaco AP, Feener C, et al. (1987) Complete cloning of the Duchennne muscular dystrophy (DMD) cDNA and preliminary genomic organization of the DMD gene in normal and affected individuals. Cell 50: 509–517.

2. De Luca A (2012) Pre-clinical drug tests in the mdx mouse as a model of dystrophinopathies: an overview. Acta Myol 31: 40–47.

3. Hoffman EP, Dressman D (2001) Molecular pathophysiology and targeted therapeutics for muscular dystrophy. Trends Pharmacol Sci 22: 465–470.

4. Ducret T, Vandebrouck C, Cao ML, Lebacq J, Gailly P (2006) Functional role of store-operated and stretch-activated channels in murine adult skeletal muscle fibres. J Physiol 575: 913–924.

5. Lindahl M, Backman E, Henriksson KG, Gorospe JR, Hoffman EP (1995) Phospolipase A2 activity in dystrophinopathies. Neuromuscul Disord 5: 193–199.

6. Boittin FX, Petermann O, Hirn C, Mittaud P, Dorchies OM, et al. (2006) Ca^{2+}-independent phospholipase A2 enhances store-operated Ca^{2+} entry in dystrophic skeletal muscle fibers. J Cell Sci 119: 3733–3742.

7. Ruegg UT, Shapovalov G, Jacobson K, Reutenauer-Patte J, Ismail HM, et al. (2012) Store-operated channels and Ca^{2+} handling in muscular dystrophy. In: Groschner K, Graier WF, Romanin C, editors. Store-operated Ca^{2+} entry (SOCE) pathways: SpringerWien. 449–457.

8. Tidball JG, Wehling-Henricks M (2007) The role of free radicals in the pathophysiology of muscular dystrophy. J Appl Physiol 102: 1677–1686.

9. Shkryl VM, Martins AS, Ullrich ND, Nowycky MC, Niggli E, et al. (2009) Reciprocal amplification of ROS and Ca^{2+} signals in stressed mdx dystrophic skeletal muscle fibers. Pflugers Arch 458: 915–928.

10. Whitehead NP, Pham C, Gervasio OL, Allen DG (2008) N-Acetylcysteine ameliorates skeletal muscle pathophysiology in mdx mice. J Physiol 586: 2003–2014.

11. Dorchies OM, Wagner S, Vuadens O, Waldhauser K, Buetler TM, et al. (2006) Green tea extract and its major polyphenol (−)-epigallocatechin gallate improve muscle function in a mouse model for Duchenne muscular dystrophy. Am J Physiol-Cell Ph290: C616–C625.

12. Nakae Y, Dorchies OM, Stoward PJ, Zimmermann BF, Ritter C, et al. (2012) Quantitative evaluation of the beneficial effects in the mdx mouse of epigallocatechin gallate, an antioxidant polyphenol from green tea. Histochem Cell Biol 137: 811–827.

13. Hibaoui Y, Reutenauer-Patte J, Patthey-Vuadens O, Ruegg UT, Dorchies OM (2011) Melatonin improves muscle function of the dystrophic mdx5Cv mouse, a model for Duchenne muscular dystrophy. J Pineal Res 51: 163–171.

14. Buetler TM, Renard M, Offord EA, Schneider H, Ruegg UT (2002) Green tea extract decreases muscle necrosis in mdx mice and protects against reactive oxygen species. Am J Clin Nutr 75: 749–753.

15. Kim JH, Kwak HB, Thompson LV, Lawler JM (2013) Contribution of oxidative stress to pathology in diaphragm and limb muscles with Duchenne muscular dystrophy. J Muscle Res Cell M 34: 1–13.

16. Barbieri E, Sestili P (2012) Reactive oxygen species in skeletal muscle signaling. J Sig Transd 2012: 982794.

17. Xia R, Webb JA, Gnall LL, Cutler K, Abramson JJ (2003) Skeletal muscle sarcoplasmic reticulum contains a NADH-dependent oxidase that generates superoxide. Am J Physiol 285: C215–221.

18. Sakellariou GK, Vasilaki A, Palomero J, Kayani A, Zibrik L, et al. (2013) Studies of mitochondrial and nonmitochondrial sources implicate nicotinamide adenine dinucleotide phosphate oxidase(s) in the increased skeletal muscle superoxide generation that occurs during contractile activity. Antioxid Redox Sign 18: 603–621.

19. Bedard K, Krause KH (2007) The NOX family of ROS-generating NADPH oxidases: physiology and pathophysiology. Physiol Rev 87: 245–313.

20. Whitehead NP, Yeung EW, Froehner SC, Allen DG (2010) Skeletal muscle NADPH oxidase is increased and triggers stretch-induced damage in the mdx mouse. PLoS One 5: e15354.

21. Spurney CF, Knoblach S, Pistilli EE, Nagaraju K, Martin GR, et al. (2008) Dystrophin-deficient cardiomyopathy in mouse: expression of Nox4 and Lox are associated with fibrosis and altered functional parameters in the heart. Neuromuscul Disord 18: 371–381.

22. Kim JA, Neupane GP, Lee ES, Jeong BS, Park BC, et al. (2011) NADPH oxidase inhibitors: a patent review. Expert Opin Ther Pat 21: 1147–1158.

23. Rey FE, Cifuentes ME, Kiarash A, Quinn MT, Pagano PJ (2001) Novel competitive inhibitor of NAD(P)H oxidase assembly attenuates vascular O$_2^-$ and systolic blood pressure in mice. Circ Res 89: 408–414.

24. Vejrazka M, Micek R, Stipek S (2005) Apocynin inhibits NADPH oxidase in phagocytes but stimulates ROS production in non-phagocytic cells. Biochim Biophys Acta 1722: 143–147.

25. Kanegae MP, Condino-Neto A, Pedroza LA, de Almeida AC, Rehder J, et al. (2010) Diapocynin versus apocynin as pretranscriptional inhibitors of NADPH oxidase and cytokine production by peripheral blood mononuclear cells. Biochem Biophys Res Commun 393: 551–554.

26. Stefanska J, Pawliczak R (2008) Apocynin: molecular aptitudes. Mediators Inflamm 2008: 106507.

27. Whitehead NP, Streamer M, Lusambili LI, Sachs F, Allen DG (2006) Streptomycin reduces stretch-induced membrane permeability in muscles from mdx mice. Neuromuscul Disord 16: 845–854.

28. Khairallah RJ, Shi G, Sbrana F, Prosser BL, Borroto C, et al. (2012) Microtubules underlie dysfunction in duchenne muscular dystrophy. Sci Signal 5: ra56.

29. Ismail HM, Dorchies OM, Perozzo R, Strosova MK, Scapozza L, et al. (2013) Inhibition of iPLA$_2$beta and of stretch activated channels by doxorubicin alters dystrophic muscle function. Br J Pharmacol: In press.

30. Wang Q, Smith RE, Luchtefeld R, Sun AY, Simonyi A, et al. (2008) Bioavailability of apocynin through its conversion to glycoconjugate but not to diapocynin. Phytomedicine 15: 496–503.

31. Basset O, Boittin FX, Dorchies OM, Chatton JY, van Breemen C, et al. (2004) Involvement of inositol 1,4,5-trisphosphate in nicotinic calcium responses in dystrophic myotubes assessed by near-plasma membrane calcium measurement. J Biol Chem 279: 47092–47100.

32. Reutenauer-Patte J, Boittin FX, Patthey-Vuadens O, Ruegg UT, Dorchies OM (2012) Urocortins improve dystrophic skeletal muscle structure and function through both PKA- and Epac-dependent pathways. Am J Pathol 180: 749–762.

33. Dorchies OM, Reutenauer-Patte J, Dahmane E, Ismail HM, Petermann O, et al. (2013) The anticancer drug tamoxifen counteracts the pathology in a mouse model of duchenne muscular dystrophy. Am J Pathol 182: 485–504.

34. Kleniewska P, Piechota A, Skibska B, Goraca A (2012) The NADPH oxidase family and its inhibitors. Arch Immunol Ther Exp (Warsz) 60: 277–294.

35. Simons JM, Hart BA, Ip Vai Ching TR, Van Dijk H, Labadie RP (1990) Metabolic activation of natural phenols into selective oxidative burst agonists by activated human neutrophils. Free Radic Biol Med 8: 251–258.

36. Johnson DK, Schillinger KJ, Kwait DM, Hughes CV, McNamara EJ, et al. (2002) Inhibition of NADPH oxidase activation in endothelial cells by ortho-methoxy-substituted catechols. Endothelium 9: 191–203.

37. Kanegae MP, da Fonseca LM, Brunetti IL, Silva SO, Ximenes VF (2007) The reactivity of ortho-methoxy-substituted catechol radicals with sulfhydryl groups: contribution for the comprehension of the mechanism of inhibition of NADPH oxidase by apocynin. Biochem Pharmacol 74: 457–464.

38. Castor LR, Locatelli KA, Ximenes VF (2010) Pro-oxidant activity of apocynin radical. Free Radic Biol Med 48: 1636–1643.

39. Wind S, Beuerlein K, Eucker T, Muller H, Scheurer P, et al. (2010) Comparative pharmacology of chemically distinct NADPH oxidase inhibitors. Br J Pharmacol 161: 885–898.

40. Jiang J, Kang H, Song X, Huang S, Li S, et al. (2013) A Model of Interaction between Nicotinamide Adenine Dinucleotide Phosphate (NADP) Oxidase and Apocynin Analogues by Docking Method. Int J Mol Sci 14: 807–817.

41. Balboa MA, Balsinde J (2002) Involvement of calcium-independent phospholipase A$_2$ in hydrogen peroxide-induced accumulation of free fatty acids in human U937 cells. J Biol Chem 277: 40384–40389.

42. Luchtefeld R, Luo R, Stine K, Alt ML, Chernovitz PA, et al. (2008) Dose formulation and analysis of diapocynin. J Agric Food Chem 56: 301–306.

43. Weir EK, Wyatt CN, Reeve HL, Huang J, Archer SL, et al. (1994) Diphenyliodonium inhibits both pottasium and calcium currents in isolated pulmonary-artery smooth-muscle cells. J Appl Physiol 76: 2611–2615.

44. Riganti C, Gazzano E, Polimeni M, Costamagna C, Bosia A, et al. (2004) Diphenyleneiodonium inhibits the cell redox metabolism and induces oxidative stress. J Biol Chem 279: 47726–47731.

45. Prosser BL, Khairallah RJ, Ziman AP, Ward CW, Lederer WJ (2012) X-ROS signaling in the heart and skeletal muscle: Stretch-dependent local ROS regulates [Ca^{2+}]$_i$. J Mol Cell Cardiol 58: 172–881.

46. Boittin FX, Shapovalov G, Hirn C, Ruegg UT (2010) Phospholipase A2-derived lysophosphatidylcholine triggers Ca^{2+} entry in dystrophic skeletal muscle fibers. Biochem Biophys Res Commun 391: 401–406.

47. Chakraborty S, Berwick ZC, Bartlett PJ, Kumar S, Thomas AP, et al. (2011) Bromoenol lactone inhibits voltage-gated Ca^{2+} and transient receptor potential canonical channels. J Pharmacol Exp Ther 339: 329–340.

48. Petrof BJ, Shrager JB, Stedman HH, Kelly AM, Sweeney HL (1993) Dystrophin protects the sarcolemma from stresses developed during muscle contraction. Proc Natl Acad Sci USA 90: 3710–3714.

49. Reggiani C (2008) Between channels and tears: aim at ROS to save the membrane of dystrophic fibres. J Physiol 586: 1779.

50. Yeung EW, Whitehead NP, Suchyna TM, Gottlieb PA, Sachs F, et al. (2005) Effects of stretch-activated channel blockers on [Ca^{2+}]$_i$ and muscle damage in the mdx mouse. J Physiol 562: 367–380.

51. Selsby JT (2011) Increased catalase expression improves muscle function in mdx mice. Exp Physiol 96: 194–202.

52. Gervasio OL, Whitehead NP, Yeung EW, Phillips WD, Allen DG (2008) TRPC1 binds to caveolin-3 and is regulated by Src kinase - role in Duchenne muscular dystrophy. J Cell Sci 121: 2246–2255.

53. Reid MB (2001) Plasticity in skeletal, cardiac, and smooth muscle: Redox modulation of skeletal muscle contraction: what we know and what we don't. J Appl Physiol 90: 724–731.

54. Buetler TM, Krauskopf A, Ruegg UT (2004) Role of superoxide as a signaling molecule. News Physiol Sci 19: 120–123.

55. Ghosh A, Kanthasamy A, Joseph J, Anantharam V, Srivastava P, et al. (2012) Anti-inflammatory and neuroprotective effects of an orally active apocynin derivative in pre-clinical models of Parkinson's disease. J Neuroinflamm 9: 241.

56. Houser KR, Johnson DK, Ishmael FT (2012) Anti-inflammatory effects of methoxyphenolic compounds on human airway cells. J Inflamm (Lond) 9: 6.

57. Zheng W, Wang SY (2001) Antioxidant activity and phenolic compounds in selected herbs. J Agric Food Chem 49: 5165–5170.

58. Kondo K, Kurihara M, Miyata N, Suzuki T, Toyoda M (1999) Scavenging mechanisms of (−)-epigallocatechin gallate and (−)-epicatechin gallate on peroxyl radicals and formation of superoxide during the inhibitory action. Free Radic Biol Med 27: 855–863.

59. Nakagawa T, Yokozawa T (2002) Direct scavenging of nitric oxide and superoxide by green tea. Food Chem Toxicol 40: 1745–1750.

Permissions

All chapters in this book were first published in PLOS ONE, by The Public Library of Science; hereby published with permission under the Creative Commons Attribution License or equivalent. Every chapter published in this book has been scrutinized by our experts. Their significance has been extensively debated. The topics covered herein carry significant findings which will fuel the growth of the discipline. They may even be implemented as practical applications or may be referred to as a beginning point for another development.

The contributors of this book come from diverse backgrounds, making this book a truly international effort. This book will bring forth new frontiers with its revolutionizing research information and detailed analysis of the nascent developments around the world.

We would like to thank all the contributing authors for lending their expertise to make the book truly unique. They have played a crucial role in the development of this book. Without their invaluable contributions this book wouldn't have been possible. They have made vital efforts to compile up to date information on the varied aspects of this subject to make this book a valuable addition to the collection of many professionals and students.

This book was conceptualized with the vision of imparting up-to-date information and advanced data in this field. To ensure the same, a matchless editorial board was set up. Every individual on the board went through rigorous rounds of assessment to prove their worth. After which they invested a large part of their time researching and compiling the most relevant data for our readers.

The editorial board has been involved in producing this book since its inception. They have spent rigorous hours researching and exploring the diverse topics which have resulted in the successful publishing of this book. They have passed on their knowledge of decades through this book. To expedite this challenging task, the publisher supported the team at every step. A small team of assistant editors was also appointed to further simplify the editing procedure and attain best results for the readers.

Apart from the editorial board, the designing team has also invested a significant amount of their time in understanding the subject and creating the most relevant covers. They scrutinized every image to scout for the most suitable representation of the subject and create an appropriate cover for the book.

The publishing team has been an ardent support to the editorial, designing and production team. Their endless efforts to recruit the best for this project, has resulted in the accomplishment of this book. They are a veteran in the field of academics and their pool of knowledge is as vast as their experience in printing. Their expertise and guidance has proved useful at every step. Their uncompromising quality standards have made this book an exceptional effort. Their encouragement from time to time has been an inspiration for everyone.

The publisher and the editorial board hope that this book will prove to be a valuable piece of knowledge for researchers, students, practitioners and scholars across the globe.

List of Contributors

Na Li, Chaoyang Sun, Bo Zhou, Ding Ma, Gang Chen and Danhui Weng
Cancer Biology Research Center, Tongji Hospital, Tongji Medical College, Huazhong University of Science and Technology, Wuhan, Hubei, China

Hui Xing
Department of Obstetrics and Gynecology, Xiangyang Central Hospital, First Affiliated Hospital of Hubei University of Arts and Science. Xiangyang, Hubei, China

Min Zhang, Min Hou, Lihua Ge, Congcong Miao, Jianfei Zhang, Xinying Jing and Xiaofei Tang
Institute of Dental Research, Beijing Stomatological Hospital and School of Stomatology, Capital Medical University, Beijing, China

Ni Shi and Tong Chen
Division of Medical Oncology, Department of Internal Medicine, The Arthur G. James Cancer Hospital and Richard J. Solove Research Institute, The Ohio State University, Columbus, Ohio, United States of America

Stephan P. Frankenfeld, Igor C.C. Rego-Monteiro, Alvaro C. Leitão and Rodrigo S. Fortunato
Laboratório de Radiobiologia Molecular, Instituto de Biofísica Carlos Chagas Filho, Universidade Federal do Rio de Janeiro, Rio de Janeiro, Brazil

Leonardo P. Oliveira and Elen A. Chaves
Laboratório de Biologia do Exercício, Escola de Educação Física e Desportos, Universidade Federal do Rio de Janeiro, Rio de Janeiro, Brazil

Victor H. Ortenzi and Denise P. Carvalho
Laboratório de Fisiologia Endócrina Doris Rosenthal, Instituto de Biofísica Carlos Chagas Filho, Universidade Federal do Rio de Janeiro, Rio de Janeiro, Brazil

Andrea C. Ferreira
Polo de Xerém/Laboratório de Fisiologia Endócrina Doris Rosenthal, Instituto de Biofísica Carlos Chagas Filho, Universidade Federal do Rio de Janeiro, Rio de Janeiro, Brazil

Marcella Reale, Erica Costantini and Chiara D'Angelo
Department of Experimental and Clinical Sciences, University "G. d'Annunzio, Chieti, Italy

Mohammad A. Kamal
King Fahd Medical Research Center, King Abdulaziz University, Jeddah, Kingdom of Saudi Arabia

Antonia Patruno and Miko Pesce
Department of Medicine and Aging Science, University 'G. d'Annunzio' of Chieti-Pescara, Chieti, Italy

Nigel H. Greig
Drug Design and Development Section, Translational Gerontology Branch, Intramural Research Program, National Institute on Aging, National Institutes of Health, Baltimore, Maryland, United States of America

Gemma Flores-Mateo and Josep Basora-Gallisà
Unitat de Suport a la Recerca Tarragona-Reus, Institut Universitari d9Investigacióen AtencióPrimària Jordi Gol (IDIAP Jordi Gol), Tarragona, Spain
CIBER Fisiopatología Obesidad y Nutrición (CIBEROBN), Madrid, Spain

Mònica Bulló and Jordi Salas-Salvadó
CIBER Fisiopatología Obesidad y Nutrición (CIBEROBN), Madrid, Spain
Human Nutrition Unit, School of Medicine, University Rovira i Virgili, Reus, Spain

Roberto Elosua
Epidemiology and Cardiovascular Genetics Research Group, Institut Municipal d'Investigació Mèdica (IMIM), Barcelona, Spain
CIBER de Epidemiología y Salud Pública (CIBERESP), Madrid, Spain

Teresa Rodriguez-Blanco
Institut Universitari d'Investigacióen AtencióPrimària Jordi Gol (IDIAP Jordi Gol), Barcelona, Spain

Isaac Subirana
CIBER de Epidemiología y Salud Pública (CIBERESP), Madrid, Spain

Institut Universitari d9Investigacióen Atenció Primària Jordi Gol (IDIAP Jordi Gol), Barcelona, Spain

Miguel Ángel Martínez-González
Department of Preventive Medicine and Public Health, University of Navarra- Osasunbidea, Servicio Navarro de Salud, Pamplona, Spain

Ramon Estruch
CIBER Fisiopatología Obesidad y Nutrición (CIBEROBN), Madrid, Spain

Department of Internal Medicine, Hospital Clinic, Institut dInvestigacions Biomèdiques August Pi Sunyer (IDIBAPS), Barcelona, Spain

Dolores Corella
CIBER Fisiopatología Obesidad y Nutrición (CIBEROBN), Madrid, Spain
Department of Preventive Medicine and Public Health, University of Valencia, Valencia, Spain

Montserrat Fitó and Maria-Isabel Covas
CIBER Fisiopatología Obesidad y Nutrición (CIBEROBN), Madrid, Spain
Cardiovascular Risk and Nutrition Research Unit, Institut Municipal d'Investigació Mèdica (IMIM), Barcelona, Spain

Miquel Fiol
CIBER Fisiopatología Obesidad y Nutrición (CIBEROBN), Madrid, Spain
Institute for Health Sciences Investigation, IdISPa, Palma de Mallorca, Spain

Fernando Arós
Department of Cardiology, Hospital Txangorritxu, Vitoria, Spain

Enrique Gómez-Gracia
Department of Epidemiology, School of Medicine of Malaga, Malaga, Spain

José Lapetra
Department of Family Medicine, Primary Care Division of Sevilla, San Pablo Health Center, Sevilla, Spain

Valentina Ruiz-Gutiérrez
CIBER Fisiopatología Obesidad y Nutrición (CIBEROBN), Madrid, Spain
Instituto de la Grasa, CSIC, Sevilla, Spain

Guillermo T. Sáez
CIBER Fisiopatología Obesidad y Nutrición (CIBEROBN), Madrid, Spain

Department of Biochemistry and Molecular Biology, Faculty of Medicine, Service of Clinical Analysis, Doctor Peset University Hospital, University of Valencia, Valencia, Spain

Zhenxing Chi and Hong You
State Key Laboratory of Urban Water Resource and Environment, Harbin Institute of Technology, Harbin, PR China

School of Marine Science and Technology, Harbin Institute of Technology at Weihai, Weihai, PR China

Shanshan Ma, Hao Cui and Qiang Zhang
School of Marine Science and Technology, Harbin Institute of Technology at Weihai, Weihai, PR China

Rutao Liu
School of Environmental Science and Engineering, Shandong University, Jinan, PR China

Victor M. Victor, Susana Rovira-Llopis, Celia Bañuls, Rosa Falcón, Raquel Castelló and Milagros Rocha
Foundation for the Promotion of Healthcare and Biomedical Research in the Valencian Community (FISABIO), Valencia, Spain
Service of Endocrinology, University Hospital Doctor Peset, Valencia, Spain
Institute of Health Research INCLIVA, University of Valencia, Valencia, Spain

Vanessa Saiz-Alarcon, Maria C. Sangüesa and Luis Rojo-Bofill
Psychiatry Service, University Hospital La Fe, Department of Medicine, University of Valencia, Valencia, Spain

Luis Rojo
Psychiatry Service, University Hospital La Fe, Department of Medicine, University of Valencia, Valencia, Spain

Research Group CIBER CB/06/02/0045, CIBER actions, Epidemiology and Public Health, University of Valencia, Valencia, Spain

Antonio Hernández-Mijares
Foundation for the Promotion of Healthcare and Biomedical Research in the Valencian Community (FISABIO), Valencia, Spain
Service of Endocrinology, University Hospital Doctor Peset, Valencia, Spain
Institute of Health Research INCLIVA, University of Valencia, Valencia, Spain

Department of Medicine, University of Valencia, Valencia, Spain

Zohreh Tamanai-Shacoori
Equipe de Microbiologie, EA 1254, Université Rennes 1, UEB, Rennes, France

Fatiha Chandad
Groupe de Recherche en Ecologie Buccale, Faculté de médecine dentaire, Université Laval, Québec City, Québec, Canada

Amélie Rébillard and Josiane Cillard
Laboratoire Mouvement, Sport, Santé, EA 1274, Université Rennes 1, Université Rennes 2, UEB, Rennes, France

Martine Bonnaure-Mallet
Equipe de Microbiologie, EA 1254, Université Rennes 1, UEB, Rennes, France
Centre hospital-universitaire, Rennes, France

Lourdes Robles, Nosratola D. Vaziri, Shiri Li, Yuichi Masuda, Chie Takasu, Mizuki Takasu, Kelly Vo, Seyed H. Farzaneh, Michael J. Stamos and Hirohito Ichii
Departments of Surgery and Medicine, University of California Irvine, Irvine, CA, United States of America

Eunice Molinar-Toribio, Josep Lluís Torres and Jara Pérez-Jiménez
Institute of Advanced Chemistry of Catalonia (IQAC-CSIC), Barcelona, Spain

Sara Ramos-Romero
Institute of Advanced Chemistry of Catalonia (IQAC-CSIC), Barcelona, Spain
Biomedical Research Networking Center in Bioengineering, Biomaterials, and Nanomedicine (CIBER-BBN), Zaragoza, Spain

Laura Lluís, Vanessa Sánchez-Martos, Núria Taltavull and Marta Romeu
Unidad de Farmacología, Facultad de Medicina y Ciencias de la Salud, Universidad Rovira i Virgili, Reus, Spain

Manuel Pazos, Lucía Méndez and Isabel Medina
Instituto de Investigaciones Marinas (IIM-CSIC), Vigo, Spain

Aníbal Miranda and Marta Cascante
Department of Biochemistry and Molecular Biology, IBUB and unit associated with CSIC, Faculty of Biology, Universitat de Barcelona, Barcelona, Spain

Institut d'Investigacions Biomèdiques August Pi i Sunyer (IDIBAPS), Barcelona, Spain

Takeshi Fukushima, Hideaki Iizuka, Ayaka Yokota, Takehiro Suzuki, Chihiro Ohno, Yumiko Kono, Minami Nishikiori, Ayaka Seki and Hideaki Ichiba
Department of Analytical Chemistry, Faculty of Pharmaceutical Sciences, Toho University, Funabashi-shi, Chiba, Japan

Yoshinori Watanabe and Seiji Hongo
Nanko Clinic of Psychiatry, Himorogi group, Medical Corporation JISENKAI, Shirakawa-shi, Fukushima, Japan

Mamoru Utsunomiya and Masaki Nakatani
Public Interest Incorporated Foundation, Sumiyoshi-kaiseikai Sumiyoshi hospital, Koufu-shi, Yamanashi, Japan

Kiyomi Sadamoto
Department of Clinical Pharmacy, Yokohama College of Pharmacy, Yokohama-shi, Kanagawa, Japan

Takashi Yoshio
Department of Clinical Pharmacy, Faculty of Pharmaceutical Sciences, Toho University, Funabashi-shi, Chiba, Japan

Marta Maria Medeiros Frescura Duarte, Clarice Pinheiro Mostardeiro, Taís Cristina Unfer, Jéssica de Rosso Motta and Matheus Marcon
Biogenomic Laboratory, Federal University of Santa Maria, Santa Maria, RS, Brazil

Fernanda Barbisan and Verônica Azzolin
Pharmacology Graduate Program, Federal University of Santa Maria, Santa Maria, RS, Brazil

Eduardo Bortoluzzi Dornelles, Thaís Doeler Algarve and Karen Lilian Schott
Biochemical Toxicology Graduate Program, Federal University of Santa Maria, Santa Maria, RS, Brazil

Ivana Beatrice Mânica da Cruz
Biogenomic Laboratory, Federal University of Santa Maria, Santa Maria, RS, Brazil
Pharmacology Graduate Program, Federal University of Santa Maria, Santa Maria, RS, Brazil
Biochemical Toxicology Graduate Program, Federal University of Santa Maria, Santa Maria, RS, Brazil

Alexis Trott
Laboratory of Molecular Biology, University of Western Santa Catarina, UNOESC, Chapecó, SC, Brazil

Marta Columbaro
SC Laboratory of Musculoskeletal Cell Biology, IOR, Bologna, Italy

Silvia Ravera and Isabella Panfoli
DIFAR-Biochemistry Lab., University of Genova, Genova, Italy

Cristina Capanni
CNR-National Research Council of Italy, Institute of Molecular Genetics, Unit of Bologna-IOR, Bologna, Italy

Paola Cuccarolo and Paolo Degan
S. C. Mutagenesis, IRCCS AOU San Martino – IST (Istituto Nazionale per la Ricerca sul Cancro), Genova, Italy

Giorgia Stroppiana
Centro di Diagnostica Genetica e Biochimica delle Malattie Metaboliche, Istituto Giannina Gaslini, Genova, Italy

Enrico Cappelli
Hematology Unit, Istituto Giannina Gaslini, Genova, Italy

Jing Zhao, Kentaro Ozawa, Yoji Kyotani, Kosuke Nagayama, Satoyasu Ito, Akira T. Komatsubara, Yuichi Tsuji and Masanori Yoshizumi
Department of Pharmacology, Nara Medical University School of Medicine, Kashihara, Nara, Japan

Yuhua Fan, Lei Yu and Kun Fang
College of Pharmacy, Harbin Medical University-Daqing, Daqing, China

Meng Chen
Department of Respiratory Medicine, the Fourth Hospital of Harbin Medical University, Harbin, China

Jia Meng
Department of Geriatrics, the Second Affiliated Hospital of Harbin Medical University, Harbin, China

Yingfeng Tu
Department of Cardiology, the Fourth Hospital of Harbin Medical University, Harbin, China,

Lin Wan
Radiology Department and Key Laboratory of Molecular Imaging, the Fourth Hospital of Harbin Medical University, Harbin, China

Wenliang Zhu
Institute of Clinical Pharmacology, the Second Affiliated Hospital of Harbin Medical University, Harbin, China

Mats I. Nilsson, Lauren G. Macneil, Yu Kitaoka, Fatimah Alqarni, Rahul Suri, Mahmood Akhtar, Maria E. Haikalis, Pavneet Dhaliwal, Munim Saeed and Mark A. Tarnopolsky
Department of Pediatrics and Medicine, Neuromuscular Clinic, McMaster University Hospital, Hamilton, Ontario, Canada

Erqun Song, Juanli Fu, Xiaomin Xia, Chuanyang Su and Yang Song
Key Laboratory of Luminescence and Real-Time Analytical Chemistry (Ministry of Education), College of Pharmaceutical Sciences, Southwest University, Chongqing, People's Republic of China

Chongxiao Liu, Xiaoyu Wan, Tingting Ye, Fang Fang, Xueru Chen and Yan Dong
Department of Endocrinology, Xinhua Hospital, Shanghai Jiao Tong University School of Medicine, Shanghai, China

Yuanwen Chen
Department of Gastroenterology, Xinhua Hospital, Shanghai Jiao Tong University School of Medicine, Shanghai, China

Chengpeng Zhu, Fangyu Pan, Lianping Ge, Jing Zhou, Longlong Chen, Tong Zhou, Rongrong Zong, Xinye Xiao and Yueping Zhou
Eye Institute of Xiamen University, Fujian Provincial Key Laboratory of Ophthalmology and Visual Science, Xiamen, Fujian, China

Nuo Dong
Affiliated Xiamen Eye Center of Xiamen University, Xiamen, Fujian, China

Maomin Yang
Xiamen Kehong Eye Hospital, Xiamen, Fujian, PR China

Jian-xing Ma
Department of Physiology, The University of Oklahoma Health Sciences Center, Oklahoma City, Oklahoma, United States of America

Zuguo Liu
Eye Institute of Xiamen University, Fujian Provincial Key Laboratory of Ophthalmology and Visual Science, Xiamen, Fujian, China
Affiliated Xiamen Eye Center of Xiamen University, Xiamen, Fujian, China

David Hevia, Juan C. Mayo, Aida Rodriguez-Garcia and Rosa M. Sainz
Departamento de Morfologia y Biologia Celular, School of Medicine, University of Oviedo, Oviedo, Spain
Instituto Universitario Oncologico del Principado de Asturias (IUOPA), Oviedo, Spain

Dun-Xian Tan
Department of Cellular and Structural Biology, University of Texas Health Science Center at San Antonio, San Antonio, Texas, United States of America

Xinli Huang, Yun Gao, Jianjie Qin and Sen Lu
Center of Liver Transplantation, The First Affiliated Hospital of Nanjing Medical University, The Key Laboratory of Living Donor Liver Transplantation, Ministry of Health, Nanjing, China

Kazuma Sugahara, Yoshinobu Hirose, Takefumi Mikuriya, Makoto Hashimoto, Eiju Kanagawa, Hirotaka Hara, Hiroaki Shimogori and Hiroshi Yamashita
Department of Otolaryngology, Yamaguchi University Graduate School of Medicine, Ube, Yamaguchi, Japan

Hesham M. Ismail, Leonardo Scapozza, Urs T. Ruegg and Olivier M. Dorchies
School of Pharmaceutical Sciences, University of Geneva and University of Lausanne, Geneva, Switzerland

Index